MATERIA MEDICA OF WESTERN HERBS

MATERIA MEDICA OF
WESTERN HERBS

Carole Fisher

AEON

First published in 2009 by Vitex Medica.

This edition published in 2018 by
Aeon Books Ltd
12 New College Parade
Finchley Road
London NW3 5EP

British Library Cataloguing in Publication Data

A C.I.P. for this book is available from the British Library

ISBN-13: 978-1-91159-751-3

Typeset by Medlar Publishing Solutions Pvt Ltd, India

www.aeonbooks.co.uk

CONTENTS

ACKNOWLEDGMENTS

I would like to recognize with gratitude those herbalists, past and present, who have contributed to the knowledge of herbal medicine and from whom we all benefit.

I thank Gilian Painter for supplying botanical information for each monograph and for her help with proof reading. Thanks also to Alan Esler for his earlier permission to use his diagrams of families, Apiaceae, Asteraceae and Lamiaceae and Isabel Sutherland for her help with redrawing some of the illustrations in the text.

Most illustrations have come from botanical works from last century and I gratefully acknowledge the work of W. H. Fitch and W. G. Smith in the *Illustrations of The British Flora*, L. Reeve and Co., London, 1880; Britton, N. L., and A. Brown. 1913. *An illustrated flora of the northern United States, Canada and the British Possessions* as well as Vol. 1–3 of the USDA-NRCS PLANTS Database from the same book, *Medicinal Plants* by R. Bently

and H. Trimen, J. and A. Churchill, London. 1888. Also used were the works of older herbalists John Gerard, Leonhart Fuchs and Matthiolus.

I also gratefully acknowledge:

CRC Press Inc. Boca Raton Florida for permission to use the illustrations of *Harpagophytum* from *Handbook of Medicinal Plants* by James Duke.

The University of Hawaii for permission to use the illustration of *Serenoa repens* from *The Manual of the Flowering Plants of Hawaii* Vol. 2 by W. L. Wagner, B. R. Herbst and S. H. Sohmer.

I would especially like to thank Doreen Marshall for her invaluable suggestions, careful compilation, dedication and patience in editing and producing this text. Without her enormous effort, wise contributions and unerring support my task would have been very much more difficult.

Finally my heartfelt thanks for the tremendous love and support I have received from my family.

INTRODUCTION

Herbal medicine is the traditional medicine of all cultures and still accounts for three quarters of the remedies used throughout the world today. Although the principles and practice of herbal medicine had been largely dismissed in the west in the last several centuries, studies are increasingly supporting their age-old uses as well as discovering new properties and applications for them. The recent interest in herbs and their constituents is the result of awareness of iatrogenic diseases; side effects of allopathic medicine; the resistance that has developed to over-used antimicrobials; and the search for new and better medicines.

This book is a series of monographs of some of the most commonly used herbs in western herbal medicine. They have been arranged in a format similar to Dioscorides' original text, *De Materia Medica* written about 2000 years ago, but in a modern framework that also presents a summary of the knowledge that has accumulated in recent years for the herbs and/or their constituents. Each herb is presented with:-

- Plant name and picture
- Parts used
- Actions

- Pharmacy
- Interaction with drugs
- Botanical description
- Active constituents
- Scientific information
- Precaution and/or Safety
- Historical uses
- Habitat and geographical location
- Nutritional constituents
- Medicinal uses
- Contraindications

Unfortunately not all monographs contain information in all these areas for whilst a great deal is known about a few herbs, like *Panax ginseng* and *Hypericum perforatum*, for others virtually no research exists or what there is may be many decades old and based on using scientific tools that lack today's level of reliability.

Also included in this text is information on scheduled or restricted herbs. These have been included for information only as many countries do not allow their general use and in some cases do not allow herbalists to use them.

Scientific information (both positive and negative) from reputable journals and texts has been compiled, without personal evaluation, with the aim of providing an understanding of the scope of activity and mechanisms, as far as they are known, for each herb. Scientific methods used and conclusions drawn from this data should be assessed bearing in mind that the goals of modern science are not necessarily in harmony with the tenets of herbal medicine and the hypotheses being tested may be at odds with the herbs' traditional use. Moreover the aim of phytotherapy is not to simply treat symptoms or conditions, by suppressing biochemical reactions, and herbalists should not rely solely on this science to guide their application of these unique and complex healing agents. Their actions and effectiveness have been gleaned and refined over many thousands of years of practical use which is one of the soundest ways to evaluate their medicinal value for human health. At the same time science can provide us with important scientific information as well as ensure our method of practice is safe as well as appropriate.

Information on the botany, growing and harvesting of herbs has been provided by Gilian Painter so that those who are keen gardeners can plant and work directly with fresh herbs and the various preparations that can be manufactured from them.

GENERAL NOTES

Botanical names

The herbs are presented under their botanical names and within their botanical families. Using botanical names is necessary to ensure the identity of the herb is understood throughout the world. Common names change from place to place and have on occasion been used to identify different plants altogether e.g. colic root which can signify wild yam—*Dioscorea villosa*, true unicorn root—*Aletris farinosa* or pleurisy root—*Asclepias tuberosa*. Also throughout the scientific literature chemical differences are noted in species with the same genus name so for reasons of both safety and efficacy an exact nomenclature is necessary.

Each herb is set out in the same format and has the botanical and most used common name(s) as well as a simple drawing which can help in the identification, although a more detailed field guide may be required for this purpose.

Description

This covers the general appearance of the plant and its height in flower, or in the case of trees, when mature. It is followed by descriptions of the various parts including fruit and seeds, as well as the flowering or fruiting time of the plant. When two measurements are used together e.g. 5.5 × 2 mm, the first measurement is length/height and the second width. Herbs respond to differences of soil, light and rainfall which make their appearance different in different environments so positive identification should be made from flowers and seeds. Appendix IIIa is a botanical glossary.

Habitat and cultivation

Habitat refers to the country from which the plant originated and the conditions in which it grows wild. Cultivation of that plant is more likely to be successful if the same growing conditions are provided. However many herbs have become successful weeds regardless of their original habitat. Cultivation includes the ways in which each plant may be propagated, and the ideal soil and situation for growing it. The two other factors of drought and frost indicate whether or not the plant will succeed in a particular area on its own or will need special care.

Parts used

This refers to the part of the plant used medicinally. This may involve the whole plant but often only 1 or 2 parts are used and sometimes the part of a herb used differs with tradition. In some cases one part has medicinal value whilst another part of that same plant may be toxic. Whether the part is used fresh or dried can also be significant. In order to make safe medicine attention to these details is essential. Each part of the plant should be harvested at the appropriate time to ensure maximum levels of active constituents.

Wild crafting or gathering non-cultivated plants, particularly roots, should never deplete the habitat of the ability to produce future generations and should not be undertaken at all if the plant is an endangered species.

Plants should be gathered when not wet from dew or rain and processed as quickly as possible after picking so that they do not spoil. If they are to be dried this should be done in a warm, airy place out of direct sunlight. Too much light and/or heat can alter the active constituents and change the herb's therapeutic potential. Once dried, they should be stored, taking into account their particular requirements, some need to be stored before being made into a safe medicine and others may deteriorate if stored for too long. Herbs to be stored should be kept as whole as possible (not crumbled or powdered) because the smaller the pieces of plant material are the greater the level of oxidation that can occur. They are best ground just before processing.

The parts used may include:

- **Leaves or *Folia* (fol.)**—generally collected just as the plant comes into flower
- **Flowers or *Flores* (flos.)**—usually collected at midday when fully open but before they begin to fade
- **Aerial parts or *Herba***—consists of the whole plant above ground, usually gathered when flowers and/or buds are present as well as leaves and stems
- **Fruits or *Fructus* (fruc.)**—consists of the berries collected when just ripe
- **Seeds or *Semen* (sem.)**—usually picked as the whole seed head, still on the stalk, when most of the seeds are just ripe
- **Bark or *Cortex* (cort.)**—consists of the outer covering or "skin" of the branches, or inner bark as specified. It is usually collected in

autumn or early spring before the sap rises so that damage to the plant is minimised. If taken directly from a tree this should be done as longitudinal strips and not as a band ("ring barking" will kill the plant). If inner bark is specified it can easily be separated from the outer cork layer
- **Roots or *Radix* (rad.), rhizomes (rhiz.), bulbs** generally collected when the foliage dies back

Active constituents

This knowledge is not as simple to acquire as may be expected. Every plant is made up of many constituents some are considered active; others may become activated *in vivo*; some may simply assist for example in the absorption of "actives"; and yet others may be nutritional. Not all active constituents have been identified and the importance of some constituents may not be recognised at present.

Knowledge of active constituents should lead to a better understanding of the herb's pharmacology and possibly to new applications. It is not, however, an exact science. Even with the advantage of sophisticated technology to help separate and identify constituents, extraction procedures are not perfect. Variables that have been identified as contributing to an altered constituent profile include:-

- Geographical location—the origin of the herb and its local environment can alter the quantity and quality of constituents. Cultivated herbs too can vary from those that grow wild e.g. see *Tanacetum parthenium*
- Genetic variability like polyploidy (e.g. *Achillea* which may have 2n, 4n or 6n chromosomes) or tendency to hybridisation (e.g. *Salix* spp.). Genotypes and/or hybrids found in the wild can be hard to distinguish visually and without chemical profiling. These genetic differences may significantly alter the plants' chemistry. Profiling every plant would render manufacturing uneconomical and certain mixed species, where these are similar enough in actions, have become acceptable pharmaceutically e.g. *Barosma*

- Time of harvest and growing conditions experienced by plant in year of harvest e.g. water availability, sunshine hours, soil type, insect predator levels (some constituents help repel insect attack)
- Age of herb at time of harvest—constituents can be affected by age e.g. terpene levels are higher in younger gingko leaves
- Incorporation of other plant parts (e.g. leaves may be harvested with or without buds in the case of *Cratageus* spp.) altering the final preparation
- Conditions in which material is stored prior to extraction (e.g. temperature and light) as well as duration of storage
- Method of extraction and analysis used—the solvent system, temperature, pressure and pH. The procedure and/or solvents used can lead to artefacts or the preferential extraction of some actives at the expense of others. The process used is not necessarily intended to gain a profile of the herb as used by herbalists
- Although an active constituent has been identified in a herb, its lack of bio-availability may mean it does not necessarily have an important role in the herb's activity *in vivo* e.g. oleuropein in olive leaf
- Dosage forms may alter the bio-availability of active constituents (e.g. a commercial tablet preparation as opposed to a tea or a tincture)

These variables are perhaps academic. Herbalists in times past would not have been concerned about many of these factors, although the difference conditions made to the potency of a herb was sometimes reflected in the instructions surrounding its gathering. Lack of scientific understanding about the herbs did not mean they were any less effective in practice. It is still true, too, that the action of a herb relies on the combination of all, or many, of its constituents acting in synergy, not just the so called "actives".

For a small number of herbs a great deal of information is available about their constituents, others are only partially determined and for some very little is known. These isolated constituents have again been subjected to a variable degree of pharmacological study. The quantity of information should not indicate the relative worth of any herb.

It should also be noted that with better technology older named constituents may since have been identified and renamed and so no longer appear as listed constituents. This is especially likely to be the case with constituents that were simply identified at one time as a "bitter principle".

Appendix III lists the more commonly encountered active constituents and their known pharmacology.

Nutritional Constituents

As well as having medicinally active constituents, many herbs contain vitamins and minerals as well as other important nutritional elements such as essential fatty acids and essential amino acids. Herbs like *Avena sativa* and *Urtica dioica* may be considered nutritive because of their vitamin and mineral content whilst others like *Valeriana* have nutritional elements, glutamine in this case, that could be key to the herb's activity. It can help to be aware of the nutritional contribution a herb although this has not generally been well studied. There may be detailed evaluations for some herbs and next to no information on others. As with active constituents, the presence of a nutrient may have variable bio-availability. Any data that exists in the scientific literature has been referenced, otherwise the nutritional information is based on a variety of texts and should act as a qualitative guide to the nutritional potential of the herb.

Actions

Because of their particular mix of constituents, most herbs have a variety of actions. The constituents that occur and their relative proportions interact to give each herb its characteristic main actions. For instance the presence of tannins imparts astringency but the other constituents and/or their mode of metabolism or excretion from the body means that the astringent action is focussed at a particular site—the kidneys (*Equisetum arvense*) or the upper respiratory mucous membranes (*Glechoma hederacea*). Knowledge of this sort would have been gleaned anecdotally in the first instance. Early scientific studies relied largely on the use of live animals or their isolated tissues to establish these actions. Modern research has the advantage of being able to use human models to observe them. Definitions of actions may be found in Appendix I.

Scientific information

This section is intended to extend or verify the accepted modern uses of each herb in the practice of herbal medicine.

It begins with a brief historical profile of the herb, official pharmacopoeial uses and also those uses approved by *German Commission E.* This commission is a governmental regulatory agent established in 1978 and comprised of various scientists including toxicologists, pharmacists and doctors to critically evaluate historical and current data on a range of medicinal herbs and produce guidelines for their use in Germany. They have produced monographs for a number of herbs and these have been translated into English by the American Botanical Society.

Animal based experimental data has deliberately been excluded unless otherwise stated. With the advantage of improved scientific models there is no longer a necessity to rely on these studies which may not only be cruel but also leaves unanswered the question of whether the observed actions can be considered a true reflection of their effects in humans. The history of medicine has many examples of animal models having failed to predict drug activity in humans with serious consequences.

The scientific information used therefore comprises the following three elements:

In vitro

In which isolated human cells or metabolites are subjected to the herb, or its constituents, in a laboratory situation ("test tube") to evaluate their effects. This research attempts to predict *in vivo* outcomes. Whilst these models have the advantage of better representing human biochemistry and being more ethical than live animal models they also have some disadvantages which need to be borne in mind. Extracts of herbs, or isolated constituents, bathing human cells is not the same as ingesting them, obvious differences are:-

- *in vivo* the antimicrobial efficacy may be altered by absorption
- effective concentration around and within the cells is likely to be much higher and experimentally controlled
- absorption through the mucosa may filter out certain constituents e.g. polysaccharides
- the chemistry following ingestion of a herb is likely to be altered as it passes through the gastro-intestinal tract and/or liver and this may or may not alter what eventually reaches individual cells
- the effect the body has to direct where a herb or its constituents may accumulate and/or concentrate for excretion/secretion
- the many complex processes that may intervene to alter the herb or constituent that is ultimately presented to the living cells

There are therefore limitations in these studies and it is difficult to directly extrapolate data gleaned from them to the *in vivo* situation. However this research may give insights into mechanisms underlying a herb or a constituent's action.

Ex vivo

In which the herb or its constituents are given to live people and then cells or metabolites are isolated in a laboratory, away from the live source, to assess changes made. This method has the advantage of allowing the herb to act in a real live context although end measurements are confined to a single fixed point in time and to the one model for which the experiment was designed.

In vivo

In which the herb or constituent is given to living subjects and the effect on a clinical condition or physiological function is evaluated. This evaluation may be subjective and/or objective, stand alone or be compared to *placebo* and/or current standard pharmaceuticals. They may be:

- prospective—the outcome of a treatment protocol after a specified period of time (this includes the standard randomised, controlled, double-blind type of study) is assessed

- retrospective—looks back at a lifestyle choice of a sample group and assesses if there is a correlation between it and a particular health outcome
- epidemiological—rates likely causal links between a herb's use in the general population and the development or prevention of diseases or physiological changes for that population

These studies, particularly the epidemiological ones, which link the use of a herb to likely health outcomes can be informative but they are not routinely carried out and can be complicated by the number of confounding variables. Other types of clinical trials are all too often economically driven where a developed health product—this may be a partial extract, one standardised on one or two main constituents or a combination of extracts with or without dietary supplements—is tested and the results are quite specific to that preparation. There is little research relevant to herbalists that establishes a direct benefit for a particular plant extract.

In vivo studies can nonetheless be useful but suffer the following disadvantages:-

- trials do not reflect what happens in our clinics because we treat the whole person not just their "medical condition"
- isolated constituents, standardised extracts or fixed combinations of herbs are more likely to be examined as these **can** be patented and have commercial potential
- sample groups are usually small (some have been less than 20 people). Financial returns on herbal preparations are not great and there are fewer employed or interested scientists to carry out the research
- herbs may be assessed in the treatment of conditions for which they are not used traditionally. There are medical imperatives for new treatments of epidemic diseases for which no current remedy exists or for which pharmaceutical approaches are no longer effective e.g. antibiotics. The research is therefore driven by the need to treat these diseases, not by the desire to establish the intrinsic value of a herb.

Because traditional uses are often not being assessed research may end up distorting the perception of the medicinal benefit of that herb. It may also be that through inappropriate testing, a herb appears not to be effective for its traditional uses even though history tells us otherwise.

- delivery systems may not be relevant to the practice of herbalists e.g. injections
- biochemical processes are being unravelled and illustrate the complexities of living systems, many are still to be elucidated. A herb or constituent may block one or several biochemical processes yet this does not necessarily reflect the full extent of its action, wanted or not, in other metabolic functions. This symptomatic, mechanistic approach is also at odds with the aim of herbal medicine which tries to resolve underlying problems.

Science has come a long way in explaining mechanisms of action for some herbs. Yet it is apparent that their very complex nature means they may remain difficult to understand. Not only are there numerous active constituents for many medicinal herbs but their *in vivo* interactions are unknown. The multitude of biochemical functions they can influence may remain unknown until technology is much more sophisticated than it is today.

Herbal medicine as practised by phytotherapists is a customised process where the individual's history and needs are established and the whole person treated with tailor-made mixtures not standard formulas, isolated constituents or simples (single herbs). The medical herbalists' approach to their art is therefore difficult to measure by current standards of clinical research. Because this practice does not conform to the current belief in the overriding value of the randomised, doubleblind controlled study this should not diminish the worth of the *materia medica*.

On the other hand science can help widen our understanding of herbs.

- It regularly confirms the concept of synergy in the action of herbs, or within a herb, by its constituents

- It has highlighted subspecies differences in herbs that are used in different countries which may explain discrepancies in cultural usage
- New applications may arise from these studies
- Possible dangers and interactions to which we have previously been oblivious are being brought to the fore
- Most importantly science may help persuade a sceptical audience of the medicinal value of herbs.

Medicinal uses

It will be seen that for many herbs the record of their use dates back hundreds if not thousands of years. The current accepted use is often a narrowed or refined version of this list supported by studies undertaken to corroborate them. In many cases they were the accepted uses in pharmacopoeias, even within the last 50 years or so, and they are the accepted uses recorded in standard herbal texts like the *BHP* and *BHC*. I have used these latter two as the main guide to modern medicinal uses as well as material provided by members of the National Institute of Medical Herbalists (U.K.). Where research has unequivocally confirmed new uses I have often included them.

Pharmacy

This lists the various preparations which may be made from each herb. These may be for internal or external use. Water-based preparations include infusions and decoctions for internal use, compresses and poultices for external use. Oil-based preparations are infused herb oils and ointments for external use only. Alcohol-water preparations which includes tinctures and fluid extracts are used either as lotions or washes externally or used internally. In addition information is included on standardised extracts which have been used in clinical trials relating to that herb.

A standard infusion is made from leaves and/or flowers or seeds of a single herb or combination of herbs using the dose recommended for each herb. It is made up by adding boiling water to the herb which should then be kept covered with a lid and left to infuse for at least 10 minutes. Some constituents like mucilage are more effectively extracted if left to infuse over night. Once infused the tea should be strained and kept in a cool place if not all used at once. It may be drunk hot or cold and should be made fresh daily.

A standard decoction is used to extract the properties of tougher material such as roots, bark, twigs and some berries. Infusing will not extract well unless these parts are dried and powdered and so a more energetic extraction process is necessary. The same approach to dosage is used as for any infusion, but as some of the water is lost as steam, more water is usually added to start with. Combine water and herb in a saucepan, bring to the boil and simmer for at least 20 minutes. Strain, cool and store as for the infusion. It may be drunk hot or cold.

A compress is made using a soft cotton or linen cloth soaked in a hot or cold herbal extract. This may be made as a standard infusion or decoction or by adding 5–20 ml of tincture to 500 ml of hot or cold water. For a hot compress soak the cloth in the herbal extract until it has absorbed the herb and the heat, wring it out and apply it to the affected area. When it cools or dries repeat the process, reheating the herbal extract. A hot compress is healing for muscle injuries or wounds, spasms, cramps and tension. A cold compress (made with cold preparations rather than hot as above) is helpful for headaches, sprains, sore and tired eyes, burns or rashes.

A poultice is similar to a compress but is made from the actual herbs rather than an extract of herbs. Boil sufficient chopped herb to cover the area, squeeze out the moisture and spread the herb directly on the skin or on a piece of gauze. Cover with a cotton or gauze bandage to hold it in place. May be used hot or cold. Replace the poultice every 2–4 hours or as necessary. If applying the herb directly to the skin rub a little oil on first to protect it and keep the herb from sticking.

A succus is the juice of a fresh herb expressed using a press or juicer. It can be done with succulent herbs only and is a way of accessing the herb's constituents without the need for additional water or alcohol and without the application of heat.

Infused herb oil is made by covering the herb with vegetable oil in a container and indirectly heating it, as in a double boiler, for several hours. Strained oil can be stored for later use or combined with beeswax to give an ointment.

Tinctures are made by adding alcohol to the water in the extraction process and not using heat as in infusions/decoctions. Water is a good solvent and can dissolve out many of the chemical constituents. But water does not extract some constituents like resin, for example, and so herbs in which this is an important active constituent are not usually infused. In these cases tinctures are made by chopping or powdering the fresh or dried herb and adding a water- alcohol mixture to it. The amount of herb to water-alcohol (menstruum) gives the extraction ratio quoted as e.g. 1:10. This means one unit by weight of herb has been extracted by 10 units by volume of menstruum. The menstruum is given as a percentage which refers to the alcohol strength of the water/alcohol mixture. So that a 25% mixture would be made by diluting 25 ml of pure alcohol with water to give a final volume of 100 ml of menstruum. The alcohol content is varied according to which constituents are being extracted and how soluble they are in water and alcohol. Water extracts will not keep, so the use of alcohol is also a means of preserving the herbal extract.

Commercially produced tinctures in some countries are required to have chemical profile checks run to ensure the correct actives are present and contaminants are not.

Fluid Extracts. Strictly speaking this represents a tincture with the extraction ratio of 1:1 in other words 100 g of herb is extracted into 100 ml of water-alcohol. This represents the strongest tincture usually encountered although with new research and more sophisticated procedures tinctures that are standardised for a particular constituent may be stronger than this.

Dosages given are according to the *BHP* and *BHC* where available. Where these do not exist guidelines are offered based on other sources as indicated.

Contraindications

Contraindications should not be ignored. They indicate in which conditions it is not safe to use a particular herb. Pregnancy is an obvious case where extreme care should be taken and it is best to avoid treatment of any sort in the first trimester because at this stage the developing foetus is most vulnerable. This principle applies to any type of medication. Herbs rarely have side-effects but they do have contraindications and the safest standards of practice must be observed.

A table of conditions and the herbs that are contraindicated for them appears in Appendix IV. Note not all standard texts are in agreement over contraindications.

Pharmacokinetics

This section contains any relevant data on the study of the fate of pharmacologically significant chemicals derived from the herb. It may cover the absorption, distribution, metabolism and excretion of one or a few constituents. This information is usually only available for the most commonly used herbs and may serve as a guide to the time frame for dosing, expected effectiveness or potential toxicity.

Precautions and/or safety

These cover any safety checks that have been carried out *in vitro* or such as genotoxicity or mutagenicity tests or *in vivo* effects on particular groups of people e.g. pregnant women. It also lists reported side-effects for the herb that are either anecdotal or part of the information gathered during clinical trials. They may of course be specific for the particular preparation being tested. In general they tend to be minor, occurring at about the same rate and of the same severity as those recorded for placebos. However there have been more serious side effects reported for some herbs. They are for the most part anecdotal in nature, are limited in numbers and a direct causal link is not often established. Validation of anecdotal reports requires that scientists have access to the offending preparation for proper identification and characterisation. If the herb has been wild harvested by the person admitted for emergency treatment it is unlikely to be readily available for analysis. It may be that the wrong plant has been used or that the right herb was harvested but contained toxic contaminants. Unless verified it cannot be categorically accepted that the herb was to blame but the doubt of its safety becomes a matter of record. If the preparation is a commercial one it is possible to do the requisite analysis but this does not always seem to have been carried out and many cases of reported serious events do not report that positive identification of the herbal preparation was made, that the preparation only contained the ingredients specified and that other contaminants (toxic plants, pesticides, heavy metals) were not present. It may therefore be difficult to interpret the reality of the danger of any herb it may have purported to contain. Mixtures of herbs have their own problems in that it may be difficult to identify which is the likely culprit or if a particular constituent is to blame. However there are certainly instances of herbs having caused serious health problems and idiosyncratic reactions can and do occur.

It remains possible also that although herbs used properly are safe there is scope for individual levels of tolerance to differ just as happens with pharmaceuticals. This is accounted for by the current state of health, immune status, liver function and genetic make-up of that individual. We must therefore remain open to the possibility that side-effects exist. The precautions will indicate if there have been any earlier reported problems with the use of this herb. If encountered in practice side effects should always be reported to relevant professional bodies of herbalists for evaluation and to enable a data base of adverse reactions to be established for future reference.

Interactions

This is an area of knowledge that is growing with the choice by the public to use both herbs and pharmaceutical medicines together for their health care. There are again the two types of scientific enquiry that have been undertaken to assess the possible interactions of herbs and drugs.

In vitro—Using isolated drug metabolising enzymes or drug transport carriers which represents potential or theoretical interactions. These potential interactions are not always borne out *in vivo* but indicate caution may be necessary.

In vivo—Real live studies are limited except for the most popular herbs e.g. *Hypericum* and *Ginkgo* and may be represented by anecdotal events which often have a number of variables for consideration e.g. pharmaceuticals being used concurrently, whether the product contained what was claimed or contained constituents not disclosed on the label.

Studies have also been conducted using herbs in:

- healthy volunteers simultaneously given probe drugs, known to be metabolised by a particular route, or
- clinical trials of populations who require the use of pharmaceuticals as well. The latter are more likely to accurately reflect interactions of significance. Established interactions are indicated by bold type face of named drugs under the given herb.

Given that popular herbs are reaching many people across all ages and in varying states of health there are remarkably few actual herb/drug interactions reported. This may reflect the true state of affairs or it may be a case of under-reported events. Also those herbs that are used less frequently may be associated with interactions not recognised and/or properly reported. Knowledge of the actions of pharmaceuticals and herbs being used concurrently may help in assessing if an interaction has occurred. Again any such possibility should be reported so that proper databases can be established.

A table of clinically relevant cytochrome P450 isozymes, their substrates, inhibitors, inducers and herbs with potential to affect them has been included for reference purposes in Appendix VI.

Historical uses

The long history attached to our *materia medica* has gone through and continues, to some extent, to go through fashions. Under this heading is given abbreviated lists of past usage of each herb, where known, and which may point to applications that are worth revisiting in the future.

Therapeutic index

Lists medical conditions for which whole herb or essential oil (if this is generally available) may be beneficial and in the main is based on traditional use or scientific evidence (*in vivo*).

Isolated constituents and *in vitro* uses are not generally included in the therapeutic index as their relevance to the practice of herbal medicine is uncertain. Exceptions have been made in two areas which are major problems today and for which new treatment strategies are constantly being sought, namely cancer and drug-resistant pathogens. A single asterisk (*) besides an entry denotes data for the whole herb, whilst a double asterisk (**) denotes information on isolated constituents of a herb, all based on *in vitro* research. The reason this has been done is to suggest possible treatment strategies for conditions for which current medication is inadequate. Herbs or their constituents that have shown the ability to effect cancer cell or pathogen survival, but for which clinical trials are lacking, may still have a supportive role to play in the overall treatment strategy as indicated by these studies.

Some applications for disease conditions suggested by *in vitro* studies on a herb has also been indexed to indicate a **potential** benefit and should not be taken as an accepted therapeutic effect of the herb without further evidence.

Actions listed for within each monograph appear in the index in **bold**.

APIACEAE

[Formerly known as Umbelliferae]

There are 300 genera in this family which is plentiful in all parts of the temperate world but not in the tropics.

Many of our common vegetables belong to this family e.g. carrot, parsnip, celery and many of the seed spices e.g. dill, cumin and anise.

The general characteristics of the Apiaceae are:

- The flowers are very small, in umbels
- The sepals are tiny or lacking
- There are 5 free petals, each curved at the tip
- The 5 stamens are attached to a disc around the base of the styles
- The pistil has 2 styles and stigmas. Its ovary is inferior with 2 carpels
- The fruit is distinctive. The 2 dry carpels split apart. They separate at the base, but hang by their tops from a slender stalk. Each contains 1 seed. On their surfaces are the oil ducts which give the flavour and distinctive odour

- The leaf stalks often have sheaths which wrap around the plant stems
- Usually the leaves are much divided, even fern-like
- Outer florets are often enlarged and sterile serving only as banners to guide pollinating insects
- Nearly all members of the family are herbaceous annuals or
- biennials but *Foeniculum vulgare* is perennial

There are three sub-families:

1. **Apioideae** which contains, among others, the following genera—*Ammi, Angelica, Anthriscus, Apium, Conium, Coriandrum, Daucus, Foeniculum, Petroselinum*
2. **Hydrocotyloideae** which contains the genus *Centella*
3. **Saniculoideae**

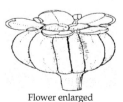

Flower enlarged

Fruit splits into
2 sections
(mericarps)

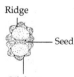

Ridge

Seed

Oil duct

Angelica archangelica

Angelica

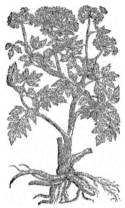

Family Apiaceae

Description
Angelica archangelica is a robust biennial with a stout taproot grown from seed. In the first year it forms a clump of large, matt green leaves borne on round, hollow, green stems 0.5–1 m long, depending on the season and distance from the equator. It dies back in winter and in the second year grows larger and sends up one or more flowering stems. It blooms in early spring and dies after seeding. *Basal leaves* large, 30–60 cm, 2–3 times pinnate, lobes oval lance-shaped and toothed. Stalk leaves smaller or reduced to inflated sheaths enclosing flower buds. *Flower* stems stout, grooved, round and hollow, 1–2 m high with branches topped by green or greenish-white flowers in globular umbels. *Fruits* 5–6 mm with ribs which become corky. All parts are aromatic.[†]

Odour—intensely spicy; taste—at first aromatic then acrid, bitter and lastingly pungent.

Habitat and cultivation
Angelica is native to parts of Europe and Asia and is naturalised in damp situations, blooming in spring/summer of its second year. Cultivated from fresh seed in cooler climates, in sun with well-drained soil. Frost and drought resistant.

[†]The shiny leaved *Angelica pachycarpa* is widely grown as an ornamental plant but has little fragrance and no medicinal use.

Parts used
Leaves—harvested at the end of the first year and as the plant comes in to flower.

Roots and rhizomes—harvested in the autumn of the first year or early spring of second year before flowering. The oil content is highest in roots greater than 5 mm in diameter.[1]

Seeds—harvested when ripe (use of the seeds appears to be a modern adaptation).

Culpeper favoured the root over the leaves.

Active constituents
1) Volatile oil including α- and β-phellandrene, pinene, linalool, borneol, β-bisabolene, β-caryophyllene, limonene[2]
2) Coumarins (at least 15 have been identified) including
    a) furanocoumarins—bergapten (5-methoxypsoralen), oxypeucedanin, isopimpinellin, xanthotoxin, imperatorin, marmesin and apterin
    b) simple coumarins—osthol and umbelliferone[3,4]
3) Phenylpropanoids including angelic and valerianic acids. Also amino-acid amides of N-phenylpropenoyl[5]
4) Flavonoids including archangelenone

In addition the root has resin, tannins and sterols.

Nutritional constituents
Vitamins: E
Minerals: Calcium

Actions
1) Expectorant
2) Diaphoretic
3) Carminative
4) Bitter (root)
5) Spasmolytic
6) Diuretic
7) Anti-inflammatory

Scientific information
Roots, rhizomes and seeds have been officially used as expectorants[22] in a number of countries. *German Commission E* has approved use of the root

to treat loss of appetite, gastro-intestinal spasms, feeling of fullness and flatulence.

The mode of action of *A. archangelica* is largely unexplained. The furanocoumarins, psoralen and its derivatives, are like those now used in treating psoriasis and vitiligo in orthodox medicine. Psoralen is the most phototoxic of the furanocomarins found in the Apiaceae followed by bergapten then xanthotoxin.[6]

In vitro—the seeds inhibit acetylcholinesterase[7] and whole extract, furanocoumarins and essential oil are cytotoxic to cancer cells from the pancreas.[8,9]

Several of the main constituents and the herb itself have anti-oxidant[10] and anti-inflammatory activity[11] and the root oil is antibacterial.[12]

The N-phenylpropenoyl-L-amino acid amides stimulate proliferation of hepatocytes and keratinocytes and reduce adhesion of *H. pylori* to stomach tissue.[5]

In vivo—a herbal combination which included *Angelica* was effective in the treatment of functional dyspepsia with equivalent efficacy to cisapride.[13]

Witchl[14] states *Angelica* is contraindicated in peptic ulceration due to its stimulation of gastric and pancreatic secretions. However this warning is not found elsewhere and *Angelica* was used in combination with 7 other herbs that proved to be anti-ulcerogenic in animal-based studies.

Medicinal uses
Cardiovascular system
- fever
- peripheral vascular disease

Respiratory tract
Used for treating a variety of respiratory problems of varying origin including nervous respiratory conditions, infections and chronic mucus problems:

- coughs
- colds
- pleurisy
- bronchitis
- respiratory catarrh
- psychogenic asthma

Gastro-intestinal tract
The volatile oil aids the digestive process, stops cramping and eases gas build-up. The herb is ideal for treating:

- flatulent dyspepsia
- indigestion
- anorexia
- nervous dyspepsia
- colic

Externally
Angelica oil has been used as a rub in the treatment of:

- rheumatic conditions (*Weiss*)

Pharmacy
Three times daily

Leaf
Infusion of dried herb	–	2–5 g
Tincture 1:5 (45%)	–	2–5 ml
Fluid Extract (25%)	–	2–5 ml

Root
Decoction of dried root	–	1–2 g
Tincture 1:5 (50%)	–	0.5–2 ml
Fluid Extract (25%)	–	0.5–2 ml

Precautions and/or safety
The furanocoumarins in *Angelica* can cause photosensitivity if taken in large doses. (This same light-induced sensitivity gives the herb use as an insecticide as this process is fatal to insects).

Historical uses
Internally for epidemic diseases like the plague; an antidote to poison; for "cold stomachs"; strangury; urinary obstruction; an aid to menstruation and to expelling the afterbirth; overeating; typhoid fever. Externally for poor sight or hearing (drops); toothache; bites of mad dogs or venomous creatures; old filthy ulcers; gout; sciatica; lung and chest complaints (poultice). Used in liqueurs and cordials e.g. Bénédictine and Chartreuse and in Eau de Mélisse de Carmes.

Apium graveolens

Celery, smallage

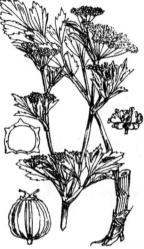

Family Apiaceae

Description
A leafy, much-branched, erect biennial, 0.8–1 m, smelling strongly of celery. *Root* fleshy and bulb-like. *Stems* deeply grooved, hollow and branching at top. *Flowers* about 0.5 mm across, greenish-white petals, entire, acute, in compound umbels 2–4 cm across, more or less sessile and leaf opposed. Primary rays unequal, 4–15, bracts and bracteoles absent. *Basal leaves* once pinnate, with three-lobed leaflets 0.5–3 cm, lower leaves stalked, upper leaves sessile, three-lobed, all shiny green. *Fruits* dark brown, 1–2 mm long, ribs light brown, filiform. Flowers from early summer to late autumn.

Odour—characteristic, spicy; taste—spicy, somewhat bitter.

Habitat and cultivation
Native to Southern Europe growing wild in salt marshes or salt rich ground. Introduced, naturalized and cultivated elsewhere from seed in open, sunny situations with adequate moisture. Frost resistant, drought tender. Celery and celeriac are vegetable forms of this species.

Parts used
The seeds collected when dry and ripe.

Active constituents
1) Volatile oil (1.5–3.0%):-
    a) mainly limonene and β-silinene, also apiol, sesquiterpenoid glucosides[15] viz. celerioside (A–E)[16,17]
    b) phthalides including sedanolide, 3-n-butyl-4,5-dihydrophthalide, senkyunolides[18,19] and celephthalide (A–C).[15] It is these constituents that give celery its characteristic smell
2) Furanocoumarins including bergapten
3) Fixed oil including petroselinic acid[16,20]
4) Flavonoids including derivatives of luteolin, chrysoeriol and apigenin[21]

Also a lignan[15] and L-tryptophan.[18]

Actions
1) Carminative
2) Urinary antiseptic
3) Spasmolytic (mild)
4) Diuretic
5) Hypotensive
6) Anti-inflammatory
7) Antirheumatic

Scientific information
Celery has been grown for around three thousand years and used as a spice and vegetable. The seeds have been an official medicine reputed to have a sedative effect on the nervous system, whilst their oil was considered antispasmodic, a nerve stimulant and useful for treating rheumatoid arthritis.[22] It is used in India to treat liver dysfunction and in Germany to improve bowel function and treat loss of appetite, exhaustion, hysteria and restlessness.

In vitro—The seeds have mosquito repellent activity.[23]

Constituents of the seeds are effective against *Candida* spp.[16,19] and some nematodes,[16,19] antioxidant[17,18] and can inhibit COX1, COX2[18] and topoisomerase I and II.[16,18]

Medicinal uses
Gastro-intestinal tract
- flatulence
- colic
- indigestion

Urinary tract
* cystitis
* urinary stones
* urinary tract inflammation

Musculoskeletal

The herb is nutritious and aids the excretion, through the kidneys, of waste metabolites.

* rheumatism
* arthritis
* gout

The *BHP* gives the specific application for *Apium* as rheumatoid arthritis with mental depression.

Pharmacy

Three times daily

Decoction	–	0.5–2 g
Tincture 1:5	–	2–8 ml
		(suggested guidelines)
Fluid Extract (60%)	–	0.3–1.2 ml

CONTRAINDICATIONS—Kidney disorders—apiol is toxic to kidneys. **Pregnancy**—in large doses the herb (apiol) can cause uterine contractions that may lead to abortion.

Precautions and/or safety

May cause allergic reaction, though this is rare. The furanocoumarins, as in *Angelica*, can lead to photosensitivity. Ingestion of normal amounts of psoralen-containing foods do not increase UV-induced skin erythema.[24] At recommended doses *Apium* is a safe herb.

Historical uses

Insomnia; opens liver and spleen; expectorant; agues; worms. As a gargle for mouth, throat sores and ulcers; bad breath. As a lotion for sores and cankers. Melancholy.

Carum carvi

Caraway

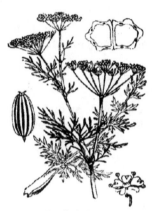

Family Apiaceae

Description

An erect, hairless, much-branched biennial, 25–60 cm tall. *Flowers* white, 2–3 mm in umbels 2–4 cm across. Primary rays very unequal, 5–12. Flower stems hollow, furrowed, branched. Bracts and bracteoles bristle-like or absent. *Leaves* twice-pinnate with segments further deeply cut into narrow lance-shaped or linear lobes. Upper leaves have a sheathing petiole. *Root* spindle-shaped. *Fruits* dark brown, 3–4 mm, oblong with low ribs, strong smelling when crushed. Flowers in late spring to early summer.

Odour—aromatic; taste—spicy and aromatic.

Habitat and cultivation

Originally introduced from Arabic countries, caraway is naturalized in Europe being cultivated there and elsewhere from seed sown in rows in open, sunny situations in moist well-drained soil. Drought and frost tender.

Parts used

The seeds collected when dry and ripe.

Active constituents

1) Volatile oil (up to 7%) predominantly comprised of (+) carvone and (+) limonene.[25,26] Also carvacrol, germacrene B and D, derivatives of carvone and anethofuran[27–29]

2) Flavonoids including isoquercetin and derivatives of quercetin and kaempferol[30]
3) Fatty oil
4) Polyacetylenes[31]

Also contains protein (around 20%).

Nutritional constituents
Vitamins: B
Minerals: Magnesium, silica, phosphorous, sulphur, potassium, calcium, manganese, iron, copper and zinc[32]

Actions
1) Carminative
2) Antimicrobial
3) Emmenagogue
4) Expectorant
5) Astringent
6) Spasmolytic

Scientific information
Caraway is used as a spice and was an official medicine in many countries, as a carminative for flatulent colic in young children.[22] The essential oil is still used for flavouring liqueurs and toiletries.

In vitro—Aqueous extracts have strong antioxidant activity, being more than twice as strong as ascorbic acid.[33] The herb and/or its constituents also have anti-proliferative,[32] anti-mutagenic[34] and anti-carcinogenic activity.[35] The monoterpene, limonene, and its metabolite perillyl alcohol found in both celery seeds and caraway have shown potential as a preventative, and treatment, for breast, colon and prostate cancers.[36,37]

Carum has only mild antibacterial activity against *Helicobacter pylori*[38] but the essential oil is active against *Escherichia coli*.[27] Its action in helping with gastro-intestinal dysfunction may be primarily through its anti-oxidant and therefore anti-inflammatory activity.[39]

A model simulating the gastro-intestinal environment and mucosa indicates that the essential oil profile may change with pH but constituents can cross the cell membrane barrier.[40]

In vivo—A number of studies have been carried out on the treatment of functional dyspepsia using *Carum* extracts in conjunction with other herbs. Symptoms improved in all studies, whether *Helicobacter pylori* was present or not.[41-45]

Isolated caraway oil relaxes the gall-bladder[46] and smooth muscle of the stomach and duodenum.[47]

Medicinal uses
Respiratory tract
A less strong expectorant than either *Pimpinella* or *Foeniculum* it is still used for:

• bronchitis

Gastro-intestinal tract
• flatulent dyspepsia
• intestinal colic
• cramps
• hiccoughs
• flatulence/bloating
• dyspepsia
• diarrhoea
• anorexia

Reproductive tract
• dysmenorrhoea

Externally
• laryngitis (gargle)

Pharmacy
Three times daily
Decoction   –   0.5–2 g
Tincture 1:5 (45%) –   0.5–4 ml

Precautions and/or safety
The above clinical trials did not record any adverse events from the preparation containing *Carum*. As an emmenagogue one might expect the herb to be contra-indicated in pregnancy. This has not been the case historically and presumably this action is encountered only with large doses.

Based on skin prick tests some individuals could have allergies to caraway.[48-50]

Historical uses
Diuretic; to clear head; improve eyesight. *Culpeper* recommended the root as a vegetable "to strengthen

the stomach of old people exceedingly" and also includes in the medicinal actions the promotion of urine and benefits for eyesight. Externally as a poultice for bruises; earache.

Centella asiatica

Gotu kola, hydrocotyle

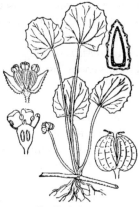

Family Apiaceae

Description
Centella asiatica is a creeping perennial of tropical climates whose appearance varies depending on wet/dry conditions. *The roots* form at the leaf nodes with 3–4 leaves growing up on individual, long stems. The plant spreads by reddish stringy stolons from the nodes to form a large patch. *The leaves* are round-kidney shaped, brown-green, about 3 cm wide and can have smooth, crenate or lobed margins. The petioles are up to 15 cm tall and green at the top but purplish-pink at the sheathing base. *Flowers* are small and purple, usually 3–6, appearing in summer in axillary umbels on 2–8 mm tall stems. They are below the upper leaves and are insignificant or difficult to see. *Fruit* forms throughout the growing season. It is compressed sideways, about 3–5 mm long with 7–9 ribs and a curved strongly thickened pericarp.

Odour—characteristic; taste—slightly bittersweet.

Habitat and cultivation
Native to tropical and subtropical parts of Africa, Australia, Cambodia, China, India, Indonesia, Madagascar, Central and South America and Southern USA growing in damp or swampy areas. Also grows less lushly in rocky areas in India and Sri Lanka. Propagated by division. It may be grown in containers in warm, temperate climates but is frost tender.

Parts used
Leaves or whole herb, fresh or dried, harvested as needed throughout the year.

Active constituents
1) Triterpenoids including asiaticoside, madecassoside, asiaticoside-B and free asiatic, madecassic and terminolic acids.[51,52] (The triterpene ester glycosides constitute not less than 2% of the herb.[53]) Asiatic acid level increases *in vivo* by conversion from asiaticoside[54]
2) Volatile oils including β-caryophyllene, β-farnesene and germacrene[55]
3) Flavonoids including apigenin, rutin, kaempferol and quercetin[56,57]

Also an alkaloid (hydrocotyline), pectin[58] polyacetylenes,[59,60] phenolic acids[56] and tannins.

Nutritional constituents
Vitamins: B and C
Minerals: Calcium, magnesium and sodium

Actions
1) Vulnerary
2) Anti-inflammatory
3) Venous tonic
4) Antimicrobial
5) Anxiolytic
6) Dermatological agent

Also used in India as an alterative tonic and a diuretic.[22] Its long list of historical uses may have lead to it being described as an adaptogen.

Scientific information
Centella is a geographically widespread herb with traditional uses in many cultures and it is currently enjoying a resurgence of interest. It has been attributed with the longevity of a Chinese healer who lived to 256 years of age! Much of the recent scientific data relates to the use of the triterpenoids

to treat venous hypertension and insufficiency and the whole herb's and/or triterpenoid's ability to promote tissue healing.

Vulnerary

Research has provided some insight into the use of *Centella* as a vulnerary.

In vitro—Constituents (triterpenoids) through modified gene expression stimulate fibroblast activity and collagen production,[61-65] increase extracellular matrix synthesis,[61,66] including fibronectin[67] and stimulate angiogenesis.[66] The herb also inhibits keratinocyte replication suggesting a possible mechanism for its use in psoriasis.[68]

In vivo—*Centella* and/or its constituents reduced inflammation including during the formation of scar tissue,[69,70] accelerated cicatrisation in wounds and ulcers,[71] helped reduce stretch marks in women prone to develop them[72] and aided in the treatment of second and third degree burns.[73]

Madecassol, a combination of the triterpenes of *Centella*, has also been used orally and topically in the treatment of patients with systemic and focal scleroderma with improvement in indurated lesions, hyperpigmentation, vascular trophic disorders and in the general condition of patients.[74] However, the preparation was less promising in patients with progressive disease and where skin lesions were diffuse. There is also an anecdotal report of this preparation benefiting the treatment of focal elastosis.[75]

Circulation

In vivo—*Centella* triterpenoids have also been used in a series of clinical trials to treat impaired venous circulation. Positive outcomes were apparent from subjective and objective assessments. Results have indicated:-

- improved circulation[76-80]
- protection and healing of the endothelium[81]
- reduced oedema[77-79,81,82]
- reduced thrombosis risk through stabilisation of arterial plaques[83,84]
- improved microcirculation[85] and neuropathy[86] in diabetics, with protection against further damage

- improved outcome in patients with venous disease who undertook air travel (DVT)[87]
- improved outcome in patients with post-phlebitic syndrome[88]

It should be noted that the above studies were conducted using a standardised form of a partial extract of the herb.

Centella should, through its ability to improve microcirculation and connective tissue in blood vessel walls, aid the treatment of haemorrhoids and varicose veins.[89,90] The herb combined with vitamin E, rutin and *Melilotus* reduced oedema and cramps in chronic venous insufficiency.[91]

Nervous system

In vitro—*Centella* stimulates neurite growth[92] and inhibits acetylcholinesterase.[93]

In vivo—The herb has a traditional reputation of improving cognitive function and this was demonstrated in healthy elderly people who also reported mood improvements after 1–2 months use.[94] A German pharmaceutical company has patented a medication based on asiatic acid to treat dementia and enhance cognition.

The whole herb has anxiolytic activity.[95]

Antimicrobial

In vitro—*Centella* and/or its constituents have a range of antimicrobial activity including:

- antiviral against HSV-1 and 2[96,97]
- antifungal against several pathogenic fungi[98]
- antibacterial against a range of enteric pathogens including *Vibrio cholerae*, *Shigella* spp. and *Staphylococcus aureus*.[99] The triterpenes cause dissolution of their cell walls.

The herb and various fractions may have some immunostimulatory potential.[58,100]

In vivo—The herb has been known as a treatment for leprosy.[22] Oral administration of capsules containing *Centella* or asiaticoside and potassium chloride compared favourably with dapsone, one of the pharmaceutical preparations used to treat this condition.[101] It has been used as a topical treatment for leprous ulcers also.[99,102]

Other
In vitro—*Centella* inhibits tumour cell growth,[103,104] induces apoptosis in melanoma cells[105] and protects cells in contact with genotoxins.[106]

In vivo—Initial studies undertaken in 1979 suggested that *Centella* may be of benefit in the treatment of chronic liver disorders,[107] however no further data has emerged. Oral use of madecassol has been a very effective treatment for peptic and duodenal ulcers.[108]

Local application of *Centella* and *Punica granatum* improved the symptoms of chronic periodontitis[109] and in Thai medicine to treat herpes infections.[96]

Medicinal uses
Cardiovascular system
- venous insufficiency
- phlebitis
- varicose veins
- thrombosis
- diabetic angiopathy

Nervous system
Centella has been used traditionally to improve mental performance, to treat depression and anxiety.

- anxiety
- cold sores
- genital herpes

Musculoskeletal
It has been used both internally and topically as a vulnerary to treat a number of skin conditions and is also listed in the *BHP* as an antirheumatic.

- psoriasis
- wounds
- scleroderma
- ulcers
- cellulitis
- leprosy
- keloids
- stretch marks
- burns
- arthritis

Pharmacy
Based on traditional use.
Three times daily

Infusion of dried herb − 0.33–0.68 g
                            (suggested guidelines[110])
Tincture 1:2 (45%)   − 0.6–1.5 ml

Centella can be used internally and externally, both being indicated by tradition and recent clinical trials. Madecassol is a trade name preparation which contains 0.5% triterpenes in ointment and 2% in powder form.[22]

Precautions and/or safety
No adverse effects were reported from trials using the triterpenoids or herb. Large doses are said to have a narcotic action[22] and may cause headache, stupor, vertigo or coma (*Grieve*).

There are a small number of people who may develop contact dermatitis on exposure to the herb.[111] The *BHP* further cites a potential for the herb to cause photosensitisation when used in tropical areas.[112] However some reported cases of dermatitis may have been due to ingredients other than *Centella* in the preparation responsible.[113]

There is a report of hepatotoxicity in three patients who were using *Centella* weight-loss tablets, the condition was reversible but recurred on rechallenge with the same tablets. These tablets do not appear to have been characterised so their actual chemical make-up is unknown.[114]

Historical uses
Uses include treatment of albinism, anaemia, asthma, bronchitis, measles, constipation, dermatitis, diarrhoea, dysentery, dysmenorrhoea, dysuria, epistaxis, epilepsy, haematemesis, jaundice, leucorrhoea, nephritis, neuralgia, rheumatism, smallpox, syphilis, toothache, tuberculosis, urethritis, fever, pain, inflammation, brain tonic. Externally fractures, sprains and furunculosis.

Foeniculum vulgare var. *dulce*

Fennel

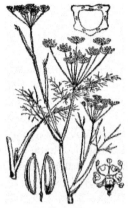

Family Apiaceae

Although it is only 1 genus, fennel has been in cultivation for more than 2000 years and there are a number of forms of it. The one used in herbal medicine is *Foeniculum vulgare* var. *dulce* and the bronze-leaved form of this is called *F. vulgare* var. *dulce* *"Purpureum"*. The fennel with the swollen basal stems that is used as a vegetable is known as *F. vulgare* var. *azoricum*. There is another vegetable type known in Europe as *Carosella*, with large fleshy stalks. Wild fennel, which grows in some parts of Europe, is named *F. vulgare* spp. *piperitum*. The flavour of the seeds is acrid and there only 4–10 rays in the umbel as opposed to the 12–25 rays in umbels of *F. vulgare* var. *dulce*. This fennel does not appear to have been introduced into the Southern Hemisphere.

Description
A stout, aromatic, erect perennial, smelling strongly of anise. *Stems* solid, striate, polished, about 2 m high. *Basal leaves* 3–4 pinnate, petiolate, ultimate segments filiform, acuminate, 3–50 mm long, not all in one plane. Stem leaves similar but petiole extended along whole length into a thin, closely-ribbed sheath. *Umbels* 2–5 cm in diameter, rays 4–25, usually slightly incurved at fruiting. *Flowers* numerous, yellow, 1–2 mm in diameter. *Fruits* dark brown, 3–6 mm long, ribs pale brown. Flowers from summer to autumn.

Odour—spicy; taste—like aniseed, aromatic and spicy.

Habitat and cultivation
Originally from Southern Europe and the Mediterranean, fennel is naturalised world wide, growing from seed in waste places in cities and in any sunny situation in the countryside Drought and frost resistant.

Parts used
The seeds collected when dry and ripe. Some traditions have also used the aerial parts.

Active constituents
1) Volatile oil (up to 6%) including trans-anethole (max. 80%), fenchone (max. 7.5%), methyl chavicol (also called estragole—max. 10%), limonene, phellandrene, pinene, p-anisaldehyde, thymol[115-119]
2) Flavonoids including rutin, quercitin and kaempferol glycosides[30]
3) Coumarins including the furanocoumarins bergapten (5-methoxypsoralen)[120] and psoralen[121]
4) Phenolic compounds including chlorogenic acid[122,123]

Also fixed oil,[124] protein (20%), trans-resveratrol and other sterols.[125]

The content and composition of the volatile oil varies with subspecies, geographical and environmental conditions.[126,127]

Nutritional constituents
Minerals: Potassium, calcium, sulphur and sodium

Actions
1) Carminative
2) Anti-inflammatory
3) Diuretic
4) Galactagogue
5) Orexigenic
6) Stomachic
7) Antimicrobial

Scientific information
Foeniculum has been a spice, food and medicine for hundreds of years and the seeds have been an official medicine in many countries, being used for the same purposes as *Carum*.[22] The seeds have been

approved for internal use by *German Commission E* for spasms of the gastro-intestinal tract, fullness and flatulence and for treating upper respiratory catarrh.

In vitro—*Foeniculum* essential oil is:

- antibacterial against a range of pathogens including *Listeria monocytogenes, Staphylococcus aureus, Salmonella typhimurium, S. enteritidis, Escherichia coli,*[128,129,135] *Helicobacter pylori*[38] and *Streptococcus haemolyticus*[130]
- antifungal including against *Candida albicans,*[131] *Trichophyton mentagrophytes* and *Aspergillus niger*[115]
- acaricidal—toxic to house dust mites

Foeniculum and its constituents are anti-oxidant,[123,132–135] the aqueous extract being stronger than ascorbic acid.[136]

A model simulating the gastro-intestinal environment and mucosa demonstrated that the essential oil profile may change with pH but the constituents can pass through the cell membrane barrier.[40]

In vivo—*Foeniculum* like *Pimpinella*, has oestrogenic properties,[137,138] both having been explored in the 1930's with a view to developing synthetic oestrogens. Anethole was considered to be the constituent responsible but the activity is likely due to its polymers.[139] Creams containing either 1% or 2% ethanol extract of *Foeniculum*, applied topically, reduced hair diameter in women with idiopathic hirsutism due to an oestrogenic effect.[140] An oral preparation of the essential oil (2%) compared favourably with mefenamic acid in the treatment of primary dysmenorrhoea.[141,142]

Colic in infants 2–12 weeks old was improved by a preparation of the essential oil[143] and also, within a week, on a combination of *Foeniculum, Matricaria* and *Melissa*.[144] *Foeniculum* as part of a herbal mixture helped to regulate bowel motions and significantly reduce abdominal pain in non-specific colitis.[145]

The essential oil is a repellent to mosquitoes.[146]

Medicinal uses
Respiratory tract
As for *Pimpinella*, it is used as an expectorant though it is milder in this action:

- coughs
- bronchitis

Gastro-intestinal tract
- colic[†]
- flatulent dyspepsia
- flatulence
- indigestion
- anorexia
- intestinal cramps
- hiccoughs
- bloating

Urinary tract
In combination with other herbs to treat:

- cystitis

Reproductive tract
- to increase milk flow in lactating mothers
- primary dysmenorrhoea

Externally
As an anti-inflammatory it is used as an eyewash and a gargle for:

- blepharitis
- conjunctivitis
- pharyngitis
- idiopathic hirsutism

Pharmacy
Three times daily
Dried herb   – 0.3–2 g
Fluid Extract (70%) – 0.8–2 ml

Precautions and/or safety
No safety issues have arisen from using *Foeniculum* or its essential oil although an allergy like that

---

[†]Especially suitable for children.

found for celery has been reported.[147] *German Commission E* recommends that the herb only be used for short periods due to the estragole content which is carcinogenic in rodent studies. The metabolism of estragole in humans is however different to that in rodents, it is not used as an isolated constituent and it does not appear to be a concern when the herb is used at recommended doses.[148] Extreme caution should be exercised in using essential oils internally.

Interactions
In vitro bergapten can inhibit CYP3A4[120,149] and an animal study has indicated a possible interaction with the antibiotic ciprofloxacin.[150]

Historical uses
A diuretic; urinary stones; nausea; opens obstructions of liver, to clear the body of poisons, spleen, gall bladder; jaundice; gout; dyspnoea; wheezing; aids menstruation and delivery of placenta; makes fat people lean; for longevity; to clear the eyes. To deter fleas.

Lomatium dissectum

Biscuit root, fern-leaved desert parsley

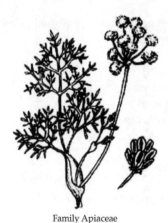

Family Apiaceae

Description
A perennial with thickened roots reaching about 1½ m in flower. *Roots* are grey externally and creamy-white and fleshy internally, containing a milky sap. *Stems* long, glabrous, hollow and chocolate coloured. *Leaves* bright green and ternately compound with 2–4 linear pinnae, clothed with fine hairs or glabrous. The stem base has a purple hue. *Flowers* small, yellow or purple in compound umbels. *Fruit* oblong ovoid about 1½ cm long flattened and with broad wings, inconspicuous.

Habitat and cultivation
Native to western North America from Vancouver Island to California, growing in sun or semi-shade in rocky/talus conditions. Not normally cultivated. There are 80 species or varieties of this genus with similar medicinal uses. Previously named *Leptotaenia multiflora*.

Parts used
The root, harvested in spring or autumn used fresh or dried; leaves have been used to a lesser extent.

Active constituents[151]
1) Flavonoids including luteolin[152]
2) Coumarins—pyranocoumarins and furanocoumarins including nodakenetin, columbianin and columbianetin[152]
3) Tetronic acids[152]
4) Volatile oil including terpenes and sesquiterpenes
5) Resin

Nutritional constituents
Vitamins: C

Actions
1) Antimicrobial
2) Immunostimulant

Scientific information
To date there is not a great deal of scientific evidence for the efficacy of *Lomatium* but there is extensive traditional use amongst the native Indians of North America. The herb came to western attention during the influenza epidemic of 1917 where it was credited with successfully limiting mortality.[153]

In vitro—*Lomatium* completely inhibited a bovine rotavirus,[154] but human pathogen studies are lacking.

Suksdorfin isolated from the fruit of a related species, *L. suksdorfii*, was effective at inhibiting the replication of HIV-1.[155] The role for *L. dissectum* in the treatment of AIDS is yet to be determined.

The tetronic acids are ichthyotoxic, (some American Indians used the immersed roots to catch fish in streams), and there is some scientific evidence of their antimicrobial and antineoplastic actions.[156]

In vivo—As an antiviral and immune stimulating agent, *Lomatium* has been used as an important herb in the treatment of chronic fatigue or post viral syndrome.[153]

Medicinal uses
Respiratory tract
All infections of the upper and lower respiratory tract:

- sore throat
- colds and influenza
- coughs
- pneumonia
- sinusitis
- bronchitis
- tuberculosis

Externally
As a wash for:

- gingivitis
- periodontitis
- tonsillitis
- cuts/abrasions
- *Candida/Gardnerella* infections

Pharmacy
Three times daily
Decoction	–	2–4 g
Tincture 1:5 (70%)	–	0.5–2.5 ml
Fluid Extract of fresh root (95%)	–	0.5–2.5 ml

Precautions and/or safety
The use of tinctures in Western herbalism has highlighted a hot, itchy rash that occurs within 5–7 days from the start of taking *Lomatium* in perhaps 10% of the population.[153,157] The rash does not respond to steroid or antihistamine treatment and is believed to be either a result of viral die-off, in those with a systemic infection, or a result of excess immune stimulation. It is also possible that as tinctures involve ethanol extraction, they may contain a constituent not found in traditional aqueous preparations where the problem did not seem to arise. However *Alstat* reports that the original symptoms often seem to improve with onset of the rash. Once the rash has resolved, this takes several days, further ingestion of *Lomatium* does not result in its recurrence.

Historical uses[158]
The root eaten as a vegetable or dried and powdered and made into biscuits hence its name. American Indian use was wide ranging and included the treatment of chest problems, hayfever; stomach complaints; rheumatism; as a tonic for convalescence and weight loss; venereal disease. The smoke of the root inhaled for asthma; poultice for bruises, boils, fractures and rheumatic joints; as a wash for dandruff. The root oil was used as an eye wash for trachoma.

Pimpinella anisum

Anise, aniseed

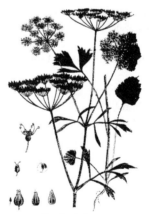

Family Apiaceae

Description
A lax, short-lived annual to 60 cm. *Basal leaves* simple, pinnate or ternately compound, deeply and irregularly toothed. Stem leaves 1–2 pinnate or ternately

compound, entire. *Flowers* white, in large, loose compound umbels. *Fruits* greyish-green to dull yellowish-brown from 2–5 mm. They have short, stout hairs and 10 light-coloured stout ridges. The fruits, with mericarps united and the pedicels attached, are usually complete when harvested and sold.

Habitat and cultivation

Native to North Africa and some Mediterranean islands, anise is cultivated elsewhere growing only from seed in light, rich, weed-free soil. It needs a cool germination period and a hot dry summer to ripen the seeds. Frost tender, drought resistant.

Parts used

The seeds collected when dry and ripe.

Active constituents

1) Volatile oil (2–6%) including mainly anethole (70–90%) also γ-himachalene (2–4%), p-anisaldehyde (less than 1%), estragole (methylchavicol 0.9–3.1%), limonene (2.6%)[124,159-162]
2) Flavonoids including rutin, quercetin, apigenin, luteolin, isovitexin and isoorientin[30]
3) Coumarins including bergapten
4) Fatty oil (8–11%)[124,159]
5) Phenylpropanoid glycosides including derivatives of pseudoisoeugenyl 2-methylbutyrate (approx 4.3%)[159,163,164]

Also contains choline and protein.[159]

Nutritional constituents

Vitamins: B and E[165]
Minerals: Potassium, calcium, iron, sulphur and magnesium[166]

Actions

1) Expectorant
2) Carminative
3) Spasmolytic
4) Parasiticide

Scientific information

Pimpinella has a long history of use both in food flavouring and as a medicine. It is still in demand for flavouring and in the manufacture of perfumes. Aniseed was an official medicine in a number of countries, mainly as an oil preparation, for use as a carminative and mild expectorant.[22]

In vitro—Pimpinella is a good anti-oxidant.[124] Both the extract and the essential oil have limited antibacterial activity[130,167,168] although an extract did have some capacity to inhibit *Helicobacter pylori*.[38] The essential oil is strongly antifungal to a number of pathogenic strains including *Candida* and *Trichophyton* species,[169] is acaricidal for dust mites,[170] repellent and insecticidal to mosquitoes[171,172] and is a very safe and effective pediculocide.[173,174]

As in *Foeniculum* anethole is a main constituent of the essential oil and it and/or its derivatives have shown oestrogen receptor binding activity.[139] The whole extract exhibited oestrogen-antagonist activity, suppressed the growth of breast cancer cell lines but stimulated (animal derived) osteoblasts without inducing uterine cell proliferation.[175] It may have use as a preventative of osteoporosis post-menopause.

In vivo—There are no clinical studies on *Pimpinella* alone but a combined preparation with ivy, thyme and marshmallow was effective in the treatment of irritable coughs.[176]

It has a pleasant taste and can be used in children's remedies and to improve the taste of other herbal medicines.

Medicinal uses

Respiratory tract
• hard, dry coughs
• pertussis
• infantile catarrh
• tracheitis with persistent cough
• bronchial catarrh
• asthma
• spasmodic coughs

Gastro-intestinal tract
• flatulence
• colic
• cramps
• to allay griping of strong laxatives

Externally
The volatile oil is used topically for:

- pediculosis (lice)
- scabies

Pharmacy
Three times daily
Decoction of dried herb   –   0.5–1 g
Tincture 1:5   –   0.5–2 ml

Precautions and/or safety
Standard tests failed to find mutagenic activity in this herb.[166] There is a potential for allergy to *Pimpinella* either through its inhalation[49,177] or ingestion.[178,179] Furthermore allergy to one member of the Apiaceae can lead to a sensitivity to other members.[180]

Historical uses
Hiccoughs; epilepsy; to counter poisons and venom; headaches (snuff); uterine pain (locally applied); galactagogue, to facilitate childbirth, increase libido; breath freshener (chewed); smoked to promote expectoration.

APOCYNACEAE

A Dicotyledon family of about 130 genera of herbs, shrubs and trees, some poisonous and/or with milky juice. Distribution world wide but *Vinca* is the only genus native to Europe. It is often used as an ornamental ground cover, and there are varieties with pink, purple and/or white flowers, some double.

Vinca major

Greater periwinkle

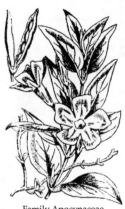

Family Apocynaceae

Description
A robust perennial trailing plant spreading 1–2 m with herbaceous stems rooting at the tips. *Leaves* 2–4 cm, dark shining green, oval with a rounded or heart-shaped base and a finely hairy margin. *Flowers* large, axillary, solitary, blue, 4–5 cm across, corolla lobes blunt, radially asymmetrical, calyx linear and hairy. Stamens fused to the corolla tube. Stigma enlarged above with a tuft of hair at the apex. (If the flower is pulled apart and the stigma detached it looks like a tiny ice cream cone.) Blooms from mid spring to summer.

Habitat and cultivation
Native to Mediterranean Europe and introduced elsewhere, *Vinca major* grows in woods, along hedges and stream banks. It is cultivated in gardens and shrubberies as an ornamental ground cover, and often naturalised.

Parts used
The leaves, harvested when the plant is in flower.

Active constituents
1) Alkaloids of the indole type, at least 40 have been isolated including majdine, isomajdine,

majoridine, reserpinine (pubescine), vincama-joridine and vincamajoreine[1-6]
2) Tannins
3) Flavonoids including a derivative of kaempferol[7]

Also cholorgenic and ursolic acids, robinin and saponins.[6] Tannins were not detected in one analysis.[6]

Actions
1) Antihaemorrhagic
2) Astringent

Scientific information
There has been very little investigation of this herb and much of what exists was carried out some time ago.

Since the discovery of the indole alkaloids vin-cristine and vinblastine (found in *Catharanthus roseus*, formerly *Vinca rosea*), which are used in the treatment of cancer, other *Vinca* species have been analysed for their cytotoxic potential. *V. major* has not been found useful in this context.

The use of *V. major* is less well studied than that of *V. minor*. It seems to have been used traditionally for its tannin dependent actions.

Medicinal uses
Gastro-intestinal tract
• diarrhoea
• bleeding haemorrhoids

Urinary tract
• enuresis

Reproductive tract
• menorrhagia
• leucorrhoea

Externally
• haemorrhoids
• mouth ulcers
• sore throat
• epistaxis

Pharmacy
Three times daily
Infusion   –   2–4 g
Fluid extract (25%)   –   2–4 ml

Precautions and/or safety
V. major may aggravate constipation due to its ten-dency to "bind" and should not be used if this is a problem, however the fresh flowers were consid-ered a gentle laxative (*Grieve*).

Historical uses
The English name "periwinkle" is derived from the Latin "to bind" because the long runners of the plant were plaited into wreaths and used as string. Known as Sorcerer's Violet used as plant of love and fertility; associated with death and immortal-ity; to treat hysteria, fits, diabetes. Externally for cramps.

Vinca minor

Lesser periwinkle

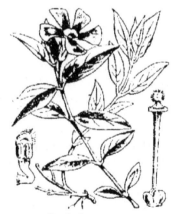

Family Apocynaceae

Description
A similar but smaller perennial with trailing stems 30–60 cm long, rooting at the nodes. *Leaves* oppo-site, dark glossy green, glabrous. *Flowers* regular, solitary, axillary. Corolla purplish blue, mauve or white, with a conical tube and 5 asymmetrical

lobes. Does not often set seed. Blooms early spring to summer.

Habitat and cultivation
Similar to that of *V. major*. Growing as a ground cover in woods, hedgerows and stream banks it is easily propagated by planting rooted runners.

Parts used
The leaves, harvested when the plant is in flower.

Active constituents
1) Alkaloids
   a) indole type including vincine, apovin-camine, vincamine and many others[8–13]
   b) bisindole alkaloids including vincarubine[14]
2) Flavonoids including kaempferol, quercetin and isorhamnetin[15]
3) Tannins

Also a lignan,[16] ursolic acid,[17] ornol,[18] β-sitosterol[18] and triacontane.[18]

Actions
1) Antihaemorrhagic
2) Astringent

Scientific information
As is the case for *V. major* there has been very little recent investigation into this herb. There is evidence accumulating to support this species' action as a circulatory stimulant, although it is largely based on the isolated alkaloids.

In vivo—The alkaloid vincamine and a synthetic derivative of apovincamine have been used in patients with dementias, they show potential in improving cognitive function.[19,20] Vincamine improved cerebral blood flow and brain metabolism,[21] may be hypotensive[22] and improved recovery of stroke patients when used in the acute phase.[23]

Extrapolating the actions of the whole plant to those of the isolated alkaloids is speculative although mediaeval uses for *V. minor* indicate that the whole plant has an action on cerebral circulation.

Further evidence is required to confirm the efficacy of *V. minor* for uses other than those for which *V. major* is used.

Medicinal uses
Cardiovascular system
Based on the studies of the isolated alkaloid, may find a use in the future treatment of:

• hypertension
• cerebral arteriosclerosis

Nervous system
Based on the studies of the isolated alkaloid, may find a use in the future treatment of:

• impaired memory
• brain injury
• vertigo
• Ménière's disease
• headaches
• tinnitus
• strokes

Pharmacy
Three times daily
Infusion   –   2–4 g
Fluid extract (25%)   –   2–4 ml
Treatment with vincamine may take between 3–6 weeks to show results (*Weiss*).

Precautions and/or safety
As for *V. major*. On the basis of studies on vincamine it may be assumed that *V. minor* should not be used in cases of brain tumour or where intracranial pressure is raised. Vincamine is considered safe and well tolerated although *Weiss* mentions mild and reversible gastro-intestinal symptoms are possible.

Historical uses
Headaches, vertigo, to aid the memory.

ARACEAE

A monocotyledon family of about 15 genera and 2,000 species of mainly tropical perennials which grow in water or as epiphytes as well as in the ground.

- Leaves arise from corms or rhizomes and are generally stemless
- Inflorescence is a densely flowered spadix subtended by a showy spathe, e.g. the arum lily
- Individual flowers very small or reduced, bisexual or unisexual
- Plants monoecious with female flowers at the base and male flowers above

Acorus calamus

Calamus, sweet flag

Description
A perennial plant of marshy places. *Leaves* green, and iris-like, about 2 cm wide, growing in a fan from a stout pinkish rhizome and from 50–125 cm tall. Leaves and rhizome aromatic when crushed. *Peduncle* and spathe a flattened triangular leaf-like unit, bearing a stout, round, green spadix, about 10 cm long jutting out on one side and above the

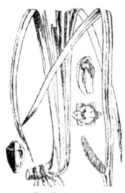

Family Araceae

middle. *Flowers* tiny, yellowish and bisexual with a 6-parted perianth. Flowers from late spring to mid summer. Does not set fruit in cooler climates. A variegated green and white leafed variety is sometimes seen. The plant occurs in diploid, triploid and tetraploid varieties.

Odour—sweet and aromatic; taste—aromatic, pungent and bitter.

Habitat and cultivation
Native to Asia and North America, calamus has been introduced elsewhere. It grows in shallow water along margins of lakes, ponds and streams

and dies back in winter. It is propagated by separating and replanting pieces of rhizome with a crown when dormant.

Parts used
The dried rhizome, harvested in autumn and the cortex removed.

Active constituents
1) Volatile oil (1–3%). There are different chemotypes one in which the predominant constituents of the volatile oil are mainly the phenylpropanoids, predominantly β-asarone (synonym Z-asarone), with small amounts of α-asarone, and a second in which they are predominantly sesquiterpenoids, shyobunone and epishyobunone. Intermediate chemotypes contain varying ratios of these two main constituent groups. Also contains to differing levels, acorenone, iso-acorone, acorone, isoeugenol, α-terpineol and limonene[1-5]
2) Flavonoids including quercetin and kaempferol[6]
3) Phenolic acids including caffeic, ferulic and p-coumaric acids[6]

The constituents of the rhizome differ quite markedly from that of the root.[7]

Nutritional constituents
Minerals: Calcium, magnesium, potassium, zinc and iron

Actions
1) Aromatic bitter
2) Diaphoretic
3) Carminative
4) Spasmolytic
5) Digestive tonic

Older studies have also shown anti-arrhythmic, hypotensive, antitussive and expectorant actions for the herb.

Scientific information
Acorus has been an official medicine[8] and is listed in the pharmacopoeias as an aromatic bitter, although traditionally its uses have been much more extensive. In India it is used to treat insomnia, melancholia, neuroses, epilepsy, hysteria, loss of memory and remittent fevers. It has been used as a food flavouring too.

In vitro—Research into the whole extract and/ or its essential oil has identified:-

* an antiproliferative and immunomodulatory activity[9]
* high anti-oxidant activity[6,10]
* antibacterial activity including against *Bacillus subtilis*,[11] *Pseudomonas aeruginosa* and some resistant strains of *Escherichia coli*,[12] *Shigella* species[12] and *Staphylococcus aureus*[13]
* antimycobacterial activity against *Mycobacterium tuberculosis*[14]
* fungistatic activity against *Candida albicans* and *Cryptococcus neoformans*[15]
* interaction with activators that are involved in lipid and glucose homeostasis[16]

Traditionally Asian cultures have used *Acorus* to improve memory and cognitive function in the elderly, a possible explanation is suggested by its strong inhibition of cholinesterase activity.[17]

Both isomers of asarone were studied decades ago as they are pharmacologically active. Current research indicates they are nematocidal and larvicidal against *Toxocara canis*.[18] A-asarone also has activity against cancer cells.[9]

Medicinal uses
Gastro-intestinal tract
It is in this system that *Acorus* is used in Western practice.

* dyspepsia
* gastritis
* colic
* flatulence
* gastric ulcers
* anorexia of any origin

Weiss comments that it is useful in the symptomatic treatment of gastric cancer where surgery is not an option. The use of the herb in the treatment of gastric ulcers may seem contradictory given that one would probably wish to avoid stimulation of digestive secretions and more particularly stomach acid in this condition. Low dose *Acorus* is reputed to reduce hydrochloric acid secretions and this may be the rational for its inclusion in the *BHP* for hyperacidity. It may also relate to some herbalists' viewpoint that gastric ulcers are more often a result of a sluggish digestive process prolonging the exposure of the gastric mucosa to acid and not over-secretion of acid *per se*.

Externally

Weiss recommends chewing the chopped rhizome to aid cessation of smoking and bits of rhizome, wrapped in cloth, to help teething children. The bitter taste is softened by the aromatic nature of the herb and according to Cree Indian tradition it is also analgesic.

Pharmacy

Three times daily

Decoction dried herb	–	1–3 g
Tincture 1:5 (60%)	–	2–4 ml
Fluid extract (60%)	–	1–3 ml

Should be used prior to a meal as an aid to appetite stimulation.

Precautions and/or safety

Acorus has been used throughout the world from early times and no adverse effects have been noted. In the 1980s β-asarone was shown to be carcinogenic and to cause chromosomal abnormalities when fed in large doses to rats. This resulted in the FDA banning *Acorus* in foodstuffs and also led to a threat to the continued use of the rhizome as a medicinal herb.[20]

Further analyses of the different varieties of *Acorus* established that the North American rhizome, a diploid variety, contained almost no β-asarone, the triploid content is between 9–19% of the essential oil fraction and it comprises 89–95% of the essential oil in the tetraploid Asian variety.[2,19] The European *Acorus* varieties are probably derived from Asia but appear to have much lower levels of β-asarone.[20]

Historical uses

Appears in the Bible as a strewing herb and used in "anointing" oil. Analgesic for toothache and headache, as a stimulant to stave off fatigue; diabetes; constipation; fevers; asthma and bronchitis; sedative; as a gargle for oral hygiene; calamus oil as a rub for tired feet and as a skin stimulant. Also used to flavour food and drinks; as a snuff.

ARALIACEAE

About 700 species of widely distributed herbs, shrubs, trees and vines found throughout temperate and tropical regions. Some genera have prickles and in some, juvenile leaves and habit of growth are different from the adult plant. Flowers small, greenish white or yellow in umbels or heads often massed in compound inflorescences.

Eleutherococcus senticosus
[Also known as *Acanthopanax senticosus*]

Siberian ginseng

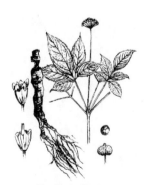

Family Araliaceae

Description
Siberian ginseng is a shrub growing from 1–5 m tall. *Stems* are erect, clothed with thin, sharp-pointed bristle-like prickles which curve backwards. *Leaves* are palmate, grow on prickly stems, 1–10 cm long; each leaf has 3–5 elliptical-ovate to obovate leaflets with serrate margins, and sometimes the veins on the back of the leaves are also covered with tiny bristles. *Flowers* are five-petalled, very small and grow in terminal umbels on long stalks, alone or in groups of 3–4. *Fruits* small, ovoid and blackish.

Habitat and cultivation
Siberian ginseng grows abundantly as an under shrub in thickets in mixed deciduous and evergreen forests throughout mountainous regions, up to 800 m, of North East China and from the mid-Amur river area in Russia across to Sakhalin, parts of Korea and Hokkaido. It is hardy, growing in full sun or semi-shade preferring a cool climate, and a moderately well-drained soil. Propagation is either by seed sown in spring or autumn, cuttings of old wood in autumn or by root division. In China plants are spaced about 1 m apart in fields or terraces.

Parts used
The roots.

Active constituents[1,28]
1) Phenylpropanoids including syringin
   (Eleutheroside B) and its aglycone sinapyl
   alcohol also confineraldehyde, dicaffeoylqui-
   ninic acids[2] and cholorogenic, protocatechuic,
   p-hydroxybenzoic, caffeic, vanillic, syringic,
   p-coumaric and ferulic acids[3]
2) Lignans including those derived from syrin-
   gasresinol (Eleutheroside D), Eleutheroside E, Eleutheroside E_1, Eleutheroside
   E_2[4] and free (-)-syringaresinol; (-)-sesamin
   (Eleutheroside B_4)
3) Sterols including daucosterol (Eleutheroside A)
   and β-sitosterol
4) Coumarins including isofraxidin and its glucoside—Eleutheroside B_1
5) Sugars including methyl-α-D-galactoside
   (Eleutheroside C), and polysaccharides or gly-
   cans including eleutherans A–G

Also contains Eleutherosides B_2, B_3, F and G (all
as yet unidentified), oleanolic acid and a small
amount of volatile oil. The constituent content
varies with the geographical location, for instance
eleutheroside B is not found in the Korean grown
herb.[1]

Nutritional constituents
Vitamins: E and β-carotene
Minerals: Calcium, magnesium, phosphorous,
potassium, sodium, iron, boron, copper, zinc,
manganese and chromium

Actions
1) Adaptogen
2) Immunomodulator

Scientific information
Siberian ginseng has been used for thousands of
years in the East. Western interest was stimulated
by recognition of the medicinal value of *Panax
ginseng* which, due to its great expense, prompted
a search for substitutes. In the 1960–80's Russia

conducted the largest clinical trials on *Eleutherococcus* and this research forms much of the basis of our
understanding of the herb's use in modern practice. *German Commission E* has approved its use as a
tonic for fatigue and debility, declining capacity for
work and concentration and to aid convalescence.
Whilst there are many studies using animal models their applicability to humans is unpredictable.

Immune support
The studies to date suggest a complex mechanism
in the action of the herb on immune function.

In vitro—In whole blood from healthy volunteers, some immune factors are stimulated in a
dose-dependent manner whilst others respond
biphasically being inhibited at higher doses and
stimulated at lower doses.[5] The action can be seen
as being immunomodulatory.

The polysaccharides are water-soluble and have
strong immunostimulating properties.[6]

In vivo—*Eleutherococcus* increased immuno-
competent cell numbers in healthy people, especially T-lymphocytes and natural killer cells,[7] and
raised levels of interferon.[8] The acute immune
phase stimulation is associated with the whole
extract rather than due to individual eleutherosides.[9] This immune-enhancing activity has been
demonstrated in studies where *Eleutherococcus* was
used in combination with other immune-modulat-
ing herbs both *in vivo*[10–12] and *in vitro*.[13]

Anticancer
In vitro—*Eleutherococcus* is a strong anti-oxidant
and a significant cytotoxic agent to human cancer
cells.[14]

In vivo—The Russians have used this herb extensively to assist in the treatment of cancer where it
is considered to enhance immune function, act as a
radioprotectant and help the body to recover from
toxicity and damage caused by radio- and chemotherapy treatment. The herb given before and during treatment helped the recovery of leucocytes
and lymphocytes, even increasing the immune
response index (as measured by levels of active
and total T-cell and B-cell populations) and raised
patients' tolerance to therapy.[8]

Antimicrobial

In vitro—The herb has antiviral activity against a range of RNA viruses such as human rhinovirus, respiratory syncytial virus and influenza A virus.[15] It also increases phagocytosis of *Candida albicans*.[16]

In vivo—A combination of *Rhodiola rosea*, *Schisandra chinensis* and *Eleutherococcus* improved the recovery time of patients with non-specific pneumonia.[17]

Adaptogen

In vitro—*Eleutherococcus* has a protective effect on cells subjected to γ-radiation[18] and increases the motility of sperm from men with asthenospermia.[19]

In vivo—In terms of its adaptogenic properties the herb improved:-

- aspects of mental perfomance and social function in the elderly[20]
- athletic performance—work output, oxygen uptake and exhaustion time,[21] also improving iron levels[22] (not corroborated[23-25])
- the circulation of children with neurocirculatory hypotension[26]
- oxygen intake with normal activity[30]
- visual[27] and auditory acuity[28]
- the incidence of general illness—reduced by around 30% over 12 months[28]
- the incidence of influenza—over a 7 year period estimated reduction of 90%[28]
- the incidence of hypertension and reduced the consequences associated with ischaemic heart disease[28]
- physical and mental stamina[28]
- stress factors associated with surgery[29]

It also decreased levels of low density lipoprotein, triglycerides, cholesterol and glucose and increased immune competent cells.[30]

Eleutherococcus appears to normalise the stress response, possibly by modulating relevant hormone catabolism which may also increase energy levels and stamina.[31] In endurance tests it raised cortisol levels.[32] Whilst the adaptogenic effect appears to occur via the hypothalamic-pituitary-adrenal axis in long-term stress, the immediate response is governed by stimulation of the sympatho-adrenal system.[33]

Medicinal uses

Cardiovascular system
- improving heart function
- hyperlipidemia

Respiratory tract
- prevention of infections
- chronic infections
- low immune function

Nervous system

Eleutherococcus may be used for acute or chronic conditions.

- fatigue
- stress
- insomnia
- debility
- convalescence

Musculo-skeletal system
Indicated for:

- chronic inflammation

Endocrine system
- diabetes

Cancer
- adjunct in cancer treatment
- prophylaxis for cancer

Pharmacy

Three times daily

Decoction of dried root	– 0.5–1.3 g
Tincture 1:2 (30%)	– 0.8–2.5 ml

Eleutheroside B and E have been thought of as the most important constituents for the actions of *Eleutherococcus* and, as a consequence, some preparations have been standardised on them.

Russian trials of the herb as a prophylactic against general illness used the extract for 2 months in a 12 month period, one month in spring and one in autumn.

Precautions and/or safety

The *BHC* recommends that the herb is not used continuously and that after a 1-month long course a rest interval of 2 months should follow. *German Commission E* suggests the herb may be used for up to 3 months at a time, but that it not be used in cases of very high blood pressure. In elderly hypertensive patients *Eleutherococcus* did not alter blood pressure.[20]

High doses for long periods of time may cause insomnia, irritability, anxiety and melancholy. Clinical studies have highlighted a low incidence of insomnia, arrhythmia (tachycardia and extrasystole) and hypertonia in atherosclerotic patients[34] and hypertension, pericardial pain, palpitations and pressure headaches in patients with rheumatic heart disease who used the herb.[35]

Interactions

No interactions are known. A study showed that CYP2D6 and CYP3A4 are unaffected by *Eleutherococcus*.[36] There was a report of a patient having raised blood levels of digoxin following concurrent use with the herb that raised concern over a possible interaction.[37] It is now suspected that the supplement involved contained *Periploca sepium* not *Eleuthrococcus*. Indeed a more recent study of patients on both medications found no interaction.[18,20] (See also under *Panax*)

Historical uses

As a tonic; to increase "Qi"; in yang deficiency of spleen and kidney; to increase sexual function; for bronchitis; heart ailments; rheumatism; to improve general health; restore memory; promote appetite; for longevity; as a general tonic; considered to be sedative.

Panax ginseng

Ginseng, Korean ginseng

Description

A glabrous perennial growing up to 60 cm. Only 1 stalk grows from the roots and it bears a single palmate leaf dividing into 3–5 fronds, each of which produces 3–5 leaflets. The *leaflets* have finely serrated margins and tiny bristly hairs on the veins.

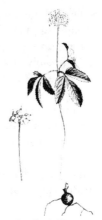

Family Araliaceae

The middle leaflet of each frond is the largest with 2 smaller leaflets on either side, and 2 even smaller leaflets beneath those. The *flowering stem* arises from the leaf and is 6–20 cm long and bears an umbel of small pale yellowish-green flowers which later become red berries each enclosing 2 hard seeds.

Odour—faintly aromatic; taste—sweetish.

Habitat and cultivation

Ginseng grows in similar mountainous regions with cool climates to *Eleutherococcus* in North-east China, Korea and Russia. Most of the cultivated crop is grown from seed in Jilin and Liaoning. Seeds take up to 2 years to germinate.

Parts used

The roots, harvested after the fourth year of growth.[38] Western use of *Panax* is confined to "white ginseng", the unprocessed roots. Eastern herbal medicine also uses "red ginseng" which is the steam treated roots. This alters the chemical constituents so that the two are not identical.[39]

Active constituents

1) Triterpene saponins commonly called ginsenosides (up to 3%). The majority (over 30) are based on the dammarane structure and these in turn are derived from one of two different aglycones:-
   a) protopanaxadiol—this group includes ginsenosides Ra_{1-3}, Rb_{1-3}, Rc, Rc_2, Rd, Rd_2, Rh_2,

Rg_3.[40] Rb_1 is the predominant ginsenoside in this series, comprising a minimum of 1.5%

b) protopanaxatriol—this group includes Re, Re_2, Re_3, Rf, Rg_1 (mainly), Rg_2, Rh_1, Rf; (20R) ginsenosides—Rg and Rh.

Also ginsenoside Ro which alone is derived from oleanolic acid. The concentration of the ginsenosides in the lateral roots and root hairs is greater than that in the main root[41] however the percentage of Rg_1 is greatest in the main root and this could account for its preference in medicinal preparations[42]

2) Peptidoglycans known as panaxans A–E
3) Volatile oil (up to 0.05%) comprised of:
   a) sesquiterpenes including β-elemene[43]
   b) monoterpenes including α- and β-pinene[43]
   c) polyacetylenes including panaxynol, panaxytriol, panaxydol and epoxyheptadecn-4,6-diyn-3-ones[44,45]
4) Polysaccharides including ginsenans PA and PB[46]

Also contains salicylic and vanillic acids, volatile alcohols,[39] a protein "panaxagin"[47] and the sterol daucosterol.

Nutritional constituents
Vitamins: C, B_1 and B_2

Actions
1) Adaptogen
2) Thymoleptic
3) Stomachic
4) Immunomodulator
5) Cancer preventative

Scientific information
Panax ginseng is one of the most studied herbs, particularly in the Far East where it has a very long traditional use and is highly esteemed. It is just one of a number of medicinal *Panax* species, their actions having much in common. The ginsenosides are considered the main active constituents. Individual ginsenosides, on analysis, often have conflicting actions possibly explaining how *Panax* behaves in an amphoteric/adaptogenic way.

Anti-oxidant
At least some of ginseng's benefits may be explained by its anti-oxidant potential.[48] Different ginsenosides have contradictory abilities to promote or prevent oxidation. The descending order of anti-oxidant potential is Rc, Rb_1, Re, Rd, Rg_1, Rb_3, Rh_1.[49-51]

In vitro—The herb and/or its constituents strongly induce major anti-oxidant enzymes, super oxide dismutase-1 and catalase, involved in the initial defence response to reactive oxygen species[52] and increase nitric oxide levels.[53]

In vivo—*Panax* raised serum superoxide dismutase and catalase levels in young healthy adults.[121]

Immune support
A second important area of research into *Panax* is associated with its immunomodulatory properties.

In vitro—*Panax* and/or its constituents:-

• stimulate non-specific proliferation of lymphocytes,[54-56] (because the different ginsenosides can either stimulate or inhibit lymphocytes the overall effect of the herb is likely to be one of immunomodulation[57])
• enhance the levels of natural killer cells and antibody activity in cells obtained from normal, chronic fatigue syndrome and AIDS subjects[58]
• enhance immune responses associated with chronic infections through cytokine modulation and increased interferon production[59]
• aid proliferation and differentiation of bone marrow stem cells[60]
• hasten T-cell mediated immune responses[61]
• inhibit TNF-α[62]

Antimicrobial activity has been shown for isolated constituents including inhibition of HIV reverse transcriptase[47] and *Helicobacter pylori*.[63]

The polysaccharide fraction has both direct and indirect antibacterial activity[64-66] as well as altering cytokine levels[67,68]

In vivo—In healthy people *Panax* (200 mg/day) increased levels of phagocytosis, chemotaxis, lymphocytes and T-helper cells,[69] although in another study using slightly higher doses (300 mg/day) levels of leucocytes or lymphocytes were not altered.[70]

Panax co-administered with an influenza vaccine resulted in significantly fewer people developing infections, their antibody and natural killer cell levels being higher than in the placebo group.[71]

Cancer

This effect would probably involve *Panax*'s antioxidant and anti-inflammatory potential and its ability to influence apoptosis, neurotransmission and immunosurveillance[72] in addition to the above immunomodulatory properties.

In vitro—*Panax* protects cells from radiation damage[73] including that caused by γ-radiation.[74] This may have significance not only for cancer prevention but for preventing cellular damage during radiotherapy. Various of the ginsenosides have anticancer effects in different cancer cell lines including neuroblastoma,[75] melanoma,[76,77] hepatoma,[78,79] colon cancer,[80] leukaemia,[81,82] myeloma,[83] prostate,[84] kidney,[85] breast[86–88] and gastric cancer.[89] Ginsenosides may increase the susceptibility of cancer cells to chemotherapy[90–93] and ginsenoside metabolites, produced by intestinal flora, protect chromosomes from potential chemical carcinogens[94] and are strongly antitumourigenic.[95]

In addition to the above effects on cancer cells some constituents can encourage cell differentiation.[96,97]

In vivo—To date no studies have proven *Panax* has an anticancer effect[98] although patients with nasopharyngeal cancer who were treated conventionally had better survival rates if they also received injections of the polysaccharide fraction.[99]

Epidemiological studies into the incidence of various cancers and the regular use of *Panax*, however, suggests that it may have a prophylactic effect,[100,101] and for example reduce the risk of lung cancer development in smokers. The protective effect appears to be dependent on the amount of *Panax* consumed[102] and the frequency of its use.[103] Furthermore ginseng use prior to getting cancer

was associated with increased survival and disease-free time and better quality of life.[104] In these studies red ginseng seemed to offer the best protection[105] whilst the extract and dry powder were more efficacious than fresh or juiced root and infusions. These studies have been on-going in Japan, Korea and China.[106]

Adaptogen

The numerous other studies carried out on *Panax* or its constituents may be viewed as an expression of the herb's adaptogenic potential as it enables cells or the whole individual to achieve a more favourable state. Most body system functions have been subjected to some analysis in terms of these effects.

Circulatory

In vitro—Fractions of *Panax* inhibit the enzymes involved in cholesterol absorption and storage,[107] this may give the herb a role in the treatment of atherosclerosis and hyperlipidaemias. Ginsenosides and/or the saponins protect endothelial cells from damage due to hypoxia/re-oxygenation (crude extract was inactive)[108] and erythrocytes from lysis in a hyperosmotic environment.[109] Apart from the directly protective effects, the saponins may also act as calcium channel blockers.[110]

Saponins stimulate bone marrow production of progenitor cells[111] and the proliferation and differentiation of granulocytes, mononcytes[112] and erythrocytes[113,114] whilst the non-saponin fraction has antithrombin properties, inhibiting the aggregation of platelets.[115,116]

In vivo—*Panax* alone, or as part of a combination, improved the condition of patients with coronary disease—angina pectoris[117] and congestive heart failure[118]—in the latter condition thyroid hormone levels were normalised as well.[119] The isolated ginsenosides were used in a group of mitral valve surgical patients with apparent protection from ischaemic and reperfusion damage.[120]

The herb may have additional benefits to circulatory health by reducing serum lipid levels including cholesterol, triglycerides and LDL whilst increasing HDL.[121] It also decreased diastolic blood pressure when used alone[122] or with ginkgo.[123]

Respiratory

Panax relaxes bronchial smooth muscle via increased nitric oxide production.[124] Constituents can stimulate the growth and proliferation of two types of bronchial cells, without changing their morphology or showing any cytotoxicity.[125,126]

In vivo—The herb improved pulmonary function in patients with moderate to severe chronic obstructive pulmonary disease (COPD).[127,128]

Gastro-intestinal

In vitro—The polysaccharide fraction inhibits the binding of *Helicobacter pylori* to gastric adenocarcinoma epithelial cells.[129]

In vivo—*Panax* hastened the healing of anal fistulas in infants who had not received surgery.[130] A hepatoprotective effect was demonstrated in elderly patients with drug or alcohol-induced liver damage when combined with supplements[131] and alone it helped improve the blood alcohol clearance in young healthy volunteers.[132]

Nervous system

In vitro—*Panax* may play a role in nerve repair by stimulating nerve growth.[133,135] It protects neuronal cells from damage by a chemical neurotoxin,[134,135] inflammation,[136] hypoxia[137] and high dose radiation.[138] A number of ginsenosides improved inter-cellular communication too which may help prevent and/or treat acquired or inherited nervous system diseases.[139] Constituents of *Panax*, (not the ginsenosides), bind to those receptor sites in brain tissue, that appear to be affected by old age, dementia and in impaired cognitive function.[140]

In vivo—This is one of the areas where *Panax* can ethically be tested. The results are mostly in accord and positive regarding its effect on quality of life.[141]

A number of studies used the combination of *Ginkgo biloba* and *Panax* to assess changes in mental function and they have shown:

- an improvement in memory tests notably in working and long term memory[142] (not verified[143])
- an improvement in neurasthenia (specifically associated with fatigue on activity and

sleep issues) measured both subjectively and objectively[144]

- a beneficial effect in brain activity in young well volunteers after a single dose[145]
- an improvement in healthy adults in response frequency, speed and accuracy on repetitive and memory tasks[146,147]—also occurs with *Panax* alone[143]

Panax used alone improved mental processing, attention and reaction time to auditory and sensory stimulii,[148] improved reaction time in athletes at rest and during exercise, without affecting maximum oxygen or lactate levels[149] and markedly improved cognitive function in healthy adults after a single dose.[150] More recently a study comparing cognitive changes due to single doses of *Paullinia cupana* (guarana), *Panax ginseng* or a combination of the two showed that whilst guarana increased attention it did so with deterioration in accuracy levels whilst ginseng improved both attention and accuracy.[151]

Over half of unexplained chronic fatigue sufferers, including those with chronic fatigue syndrome, report that ginseng has been beneficial to their condition.[152]

In a pertinent study into the effect of mental and physical stresses due to large city living two groups of people were given a supplement of minerals and vitamins either with or without *Panax*. Only the *Panax* group recorded a significant improvement in their quality of life, achieved without weight gain or increases in diastolic pressure.[153] Further evidence of the benefit of *Panax* for modulating stress comes from a study on night duty nurses who reported it improved their mood and ability to perform tasks.[154]

Negative studies have also been reported. *Panax* did not improve the mental or emotional well-being of otherwise healthy volunteers[155,156] or mental and/or physical state of elderly people when used in combination with supplements.[157,158]

Reproduction and hormones

In vitro—There has been speculation that *Panax* may be oestrogenic (see Precautions). The studies to-date are inconsistent. Isolated ginsenosides have variously shown weak oestrogen binding activity,[159,160] weak oestrogen-like activity not involving direct interaction at receptor sites,[161] inhibition of oestrogen production[93] and no oestrogenic effect (this latter effect is true of *Panax* itself).[162,163] One model even found that *Panax* stimulated the growth of a particular line of breast cancer cells in the absence of any apparent oestrogenic effect.[164] There is some evidence that the conflicting results concerning hormonal activity of *Panax* may be due either to the method of its extraction and/or the presence of a fungal contaminant[165] and/or that microflora in the gut alter ginsenosides into oestrogenic metabolites.[166]

Ginsenosides reversed, at least in part, the effect of dexamethasone, a steroidal drug, on glucocorticoid receptors.[167] *Panax* appears to have a cortisone-like effect,[168] having a particular affinity for glucocorticoid and also for mineralocorticoid and progestin receptor sites.[169] As appears to be the case for *Eleutherococcus*, *Panax* may preserve levels of stress hormones by inhibiting their breakdown effectively enhancing their serum levels, thereby improving energy utilisation and stamina.[31]

The herb reduces the uptake of glucose and maltose in human duodenal mucosal cells[170] and through its anti-oxidant activity prevents the formation of glycated haemoglobin.[171]

In vivo—*Panax* used in combination with *Ginkgo biloba* in post-menopausal women did not relieve the mental and emotional symptoms associated with reduced hormone levels.[172] A literature survey likewise revealed no discernible benefit for the use of *Panax* in relieving any symptom of menopause.[173] However it may improve some aspects of these women's health like depression and general well-being and it did not cause changes in reproductive tissue or hormone levels.[174]

Pregnant women diagnosed with intrauterine foetal growth retardation and treated with a saponin extract delivered babies with near normal birth weight and size.[175]

Abnormal spermatozoa count and motility where the cause was of an idiopathic nature or due to varicocoele was improved in men given *Panax*.[176,177] Plasma levels of total and free testosterone, DHT, FSH and LH also rose suggesting that this effect occurs at the hypothalamic-pituitary-testis axis.[177]

Red ginseng has proved to be a very effective treatment for erectile dysfunction but this action may not extend to untreated root. However a cream containing 9 constituents, including *Panax*, improved premature ejaculation in a dose-dependent manner.[178]

American ginseng (*P. quinquefolius*) lowers blood glucose levels,[179] although *P. ginseng* has gluco-modulating activity[180] its significance for diabetic control is uncertain.[181]

Musculo-skeletal and skin
In vitro—*Panax* has been esteemed for its ability to aid wound healing and this has been supported by the finding that constituents can stimulate epidermal growth and increase factors associated with tissue healing[125,182,183] and ginseng itself stimulates collagen synthesis.[184] It may also protect muscle cells from injury.[185]

In vivo—Much work has focused on the potential of *Panax* to improve athletic performance. Studies conducted between 1980 and 1990 had shown it benefited physical performance in terms of circulation, respiration and metabolism following strenuous exercise[186] and the ability to perform aerobic activity with reductions in heart rate and lactic acid levels.[187–190]

More recently standardized extracts have mainly shown no significant benefit in their effect on immune status, hormone levels, performance or recovery rate after repeated strenuous exercise[191,192] or after acute exercise[193–196] although one study did find it gave better recovery from exhaustive exercise.[197]

Possible explanations for the discrepancy in results are variation in dose, duration of trial, size of study group and age of subjects.[198]

Urinary
In vivo—Subjective and objective assessment of chronic renal failure patients given either a combination of Chinese herbs including *Panax* or standard western medical treatment did markedly better on the herbs.[199]

Aging
In Eastern countries ginseng has a particular application for the elderly and in a clinical study on older people using a standardized extract there was evidence of improved memory, immune status and circulation, the "antisenility" activity of the herb being postulated to occur via the pituitary/adrenal/gonad axis.[200]

Medicinal uses
Cardiovascular system
• anaemia
• leucopenia
• hyperlipidaemia

Respiratory tract
• chronic obstructive pulmonary disease

Gastro-intestinal tract
• ease digestive pain (stomachic)
• control blood glucose

Nervous system
This is the system for which western use of *Panax* is best known. It is likely to benefit these conditions irrespective of the initiating factors. Indications for use are:-

• stress
• neuralgia
• physical/mental exhaustion
• fatigue
• neurasthenia
• impaired cognitive function

Reproductive tract
Although *Panax* is unlikely to have direct hormonal activity as an adaptogen it may help:-

• menopausal symptoms
• oligospermia

Skin
• healing of wounds

Endocrine system
May be of use in the treatment of:

• diabetes
• adrenal insufficiency

Immune system
• low immune function
• aids recovery from chemo/radiotherapy

Possible use for cancer prophylaxis.

Pharmacy
Three times daily
Decoction of dried root   – 0.5–2 g
Tincture 1:2 (30%)   – 1–4 ml
   CONTRAINDICATIONS—In   Traditional Chinese Medicine, *Panax* should not be used in patients with hot conditions. This includes **hypertension, menorrhagia, nosebleeds** and **acute infections**.

Pharmacokinetics
Studies suggest that the ginsenosides may be altered by bacterial flora prior to absorption from the gut.[201] 20(S)protopanaxatriol and 20(S)protopanaxadiol glycosides are excreted in urine following oral administration.[202]

Precautions and/or safety
Ginseng is a highly sought after and expensive herb and as a result it is often adulterated or misrepresented in consumer products. This can give rise to erroneous reports of adverse reactions and unless the ginseng has been authenticated it is hard to draw firm conclusions as to its real side-effects. However the herb has a very long history of use and given the likely frequency of exposure to it by a very large number of people, some of them in fragile health, there are very few adverse reports and it is considered to be a safe herb. An extensive literature survey concluded that high quality single preparations of *Panax* are rarely associated with either adverse effects or drug interactions. The most common side-effects are as for placebo viz. headache, sleep and gastro-intestinal upsets.[203]

There is a "syndrome" associated with over consumption of ginseng (Ginseng abuse syndrome—GAS) leading to hypertension, nervousness, irritability, diarrhoea, skin eruptions and/or insomnia.[204] A literature survey looking at pharmacodynamic and pharmacokinetic information available suggests ginseng could potentially cause bleeding and hypoglycaemia which may have implications for peri-operative care.[205] These effects have not yet been reported.

Isolated adverse reactions have been reported and these include:

* menometrorrhagia with the simultaneous internal and external use of *Panax*. Tachycardia and arrhythmia also occurred but this was probably indirectly due to the resultant anaemia. Cessation of ginseng use and life style changes resolved the symptoms[206]
* mastalgia, and vaginal bleeding, post-menopause, associated with a topical ginseng preparation[207]
* erythematous rash due to a supplement which included *Panax*, this resolved on discontinuation of the product[208]
* cerebral arteritis following ingestion of large amounts of ginseng extracted in ethanol[209]
* two cases of "ginseng poisoning" causing mydriasis and poor accommodation in both eyes, dizziness and semiconsciousness[210]

Interactions

There are two reports of *Panax* suspected of interacting with phenelzine (monoamine oxidase inhibitor), one causing headache, insomnia and tremor[211] and the other mania,[212] one interaction with clomipramine and haloperidol causing onset of mania[213] and one with antibiotics causing reversible Stevens-Johnson syndrome.[214]

A study of the effect of *Panax quinquefolius* on warfarin intake on a small group of healthy individuals showed that it reduced the blood levels of warfarin[215] however when *Panax ginseng* was co-administered with warfarin there was no effect on levels of warfarin or blood platelet aggregation.[216,217]

There is a warning that ginseng may effect the metabolism of chemotherapeutic drugs, making them less effective, because some of the ginsenosides are able to affect cytochrome P450 isozymes[218] but the whole herb *in vivo* has not been found to have any clinically significant effect on drug levels.[219-221]

The glycosides of *Panax* and *Eleutherococcus* are similar structurally to digoxin and it has been shown that they can falsely elevate digoxin levels measured by immunoassay.[222,223] This could give a spuriously high reading of blood drug levels, a problem exacerbated by the fact that digoxin has a narrow therapeutic index.

Historical uses

The botanical name of ginseng, *Panax*, is derived from the Greek word "panacea" and this reflects its use historically as a "cure all". It was described in detail in Chinese texts dating back to AD 196. The list of uses is extensive, the herb was considered miraculous and used for a very wide range of physical and mental problems. Main uses traditionally were for digestive problems and to revitalise the elderly.

ARECACEAE

Arecaceae, formerly Palmae, are a mono-cotyledon family of about 200 genera consisting of evergreen shrublike or tree-like plants or vines, mainly of tropical or subtropical regions.

- Stems are woody, solitary or clustered, or in colonies from elongated rhizomes. They are rarely branched but may be erect, prostrate, creeping or climbing, slender, thick, smooth, prickly or covered in persistent leaf sheaths
- Leaves alternate, and very variable and the inflorescence may be among, below or above the leaves and equally variable

Important palms include the coconut and the African oil palm.

Serenoa serrulata

Saw palmetto, sabal

Description
Small palm tree from 1–4 m high with prostrate, creeping and branching stems. *Leaves* deeply divided to 20 segments, swordshaped leaf blades

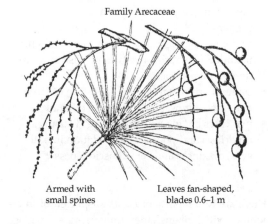

Family Arecaceae

Armed with small spines

Leaves fan-shaped, blades 0.6–1 m

radiating from a central stem, in a circular fan-shape, green-glaucous. Leaf stalks have saw-like teeth. *Flowers* inconspicuous, whitish green with 3–5 petals, blooming from May–July in the Northern Hemisphere. *Fruit* berries black, fleshy, growing in clusters each with 1 large wrinkled, oblong seed 2.5 × 1 cm.

Habitat and cultivation
Native to the West Indies and East coast of USA from South Carolina to Florida growing in sunny savannas and thickets, in moist rich soils. It is

drought and frost tender and will grow in other tropical locations.

Parts used
The ripe berries.

Active constituents
1) Fixed oil of which 9–25% is fatty acids consisting of free fatty acids (FFA)—oleic (min. 3%); lauric (min. 2%); myristic (min. 1.1%); linoleic, caphoic, caprylic (min 0.2% each); capric, palmitoleic, stearic, linolenic[1] (min. 0.1% each) and myristoleic acids and esters of FFA. The remaining fixed oil is comprised of neutral fats[1,2]
2) Volatile oil (about 1.5%)
3) Sterols including β-sitosterol, stigmasterol, daucosterol and campesterol[3]
4) Phenolic acids including ferulic and vanillic acids

Also contains resins, flavonoids,[3] tannins and polysaccharides of high molecular weight.

Nutritional constituents
Vitamins: A

Actions
1) Diuretic
2) Urinary antiseptic
3) Endocrine agent

Scientific information
Serenoa was used traditionally by the indigenous North Americans in the treatment of urinary tract problems. Scientific investigation of the herb began in the 1870s and many studies and clinical trials have and are proving its effectiveness. The herb has been an official preparation in the USA and it is approved by *German Commission E* for use in stages I and II of benign prostatic hyperplasia to aid dysuria.

The most active constituents of *Serenoa* appear to be the lipid and sterol fractions. These have been preferentially extracted into what is referred to as a liposterolic extract of *Serenoa repens* (LSESr), standardised to contain between 70–95% free fatty acids and their corresponding esters. Research most frequently is based on these standardised extracts, however the quality of preparations is variable[4] and this may account for some of the discrepancies across trials.

Benign prostatic hyperplasia
Much of the study has centred on the effectiveness of *Serenoa* and/or its constituents in treating benign prostatic hyperplasia (BPH) and, to a lesser extent, cancer of the prostate.

In older men the incidence of BPH rises so that after the age of 75 years around three quarters of the male population are likely to be affected. The enlarging prostate gland obstructs the urethra and results in problems with urination. Some of the features underlying the pathology of BPH have been elucidated as follows:-

- hyperplasia (and prostate cancer) involves the activity of iso-enzymes of 5 α-reductase and 17β-hydroxysteroid dehydrogenase[5]. In the prostate 5 α-reductase converts testosterone to the highly active steroid, dihydrotestosterone (DHT) and 17β-hydroxysteroid dehydrogenase converts testosterone to androstenedione both appear to contribute to changes in prostatic growth
- oestrogens may contribute to the development of BPH, androgens are converted to oestrogens by the "aromatase" complex[6]
- there is an observed increase in some immune cells and inflammatory markers in BPH, although the reason for this is uncertain, it is possible that inflammation is part of the pathogenesis[7]

Conventional therapeutic strategies used so far have been to inhibit the production of DHT using 5 α-reductase inhibitors like finesteride and more recently α-adrenoreceptor antagonists like tamsulosin which work by contracting the prostate gland, proximal urethra and bladder thus reducing bladder pressure and increasing urine flow. In Europe the vast majority of men who suffer with BPH are treated with phytotherapy so that interest has been focused on clinial aspects of efficacy, safety and drug interactions, especially in the case of *Serenoa*. Indeed researchers acknowledge that the phytotherapeutic treatment of BPH has been subjected to more experimental and clinical evaluation then either finasteride or tamsulosin.[3,8]

In vitro—*Serenoa* extracts inhibit both forms of 5 α-reductase,[9–11] reduce cell growth/increase apoptosis specifically in hyperplastic prostate tissue[12,13] and are anti-androgenic acting at several different receptor sites.[14,15]

In vivo—The mechanism of action of *Serenoa* in prostate diseases is likely to be several-fold. Not only does it inhibit both 5α-reductase enzymes and reduce inflammation, in prostate cells it also competitively binds to androgen receptor sites,[16] is anti-oestrogenic[17] and decreases DHT and epidermal growth factor.[18]

There are many well-conducted clinical trials, meta-analysis and/or reviews which confirm the objective and subjective benefits of LSESr for BPH.[19–25,56,57] *Serenoa*:-

- improves urinary peak flow rate
- decreases detrusor pressure
- reduces nocturia
- slows down progression of BPH
- reduces residual urine volume
- decreases prostate size
- improves the quality of life of affected men
- improves sexual function

LSESr has been tested over variable periods of time, from months up to 5 years of continuous use. It has been effective after as little as 3 months.[24] *Serenoa* does not alter serum levels of testosterone, follicle-stimulating hormone (FSH) or luteinising hormone (LH)[25,26] but does alter androgen levels in prostatic tissue.[18] There are also signs the herb may increase apoptosis in prostatic tissues of men with BPH.[27]

These extracts have been compared with current pharmaceutical medications. Whilst finasteride only inhibits one of the isoforms of 5 α-reductase,[28] LSESr has the advantage of inhibiting both. LSESr is also as effective,[29] or more so, than tamsulosin (considered to be the fastest way to achieve symptomatic relief from BPH), even for men with severe BPH.[24]

Reviews conclude that the herb is an effective treatment for BPH and/or lower urinary tract symptoms,[19,30–33,36] that the results are comparable with finasteride[28,32,34–36] when used alone[28,34,36] or with *Urtica dioica* root[35] and that it does in fact have less side effects than conventional treatment.[28,35,36]

There are a few studies that have failed to verify some of *Serenoa*'s effects *in vitro*[37] and *in vivo*.[38] There may be no added benefit in using *Serenoa* together with tamsulosin.[39,40]

Serenoa also has benefits for:-

- recovery from trans-urethral resection of the prostate (TURP) as a pretreatment[41]
- chronic prostatitis, a condition with a poor resolution rate in orthodox treatments[42–44]

Anticancer
In vitro—*Serenoa* and its constituents can inhibit prostate cell growth directly[45] and reduce the invasive ability of prostatic tumour cells.[46] The extract and/or constituents have cytotoxic activity against hormone therapy resistant[2] and hormone-dependent[37] prostatic cancer cells as well as cytotoxicity to other tumour cell lines.[47]

LSESr inhibits the metabolic activation of testosterone via both 5α-reductase and 17β-hydroxysteroid dehydrogenase from prostatic cancer tissues.[48]

Anti-inflammatory
In vitro—*Serenoa* has an anti-inflammatory activity, inhibiting the metabolism of arachidonic acid by 5-LOX and COX.[49,50]

The polysaccharide fraction is immunostimulatory.[51]

In vivo—Inflammatory markers were reduced in men with BPH treated with LSESr.[52]

Other
In vitro—LSESr reduces different tissues uptake of testosterone and DHT so conditions due to excessive androgen production may benefit.[53]

In vivo—LSESr was effective in treating mild to moderate androgenic alopecia.[54]

Medicinal uses

Genitourinary tract

- benign prostatic hyperplasia
- cystitis
- prostatic enlargement
- impotence
- infertility
- prostatitis of any origin
- virilism
- testicular atrophy
- urethritis
- catarrh

Serenoa has promise as a supportive herb in the management of prostatic cancer.

Skin

Conditions associated with raised DHT that respond are:

- androgenic alopecia
- hirsutism

Pharmacy

Three times daily

Decoction dried herb	– 0.5–1 g
Tincture 1:5 (45%)	– 1–2 ml (suggested guidelines)
Fluid extract *BPC* (1934)	– 0.6–1.5 ml

The minimum standardised dose (containing the lipid and sterol fractions) that has been used in clinical trials contained 160 mg of liposterolic extract given twice daily. Daily dosages from 320 mg LSESr and up were equally effective in the treatment of BPH, whether taken as a single or divided dose.[56,57]

Precautions and/or safety

The improvements appear to be long-lasting and the extract well-tolerated, safe and considered highly effective.[55–57] The herb does not interfere with prostate specific antigen (PSA) production—this antigen is used as a marker for prostatic cancer screening and disease progression.[25,55]

No safety issues arose even after 5 years of treatment with LSESr.[55] From the many trials conducted the only side-effects noted were minor gastro-intestinal irritations.[16] Ejaculation disorders were reported to be much less than with tamsulosin treatment.[29]

Interactions

Serenoa had no effect, *in vivo*, on CYP isozymes and is deemed to pose little risk of provoking this type of herb/drug interaction.[58,59] There has been no drug/herb interactions noted in the extensive studies so far undertaken.

Historical uses

Tonic and nutritional agent; to increase sexual function in men; mammary gland disorders; as an aphrodisiac; chronic catarrh; as a mucous membrane tonic, stomach ache and dysentery.

ASCLEPIADACEAE

This family consists of 1,700 species, in about 220 genera, of perennial plants, (often climbing shrubs), with milky sap. They are mostly tropical, especially those in Africa, but there are also a few temperate species of which a common one is the swan plant, *Gomphocarpus fruticosus*, grown in many primary schools to feed monarch butterfly caterpillars.

Leaves usually opposite, sometimes spiral, simple, entire and without stipules.

Flowers usually in many-flowered cymes, racemes or umbels, regular and perfect, with parts in 5's—sepals free, petals joined, stamens 5, carpels 2, united into a gynostegium. Insect pollinated.

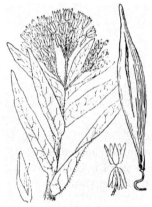

Family Asclepiadaceae

Asclepias tuberosa

Pleurisy root, butterfly weed

Description
Perennial growing 30 cm-1 m × 1 m with round, stout, hairy stems almost or entirely devoid of milky juice and a fleshy, spindle-shaped rhizome with a knotted crown. *Leaves* more or less spiral and crowded, lanceolate-oblong, to 10 cm long, sessile, dark green. *Flowers* in many flowered, flat-topped umbels in upper leaf axils, bright orange, sometimes red or yellow, blooming in summer. *Fruit* a long pod containing many dark seeds each with a silky pappus.

Habitat and cultivation
Native to North America from New England to North Dakota and south to Florida, Arizona and North Mexico, growing from seed in open, sunny areas of rich, peaty soils. It blooms from spring to autumn and is frost resistant but drought tender.

44

Parts used
The root.

Active constituents
1) Steroidal glycosides:-
   a) an adrostane—ascandroside
   b) cardenolides including glycosides of δ-5-calotropin, uzarigenin, coroglaucigenin and corotoxigenin[1]
   c) pregnane glycosides including ikemagenin, lineolon and pleurogenin[2]
2) Flavonoids including rutin, kaempferol and quercitin
3) Essential oil

Also contains friedalin, triterpenes (α- and β-amyrin, lupeol), viburnitol, choline sugars and amino acids.

The constituents of this herb are not well characterised.

Actions
1) Diaphoretic
2) Expectorant
3) Antispasmodic
4) Carminative

Scientific information
The root, which was an official drug in the *US Pharmacopoeia* from 1820–1890, was used for the treatment of asthma and bronchitis.[3]

The pharmacology of this herb is not well studied but it does achieve clinical results. Pregnane glycosides can affect fat metabolism and they are being studied in this context albeit from other plant sources.

Potter's states that it has been used for uterine disorders. However its folklore name gives the main current usage.

Medicinal uses
Respiratory tract
All actions are ideal for the treatment of lung problems and any associated fever:

- pleurisy (*BHP* specific)
- bronchitis
- pneumonia
- influenza

Pharmacy
Three times daily
Decoction dried root   – 1–4 g
Tincture 1:10 (45%)   – 1–5 ml
Fluid Extract (45%)   – 1–4 ml

Precautions and/or safety
Large doses may cause diarrhoea and vomiting.

Historical uses
Also used for pulmonary catarrh and consumption; diarrhoea and dysentery; infantile colic; headaches; mumps and measles; acute and chronic rheumatism; typhoid; eczema. Externally a poultice of the root was used traditionally to treat bruises, swelling, rheumatism and lameness.

ASTERACEAE

[Formerly known as Compositae]

This is the largest plant family with some 25,000 species worldwide.

Asteraceae are distinguished by the uniformity of the inflorescence in which many tiny flowers, called florets, are clustered together to form a flower-like head or capitulum, surrounded by calyx-like bracts called involucral bracts.

The florets are arranged on the apex of the stem, the receptacle, which may be flat, conical or concave, with or without scales subtending each floret.

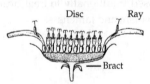

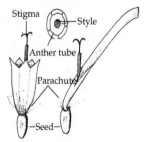

Disc floret   Ray floret

The florets are usually bisexual and complete; possessing calyx, corolla, stamens and ovary, but one or more of these organs may be absent.

The calyx is often reduced to a ring of simple or branched hairs, bristles or scales and becomes the pappus in the fruit.

The five stamens are fused by their bases to the corolla, and the anthers are fused together to form a tube around the style.

The ovary is inferior and one-seeded. There are two stigmas.

The fruit is a one-seeded nutlet, usually crowned by a pappus of scales, simple hairs, or branched feathery hair, or the pappus may be absent.

The corolla is of two basic types:

a) bell-shaped with 5 short teeth—this type of floret is called a disc floret or tubular floret
b) strap-shaped with a long narrow limb—this type is called a ray floret or ligulate floret.

Flower heads may be composed of disc florets only e.g. *Tanacetum vulgare*; or of a central group of disc florets surrounded by a peripheral row of ray florets, e.g. *Tanacetum parthenium*; or all florets may be ray florets e.g. *Taraxacum officinale*.

The Asteraceae are a highly successful family because of their high reproductive rate and ability to adapt. They occur in all habitats and every continent except Antarctica.

Because it is such a large family it is divided into two subfamilies, the Lactucoideae with 7 tribes and the Asteroideae with 6 tribes.

Medicinal plants in the Asteraceae include:

Tribe Lactuceae
The lettuce tribe, which all have a basal rosette of leaves, differ from other Asteraceae in having latex, a white fluid, which exudes from cut ends of leaves and stalks. The flowers are all ligulate (ray florets) and mostly yellow.

Cichorium intybus	chicory
Sonchus oleraceus	sow thistle
Lactuca virosa	wild lettuce
Taraxacum officinale	dandelion

Tribe Cynareae
Most of this tribe are thistle-like with spiny bracts and leaves. The flower heads consist of only disc florets which are mostly purplish or pink.

Arctium lappa	burdock
Cynara scolymus	globe artichoke
Cnicus benedictus	blessed thistle
Silybum marianum	Mary's milk thistle

Tribe Eupatorieae

Eupatorium cannabinum	hemp agrimony
E. perfoliatum	boneset
E. purpureum	gravel root

Tribe Senecioneae
This is one of the largest groups. They have alternate leaves, the flowers are usually yellow, and fruits usually have a hairy pappus.

Senecio jacobaea	ragwort
Senecio aureus	life root
Petasites hybridus	butterbur
Tussilago farfara	coltsfoot

Tribe Heliantheae
Most of these have opposite leaves and are not scented. Flowers are usually yellow or white, *Echinacea* being an exception.

E. angustifolia	purple coneflower
E. pallid	pale purple coneflower
Arnica Montana	arnica
E. purpurea	purple coneflower

Tribe Inuleae

Inula helenium	elecampane

Tribe Anthemideae
Most of these have alternate leaves and are strongly scented. The flowers are generally yellow or white and there may or may not be ray florets. The disc florets have short corolla lobes and the flower head is surrounded by two or more rows of bracts.

Achillea millefolium	yarrow
Artemisia abrotanum	southernwood
A. absinthium	wormwood
A. vulgaris	mugwort
Chamaemelum nobile	perennial chamomile
Matricaria recutita	annual chamomile
Tanacetum parthenium	feverfew
T. vulgare	tansy

Tribe Calenduleae
This tribe usually has alternate leaves and the plants are strongly scented. There are no scales on the receptacle, no pappus and no latex.

Calendula officinalis	marigold

Tribe Astereae
These plants mostly have alternate leaves, and are without scent. Most members have both ray and disc florets.

Bellis perennis	lawn daisy
Grindelia camporum	Grindelia, gumplant
Solidago spp.	golden rod

Asteraceae—general precaution
Allergic reactions from using medicinal members of the Asteraceae such as asthma, urticaria and rhino-conjunctivitis are possible in people with sensitivity to the daisy family.[1-6]

Standard tests carried out on allergic individuals have shown a low incidence[7]—around 1.4%—to Astercaeae this occurring mostly in older people or those who suffer extrinsic atopic dermatitis to other agents. However a person with sensitivity to one member has a fairly high probability of reacting to others.[2-9] The sesquiterpene lactones are considered highly likely to contribute.

Achillea millefolium

Yarrow

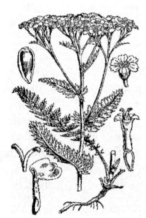

Family Asteraceae,
Tribe Anthemideae

Description
Perennial rhizomatous herb, with short non-flowering rosettes often forming dense mats. Strongly scented. *Stems* usually erect up to 80 cm tall, ribbed and striate, hairy especially above, usually not branched except to form the inflorescence. *Basal leaves* petiolate, lanceolate, moderately hairy, 2-pinnate with segments again 1–2 pinnatisect, usually 6–15 × 1–2 cm. Primary leaflets in 18–30 pairs; ultimate segments subulate, not all in one plane giving a feathery appearance to leaf; rachis c. 1–2 mm diameter, flattened, sometimes slightly winged, not toothed. *Cauline leaves* similar to basal, but above

becoming apetiolate, less divided, smaller and with fewer leaflet pairs. *Corymbs* usually more or less flat-topped or slightly convex, to 15 cm across, with numerous, closely packed capitula. Involucral bracts glabrous to sparsely hairy, 1.5–4 mm long; margin brown, hairy. Capitula 5–10 mm in diameter. *Ray florets* 4–7; ligule and disc florets usually white, sometimes pink to deep red. Flowers from summer to autumn. *Achenes* grey-brown, c. 2 mm long; wings narrow pale brown.

Odour—aromatic; taste—bitter and faintly aromatic.

Habitat and cultivation
Originally from Europe, SW Caucasia, Iran, Siberia and the Himalayas, *Achillea* is naturalised elsewhere in waste places. Grown from root division or seed; prefers deep, friable lime soil in a sunny situation. Drought and frost resistant.

Parts used
The flowering herb gathered just as the flowers begin to open, from late spring to autumn. In Switzerland both herb and flowers are used officially.

Nutritional constituents
Vitamins: A, C, E, and K
Minerals: Manganese, copper, potassium, iron and iodine

Active constituents
Achillea is geographically widespread and variable as it displays polyploidy,[10] the chromosome number can be diploid, tetraploid or hexaploid, the latter being the most common form. The chemical make-up can vary significantly according to the chromosome number, habitat,[11] level of maturation of the plant[12] and the method used to analyse these constituents.[12] This makes it very difficult to characterise precisely the constituents of any one preparation.

1) Volatile oil (max. 1.5%) present in all parts of the plant and highest during flowering. The colour of the oil varies with the quality, increasing from light to dark blue. More than 60 volatile components have been identified.[13]

Monoterpenes in the oil increase relative to sesquiterpenes as the plant matures.[12] The monoterpenes α- and β-pinene and sabinene occur in most *Achillea* samples.[14] The hexaploid plant oil is mainly made up of oxygenated monoterpenes of which either linalool (26%) or camphor (18%) predominate, with 1,8—cineole and borneol also being significant.[15,16] The tetraploid oil is mainly comprised of sesquiterpenes of which chamazulene may be an important one, representing around 25%.[15] *Achillea millefolium* L. ssp. *collina* Becker has a high level of chamazulene reported at 53%,[16] however the chamazulene content has also been reported as insignificant where steam distillation was not used[12] and here there were instead significant amounts of β-bisabolene, α-bisabolol and δ-cadinene. Also present in the tetraploid oil are β-caryophyllene, sabinene, α- and β-pinene and trace amounts of thujone.[15] Eucalyptol and α-terpineol were identified in *A. millefolium* ssp. *millefolium* Afan as well as camphor, β-pinene and borneol[17]

2) Sesquiterpene lactones including the guaianolides achillicin (considered a prochamazulene), achillin, leucodin and their 8 α-angeloxy-derivatives, desacetylmatricarin,[18,23] α-peroxyachifolids[19,20] (up to 0.6% in dried flowers and 0.05% in leaves[21]) and β-peroxyisoachifolid,[20] achimillic acids A, B and C[22] and germacranolides

3) Bitter glyco-alkaloid called achilleine. Also stachydrine, choline and betaine

4) Tannins (up to 4%)

5) Flavonoids (0.5–1.8%) including free aglycones apigenin, luteolin and centaureidin,[23] and their glucosides, also rutin,[24] artemetin and casticin[25]

6) Cyanogenic glycosides

7) Sterols including β-sitosterol, stigmasterol, campesterol, cholesterol and triterpenes—α- and β-amyrin, taraxasterol and pseudotaraxasterol[26]

8) Hydroxycoumarins

9) Phenolic acids including caffeic, salicylic and isovalerianic acids[25]

Saponins have also been reported.[26]

Nutritional constituents
Vitamins: Folic acid and C

Actions
Achillea has a wide range of actions.

1) Astringent
2) Antimicrobial
3) Diaphoretic
4) Hypotensive
5) Antipyretic
6) Spasmolytic
7) Antispasmodic
8) Anti-inflammatory
9) Haemostatic
10) Diuretic
11) Antiseptic

Scientific information
The medicinal use of *Achillea* dates back to before 1000 BC and its use has been commonly associated with Achilles who used it to staunch bleeding in his soldiers on the battlefield. Chemical analyses of the herb were undertaken over a 200 year period but much less interest has been shown in it recently. *German Commission E* has approved internal use of the flowers to stimulate appetite and for dyspepsia and its external use, as a sitz bath, for cramps of psychosomatic origin in the pelvic area.

In vitro—The volatile oil has strong anti-oxidant properties and antimicrobial activity against *Streptococcus pneumoniae, Clostridium perfringens, Candida albicans, Mycobacterium smegmatis, Acinetobacter lwoffii* and *Candida krusei*.[7] The herb however was inactive against *Staphylococcus aureus, Bacillus subtilis, Pseudomonas aeruginosa, Escherichia coli* and *Candida albicans*.[27]

Achillea is cytotoxic to a number of different liver cancer cell lines.[28]

In vivo—Recent investigations of *Achillea* have been largely associated with its chemical constituents. A combination of *Achillea, Eleutherococcus senticosus* and *Lamium album* as a topical treatment for atopic dermatitis gave improvements, both subjective and objective, but they were not significantly different from placebo.[29]

Medicinal uses
Cardiovascular system
- varicose veins
- venous stasis
- hypertension
- haemorrhoids (internal and external)
- varicose ulcers
- phlebitis
- palpitations
- fever

BHP specific for thrombotic conditions with hypertension including those affecting coronary and cerebral circulation.

Respiratory tract
As an astringent it is used in all catarrhal conditions:

- colds
- influenza
- asthma
- rhinitis
- bronchitis

Gastro-intestinal tract
- internal bleeding
- acute and chronic gastritis
- anorexia
- general indigestion
- intestinal colic
- acute or chronic dyspepsia
- diarrhea

Urinary tract
- cystitis
- urethritis

Reproductive tract
Achillea is considered a menstrual regulator. Used for:

- dysmenorrhoea (especially chronic)
- amenorrhoea
- menorrhagia
- menstrual cycle regulation

- pelvic atonia
- leucorrhoea

Musculoskeletal
- rheumatism

Pharmacy
Three times daily
Infusion of dried herb   – 2–4 g
Tincture 1:5 (45%)   – 2–4 ml
Fluid Extract (25%)   – 1–2 ml

As the flowers contain more volatile oil, if they are used on their own the anti-inflammatory, antispasmodic and diaphoretic activity is amplified, whereas the whole herb has a relatively higher tannin and bitter content and therefore greater astringency and choleretic activity.

To generate azulene as described above, the plant must be subject to steam distillation and this may be achieved by adding boiling water to it and using as a steam inhalation e.g. in asthma, or by covering the cup so that steam condenses back thus preserving the azulene that is formed.

Precautions and/or safety
Achillea is used in cosmetic products and at a concentration of 2% is non-irritating and does not produce phototoxicity.[30] **Rarely,** an allergic dermatitis has resulted from lying on new mown grass in which *Achillea* has been growing, and if skin is wet a rash may develop with pustules and hive-like lesions. The sensitiser of extrinsic dermatitis to *Achillea* is believed to be α-peroxyachifolid, although other sesquiterpene lactones probably also contribute[19,20] (see General Precaution p. 25).

Large doses of the fresh herb can cause vertigo and headache or those conditions for which it is generally used.

Historical uses
Heal-all; for melancholy; blood purifier; kidney disorders. Externally inserted into nose to relieve migraine; nose bleeds; toothache; baldness (as a wash); mouth and eye wash; healing agent for all kinds of wounds and ulcers.

Arctium lappa

Burdock

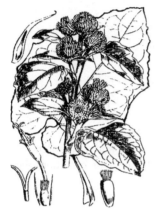

Family Asteraceae, Tribe Cynareae

Description

A biennial which dies down in winter. In the first year it forms a basal clump with long peduncles. *Basal leaves* broadly deltoid to ovate, green and sparsely hairy above, whitish and densely hairy beneath, 20–40 × 20–35 cm; base truncate to cordate; apex sub-acute to obtuse; margin dentate with apiculate vein endings; petioles solid. Upper leaves, (2nd year), alternate, similar to basal, becoming smaller. In the second year plants become openly branched, 1–1.5 m tall. *Stems* grooved, glabrous or with cobwebby glandular hairs. *Inflorescence* corymbose; peduncles 4–9 cm long. Capitula 20–25 × 30–40 mm, broadly ovoid. Involucral bracts in several series, straw yellow or yellow-green, linear, imbricate, glabrous or with sparse cobwebby hairs, the outer recurved at fruiting; margins smooth, apex spinous, inwardly hooked. Florets male and female, all tubular, corolla five-lobed, reddish purple. *Achenes* 6–7 mm long; pappus 1.5–3.5 mm long. Flowers in summer; fruits late summer to autumn.

Taste—the root becomes soft on chewing and tastes sweet and mucilaginous at first, becoming bitter later.

Habitat and cultivation

Originally from Europe, burdock is naturalised elsewhere along roadsides and waste places. It grows only from seed, likes deep, friable soil and flowers in its second year. It is a noxious weed in pasture because its burrs ruin sheep fleeces. Drought tender and frost resistant.

Parts used

The roots harvested in autumn of the first year or spring of the second year before the flowering stem develops. Leaves, heads and seeds have also been used. The leaves are gathered in the first year.

Active constituents

Root

1) Inulin (up to 45%) including a low molecular weight fructofuranan,[31] and a xyloglucan consisting of repeating units of hepta-, nona- and deca-saccharides[32]
2) Phenolic acids including chlorogenic, isochlorogenic and caffeic acids[47]
3) Polyacetylenes some containing sulphur (0.1%–0.002%)[33]—including arctinone-a, arctinols and arctinal
4) Essential oil (up to 0.4%) comprising a large number of constituents[34]
5) Bitter glycosides—arctiopicrin—a germacranolide
6) Flavonoids including baicalin[35]

Additional constituents include condensed tannins, resin, PABA, amino acids including γ-guanidinobutyric acid and mucilage.

Leaf

1) Sesquiterpenes including fukinone, arctiol and taraxasterol
2) Arctiopicrin, a germacranolide
3) Lignans including arctiin and its aglycone arctigenin[36]

Also contains mucilage, tannins and inulin.

Fruits/seeds

These are used in traditional Chinese medicine and have not been part of modern western use.

1) Lignans including arctiin[37] (around 49%),[38] arctigenin, neoarctin, mataiesinol, lappaol[39] and dilignans[40]
2) Phenolic acids including chlorogenic acid[41]

Additional constituents include daucosterol, gobosterin, essential and fatty oils.

Nutritional constituents
Vitamins: A, B_2, B_3, C, E and P
Minerals: Iron, calcium, copper, iodine, silicon, sulphur and zinc 12% protein, 70% carbohydrate.

Actions
1) Depurative
2) Diuretic
3) Orexigenic
4) Antibacterial (fresh root preferable)

The seeds have a reported hypoglycaemic action and are used in the Chinese tradition to cool and decongest.

Scientific information
The roots have been an official medicine in some European countries as a diuretic and diaphoretic.[42] They are eaten in Japan as they are a good source of dietary fibre and are also very nutritious. There has not been much recent research into their constituents or pharmacological activity.

In vitro—The root is anti-inflammatory and anti-oxidant[43,44] and one of its constituents is anti-mutagenic.[45] Chlorogenic acid is a strong anti-oxidant,[46] its presence in the root is concentrated in the skin.[47]

Arctium's use in Brazilian traditional medicine prompted its screening as an antimicrobial. It has activity against *Staphylococcus aureus, Bacillus subtilis, Escherichia coli* and *Pseudomonas aeruginosa* and also antifungal activity against *Candida albicans*.[48] It has apparently been used by some traditional healers to treat AIDS, it inhibits the integration of HIV into cells.[49] The herb also has a moderate inhibitory effect on tumour growth.[50]

Recent studies indicate that arctiin's conversion to metabolites with phyto-oestrogenic potential may occur via transformation by gut flora.[51]

Inulin offers a number of potential health benefits including enhanced immune function, improved bowel flora[52,53] and decreased inflammation of the intestinal mucosa (see *Cichorium*).[54]

Medicinal uses
Arctium is believed to achieve its main actions through its ability to help the body detoxify.

Gastro-intestinal tract
• anorexia

Urinary tract
• cystitis

Musculoskeletal
As a depurative and diaphoretic the herb may open up channels of excretion—bowel, kidney, lungs and skin:

• rheumatism
• gout
• arthritis

Skin
• eczema
• boils
• psoriasis
• acne
• cutaneous eruptions

Externally
Used topically for the treatment of the above skin conditions as an ointment, it seems to increase the skin's ability to repair itself. Used as a poultice for:

• abscesses
• boils

Pharmacy
Three times daily
Decoction of dried root   – 2–6 g
Infusion of dried leaf   – 2–6 g
Tincture 1:10 (45%)   – 8–12 ml
Fluid Extract (25%)   – 2–8 ml

The depurative action of *Arctium* may best be achieved by use of infusions or decoctions as this aids kidney elimination.

Precautions and/or safety
Side-effects are rare, there is reference to a case of contact dermatitis[55] (see General Precaution p. 25) and also a case of poisoning with burdock tea,[56] the latter has since been attributed to contamination of the root with *Atropa belladonna* root.[57]

Interactions
Animal studies suggest *Arctium* may exacerbate diabetes however the root is in common use in Italy as an aid to the treatment of this disease[58] and in countries where the root is eaten no interactions have been reported.

Historical uses
In the Middle Ages it was used for stones (*Grieve*) though whether this refers to gall-bladder or urinary tract is not clear. To cure old ulcers and sores; to help with "serpent bites" or the bites of mad dogs; to relieve sciatica; aid the healing of burns.

Arnica montana

Arnica

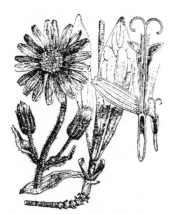

Family Asteraceae, Tribe Heliantheae

Description
A perennial mountain plant with a stout creeping rhizome and a flower stalk reaching 20–60 cm tall. *Basal leaves* in a rosette, slightly toothed, oval to lance-shaped, 5–17 cm long, glandular hairy and aromatic. *Stem leaves* much smaller, downy, in one to two opposite pairs. *Flower heads* rich yellow, large, 4–8 cm across, usually solitary but may be up to 4 on stout erect stems. Ray florets, female, toothed, wide spreading, in a single row, as long as or longer than the width of the disc; disc florets, hermaphrodite, the same yellow; involucral bracts equal in 2 rows. *Fruit* an achene, 7–9 mm long, ribbed; hairy; pappus a row of long hairs. Flowers in Europe from spring to mid-summer.

N.B. *Arnica* may be distinguished from the similar *Doronicum* by its **opposite** stem leaves. Stem leaves of *Doronicum* are alternate.

Habitat and cultivation
Arnica is native to mountainous regions in Europe, growing in pastures, heaths and wastelands from Latvia and Norway south to Portugal. It is propagated by seed sown outside in autumn or root division in spring and prefers a mix of peat, loam and sandy soil.

Parts used
The whole flowers are harvested in full bloom and used fresh or dried. The rhizomes have also been used, though less commonly, and these should be harvested in spring or autumn.

Active constituents
1) Sesquiterpene lactones (0.4%) including predominantly the pseudoguaianolides helenalin and its derivatives (approx. 50%), dihydrohelenalin and its derivatives[59] and arnifolin.[60] This fraction is considered largely responsible for the action of *Arnica* however the content of the 2 major lactones have been found to vary with time of harvest and part of flower used. Helenalin is highest in the disc florets descending in amount through ray florets, receptacle and stem, whereas dihydrohelenalin is highest in stems. Lactones increase in amount as the flowerheads mature, the total content being highest in withered flowers[61]
2) Essential oil including thymol and esters of arnidiol, faradiol, maniladiol and calenduladiol[60,62]
3) Flavonoids including eupafolin, patuletin and spinacetin

Also contains mucilage, carotenoids,[63] a bitter principle (arnicin), resins, tannins and polysaccharides.

Actions
1) Anti-inflammatory
2) Counter-irritant

Scientific information
Arnica is a well recognised anti-inflammatory and has been an official medicine in many countries in Europe. The pharmacopoeia uses listed for both flowers and rhizomes are for bruises and sprains.[42]

Anti-inflammatory
In vitro—The sesquiterpene lactones are considered central to the anti-inflammatory effect of *Arnica*. They inhibit transcription factors that initiate inflammation, even at low concentrations,[64] in a dose-dependent manner.[65] Helenalin has the strongest anti-inflammatory effect its mode of action being different from that of non-steroidal anti-inflammatory drugs, indomethacin and acetyl salicylic acid.[66] Both helenalin and dihydrohelenalin inhibit platelet aggregation, thromboxane and 5-hydroxytryptamine secretion, probably by reducing phospholipase A2 activity.[67]

In vivo—Topical application of *Arnica* and hydroxyethyl salicylate gave a greater analgesic effect than either substance alone.[68] *Arnica* gel did not significantly improve bruising after laser surgery[69] but it reduced pain and stiffness in mild to moderate osteoarthritis of the knee[70] (6 weeks applications).

A combination of homeopathic *Arnica* internally and *Arnica* ointment topically used post-operatively for carpal tunnel release surgery reduced pain but had no affect on swelling and/or muscle strength.[71]

Other
In vitro—The sesquiterpene lactones have significant activity against *Plasmodium falciparum*, the organism causing malaria, helenalin was stronger than artemisinin[72] from *Artemisia annua* currently being used to treat resistant forms of the disease. They also have activity against the African

Trypanosoma brucei rhodesiense and American *T. cruzi*.[73] *Arnica* itself has long been considered an antimicrobial and shows good antibacterial activity against most periodontal organisms.[74]

The polysaccharides stimulate phagocytosis[75,76] and TNF-α secretion from macrophages.[77]

Helenalin is cytotoxic to small lung carcinoma and colorectal cancer cells.[78]

Medicinal uses
Externally
- bruises
- sprains
- joint/muscle inflammation
- strains
- chilblains (skin unbroken)
- alopecia neurotica (BHP)

Pharmacy
ARNICA IS NOT USED INTERNALLY OR ON BROKEN SKIN
Applied as required
Tincture BPC (1949) 1:10 (45%) as a compress
Cream or ointment up to 25% v/w.
Some pharmacopoeias recommend an extraction medium of ethanol:water of 60–70%.[42]

Precautions and/or safety
Internally—*Arnica* can irritate mucous membranes causing severe gastroenteritis, hypotension, tachycardia, dyspnoea, coma and possibly death.

Externally—there is the potential for allergic dermatitis reactions (see General Precaution p. 25)[7] probably due to the sesquiterpene lactones[79-81] which are well absorbed through the skin.[82] The estimated level of allergy to *Arnica* could be just over 1%.[83]

A review into its safety has concluded that there is insufficient data available of the effects of long term exposure to topical preparations. Standard animal based safety tests undertaken by this review found no cause for concern from short term use.[84]

Historical uses
Arnica is mentioned by Hildegarde of Bingen (12th century) and has been used extensively in European folk medicine. *Weiss* states its use, like that of

Crataegus, is as a circulatory stimulant but for acute conditons i.e. for senile heart and heart disease. [Goethe (1749–1832) apparently drank *Arnica* tea to ease angina pain.] Also for fevers; paralytic affections; slow healing wounds; leg ulcers. As a gargle for sore throat, pharyngitis; smoker's cough.

NB It is no longer recommended for internal use.

Artemisia absinthium

Wormwood

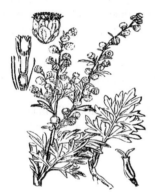

Family Asteraceae, Tribe Athemideae

Description
Herbaceous perennial, dying back more or less to woody stem bases each winter. *Stems* numerous ascending to erect, densely sericeous, becoming glabrous below, ribbed, up to about 1 m long, much branched towards the base. *Leaves* scattered along stems, densely sericeous on upper and lower surface, appearing silvery-white. Lower cauline leaves petiolate, 1-pinnate with leaflets usually 2 pinnatisect, up to about 30 × 20 cm in lower leaves; ultimate segments oblong-ovate, obtuse, 5–10 × 2–4 mm, with only the central vein evident. *Inflorescence* paniculate, with leaves similar to cauline leaves but becoming apetiolate and 1-pinnatisect, finally reduced to less than 1 cm long and not lobed. *Flowers* arranged in a panicle, outer involucral bracts herbaceous or with a membranous apex, sericeous; inner bracts sparsely hairy, with broad membranous margins and apex. Capitula 2–4 mm in diameter; receptacle pilose; florets many, dull yellow, glabrous. *Achenes* 0.8–1.3 mm long, brown, ovoid, more or less terete, smooth; no pappus. Flowers from mid-summer to autumn. Cultivars of *A. absinthium* e.g. "Powis Castle" are not used medicinally.

Odour—aromatic, sweet and bitter; taste—aromatic and intensely bitter.

Habitat and cultivation
Native to Eurasia and North Africa, wormwood grows in waste places and rocky screes. It is naturalized elsewhere in dry, sunny situations. It is grown from seed or cuttings and is frost tender and does not survive prolonged drought.

Parts used
Leaves and flowering tops collected as the plant comes into flower.

Active constituents
1) Essential oil (max. 1%) predominantly monoterpenes, including, α- and β-thujone, epoxyocimene, linalool, sabinene, 1,8-cineole, chamazulenes and their derivatives.[85-87] There is considerable variation in the constituent make-up according to origin.[88] Immature leaves contain a high level of sabinyl acetate as well as α-thujone and sabinene[89]
2) Bitter sesquiterpene lactones including absinthin, matricin, anabsinthin, artabsin, absintholide[90] and santonin
3) Terpenoids including homoditerpene peroxides[91]
4) Triterpenoids
5) Flavonoid glycosides (many)
6) Hydroxycoumarins
7) Polyacetylenes

Also tannins, resin, choline and organic acids including chlorogenic acid and amino acids (significant levels of histidine[92]) have also been identified.

Nutritional constituents
Vitamins: B complex and C
Minerals: Manganese, calcium, sodium, potassium and silicon

Actions
This is a herb with an enormous number of active constituents that give it a wide range of actions.

1) Bitter tonic
2) Stomachic
3) Choleretic
4) Anthelmintic
5) Anti-inflammatory

Scientific information
Wormwood has been a recorded medicine since at least 1552 BC and its common name gives a clear indication of its anthelmintic properties. It has been an official medicine, its bitter properties being used to stimulate appetite and improve digestive function.[42]

In vitro—The herb and/or its constituents have:-

- good antimicrobial properties against a range of bacteria including *Escherichia coli, Staphylococcus aureus, Klebsiella pneumoniae, Salmonella enteritidis, Pseudomonas aeruginosa;* fungal pathogens including *Candida albicans* and *Aspergillus niger;*[87,88,93,94] viruses, by protecting cells from their invasion, including herpes, cytomegalovirus and Epstein Barr viruses.[95] A constituent also induces interferon production[95]
- moderate anti-oxidant activity[85]
- cytotoxic activity, particularly the germacranolide sesquiterpene lactones[96]
- anti-inflammatory activity (azulenes)[97]
- cholinergic activity—not due to the presence of choline alone[98]—this activity lends support to its traditional use for impaired memory
- cell-protectant action against osmotic damage[99]
- antimalarial activity[91]

Thujone was identified as the constituent that caused absinthe "intoxication". It was believed at one time to act via cannabinoid receptors, however animal studies indicate this is unlikely.[100] A-thujone (which is the more toxic of the two thujones) may affect the nervous system by:

a) blocking the inhibitory effect of γ-aminobutyric acid leading to excitation of neurones

b) inhibiting serotonin receptors[101]
c) causing a porphyric crisis in cases where its metabolic breakdown is too slow[101]

It is, however, unlikely that either thujone isomer was responsible for the observed effects of "absinthism" (see Precautions).

Santonin is listed as an official vermifuge.[42]

In vivo—A combination of herbs predominantly composed of wormwood improved the standard medical treatment of patients with Crohn's disease, enabled a reduction and/or cessation of steroid treatment and improved mood and quality of life.[95]

Thujone at high enough levels can reduce mental performance and negate the anxiolytic effect of alcohol.[102]

Old research had demonstrated that wormwood stimulated digestive secretions from both pancreas and liver.[103]

The herb is used traditionally in the West Indies to treat worms[104] and it is a frequently used agent in rural Italy against parasites and as an insect repellent.[105]

Medicinal uses
Gastro-intestinal tract
It has a reputation for use in poor digestion and lack of energy resulting from inadequate nutrition.

- anorexia
- atonic dyspepsia
- *Enterobius* (BHP)
- malabsorption
- indigestion
- biliary disorders
- nausea
- chronic gastritis
- *Ascaris* (BHP)
- flatulence
- colic

Reproductive tract
Regarded as a stimulant of uterine muscle and antispasmodic the herb is used for:

- amenorrhoea or delayed menstruation
- aid to childbirth for pain relief
- dysmenorrhoea

Musculoskeletal
- arthritis
- rheumatism

Pharmacy
Three times daily
Infusion of dried herb   – 1–2 g
Tincture 1:5 (45%)   – 1–2 ml   (suggested guidelines)
Fluid Extract (25%)   – 1–2 ml

The herb is used in small doses to tone the digestive tract and stimulate the appetite and in larger doses to act as a vermifuge and toxin cleanser. The powder is used in 4–10 g doses for intestinal worms.

Artabsin, like achillin in *Achillea* and chamazulene in *Matricaria recutita*, will generate azulene on steam distillation and should be prepared accordingly (see *Achillea*) if the anti-inflammatory properties are required. Diluted oil may be used externally for local pains.

Extracts may be standardised on absinthin content. Available commercially in wine and aperitifs e.g. Vermouth.

CONTRAINDICATIONS—Pregnancy.

Precautions and/or safety
The essential oil of *Artemisia absinthium* was the basis of the French liqueur absinthe which had a narcotic and hallucinogenic effect attributed to thujone. It was banned because it was deemed to cause damage to the central nervous system. Interestingly due to the recent re-instatement of absinthe to the market, an analysis of the content of thujone in vintage absinthe and absinthe made according to old recipes was undertaken using sensitive tests. The amount of thujone present was well below current maximum allowable levels. The authors' deduced thujone at most would have made a very minor contribution to the symptoms of absinthism.[106] They speculate that this phenomenon was a result of adulterants in the spirit e.g. colouring agents or chronic alcoholism possibly (it was extracted into high strength alcohol[101]).

In excessive amounts the herb may cause insomnia, nightmares, vomiting and convulsions. It should therefore not to be used for long term therapy and the maximum weekly dosage must not be exceeded. Toxicity due to thujone is rare[101] and used properly wormwood is a valuable and safe herb.

There is a possibility of allergy (see General Precaution p. 25), which could also be linked to the high levels of histidine.[100]

Historical uses
Counteracting the effects of poisons including hemlock and toadstools. Cancer; colds and fevers; rheumatism; to deter insects; epilepsy; melancholy; nervine; colic; jaundice (for which Culpeper rates this herb most highly), hepatitis and congestive states of the liver; diuresis; for treating bruises and contusions; scabs and itches; as a face wash to make the face "fair". There has been some speculation that Vincent van Gogh did not suffer from a psychosis but an overuse of absinthe and liking for terpenes of the thujone type (camphor and pinene).[107]

Artemisia vulgaris

Mugwort, cronewort

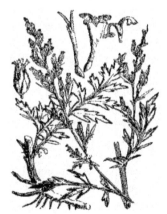

Family Asteraceae, Tribe Anthemideae

Description
An erect, aromatic, much branched perennial, 60–120 cm high, dying back every winter. Rhizomes branched, nodular. *Stems* grooved, reddish, erect

but tending to flop as flowering begins. *Basal leaves* 5–8 cm long, stalked, pinnately lobed, stem leaves stalkless and clasping the stem, once or twice pinnate with ultimate segments lance-shaped, dark green and glabrous above, very white underneath. *Inflorescence* erect, forming a long, leafy terminal panicle, each head containing 12–20 complete florets and a few female ones, all fertile. *Florets* ovoid 3–4 mm reddish-brown, with cottony involucres. *Achenes* obovate without any pappus. Flowers mid-summer to autumn.

Odour—aromatic; taste—spicy and a little bitter.

Habitat and cultivation
Native to all Europe and much of Asia from the Arctic Circle to the Tropics in waste places. Cultivated elsewhere from seed or root division, forming large clumps in sunny places. Drought and frost resistant.

Parts used
The flowering herb.

Active constituents
1) Volatile oil which varies with geographical location and time of harvest.[108,109] In Europe the oil appears to be predominantly comprised of camphor (up to 47%) with significant amounts of myrcene, 1,8-cineole, borneol, terpinen-4-ol, sabinene, caryophyllene and β-thujone;[87] Indian and Moroccan oil is mainly camphor but also α-thujone (max. 56%) and β-thujone; Cuban oil mainly caryophyllene oxide (up to 31%), Vietnamese mainly 1,8-cineole, α-terpineol and camphor with increasing levels of α- and β-pinene as the plant reaches flowering. Previously β-caryophyllene, β-cubebene and β-elemene had been identified. Camphor and α-terpineol levels were found to be fairly constant through maturation of the flowers but other constituents such as borneol, myrtenol and carveol decrease with flowering. Leaf and flower oil are similar
2) Sesquiterpene lactones—vulgarin[110]
3) Coumarins including scopoletin[111]
4) Triterpenes including β-sitosterol

5) Phenolic acids including hydroxycinnamic, chlorogenic, dicaffeoylquinic and eudesmane acids[112–114]
6) Cyanogenic glucoside—prunasin[115]

Also contains flavonoids, tannins, polyacetylenes,[116,117] eudesmane dialcohol[112] and fernenol.[118] The species of *Artemisia* from which vulgarin was first isolated has more recently been identified as *A. verlotorum* Lamotte.[119]

Nutritional constituents
Vitamins: Niacin and C
Minerals: Chromium, iron, manganese, phosphorous and potassium

Actions
1) Emmenagogue
2) Orexigenic
3) Choleretic
4) Stomachic
5) Anthelmintic

Scientific information
There is not a great deal of modern research on this herb however it has been used in both western and eastern traditions of herbal medicine. In the west it was used as an insect repellent and flavouring for drinks, in the east it is used for the preparation "moxa".

In vitro—The essential oil of mugwort has a similar antimicrobial activity to that of wormwood.[87] Extracts of the whole herb and the volatile oil, in particular, have the following activities:-

• antimutagenic[120]
• strong anti-oxidant[121]
• inhibition of xanthine oxidase—used in Vietnam for the treatment of gout[122]
• cytotoxic to various cancer cell lines—oral squamous cell carcinoma, salivary gland, melanoma and leukaemia[123]
• antibacterial activity against the cariogenic bacterium *Streptococcus mutans*[124]

Prunasin is an inhibitor of DNA polymerase.[115]

In vivo—*Artemisia vulgaris* in combination with 7 other herbs was used as an irrigant following prostatectomy and effectively reduced the incidence of bladder infection and bleeding without side-effects.[125]

The obvious similarities to *A. absinthium* indicate similar medicinal uses for this herb but generally mugwort is considered weaker and with a more specific application for the female reproductive tract. In the Philippines it is used as an anti-inflammatory.

Medicinal uses

Gastro-intestinal tract

Mugwort has a similar effect on the digestive tract to wormwood and is used for the same conditions, as a bitter tonic to stimulate the appetite, improve digestive function and as an anthelmintic. It is considered to be carminative.

- anorexia
- indigestion
- round worms
- thread worms
- colic
- nervous dyspepsia

Nervous system
- depression
- tension
- convulsions

Reproductive tract

It seems to be able to exert a toning, as well as stimulating effect, on the uterus:

- menorrhagia
- functional amenorrhoea
- scant but prolonged menstruation
- delayed menstruation
- hasten labour
- dysmenorrhoea
- help expulsion of the placenta
- irregular menstruation

BHP specific for mugwort are for functional amenorrhoea and dysmenorrhoea.

Pharmacy

Three times daily

Infusion of dried herb	–	0.5–2 g
Tincture 1:5	–	2–4 ml (suggested guidelines)
Fluid Extract (25%)	–	0.5–2 ml

CONTRAINDICATIONS—Pregnancy.

Precautions and/or safety

Mugwort pollen seems to be commonly implicated in allergic rhinitis and/or asthma. Large doses of the herb should be avoided (see also General Precaution p. 25).

Historical uses

Used in beer making before being replaced by hops. To treat urinary stones; dropsy and jaundice; expel poisons including those from an over indulgence of opium and from infections e.g. boils; sciatica; "hysterical fits"; palsies. Fevers. Externally to treat wens and hard knots and kernels around the neck and throat; as a warm wash to treat pains of the sinews and cramps.

Calendula officinalis

Marigold, pot marigold

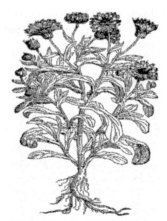

Family Asteraceae, Tribe Calenduleae

Description

Erect or ascending annual or short-lived perennial, sometimes with a woody base, 15–50 cm tall.

Stems clothed in short erect glandular hairs usually becoming glabrous below, much branched. *Leaves,* basal and lower cauline sparsely to moderately hairy, ciliate, usually narrow-obovate, sometimes elliptic/orbicular, entire with a few minute, scattered teeth, obtuse to acute and mucronate, apetiolate and long-cuneate, 6–20 × 1.5–5 cm. Upper cauline leaves similar but becoming smaller, oblong to lanceolate, broad-based and often amplexicaul. *Capitula* solitary, 35–85 mm diameter. Involucral bracts in 2 rows, glandular and ciliate, lanceolate, acuminate 10–15 mm long, the inner with more conspicuous margins. Ray florets 40–60, in 1-several rows; ligules usually orange or shades of yellow, clearly exceeding bracts, 12–30 mm long. Disc florets numerous, usually orange or shades of yellow, rarely brownish-black. *Achenes* glabrous or sparsely hairy, usually of 3 types:

a) outermost achenes strongly incurved, long-beaked, 12–18 mm diameter, with small stout spines on back, usually alternating with
b) shorter, short-beaked, broadly 3-winged, tuberculate or smooth-backed achenes
c) inner achenes enclosed by outer, tuberculate on back, 4–7 mm diameter.

Flowers all year in many areas with the main season late spring to late autumn.

Odour—faint but characteristic; taste—somewhat bitter and salty.

Habitat and cultivation
Native to Mediterranean Europe and grown in other countries from seed. Self-sows freely in sunny open situations with adequate water. Removing dead flower heads encourages more flowers and sturdy plants. Humidity can cause mildew. Drought and frost resistant.

Parts used
Flowers or ray florets gathered when fully opened. May be used fresh or dried.

Active constituents
1) Triterpenes:-

a) alcohols and esters which are based on monol, diol and triol alcohols.[126] Faradiol (85%) monoesters and calenduladiol are the main diols,[127,129] arnidiol and maniladiol are present in much smaller quantities.[128] The triterpendiols are the main lipophilic constituents[128,129] and the diol esters make up between 2–4% of the dry mass of flower. Monols include ψ-taraxasterol,[130] taraxasterol, helianol,[131] α- and β-amyrin and lupeol, and triols include heliantriol, ursatriol and longispinognine. The levels of esters are highest in the ray florets, present to a lesser extent in the disc florets and lower still in the involucral bracts. None are present in the receptacle[132]
b) triterpenoid saponins including calendulosides A–F, based on oleanolic acid and representing 2–10% of the dry mass of flowers[126,133]
2) Carotenoids—(1.5–3%) mainly flavoxanthin and auroxanthin.[134] The constituents differ with petal colour[135] and in quantity with geographical origin[136]
3) Essential oil—(0.02%) including ionone glucosides and sesquiterpene oligoglycosides (officinosides)[137]
4) Flavonoids—(0.3–0.8%) derivatives of isorhamnetin and quercetin including astragalin, hyperoside, isoquercitrin and rutin[126]

Also contains sterols, mucilage, resin, chlorogenic acid and polysaccharides.[138]

Nutritional constituents
Vitamins: A, C, E and coenzyme Q10
Minerals: Phosphorus and calcium

Actions
1) Anti-inflammatory
2) Vulnerary
3) Spasmolytic
4) Emmenagogue
5) Antihaemorrhagic
6) Antiseptic[†]
7) Styptic

[†] Active against bacteria, fungi, viruses and protozoa.

In addition this herb is also credited with being a mild diaphoretic, a circulatory stimulant and a sedative.

Scientific information
Calendula was once an official medicine and has been used in the west as well as in Asia. It is approved by *German Commission E* for the treatment of oral mucosa inflammation and topically as a cicatrizing agent for healing skin injuries. Although recent research has gone into identifying the constituents of *Calendula* not a great deal of new information has emerged to support the traditional use of this effective and frequently used herb. It is also used in the food industry as a colouring agent.

Antimicrobial
In vitro—The contstituents of *Calendula* and, to a limited degree, the whole extract have antimicrobial activity including:-

- antibacterial—*Bacillus subtilis, Escherichia coli, Staphylococcus aureus, Pseudomonas aeruginosa, Sarcina lutea, Klebsiella pneumoniae* and anaerobic and aerobic periodontal organisms.[139–141] Although the whole herb has been used to treat periodontal disease like chronic catarrhal gingivitis[142] a dentifrice, containing *Calendula* extract, failed to inhibit organisms isolated from saliva and dental plaque[143]
- antifungal—*Candida monosa,*[144] *C. albicans*[139] and *Trichomonas vaginalis*[145]
- antiviral—HIV-1 (and significantly inhibited reverse transcriptase),[146] herpes simplex and the influenza viruses A2 and APR-8[140]

The herb also has potential immunomodulatory activity.[147,148]
In vivo—*Calendula* used clinically with acyclovir in treating herpetic keratitis (the result of HSV-1 infection affecting the cornea) was more effective at healing ulceration then acyclovir alone.[149]

Anti-inflammatory and vulnerary
In vitro—The triterpenoid esters are considered to be largely responsible for the anti-inflammatory activity of the herb,[128] especially faradiol which is present in high levels.[129] The flavonoids based on isorhamnetin inhibit LOX.[150]

In vivo—*Calendula* was one of a combination of herbs used to successfully treat:-
Internally:-

- chronic colitis—reduced pain and normalised bowel function[151]
- duodenal ulcers and gastroduodenitis, with or without the use of antacids—reduced pain levels and dyspepsia, encouraged healing of ulcers (confirmed by gastroscopy)[151]

Externally:-

- contact dermatitis—reduced signs and symptoms[152]
- acute inflammation from radiotherapy—reduced dermatitis and pain levels more effectively than the standard treatment, Trolamine[153]
- 2nd and 3rd degree burns—better tolerated and more effective than petroleum jelly[154]

Apart from a number of animal based experiments which have examined the wound healing properties of *Calendula* its use for this purpose is based on tradition and anecdotal evidence.[140]

Other
In vitro—*Calendula* has significant anti-oxidant activity,[155] aqueous extracts being superior to methanolic ones.[156]

The herb and some constituents are cytotoxic to a range of cancer cells including colon, melanoma and leukaemia lines.[126,148]

The polysaccharides have a strong immunostimulatory activity, enhancing phagocytosis.[138,139,157]

Medicinal uses
Cardiovascular system
Calendula has a reputation for improving varicose veins and is used both internally and externally. It also benefits the lymphatic system.

- varicose veins
- haemorrhoids
- crural ulcers

- lymphoma
- lymphadenopathy
- fevers

Respiratory tract
- epistaxis

Gastro-intestinal tract
The local healing, anti-haemorrhagic and bitter properties give the herb a broad use in the GIT:

- gastric ulcers
- duodenal ulcers
- gastritis
- enteritis
- proctitis
- jaundice
- haematemesis
- biliary insufficiency
- liver congestion
- indigestion
- anorexia
- hepatitis
- gallstones
- constipation

Reproductive tract
- functional amenorrhoea
- dysmenorrhoea
- mastitis
- leucorrhoea
- cervical dysplasia
- vaginal thrush
- vaginitis
- *Trichomonas vaginalis*

Externally
The combination of *Calendula's* actions make it applicable for the treatment of many skin problems:

- wounds/inflamed skin conditions
- bruises
- boils
- broken capillaries
- chilblains
- fungal infections e.g. athlete's foot

- acne
- eczema
- sebaceous cysts
- sore nipples
- periodontal disease (mouthwash)
- sunburn
- blepharitis
- conjunctivitis
- nappy rash
- herpes simplex including cold sores

The specific action according to the *BHP* is for enlarged and inflamed lymph nodes, sebaceous cysts, duodenal ulcers and acute and chronic inflammatory skin lesions.

Pharmacy
Three times daily
Infusion of dried herb   – 1–4 g
Tincture 1:5 (90%)   – 0.3–1.2 ml
Fluid extract (40%)   – 0.5–1 ml

The oleoresin, containing the triterpenes, is considered to contribute significantly to *Calendula's* beneficial effects but it requires 90% alcohol to solubilise it.

Internally—infusion and tincture. Externally—infusion as a wash or applied as an oil, ointment or cream.

Precautions and/or safety
There is potential for *Calendula* to cause allergic reactions[79] (see General Precaution p. 25) with an estimated incidence of around 2% in sensitive individuals.[158]

The tincture is usually prepared at high alcohol concentrations so care is needed when using it on abraded tissues such as peptic ulcers. An alternative in the acute phase of therapy may be to use infusions.

Calendula extracts have been tested for irritant effects and safety according to the standards used by the cosmetic industry and are classified safe. Human safety is based on tradition.[159] It is both genotoxic and anti-genotoxic as well as displaying cytotoxicity in some standard non-human models. However it is not mutagenic.[160–162]

Historical uses

Bites of wild animals; liver and spleen congestion; stomach complaints; cancer treatment. The juice was used externally for psoriasis; swollen glands; warts; contusions and bruises. To strengthen the heart; smallpox; measles; headaches; jaundice; red eyes; toothache; ague; plague. Leaves eaten fresh for scrofula in children.

Cichorium intybus

Chicory, succory

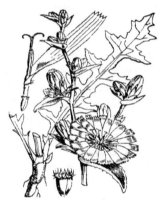

Family Asteraceae, Tribe Lactuceae

Description

Perennial rosette herb. *Stems* erect, 40–120 cm tall, branched above, finely ribbed, glabrous or with short crisped hairs. *Leaves*, rosette and lower stem leaves petiolate, oblanceolate, simple, toothed, shallowly or deeply pinnatifid, 10–30 × 2–7 cm, margin dentate. Upper leaves alternate, sessile, smaller than lower leaves, becoming less lobed, lanceolate with amplexicaul base, distantly toothed. *Capitula* in sessile clusters or terminal on short peduncles 2–6 cm long. Involucre 11–13 mm long: bracts with sparse, long, glandular hairs or glabrous, enclosing achenes tightly at fruiting. Florets few, corolla usually blue, sometimes white, about twice the length of the involucre, tube less than ligule. *Achenes* angular-obconic, flat at apex, glabrous, pale or mottled 2.5–3 mm long. Flowers mid-summer to autumn. Flowers open with the morning sun and close about midday.

Habitat and cultivation

Originally from Europe, West Asia and North Africa *Cichorium* is naturalised in other countries in cultivated and waste lands. It is an important permaculture crop. Grown from seed set 30 cm apart and transplants easily when young. Cut flowering stems back in autumn. Clumps can be dug in autumn and roots with a crown divided and replanted. Drought and frost resistant.

Parts used

Root harvested in autumn, in the second year of growth or thereafter.

Active constituents

1) Sesquiterpene lactones of the guaianolide group including lactucopicrin (intybin), lactucin and 8-deoxylactucin,[163–165] these are the predominant sesquiterpene lactones. Also present are eudesmanolides including magnolialide and germacranolides[165,166]
2) Triterpenes including α-amyrin, taraxerone, β-sitosterol,[167] taraxasterol and daucosterol[170]
3) Coumarins including cichoriin and glycosides of esculetin
4) Flavonoids including apigenin and quercitin
5) Pseudotannins
6) Inulin (up to 58%) consisting of linear fructan polymers, 2–60 units (average 12 units) in β (2,1) linkage[168]

Other constituents isolated from *Cichorium* include furofuran lignans,[169] phenolics including syringin, chlorogenic and cichoric acids,[164,169] azelaic and other carboxylic acids,[170] mannitol and the alkaloids harman and norharman.

Nutritional constituents

Vitamins: A, B, C, K and P
Minerals: Calcium, potassium, sodium and magnesium

Actions

1) Bitter tonic
2) Diuretic
3) Laxative

Scientific information

The herb has been recorded as a medicine since 1550 BC although today it is perhaps better known as a food. The leaves are eaten in salads or as a cooked vegetable and the roots, roasted and ground, are used in coffee powders. It is used in the East as an anti-inflammatory. In Turkey *Cichorium* is a traditional treatment for stomach pain whilst in India[183] and Peru[185] it is used for treating gastro-intestinal infections.

Similarities exist between its constituents and those of *Taraxacum* but *Cichorium* does not have the stature in the British herbal tradition that dandelion enjoys, although it is more highly valued in Europe. There are many varieties of *C. intybus* used commercially.

Anti-oxidant

In vitro—The leaves[171,172] and root extract[173] have both demonstrated anti-oxidant activity.

Digestive tract

In vitro—Current research has focussed on the benefits of inulin, derived mainly from *Cichorium* root, as a functional food. Inulin is water-soluble but it is not amenable to digestion in the gut due to the way the fructose units are linked.[168] It ferments in the digestive tract forming short chain fatty acids and lactic acid which are absorbable.[174] Inulin is described as a "prebiotic", because it has the potential to make improvements to gut flora, without containing any flora itself and without being absorbed. This leads to improvement in metabolic function, stimulation of the growth of beneficial bacteria, like bifidobacteria, and a reduction in the levels of harmful organisms.[175] The short chain fatty acids may play a role in this action.[168]

The sesquiterpene lactones are bitter.[164]

In vivo—Inulin enhances the absorption of calcium, reduces blood lipid levels including triglyceride and cholesterol.[168] Human faecal flora show increased levels of bifidobacteria after supplementing with partially hydrolysed inulin.[175] However all fructans, including inulin itself, are bifidogenic.[176] In addition as a soluble fibre it bulks out stools, increasing their water content and improving bowel function with less associated discomfort than lactulose.[177]

Inulin may also help to regulate food intake and blood glucose levels though this is yet to be established in humans.[178]

Other

In vitro—The root extract and/or the main sesquiterpenoids inhibit acetylcholinesterase,[179] have potential to be anti-inflammatory (through inhibition of COX-2 induction and activity)[180] and also to be immunomodulatory.[147]

Inulin fructans and magnolialide inhibit the growth of several tumour cell lines, modulate differentiation and reduce metastatic activities.[174,181]

Cichorium has been used traditionally as a treatment for malaria in Afghanistan and lactucin and lactupicrin are antiplasmodial against *Plasmodium falciparum*.[182] The herb has antimicrobial activity against a variety of bacteria including a multi-drug resistant species of *Salmonella typhi*[183,184] (but not against *Vibrio cholerae*[185]) and antifungal activity against the dermatophytes *Trichophyton rubrum* and *T. tonsurans*.[164]

In vivo—Inulin's various actions on the bowel include its potential, through the short chain fatty acids like butyrate, to reduce colon cancer and a project was due to assess its protective benefits to patients at high risk of developing this disease.[186]

A meta-analysis spanning 30 years of clinical trials found an Ayurvedic formulation containing *Cichorium* was beneficial in the treatment of hepatitis A.[187] This same formulation was also hepatoprotective in patients with liver cirrhosis.[188]

Medicinal uses

Gastro-intestinal tract
- indigestion
- anorexia
- constipation
- hepatitis
- cholelithiasis

Urinary tract
- fluid retention

Musculoskeletal

The herb encourages the excretion of metabolic waste through increased bile secretion and is also attributed with the ability to increase uric acid excretion. Used in the treatment of:

• rheumatism
• gout

Pharmacy
Three times daily
Decoction   – 8–12 g (suggested guidelines)
Tincture 1:5   – 2–4 ml

The root may be juiced when fresh and a suggested dosage is 10–15 ml three times daily. Trials on the benefits of inulin used 4–20 g daily.

Note: Inulin is extracted from the root in hot water, it is only slightly soluble in cold water or alcohol, and therefore it is not a major active constituent in the tincture.

Precautions and/or safety
For allergic potential see General Precaution p. 25. *Cichorium* leaves have caused a few cases of oral, cutaneous and respiratory allergy.[189,190]

Historical uses
This herb has been used largely as a salad food and beverage and it is possible its addition to coffee may help counter the excitatory effects of caffeine. Anaemia and debility with weakness and fatigue.

Cynara scolymus

Globe artichoke

Description
Perennial, rosette plant, 1–2 m tall in flower. *Stems* stout, ridged, sometimes branching, with fine white hairs. *Basal leaves* deeply pinnatifid, 30–60 × 15–40 cm, with lanceolate lobes becoming smaller near the base, smooth greyish-green above, tomentose beneath, viscid. Midrib stout and ridged. *Stem leaves* similar but becoming smaller and less divided. *Capitula* usually

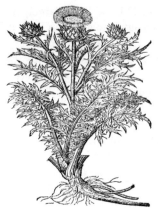

Family Asteraceae, Tribe Cynareae

solitary, 8–12 cm in diameter, in terminal heads. Involucre globose to hemispheric, with fleshy outer and middle bracts. *Corolla* 50–65 mm long comprised of all disc florets, rich lilac blue in colour. *Achenes* 6–9 × 3–5 mm, obovoid, usually pale and spotted with a 30–50 mm long pappus. Blooms and fruits in late summer.

Habitat and cultivation
Cynara is native to, and originally cultivated in, the Mediterranean region probably evolving from selected *C. cardunculus* which were not spiny and had fleshier involucral bracts. It is cultivated in many countries as a gourmet food. Grown from seed or division of clumps. Likes deep, rich, alkaline garden and dies back after flowering. Drought tender, frost resistant.

Parts used
The leaves, which are at their most bitter just before flowering.

Active Constituents
1) Sesquiterpene lactones (0.5–4%) of the guaianolide type, mainly cynaropicrin, and others including cynarascolosides A–C[191]
2) Phenolic acids (up to 2%) the main ones being mono- and di-caffeoylquinic acids including chlorogenic acid, caffeic acid and cynarin (1,5-dicaffeylquinic acid).[192–195] Cynarin may be an artefact of aqueous extraction[196]

3) Flavonoids (0.1–1%) based largely on luteolin also cynaroside and apigenin derivatives[193,195]

Also contains coumarins, alkaloids, phytosterols (taraxasterol), pseudotannins, polyacetylenes and a curdling enzyme—cynarase.

Nutritional constituents
Vitamins: Provitamin A, B_1, B_2 and C
Minerals: Iodine

Actions
1) Hepatoprotective
2) Choleretic
3) Cholagogue
4) Diuretic
5) Liver trophorestorative
6) Hypolipidaemic

Scientific information
Cynara was cultivated in ancient Rome and Greece. It has been an official medicine and was listed in a number of European countries as a diuretic and choleretic.[42] It is approved by *German Commission E* for use in dyspeptic conditions.

Anti-oxidant
In vitro—The phenols and especially luteolin and cholorgenic acid are significant anti-oxidants.[197] Both aqueous and particularly ethanolic extracts display anti-oxidant properties superior to the lipophilic fraction.[198,199]

Circulation
The action of artichoke leaves on lipid levels although newer to medicine than that of its choleretic properties has nonetheless been appreciated for some decades.
In vitro—The phenolic constituents are considered important to activity within the cardiovascular system and they may be central to the herb's apparent ability to prevent atherosclerosis. *Cynara* has the following actions:-

• strong anti-oxidant activity including preventing oxidation of low density lipoprotein[199]

• inhibition of cholesterol synthesis (so far demonstrated in animal models only)[199]
• increases endothelial production of nitric oxide which also contributes to an antithrombotic action[200]

In vivo—*Cynara* lowered cholesterol, triglycerides and soluble adhesion molecules (markers of lipid disorders) and increased flow-mediated vasodilation in hyperlipaemic people.[201–203] The juice was also beneficial in reducing lipid levels of patients with Fredrickson types IIa and IIb primary hyperlipidaemia.[204]

Isolated cynarin however did not improve the biochemistry of patients with familial type II hyperlipoproteinaemia in short-term trials.[205]

Reviews of clinical trials using *Cynara* in hyperlipidaemias conclude that although it has demonstrated good reductions in blood cholesterol the trials generally lack rigor.[206,207] However the herb has received some acceptance as a hypolipidaemic agent and as it is safe, it is suitable for long-term use, having fewer side-effects and added benefits compared to the corresponding pharmaceuticals.[208]

The herb is, in addition, a diuretic.

Gastro-intestinal
In vitro—Whilst the phenolic constituents are credited with the herb's capacity to act as a choleretic and hepatoprotective[214] the whole extract likely contributes to these activities.[209]

In vivo—Investigations of *Cynara* have shown that it is a choleretic[210] and has spasmolytic, carminative and anti-emetic activity.[211]

It was used to treat functional dyspepsia and dyspepsia due to irritable bowel syndrome with subjective improvement in gastro-intestinal function and quality of life.[212–214]

Other
In vitro—The herb has antifungal properties.[215] A number of the phenolic constituents also have activity against bacteria including *Staphylococcus aureus, Escherichia coli, Salmonella typhimurium* and *Pseudomonas aeruginosa* and against some pathogenic fungi like *Candida albicans* and *C. lusitaniae*.[193]

Cynara has anti-inflammatory properties.[216]

In vivo—It was not effective as a prophylactic for hangovers.[217]

The herb was shown in early studies to have decreased blood levels of urea and nitrogenous waste[218] and so may aid detoxification.

Medicinal uses

Cardiovascular system
- mild oedema
- arteriosclerosis
- ascites (portal hypertension)
- obesity
- hyperlipidaemia

Gastro-intestinal tract
- dyspepsia
- cholelithiasis
- cholecystitis
- nausea
- liver disease
- chronic constipation
- anorexia
- hepatitis

Urinary tract
- mild renal insufficiency

Musculoskeletal

By enhanced elimination via kidneys and liver could aid the treatment of:

- arthritis
- gout

Skin

For the same reasons as above, an aid to treatment of:

- skin conditions

Pharmacy

The *BHP* has no entry for *Cynara*.

Three times daily (*German Commission E* recommended)

Infusion of dried leaf	– 2 g
Tincture 1:5	– 6 ml
Fluid extract	– 2 ml

Clinical trials used doses ranging from 320–1920 mg daily of encapsulated standardised herb or 10 ml of the juice of leaves/buds three times daily. In the latter case results were measurable after 6 weeks.

CONTRAINDICATIONS—It has been suggested that lactating and pregnant women should use *Cynara* with caution because of the milk curdling enzyme—there are no adverse reports and it seems unlikely to be a problem.

Pharmacokinetics

Studies indicate that the main phenolics in plasma after absorption of *Cynara* are caffeic, ferulic and isoferulic acid and their hydrogenated derivatives which in the main are conjugated. The non-hydrogenated metabolites have peak plasma levels 1 hour after oral administration and the hydrogenated metabolites peak after 6–7 hours.[219]

Precautions and/or safety

From clinical trials *Cynara* seems to be safe with only mild, transient, infrequent side-effects including flatulence, hunger and weakness.[207] Also reported are contact dermatitis,[220] rhinitis and asthma[221] after handling the fresh plant and a case of anaphylaxis to inulin of *Cynara* origin.[222] For allergic reactions see General Precaution p. 25.

Historical uses

For body odour in addition to the above uses. Snakebites.

Echinacea angustifolia

Narrow-leaved purple coneflower

Description

Tap-rooted perennial, 15–50 cm tall with erect single or branched stems which are covered with stiff bristly hairs. *Leaves* lance-shaped, entire, dark

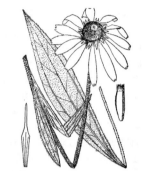

Family Asteraceae, Tribe Heliantheae

green with 3–5 nerves running the length of the blade. Basal leaves on long petioles, upper stem leaves sessile, alternate. *Flower head* solitary, with prominent, cone shaped red-brown disc florets surrounded by sterile pale to deep purple spreading rays which are about as long as the width of the disc. Involucral bracts are lance-shaped and overlapping in a series of two or more and transfer into pales as they move to the flowers themselves. (The pales are chaffy scales subtending the fruit, and extend slightly beyond the corolla of each disc flower.) They appear to be folded together lengthwise and end in sharp, blunt or slightly curved points. Once the flower head is dry the pales remain intact and this is what gave the plant its name after *echinos*, Greek for sea urchin or hedgehog. *Achenes* are four-sided and have slight teeth at each corner of the crown. Flowers mid-summer to mid-autumn.

Odour—mildly aromatic; taste—sweet becoming bitter and causing a tingling sensation on the tongue.

Habitat and cultivation
Native to barren and dry prairies in North America from Minnesota to Texas, Western Okalahoma, Kansas, Nebraska and Iowa, the Dakotas, Eastern Colorado, Wyoming and Montana and extreme Southern Saskatchewan and Manitoba. Grown from seed which needs cold and light to germinate. Also grown from root division. Slow growing and often does not flower until second or third year. Likes an open, sunny situation and slightly alkaline soil, is drought tolerant.

Parts used
The fresh or dried root harvested after flowering is over and after the 2nd year of growth.

Echinacea pallida

Pale purple coneflower

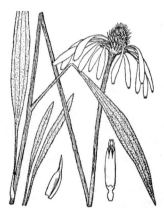

Family Asteraceae, Tribe Heliantheae

Description
A tap-rooted perennial growing up to a 1 m tall and dying back in winter. *Leaves* alternate, lower leaves lance-shaped, stiff, hairy with short petioles. Stem leaves smaller and sessile. *Flowers* solitary or few on long peduncles, ray florets, sparse, pale pinkish purple, about 10 cm long and drooping. Disc florets in cone whose scales are longer than the disc florets. *Seeds* whitish-grey and tooth-like. Blooms from late spring to late summer.

Odour—mildly aromatic; taste—sweet becoming bitter, does not cause a tingling sensation on the tongue.

Habitat and cultivation
Native to prairies and glades of North America from Michigan to Nebraska, south to Georgia and west to Texas. Can be grown commercially or in gardens from seed stratified in containers in the refrigerator for about 6 weeks or from root division in early spring. It prefers rich sandy soil and a cold winter.

Parts used
Roots of 2 year old plants harvested after the plants have gone to seed.

Echinacea purpurea

Purple coneflower

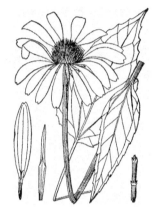

Family Asteraceae, Tribe Heliantheae

Description
Fibrous rooted perennial growing from 60–150 cm tall often branching. *Basal leaves* oval to broadly lanceolate, coarsely pubescent and coarsely dentate with irregular teeth and long petioles. Stem leaves alternate and smaller. *Capitula* large with sterile rosy-purple ray florets and bright orange-tipped pales. Flowers mid-summer to late autumn.

Odour—mildly aromatic; taste—sweet becoming bitter and causing a tingling sensation on the tongue.

Habitat and cultivation
Native to open woods thickets and prairies from Louisiana, North East Texas and Eastern Okalahoma north through Ohio, Michigan and eastward. Cultivated as an ornamental for at least 200 years. Cultivars available. Grown like *E. angustifolia* but self-sows in frosty areas, and grows faster and taller, often flowering in first or second year.

Parts used
Whole plant in flower.

Active constituents
There are not only variations in the 3 medicinal species of *Echinacea* but within the same species genetic differences occur naturally[223] though how this affects the constituents of the herb is unclear. *E. angustifolia* and *E. pallida* are more alike[224] and at one time were considered varieties of the same species.[225]

1) Alkamides, more than 20, not all have been identified. Isobutylamides are predominant in *E. angustifolia*, the main one being dodeca-2,4,8,10 tetraenoic acid isobutylamide. Isobutylamides occur also in *E. purpurea* and to a much lesser extent in *E. pallida*[226]
2) Caffeic acid esters including caftaric, chlorogenic, caffeic and cichoric acids, echinacoside and cynarin.[227] The latter is present only in *E. angustifolia* and is used as a marker for the species.[225] *E. purpurea* contains the highest concentration of these phenolic constituents (the predominant one being cichoric acid which reaches a maximum of 2.27%[228]), followed by *E. pallida* and then *E. angustifolia*.[229] Echinacoside (0.4–1.7%) is present in larger amounts in *E. pallida* (around 2%)[230] than in *E. angustifolia* (1.04%)[228] and not present in *E. purpurea*. It is however one of the main phenolic constituents in *E. angustifolia*.[228] Verbascoside is the other predominant phenolic in *E. purpurea*.[231] In *E. pallida* these constituents are caffeic glycosides or caffeic esters of quinic or tartaric acid[232]
3) Volatile oil (0.2–2.0%), including in all species acetaldehyde, dimethyl sulfide, camphene, hexanal, β-pinene and limonene.[233] Also in *E. angustifolia* humulene and in *E. purpurea* borneol, bornyl acetate, a germacrene D derivative, caryophyllene and a sesqutierpene based on eudesmane.[232,234] A-phellandrene is present in the roots of *E. angustifolia* and *E. purpurea* only. In all species butanals and propanals constitute about half of the volatile oil[233]
4) Polysaccharides, two types, an arabinogalactan-protein, rich in hydroxyproline, and a heteroxylan[225,235,236]
5) Polyacetylenes including ketoalkenes and ketoalkynes

Also resin, betaine (0.3%), trace amounts of pyr-rolizidine alkaloids (tussilagin and isotussilagin), phytosterols including β-sitosterol and inulin.

In the past *Echinacea* was often substituted with *Parthenium integrifolium* as they both have the common name in the USA of "Missouri snakeroot". *P. intergrifolium* is distinguished by its sesquiter-pene esters.[237]

Nutritional constituents
Vitamins: A, C and E
Minerals: Iron, iodine, copper, potassium and sul-phur. In *E. purpurea*:- root—iron, copper and man-ganese; aerial—calcium, magnesium and zinc[238]

Actions
1) Immunomodulator
2) Antimicrobial
3) Diaphoretic
4) Vasodilator (peripheral)
5) Anti-inflammatory
6) Vulnerary
7) Alterative

Scientific information
The historical use of *Echinacea* in the West dates back to the 19th Century when the herb was intro-duced to new settlers in North America by the indigenous peoples who used it predominantly to treat infections.[239] *E. angustifolia* was an offi-cial herb in *USA National Formulary* until 1950.[240] *E. angustifolia* and *E. pallida* were undoubtedly used interchangeably in commercial preparations in the past.[225]

Apart from the interest in the efficacy and mechanism of its action, *Echinacea* has also gener-ated a good deal of scientific enquiry into its safety and potential for interaction due to its widespread public use.[241–243] 26% of primary health care patients questioned had used, or were, using *Echinacea*[244] and it has been estimated that spending in 2005 on this one herb in the United States had reached more than US$300 million annually.[245]

The constituents responsible for its effects have not been determined although alkamides, phenolics and polysaccharides are all potentially active. (The bio-availability of the polysaccharides is questionable; they are not soluble in ethanol). The activity of this species is likely to be multi-factorial.

Anti-oxidant
In vitro—Anti-oxidant activities have been shown in all species of *Echinacea*.[231,246] The phenolic con-stituents seem to be strongly correlated with this activity and within them,[227] echinacoside has the highest anti-oxidant potential and caftaric acid the lowest.[229] However studies have shown that a number of the caffeic acid esters have low cell permeability and therefore may not cross the intes-tinal mucosa.[247]

Ex vivo—Healthy people who took *Echinacea* had an improved plasma anti-oxidant capacity.[263]

Immunomodulatory
The reputation that *Echinacea* has for immune stimulation is based on over 50 years of scientific research. *In vitro* and *in vivo*, whole extracts, as well as isolated constituents have been shown to:-

• enhance non-specific immune function includ-ing increased phagocytosis and leukocyte mobility[225,248–251,263]
• stimulate natural killer cell activity[225,249,252,253]
• increase properdin production[254]
• increase levels of various cytokines including interferon[225,253,255,256]
• increase T-cell response[257]

In vitro—The alkamides from *E. purpurea* are not only immunomodulatory[258] they also inhibit COX-1 and -2 activity.[259]

Interestingly a study using simulated-digestion extracts of various *Echinacea* preparations stimu-lated macrophages, *in vitro*, where the whole herb extract/juice did not[260] and the effect of liver metabolism on constituents is likely to alter the *in vivo* effects of the herb.[261]

In vivo—Immune function and natural killer cell activity increased, after using *E. purpurea* extracts, not only in healthy volunteers but also in patients suffering with chronic fatigue syndrome or AIDS.[262] A combined *E. angusifolia* and *E. purpurea* prepara-tion increased both immune response (including raising white blood cell count) and anti-oxidant status in healthy people.[263] However some small studies using a number of different *Echinacea* preparations orally and given over several days failed to corroborate enhanced phagocytosis in healthy subjects.[264,265]

Treatment of autoimmune based uveitis improved when *Echinacea* was used alongside standard therapy.[266]

Injections of *Echinacea* polysaccharides were found to help chemotherapy-induced leukopenia[267] however this may be irrelevant for oral use of *Echinacea* and parenteral use is no longer recommended by *German Commission E*.

Antimicrobial
In vitro—*E. purpurea* extracts have good antifungal activities against *Candida* spp., including *C. albicans*, when combined with UV light exposure, although this activity still occurs to a lesser extent without it. The ketoalkenes and ketoalkynes are considered key to phototoxicity.[268]

In all species the whole extracts and alkamides inhibit HSV-1 in UV-A and visible light.[269] Cichoric acid also inhibits the enzyme that allows the AIDS virus to integrate into host DNA but it is poorly absorbed into cells.[270]

In vivo—Most of the clinical research that has been carried out relates to *Echinacea's* most widespread application, that of treating respiratory infections including the common cold. This may involve a direct antimicrobial action but most likely is through an enhanced immune response. Results have been variable and are presented below.

Positive studies using either *Echinacea* preparations alone or in combination with other agents have shown:

- decreased risk of developing an infection[271,†]
- decreased duration of infection[271,272†,273†,274–276]
- decreased severity of symptoms associated with infection[274,275,277]
- decreased risk of relapse in chronic sufferers[272,278]
- quicker resolution of symptoms[273,275†,278,279]

---

†*Echinacea* as part of combination.

A recent meta-analysis found the herb does appear to reduce the incidence and duration of the common cold.[280] **Negative** studies using *Echinacea* alone concluded:

- no significant benefits in preventing infection[281,282]
- no reduction in duration of infections[283–285]
- no altered levels of immune response[286]
- no reduction in the severity of symptoms[245–247,287]

A number of reviews have suggested reasons for the above inconsistencies which include variability in the *Echinacea* species, type and quality of extract used, outcome measures sought and dosage regimes used (these tended to be low in negative studies).[252,288–290]

Overall the conclusion, though not unanimous,[245,291] is that *Echinacea* treatment is effective in terms of reducing duration and severity of symptoms.[248,253,292–294]

Whole extracts of *E. purpurea* administered for 6 months did not benefit patients with recurrent genital herpes.[295]

Other
In vitro—Apart from the effect of the herb on the immune system, *Echinacea* extracts and echinacoside[296] also inhibit hyaluronidase,[225] an enzyme used by invading organisms to break down host connective tissue allowing microbial entry and spread. The herb can increase fibroblast activity which would aid healing of connective tissue.[225]

Extracts of all 3 roots are cytotoxic to a number of cancer cell lines with *E. pallida* demonstrating the most effective activity.[297] However phenolic constituents of *E. angustifolia* have also increased the proliferation of some cancer cells cotreated with a chemotherapeutic drug.[298]

Alkylamides from *E. angustifolia* are inhibitors of COX-2[299] and the whole herb has potential anti-inflammatory activity.[260]

In vivo—*E. purpurea* has been used traditionally for healing wounds, a clinical trial indicates it increased the healing of purulent wounds.[300]

Medicinal uses

Cardiovascular system
- *Echinacea* is a circulatory stimulant and peripheral vasodilator and by increasing blood flow to the tissues acts as a diaphoretic—in **fevers**
- **infections** of this system e.g. **septicaemia** and **leucopenia** due to acute causes e.g. radiation therapy

Respiratory tract

All infections of this tract, for treatment and prevention e.g.:

- colds/influenza
- tonsillitis[†]
- sinusitis
- nasopharyngeal catarrh
- bronchitis
- hayfever
- otitis
- pertussis

Gastro-intestinal tract

All infections in this tract e.g.:

- food poisoning
- gingivitis
- peptic ulcers

Urinary tract

All infections of this tract e.g.:

- cystitis
- urethritis

Reproductive tract
- infections of this tract e.g. pelvic inflammatory disease

Musculoskeletal
- infections
- auto-immune diseases e.g. rheumatoid arthritis

Skin

All infections, allergic reactions, an aid to skin conditions (including those of immune origin) e.g.

[†]Including *Streptococcal* infections.

- boils
- abscesses
- infected wounds
- impetigo
- thrush
- bites and stings
- burns
- psoriasis
- athlete's foot
- varicose ulcers
- eczema
- herpes infections

Pharmacy

Three times daily

Decoction/infusion of dried herb	– 0.5–1 g
Tincture 1:5 (45%)	– 1–2 ml
Fluid Extract (45%)	– 0.25–1 ml

Echinacea has been used externally in creams, ointments or lotions to treat skin infections.

The level of essential oil is increased markedly by drying. However the active constituents of *Echinacea* are complex and the gain of essential oil on drying may be balanced by the loss of other actives. There is no clear evidence yet whether the herb is more effective when used dry or fresh and both preparations achieve satisfactory results.

The quality of commercial products inevitably has come under scrutiny, it is very variable.[301] This has no doubt contributed to the lack of consistency in clinical trials.

Pharmacokinetics

Echinacea has been used frequently by pregnant women[302] with no increased risk to foetal development.[303] Standard mutagenicity and carcinogenicity tests undertaken on the species have not raised safety concerns.[225]

Studies to date have shown that following ingestion of a combined *E. angustifolia* and *E. purpurea* tablet prepared from an ethanolic extract, the caffeic acid esters were not measurable at any time in the blood samples of healthy volunteers.

The alkamides were present in the blood stream 20 minutes after ingestion and were still detectable up to 12 hours later.[304] Alkamides from

E. angustifolia tincture were maximal in the blood stream after 30 minutes.[305]

Precautions and/or safety

Echinacea should cause a tingling sensation on the tongue and is a sialagogue. This effect is more marked in *E. angustifolia*. The fluid extract can cause excessive salivation and discomfort if taken in too large a quantity, undiluted.

Considering the very widespread use of *Echinacea* there have been very few reports of adverse reactions and these have, in the main, been mild involving gastro-intestinal upsets, rashes[240] and infrequently allergic reactions.[306,307] In 1997/8 of reported adverse events associated with herbal remedies and dietary supplements around 7% of these related to *Echinacea*, the majority of them being classed as minor.[308] *Echinacea* was reported as being safe and well tolerated in the above studies.[253,274,285,288]

See General Precaution p. 25. The risk of allergic reaction is somewhat lower for *Echinacea*.[79]

Serious adverse event reports in which *Echinacea* is cited include anaphylaxis, acute asthma, eye irritation and conjunctivitis (topical use),[309] a suspected link to recurrent erythema nodosum,[310] acute cholestatic auto-immune hepatitis[311] and possible aggravation of *pemphigus vulgaris*.[312]

A small proportion of liver transplant patients using "large amounts" of *Echinacea* had raised blood transaminase levels which returned to normal on cessation of the supplement involved.[313] There has been some speculation about the potential harm of *Echinacea* based on its content of pyrrolizidine alkaloids, a class of alkaloids associated with hepatotoxicity in the *Senecio* spp. However those found in *Echinacea* have a 1,2 saturated necine ring which are not considered hepatotoxic.[225]

German Commision E suggests *Echinacea* should not be taken for longer than 8 weeks (due to tachyphylaxis), or where the immune system is dysfunctional, such as in auto-immune conditions. (The trial on patients with auto-immune uveitis does not corroborate this caution[266]).

The above restrictions for using the herb are theoretical.

Interactions

In vitro—Studies have shown *Echinacea* and/or its constituents can inhibit CYP3A4,[314] CYP2C9[315] and CYP2E1.[316]

In vivo—*Echinacea* appears to have some effect on cytochrome CYP450. One study indicated an interaction with CYP3A substrates and those of CYP1A2.[317] In another the effects on cytochromes CYP1A2, CYP2D6, CYP2E1 and CYP3A4 (considered the most important ones) were not found to be significant.[318,319] It does not interact with P-glycoprotein mediated drug metabolism e.g. digoxin.[320]

A review of studies in 2001 found no reported drug/herb interactions.[321]

Historical uses

Fevers; infections; snake and spider bites.

Eupatorium cannabinum

Hemp agrimony

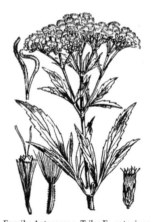

Family Asteraceae, Tribe Eupatorieae

Description

A perennial with short woody rhizomes forming clumps 1.5 × 1 m and dying down completely in winter. *Stems* round and hairy. *Leaves* opposite, divided into 3 lanceolate coarsely toothed segments, the middle segment largest 3–11 cm long, dull green. *Flowers* in dense corymbs. The involucre has 10 bracts arranged in 2 rows with purple tips, the outer row shorter than the inner. The florets are all tubular, hermaphrodite, 5–7 to each flower, white or pinkish-mauve. The *fruit* is a 5-angled achene, dotted with glands, with a whitish pappus. Flowers in late summer to early autumn.

Habitat and cultivation
Native to Europe and North Africa *E. cannabinum* grows in sun or semi-shade in rich, moist soil. It is frost resistant but drought tender and may be grown from seed or root division.

Parts used
The herb.

Active constituents
There are varieties of *E. cannabinum* which may differ in composition and proportions of constituents.[323]

1) Volatile oil (about 0.5%) including germacrene D (approx. 28.5%), α-phellandrene (approx 20%),[322] α-terpinene, thymol (up to 12%)[323] and p-cymene
2) Sesquiterpene lactones the main one being eupatoriopicrin[324]
3) Flavonoids including astragalin, kaempferol, hyperoside, isoquercitrin, rutin, hispidulin and eupafolin[325]
4) Alkaloids (pyrrolizidine) including supinine, echinatine,[326] amabiline, viridiflorine, lycopsamine, cynaustraline and intermidine

Also contains polysaccharides, euparin, eupatopicrin and lactucerol.

Actions
1) Diuretic
2) Alterative

Scientific information
This herb was well known in former times but has fallen out of modern use in the west.

In vitro—Eupatoriopicrin has antitumour activity being both cytostatic and cytotoxic,[323] the mode of action may be due to DNA damage.[327] The polysaccharides are immunostimulant and have been found to encourage phagocytosis.[328]

The pyrrolizidine alkaloids found in this herb are considered to be potentially hepatotoxic and/or carcinogenic although 80% of them are saturated at the 1,2 necine ring position which chemically makes this very unlikely.[329] There are no cases of toxicity reported in the literature.

Flowering tops have been used in Italy in an ointment as a cicatrizing agent.[330]

Precautions and/or safety
Possible allergic reaction (see General Precaution p. 25).

Historical uses
For fevers; bilious catarrh; influenza; hypocholesterolaemic, jaundice with swollen feet (portal hypertension); spring tonic to purify the blood and for scurvy. A strong infusion as a purgative and emetic; for psoriasis, eczema, fomenting ulcers and putrid sores.

Eupatorium perfoliatum

Boneset, thoroughwort

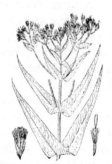

Family Asteraceae, Tribe Eupatorieae

Description
Perennial growing 50 cm–1.5 m tall, with erect, stout, round, pubescent stems growing from rhizomes and branching at the top. *Leaves* opposite, lanceolate to 20 cm long, acuminate, mostly connate-perfoliate, (stem seems to be inserted through the middle of leaf pairs) crenate-serrate, rugose. *Flowers* 10–40, in flat-topped corymbs, all tubular, bisexual, white. Blooms late summer—mid autumn.

Habitat and cultivation
Native to North America from Nova Scotia to Florida, Louisiana, Texas and North Dakota, growing in moist woods or thickets. May be grown from seed or root division. Spring growth slow. Frost resistant and drought tender.

Parts used
The herb harvested during or just prior to flowering.

Active constituents
1) Sesquiterpene lactones including eupafolin, euperfolitin, eufoliatin, eufoliatorin, euperfolide,[331] eucannabinolide and helenalin
2) Polysaccharides mainly 4-O-methylglucuroxylans
3) Flavonoids including kaempferol, quercitin, hyperoside, astragalin, rutin and eupatorin[332]

Also contains diterpenes, phytosterols, small amounts of volatile oil and some PABA.

Nutritional constituents
Vitamins: C
Minerals: Calcium, magnesium and potassium

Actions
1) Diaphoretic
2) Antipyretic
3) Aperient
4) Emetic (large doses)
5) Laxative (large doses)

Scientific information
There is very little new information available on the medicinal actions of this plant or its constituents although it was well known and well used by the North American Indians and appeared in the US Pharmacopoeia until 1916 as a stimulant as well as for above uses.[333]

In vitro—The leaves are strongly cytotoxic to normal and cancer cells and weakly antibacterial against Gram-positive bacteria like Staphylococcus aureus.[332] Eupatorin is a bitter and also has cytotoxic activity.[334]

The sesquiterpene lactones and polysaccharides increase phagocytosis.[335,336]

Medicinal uses
Respiratory tract
• influenza
• acute bronchitis
• fevers
• nasopharyngeal catarrh

BHP specific use—influenza with deep aching and congested respiratory mucosa.

Gastro-intestinal tract
The bitterness may contribute to the laxative action used in larger doses for:

• constipation

Pharmacy
Three times daily
Infusion of dried herb   – 1–2 g
Tincture 1:5 (45%)   – 1–4 ml
Fluid Extract (25%)   – 1–2 ml (2–4 ml Potter's)
    Diaphoresis best achieved with hot infusion.

Historical uses
Muscular rheumatism; intermittent fever/malaria also typhoid and yellow fevers. Dyspepsia and in old age to improve digestive function. Cutaneous diseases. Tape worm.

Eupatorium purpureum

Gravel root, Joe-pye weed

Description
Perennial up to 3 m tall with green stems hairy above, glabrous below, and tinged purple at leaf nodes. Leaves in whorls of 3–4; petiole glabrous to sparsely hairy, 15–35 mm long; lamina glabrous above but hairy beneath especially on veins; ovate-lanceolate, acute-acuminate, serrate, 80–120 × 20–60 mm, upper leaves smaller. Flowers numerous in slightly convex terminal corymbs.

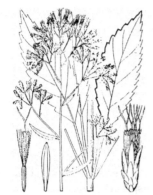

Family Asteraceae, Tribe Eupatorieae

Florets pink to purple. Flowers later summer to early autumn.

Habitat and cultivation
Native to North America, New Hampshire to Florida, Arkansas, Okalahoma, West Nebraska to Minnesota. Grown from seed or root division. Spring growth slow. Frost resistant, drought tender.

Parts used
The root and rhizomes collected in late summer or early autumn.

Active constituents
1) Volatile oil (about 0.07%)
2) Flavonoids including the benzofurans euparin, euparone and cistifolin[337]
3) Resin—eupurpurin

May also include tannins and saponins.

Actions
1) Diuretic
2) Antilithic
3) Antirheumatic

Scientific information
This species was also an official medicine but was dropped from the *US Pharmacopoeia* much earlier than *E. perfoliatum*[333] where it was listed as a diuretic, stimulant, astringent, emetic and cathartic. There is very little scientific information available for either the herb or its constituents.

In vitro—Studies were conducted on some of the herb's benzofurans which are anti-inflammatory, particularly cistifolin.[337,338] The herb and cistifolin inhibit cell-cell and cell-protein adhesion strongly and may offer a potential treatment for diseases mediated by integrin adhesion eg. thrombosis and cancer.[339]

Medicinal uses
Genitourinary tract
The herb has the reputation of being able to dissolve "solids" and soothe and tone tissues.

• cystitis
• urethritis
• prostatitis
• urinary calculus (*BHP* specific)
• dysuria
• haematuria

Musculoskeletal
• gout
• rheumatism

Pharmacy
Three times daily
Decoction of dried root   – 2–4 g
Tincture 1:5 (40%)   – 1–2 ml
Fluid extract (25%)   – 2–4 ml

Historical uses
Dropsy and chronic renal and cystic problems. Similar uses to *E. perfoliatum*. Used also as a partus praeparator and considered to tone and normalise uterine function and treat leucorrhoea. Asthma and chronic catarrh.

Grindelia camporum
[Syn. *G. robusta var. rigida*]

Gum plant, gum weed

Description
A glabrous, perennial herb growing to 1 m in flower. *Basal leaves*, petiolate, slender spoon-shaped with slightly toothed margins, pale matt green both sides.

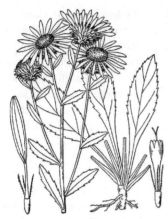

Family Asteraceae, Tribe Astereae

Stem leaves alternate, smaller, sessile and clasping. *Flowers* yellow, borne alternately on single peduncles on stout stems. Flower-heads oozing a sticky white gummy substance, noticeable in the bud and continuing in the flower, borne in a green, softly spiny cup-shaped receptacle. Blooms in summer.

Odour—balsamic, taste—aromatic and bitter.

Habitat and cultivation
Native to California in coastal areas and in central and western desert regions, also in parts of Oregon. May be grown easily in gardens from seed sown in spring.

Parts used
Dried aerial parts of the plant harvested before or during flowering.

Active constituents
1) Saponins (2%) including grindeliasapogenin D, oleanolic acid and bayogenin[340]
2) Resin (up to 20%)[341] comprising grindelane diterpenoids many based on grindelic acid,[342] also camporic, chrysolic and strictanonic acids.[343] Most are methyl esters.
3) Flavonoids including acacetin, kumatakenin and quercetin[342]
4) Volatile oil

Also contains a phytosterol, hentriacontane (a long-chain hydrocarbon), tannins, possibly an alkaloid (termed "grindeline").

Grindelia displays polyploidy and can be either diploid or tetraploid. It was at one time assumed that *G. robusta* was the main medicinal species but this is not commonly found growing and by the early 20th century it was recognised that *G. camporum* was the main medicinal although other species have also been used.[344]

Chemical constituents and their levels vary with species, variety and geographical location.

Actions
1) Antispasmodic
2) Expectorant
3) Anti-asthmatic

Scientific information
Grindelia species have been official medicines in various countries as expectorants with a spasmolytic effect.[42] The herb was introduced into official American medicine in 1875, appearing in the *U.S. Pharmacopoeia* and *National Formulary* between 1882–1960. However, it was described as having "feeble physiologic powers".[344]

G. camporum produces a great quantity of resin especially in the glands of the involucre bracts and this has attracted scientific interest for its potential use as a bio-fuel.[345]

There are no recent investigations into its pharmacology. It appears to have antibacterial and anti-inflammatory properties and is also considered a cardiac depressant as it can slow, and regulate, the action of the heart via the nervous system.[344]

Medicinal uses
Respiratory tract
The saponins are considered to have a stimulating expectorant action, helping to thin thick mucus. It is well suited to the treatment of:

- bronchial asthma
- catarrh
- bronchitis
- whooping cough
- hayfever

The *BHP* specific use of the herb is for bronchial asthma asscociated with tachycardia.

Urinary tract
• cystitis

Externally
• relief of allergic reaction to poison ivy (*Rhus toxicodendron*)

Pharmacy
Three times daily
Infusion of dried herb   –   2–3 g
Fluid Extract 1:1 (22.5%)   –   0.6–1.2 ml
Tincture 1:10 (60%)   –   0.5–1 ml
    Lotion diluted F.E. 1:10 in 10% alcohol

Precautions and/or safety
Large doses are purported to cause renal irritation, some active constituents are excreted via the kidneys.[42]

Historical uses
To treat chronic catarrh of the bladder. Topically for burns and vaginitis. Smoked to treat asthma. Roots decocted to treat lice.

Inula helenium

Elecampane

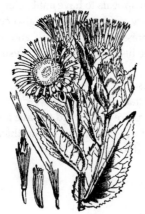

Family Asteraceae, Tribe Inuleae

Description
Erect rhizomatous perennial up to 2 m tall. Dormant in winter. *Stems* densely hairy, branched above to form the inflorescence. *Leaves*, lower cauline sparsely to moderately hairy on upper surface, tomentose on lower, ovate-elliptic, petiolate and cuneate, acute, finely denticulate, up to 60 × 20 cm. Upper leaves similar but alternate, smaller, apetiolate and usually amplexicaul. *Capitula* 6–9 cm diameter, few, in corymbs. Outer involucral bracts tomentose, herbaceous, ovate, 10–15 mm long, inner bracts glabrous or tomentose only on lamina, membranous, 15–25 mm long. Ray florets numerous; ligules yellow, c. 2–3 cm long. Disc yellow. *Achenes* glabrous 4–5 angled with faces finely ribbed, 3.5–5 mm long; pappus minutely barbellate, fused at the base. Flowers from late spring to autumn.

Habitat and cultivation
Native to Europe and Asia and cultivated elsewhere. Grown from seed or division of crowns during winter dormancy. Prefers damp, semi-shady places with deep soil. Drought tender, frost resistant.

Parts used
Roots and rhizomes gathered in early winter or early spring after 2nd year's growth.

Active constituents
1) Essential oil (1–4%) including
   a) camphor, alantol,[†] alantoic acid and thymol derivatives[346,347]
   b) sesquiterpene lactones including mainly eudesmanolides of which around 90% comprises alantolactone and isoalantolactone.[348] Also germacranes and elemanes[348,349]
2) Triterpenes including dammaradienyl acetate,[350] stigmasterol, sitosterol and friedelin
3) Polyacetylenes
4) Inulin up to 44% in autumn, 20% spring

Mucilage and resin have been reported.
   "Helenin" which is sometimes quoted as a constituent of *Inula* actually refers to a combination of

---

[†]Alantol is a breakdown product of the essential oil on distillation.

the sesquiterpene lactones, alantolactone and iso-alantolactone, produced after processing.[351]

Nutritional constituents
Vitamins: A
Minerals: Calcium, potassium, sodium and magnesium

Actions
1) Expectorant
2) Antitussive
3) Diaphoretic
4) Antibacterial
5) Anthelmintic
6) Digestive tonic

Scientific information
There are a number of medicinal species of *Inula*. *I. helenium* was an official medicine in some European countries,[347] there is however, a lack of recent research into this herb.

Many of the actions of the herb have been attributed to the sesquiterpene lactones, often to alantolactone.

In vitro—Inula and/or its constituents (helenin in particular) have shown:-

- strong cytotoxic and antiproliferative activity against several types of cancer cells[348,352-354]
- good antimycobacterial activity specifically against *Mycobacterium tuberculosis* and *M. diphtheriae*.[355,351] It also has antibacterial[351] and antifungal activity[351,356]
- good anthelmintic activity against the roundworm *Ascaris lumbricoides* (effective against both eggs and larvae)[357] and the liver fluke *Fasciola hepatica*[351]

The lactones are anti-inflammatory.[347]

Medicinal uses
Respiratory tract
- chronic coughs (particularly in elderly)
- upper respiratory tract catarrh
- irritable coughs

- bronchitis (*BHP* specific)
- pulmonary tuberculosis (*BHP* specific)
- bronchial/tracheal catarrh
- asthma

Gastro-intestinal tract
Inula is a bitter and can stimulate appetite and digestion:

- colic
- nausea
- diarrhoea
- dyspepsia
- anorexia

Pharmacy
Three times daily

Decoction of dried root	– 1.5–4 g
Tincture 1:5 (25%)	– 3–5 ml (suggested guidelines)
Fluid extract (25%)	– 1–2 ml

Precautions and/or safety
Inula can cause allergic dermatitis (see General Precaution p. 25) and anecdotal evidence suggests it may do so with relative frequency.[79,358]

German Commission E states that large doses can cause vomiting, diarrhoea, spasms and paralysis-like symptoms, however, no incidents have been reported in the literature.

Historical uses
A long history exists for the use of this herb. Described by Hippocrates as a herb to cure chronic skin eruptions and itch and used by the Prophet Job to treat chronic boils.[359] Used in Salerno and by the Welsh Physicians, who called it Marchalan. As a diuretic for dropsy; an emmenagogue; a tonic; an immune stimulant and detoxifier e.g. for snake bites. Sciatica; neuralgia (rubefacient) and gout; some women's problems; dyspepsia; asthma; cramps and convulsions. For treating skin complaints in humans (USA) and animals. Employed as a paint for diphtheria.

Matricaria recutita
[Formerly *M. chumomilla*]

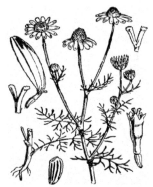

Family Asteraceae, Tribe Anthemideae

Annual chamomile, German chamomile

Description
An erect, aromatic, glabrous annual, 30 cm or more tall. *Stems* round, hollow, furrowed. *Leaves* sessile, alternate 2–3 pinnatisect, pale green. *Flowers*—capitula in terminal corymbs, pedunculate, involucral bracts in 2–3 rows, with membranous margins; receptacle conic without scales; ligules white, soon reflexed, c. 1 cm long, disc florets yellow, 5-toothed. *Seeds*—achenes 1–1.5 mm long, glandular, without a corona.

Odour—pleasant and aromatic, taste—slightly bitter and aromatic.

Habitat and cultivation
Originally from Europe and West Asia chamomile is cultivated and naturalized world-wide. Grown from seed, it may self-sow to give several crops a year in open sunny places and rich, friable soil. Does not self-sow in extremes of heat or wet. Drought and frost resistant.

Parts used
Flower heads collected at the start of flowering.

Active constituents
1) Volatile oil (0.4–2%). Four chemotypes have been identified based on the major constituent of the essential oil viz. bisabolol, bisabololoxide-A, bisabololoxide-B and bisabolonoxide.

The first type is the one that is preferred for medicinal purposes.[360] The volatile oil comprises:-
 a) sesquiterpenes[361] (-)-α-bisabolol (up to 50% of this fraction), bisaboloxides A and B, matricin (a proazulene and guaianolide lactone); trans-β-farnesene (up to 45%) and γ-cadinene;[362] and the minor constituents spathulenol and chamaviolin (guaianolide)
 b) spiroether which is comprised of cis- and trans-en-yn-dicycloethers and is highest in the centre of the flower head[363]
2) Flavonoids (up to 8%) including derivatives of apigenin, luteolin and quercetin[364,365]
3) Coumarins (0.06%) including herniarin and umbelliferone
4) Mucilage (up to 10%) consisting of polysaccharides
5) Also contains phenols, cyanogenic glycosides, salicylates, phytosterols and a spermine derived polyamine, concentrated in the pollen.[366] Matricin is converted to chamazulene by steam distillation and gives *Matricaria* oil a blue colour the deepness of which varies with the amount of azulene present.

The various active constituents of *Matricaria* require different temperatures for their stability and the level of matricin in *Matricaria's* volatile oil decreases on drying. Therefore the flowers should be processed soon after harvesting[367] or they may be preserved by freezing until ready for processing.

Matricaria displays polyploidy, diploid and tetraploid cultivars having been grown[368] in an effort to increase what is considered the more important constituents of the volatile oil. The constituents also vary with origin, growth conditions and method of preparation.[369]

Nutritional constituents
Minerals: Iodine, calcium, potassium, magnesium, iron, zinc and manganese[370]

Actions
1) Relaxant
2) Carminative
3) Antispasmodic
4) Anti-inflammatory

5) Anti-allergic
6) Bitter
7) Vulnerary
8) Antimicrobial
9) Sedative (mild)

Scientific information
Scientific interest in *Matricaria* arises from two perspectives. One is its long history of use as a medicine—it has been an official medicine in a number of pharmacopoeias worldwide (internally as an aromatic bitter and externally as a poultice for inflammation[42]) and it has the approval of *German Commision E* for many of its traditional uses. The other, as in the case of *Echinacea* spp. relates to its widespread use by the public for self-medication and the effect such a practice may have on the efficacy and safety of prescribed pharmaceuticals.

Although there is a great deal of research on *Matricaria*, most of this relates to animal experiments or the action of isolated constituents *in vitro*.

There are a large number of active constituents though much of *Matricaria's* activity is attributed to the volatile oil and flavonoid fractions. In the latter case apigenin-7-glucoside is considered to be of great importance whilst in the former it is (-)-α–bisabolol. Because of the positive actions of (-)-α–bisabolol the cultivated variety of *Matricaria recutita,* called Manzana, which is rich in this constituent has been used in commercial products and in a number of clinical trials. Manzana also has a very low potential for allergic reactions.

Anti-inflammatory
In vitro—*Matricaria* is known to be anti-inflammatory, it inhibits the action of COX and LOX.[364] A number of the constituents also inhibit leukotriene synthesis—the sesquiterpene fraction,[364] (-)-α–bisabolol;[360,364] chamazulene[371] and the spiroether component.[372] The flavonoids, particularly apigenin, not only inhibit arachidonic acid metabolism but also stabilise and inhibit calcium influx into mast cells.[360,373] Although the polyamine too was found to have good potential both as an anti-inflammatory and anti-allergic agent, it may not be absorbed *in vivo*.[366]

In addition its anti-oxidant activity has been studied as inflammation often results from oxidative stress. The herb is anti-oxidant[374] as is the volatile oil fraction[375] with chamazulene having the strongest potential.[371,376]

In vivo—Oral mucositis, a side effect of chemo- and radio-therapy, was successfully treated using a mouthwash of the herb[377,378]—not corroborated.[379] A spray applied to the cuff of endotracheal tubes prior to surgery did not however prevent subsequent inflammation of mucous membranes.[380]

Antispasmodic/spasmolytic
The relaxant effect of chamomile has been known and valued for hundreds of years. Several of its constituents display both antispasmodic activity (matricine, chamazulene, the bisabloloxides and (-)-α-bisabolol[364]) and spasmolytic activity (apigenin, apigenin-7-glucoside, (-)-α-bisabolol).[364] Apigenin is also considered an anxiolytic.[381]

In vitro—These activities have been examined for binding to benzodiazepine receptor sites in which apigenin was shown to be active.[382]

In vivo—Allergic asthma treated with a combined herbal extract which included *Matricaria* reduced associated sleep discomfort, frequency and intensity of coughing as well as significantly improving respiratory function.[383]

Antimicrobial
In vitro—*Matricaria* has antimicrobial activity against:-

- bacteria including *Staphylococcus aureus,* some *Streptococcus* spp., *Bacillus megatherium* and *Leptospira icterohaemorrhagiae*[364]
- virus responsible for tick-borne encephalitis[384] (apigenin also active against HSV-1 and 2[385])
- *Candida albicans*[386]

The polysaccharide fraction is immunostimulant.[387]
In vivo—*Matricaria* is also acaricidal against a mite pathogenic to domestic animals[388] and there is anecdotal evidence of it successfully being used to treat an unusual but persistent human infestation by poultry mite.[389]

A study found daily intake of chamomile tea over 2 weeks may increase anti-oxidant activity possibly through altered bacterial gut flora as these changes persisted for a further 2 weeks after tea intake ceased.[390]

Other

In vitro—(-)-α-bisabolol and *Matricaria* itself have antipeptic activity i.e. they inhibit the action of pepsin.[364]

Matricaria stimulates osteoblast differentiation, is anti-oestrogenic to breast cancer cells and inhibits cervical adenocarcinoma cells, actions probably mediated through binding to oestrogen receptor sites. The herb may help prevent Osteoporosis.[391]

Most studies on *Matricaria*'s flavonoids relate to apigenin which in addition to activities mentioned above, has also shown:

- stimulation of trans-membrane conductance of the type that is defective in cystic fibrosis suggesting a potential therapeutic approach to the disease. (The action was demonstrated in *in vivo* studies also on healthy volunteers[392])
- a weak progestogenic activity[393]
- some antitumorigenic activity[397] and an ability to arrest cell growth,[394,395] including that of oestradiol-stimulated breast cancer cells.[396] It may be a useful chemotherapeutic agent as well as enhancing the toxicity of radiation to cancer cells[397]
- reduced histamine release from basophils[398]

In vivo—One of the main traditional uses of *Matricaria* has been in treating gastro-intestinal problems. A combined extract, which included it, effectively treated functional dyspepsia,[399] the anti-oxidant and anti-inflammatory action of chamomile being considered valuable to the overall effectiveness.[400] A preparation containing pectin and *Matricaria* also effectively treated diarrhoea in children.[401]

A combination of *Angelica sinensis* and *Matricaria* was effective in controlling menopausal hot flushes, insomnia and fatigue.[402]

Consumption of flavonoids has been inversely related to death from coronary heart disease in epidemiological studies.[403]

Several studies have tested the value of topical applications, this being another area of traditional use for the herb. Applied externally the flavonoid fraction of *Matricaria* is able to penetrate into the deeper layers of skin.[404] The whole herb has been shown to be:-

- vulnerary on weeping wounds, drying out the area and healing skin[405]
- effective in the treatment of an induced toxic contact dermatitis[406]
- comparable in efficacy with hydrocortisone cream in treating atopic eczema, slightly superior to 0.5% hydrocortisone[407] and much better than other anti-inflammatory pharmaceuticals in treating inflamed dermatoses.[408]

Medicinal uses
Respiratory tract
- respiratory catarrh
- bronchitis
- sinusitis
- asthma
- hayfever
- mucosal inflammation

Gastro-intestinal tract
- irritable bowel syndrome
- nervous dyspepsia
- colitis including ulcerative colitis
- flatulence
- diarrhoea (from any cause)
- diverticulitis
- constipation (particularly for children)
- colic
- gastric/duodenal ulcers
- indigestion
- nausea due to nerves, travel or infection

BHP specific for gastro-intestinal disturbance with associated nervous irritability in children.

Nervous system
As a significant nervous system relaxant used for:

- insomnia
- nervous tension

- tension/digestive headaches
- vertigo
- migraine
- hyperactivity

Reproductive tract
The name *Matricaria* derives from "matrix" meaning mother or womb, it is used for:

- menopausal tension and related problem
- dysmenorrhoea
- morning sickness (safe)
- amenorrhoea due to psychological causes

Externally
- nappy rash
- cracked nipples
- acne
- conjunctivitis
- blepharitis
- varicose ulcers
- gingivitis
- eczema
- acute radiation damage
- toothache
- wounds
- sunburn
- mastitis
- acute otitis media (earache)
- haemorrhoids

N.B. The use of *Matricaria* externally to treat eczema is augmented by its internal use.

Pharmacy
Three times daily
Infusion of dried herb   – 2–8 g
Tincture 1:5 (45%)   – 3–10 ml
Fluid Extract (45%)   – 1–4 ml
Chamazulene can be developed by using the herb in steam inhalations or as hot infusions that are kept covered whilst steeping.

Precautions and/or safety
There are a number of studies that have looked into the quality of commercial chamomile flowers/teas

and these found the quality and level of contamination could pose problems.[409–411]

The effect of drinking chamomile tea with a meal may inhibit iron absorption by 47%. Black tea by comparison inhibits iron absorption by between 79–94%, adding milk does not negate this effect.[412]

(-)-α-bisabolol was tested for its potential to cause mutations as it is used in many topical preparations and it was found, in fact, to offer some protection.[413] Apigenin and luteolin have also been tested for potential genotoxicity and they have been declared safe.[414]

Matricaria is regarded as a safe herb generally. However there are a few recorded cases of allergic reactions to the external and internal use of the herb, including anaphylaxis.[415,416] There is also a degree of cross-reactivity between sensitivity to *Artemisia vulgaris* and *Matricaria in vivo* (see General Precaution p. 25).[417] Allergic conjunctivitis can result from using *Matricaria* as an eyewash—this occurred in a small number of patients (around 2%) who were suffering from hayfever although they had no reaction to the tea. The reaction is believed to be due to pollen in the flowers.[418] Considering the widespread use of this herb, allergic reactions are extremely rare.[364] There is also some speculation that at least some of the reported cases of allergic reactions to chamomile have been due to the adulteration/substitution of *Matricaria* with *Anthemis cotula* as anthecotulid, a sesquiterpene lactone found in the latter but not the former, has been specifically cited as the causative agent.[360]

Interactions
In vitro—*Matricaria*'s isolated constituents, particularly the essential oil components, inhibit cytochrome P450 enzymes CYP1A2, CYP2C9, CYP2D6 and CYP3A4 which in turn could effect the metabolism of drugs using these for their elimination.[419,420]

In vivo—As flavonoids inhibit platelet aggregation in vitro, apigenin was tested for this effect through dietary use of parsley in healthy volunteers, the results showed there was no measurable effect on platelet activity.[421] There has been speculation that *Matricaria* could potentiate the effect of warfarin,[422] perhaps due to the flavonoids, to-date no interactions between them have been reported. No drug interactions *in vivo* have been reported for chamomile.

Historical uses

For aiding problems in the head—"purge the head and to emptie it of superfluous humour and other grosse matter". For fevers; phlegm, melancholy; inflammation of the bowels; liver and spleen problems; as a bath to ease weariness and pain. It also has acquired a reputation of healing ailing plants if planted nearby.

Silybum marianum

Milk thistle, St Mary's thistle

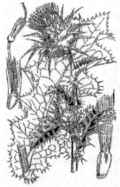

Family Asteraceae, Tribe Cynareae

Description

Annual or biennial. *Stems* erect, branched above, ridged, with sparse mealy hairs, 0.5–2 m tall, not winged. *Leaves* alternate, elliptic to lanceolate, lyrate-pinnatifid to pinnate, sinuate, coarsely dentate, green with conspicuous white markings along veins 20–60 × 10–30 cm, with sparse, short, mealy hairs on the lamina, and sparse, long, tangled multicellular hairs on midrib; base amplexicaul, auriculate, with very spinous margins; prickles marginal, yellowish, spreading, 5–12 mm long. Upper leaves alternate, clasping stems. *Capitula* ovoid, erect, 4–6 × 5–7 cm, solitary, terminal and pedunculate; and also sessile in axils of uppermost leaves; peduncles with appressed cobwebby tomentum. *Involucral bracts sparsely* covered with short mealy

hairs; margins with sparse cobwebby hairs. Outer bracts leaf-like, obovate with spinous apex and margins. Middle bracts oblong with spinous margins. Inner bracts lanceolate. *Corolla* reddish purple, 20–28 mm long, florets male and female, all tubular. Anther filaments joined at margins into a tube. Style extended 1–2 mm beyond corolla lobes. *Achenes* brown or black-streaked, obovoid, weakly transversely flattened, smooth, about 6 × 3 mm. The width of the variegated bands and the leaf length and number of spines on the leaf margin seem to be highly correlated![423] Flowers in late spring to summer. Fruits mid-summer to autumn.

Leaves taste bitter, sharp and unpleasantly salty. Seeds taste oily and bitter.

Habitat and cultivation

Originally from the Mediterranean and South Western Europe, milk thistle is naturalised worldwide in waste and cultivated land. Grows from seed in any soil but prefers open sunny situations with adequate water. It is large, with spines, and classified as a noxious weed. Drought and frost resistant.

Parts used

Seeds collected when the white pappus is visible and not too long after the head has opened. The seeds are used in medicine, the leaves and stems in cooking.

Active constituents

1) Flavolignans (1.5–3.0%)[424] including what is collectively called "silymarin", which comprises silybin A and silybin B (diastereoisomers),[425] silydianin, silychristin and diastereoisomers isosilybin A and isosilybin B (max. 5% of silymarin).[425-427] An extract comprising an equal ratio of silybin A and B is called silibinin. The more mature seeds have been shown to contain the highest content of flavolignans.
2) Flavonoids including taxifolin a 2,3 dihydroflavonol and apigenin[428]
3) Amines including tyramine, histamine and trimethylglycine (betaine)
4) Polyacetylenes

Also fixed oil of around 25% (w/w),[428] mostly linoleic and oleic acid, also myristic, palmitic and stearic acids.[429]

Actions
1) Hepatoprotective
2) Digestive tonic
3) Galactagogue

Scientific information
Milk thistle has been used in medicine for nearly 2000 years and preparations have been officially approved for use in Europe since 1969.[430] *German Commission E* has approved its use for dyspepsia and to support liver damage due to toxins, inflammation or cirrhosis.

Anti-oxidant and anti-inflammatory
In vitro—The following has been found:

- all the flavolignans have anti-oxidant potential including inhibiting LDL-oxidation[424,431,432]
- silybin has good permeability through cell membranes
- silybin inhibits xanthine oxidase[433]
- *Silybum* and silymarin strongly suppress nitric oxide production in brain cells (associated with neurone damage)[434]
- silymarin has well documented anti-inflammatory properties[424,436] and all the flavolignans are inhibitors of arachadonic acid metabolism predominantly acting by blocking LOX activity
- silymarin blocks the nuclear transcription factor NF-κB[424,435,436]

Hepatoprotective
Silybum's current prominence is based mostly on its effectiveness in the treatment of liver dysfunction, one of the main areas of traditional use and one where pharmaceuticals are not, as yet, very effective.

A good deal of the original clinical work arose from the herb's use in treating accidental poisoning with the very toxic *Amanita phalloides*—the Death Cap mushroom—which inhibits hepatocyte function, and has a fatality rate of 20%. Silymarin given up to 36 hours after toxin ingestion significantly reduced mortality and was more effective than standard orthodox therapy.[424,437,443]

Silybum and its various extracts are amongst the best studied of herbal medicines, they are commonly used by people with liver problems.[438] Most of the current research has been carried out on the flavolignan fraction or some part of it, not the whole herb. The results have been impressive enough for an extract to be registered in Belgium as a prescription only medicine.[439] *Silybum* and silymarin in particular have general recognition as a therapy for liver disease, and are recognised as hepatoprotective, anti-inflammatory and regenerative agents.[440,441] The flavolignans are assumed to achieve cytoprotection through their anti-inflammatory and anti-oxidant actions and also because they stabilise cell membranes and enhance protein biosynthesis.[435,436]

In vitro—All the main flavolignans, tested separately, protect hepatocytes from toxicity due to alcohol and carbon tetrachloride—silydianin and silychristin particularly—and were themselves devoid of toxicity.[442]

In vivo—Reviews[443-446] of over 30 trials conducted into the effects of *Silybum* on liver function have been undertaken over the last few years and although trial results have not been constistent, reviewers have concluded that silymarin may benefit the treatment of:-

- acute and chronic viral hepatitis
- hepatitis due to drugs, alcohol or chemicals
- mild alcohol induced cirrhosis, reducing mortality rates
- alcoholic cirrhosis with concomitant hepatitis C
- cirrhosis-induced diabetes mellitus, reducing both insulin requirement and blood glucose levels

The inconsistent clinical data may be due to factors commonly cited in these sorts of trials including poor design and reporting, problems with the actual aetiology and severity of the disease being treated, small sample sizes, variable duration and levels of dosing and also variations in quality of preparations used.

A recent study using silymarin to treat chronic hepatitis C patients gave only symptomatic improvement, and whilst the treatment was deemed safe, markers of the disease were unchanged after one year of treatment.[447] However further related clinical trials are due to be carried out.[448]

Anticancer
In vitro—*Silybum* and/or the main flavolignans have a range of activities that alter the growth of different cancer cell lines. Actions found to-date are:-

- inhibition of cancer cell growth—prostate (including hormone-refractory cells),[425,449–453] bladder,[454,455] breast (whether oestrogen-dependent or not),[453,456] cervix,[453] leukaemia[457] and lung[458]
- induced cell differentiation[449,457]
- reduced cell viability[453,455,459–462]
- chemopreventative ie protective against cancer development[453]
- inhibition of angiogenesis required for metastasis[461,462]
- inhibition of motility and invasiveness[463]
- enhanced action of conventional chemotherapy[462,464,465]

These actions have prompted the initiation of clinical trials into their use in the treatment of prostate cancer.[462] Their potential to aid cancer treatment is greatly supported by their lack of toxicity and compatibility in acting alongside conventional cancer therapy.

Antimicrobial
In vitro—Silybin, in particular, but also silymarin have strong antibacterial activity against Gram-positive bacteria.[466] Silybin also increases the susceptibility of resistant *Staphylococcus aureus* to antibiotic therapy.[467]

Silymarin may block the replication of some viruses, including that of HIV, by blocking nuclear transcription factor NF-κB.[436]

Other
In vitro—*Silybum* and its flavolignans stimulate lymphocytes[468] (increasing their proliferation[469])

and activate leucocytes (this has been shown to occur *ex vivo* too[470]).

In addition silymarin may be a useful agent in sunscreens in preventing photo-induced carcinogenesis[471] and was shown to protect cells from UV-induced apoptosis.[472]

Anti-allergy properties have been demonstrated by silybin via inhibition of T-lymphocyte activity[473] and through inhibition of histamine release from basophils.[424]

Ex vivo—Peritoneal macrophages from patients receiving dialysis (which tends to compromise the cells' function) had their activity restored when exposed to silymarin and silibinin.[474]

Silybum has been advocated as supportive therapy for AIDS to not only protect liver function but also because of its possible antiviral activity.[436,475]

In vivo—*Silybum* was beneficial in the treatment of gastro-intestinal ulcers.[476] Silymarin improved the lipid profile of patients with hyperlipoproteinaemias[477] and also improved the status of type 2 diabetes by reducing levels of glycated haemoglobin and fasting glucose and improving their lipid profiles.[478]

Medicinal uses
Gastro-intestinal tract
The main use of this herb is to protect and tone the liver:

- cirrhosis[†]
- drug and/or alcohol abuse
- poor digestion due to liver dysfunction
- chemical poisoning
- jaundice
- chronic active hepatitis
- hepatitis (including B and C)

Reproductive tract
- increase the milk flow of lactating women

Pharmacy
Three times daily

[†]Double blind studies show it increases survival time in this condition.

Decoction   – 2–4 g
Tincture 1:5 (25%)   – 2–4 ml

The flavolignans are commercially extracted by first defatting *Silybum* seeds to increase their yield, and then subjecting the resulting matter to high extraction temperatures not used in the preparation of herbal tinctures. They are soluble in both ethanol and hot water and are relatively stable at temperatures up to 100°C.[479–481] However silymarin in commercial tablets may be quite variable in bioavailable flavolignans.[482]

Amanita poisoning was treated with water extracts of silybin at a dose of 20 mg/kg of body weight per day.

Pharmacokinetics
Studies have shown that about half of the total intake of silymarin is slowly absorbed intestinally, blood levels peak 2 hours after oral dosing and have a half-life of around 6 hours. 5–7% of what is absorbed is subsequently excreted from the kidneys, the majority staying within the liver and being incorporated into bile before being excreted via this route.[483] Biliary levels of silybin peak within 2–9 hours and are still detectable after 24 hours.[430] Silybin appears to be well absorbed into many tissues including plasma.[462] Silybin and silychristin are not excreted in urine.[424]

Precautions and/or safety
Adverse effects reported are rare and minor including gastro-intestinal disturbances, headaches and allergic skin rashes. Allergic reactions are possible—see General Precaution p. 25.

More severe reactions reported include a single case of anaphylaxis after drinking a tea made from the herb[424] and a case of a severe reaction attributed to an encapsulated *Silybum* product.[484] However given that the herb is one of those most frequently used in a population where liver function is likely to be impaired the safety is generally accepted as very good even after long term use.[485]

Interactions
Warnings of possible drug/herb interactions have arisen from the observation of flavolignans affecting hepatocyte cytochrome enzymes CYP3A4, CYP2D6, CYP2E1, CYP2C9 and uridine diphophoglucronosyl transferase *in vitro*.[486–489] It was later found that the concentration of these constituents would not reach the levels at which they could cause inhibition *in vivo*. More recently a study looking into possible interactions with metabolism of an HIV protease inhibitor found no interaction between silibinin and indinavir *in vitro*[490] or *in vivo*.[491–493] The herb did not alter the activity of CYP1A2, CYP2D6, CYP2E1 or CYP3A4[494] in vivo either, nor did a standardized *Silybum* extract affect the metabolism of a chemotherapeutic drug that uses CYP3A4 and UGT1A enzymes.[495]

Historical uses
Eaten as a vegetable for a spring tonic. Snake bite; the plague; urinary calculus; "melancholy", antimalarial; emmenagogue, disorders of the uterus and spleen. Thought to cure rabies; for pains in the sides; internal griping. Eclectic use for varicose veins and pelvic congestion. Externally applied for cancer.

Solidago virgaurea and *S. canadensis*

Golden rod

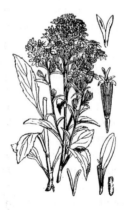

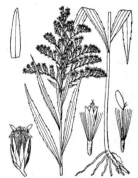

Family Asteraceae, Tribe Astereae

Description

S. virgaurea (left) is a stoloniferous perennial plant with erect, simple or branched, round, often pubescent stems to 1 m high in flower. *Leaves* alternate, mostly sessile. Basal leaves obovate from a tapering base, 2–12 cm long. Stem leaves oblong-lanceolate to elliptical, entire or slightly toothed, acute. *Inflorescence* a raceme or panicle, each short-stemmed flower head 0.5–1 cm in diameter. Involucral bracts in many rows, linear, greenish. Ray florets in one row, female, yellow. Disc florets also yellow, hermaphrodite. *Fruit* a 2.7–3.1 mm brown, pubescent achene with a greyish-white pappus. Blooms from summer to autumn.

   S. canadensis (right) is a stoloniferous perennial which forms dense clumps. *Stems* not branched, erect, green or reddish, smooth at base but slightly hairy higher up, 1–1.5 m tall in flower. New shoots reddish purple. *Basal leaves* dark green, elliptic-lanceolate and withering at flowering. Stem leaves alternate and arranged in whorls, apetiolate, usually entire, sometimes serrate, rough on the upper surface, 8–10 × 1–2 cm, upper leaves smaller. *Inflorescence* a lax, racemose panicle mostly with all flowers arranged along one side. *Flower* heads cylindrical 3.5–5 mm across. Ray florets 8–12 with yellow, linear-obovate ligules. Disc florets 3–5, yellow. Flowers in autumn.

   Odour—slightly aromatic when dry; taste—astringent and bitter.

Habitat and cultivation

S. virgaurea is native to Europe, Asia and North Africa in dry grasslands and open woods. It prefers light well-drained soil and open sunny situations. Grown from seed and root division. Drought and frost resistant.

   S. canadensis is native throughout North America and commonly grown in gardens in other countries from seed or root division. Adaptable to most soils and situations. Frost resistant and drought tender. Hybrids of the two species have been identified.

Parts used

The herb harvested during or just prior to flowering.

Active constituents

S. virgaurea

1) Triterpenoids
   a) saponins (2–6%) including bisdesmosidic polygala acid derivatives comprising a minimum of 30% of this fraction, a number of them being oleanane-type saponins called solidagosaponins and also virgaureasaponins[496-498]
   b) triterpenes based on germacrene, trans-phytol, β-amyrin[499,500]
2) Tannins (approx. 10%) of the catechin type
3) Flavonoids (1.5%) including rutin, quercetrin, isoquercetrin, astragalin, hyperoside, nicotiflorin and kaempferol[499]
4) Essential oil (0.4–0.5%) predominantly α-cadinene

Also phenol glycosides including leiocarposide (a heterodimer of salicin)[501] and virgaureoside A, phenolic acids including caffeic and chlorogenic acids,[499] diterpenoid lactones of cis-clerodane type (solidagolactones and elongatolides C and E), benzoates,[502] α-tocopherol-quinone[500] and polysaccharides.

S. canadensis

1) Triterpenoids
   a) saponins (9–12%) mainly bayogenin glycosides which are bisdesmosidic saponins called canadensis-saponins 1–8[503,504]
   b) triterpenes of lupane type and lupeol, ursolic acid, α-amyrin, stigmasterol and cycloartenol[505]

2) Tannins
3) Flavonoids (2.4%) including quercetrin, iso-quercetrin and rutin[506]
4) Essential oil including sesquiterpenes (+) and (–)germacrene D,[507] germacrene A, α-humulene and β-caryophllene[508–510]

Also phenolic acids including chlorogenic, hydroxycinnamic and caffeic acids, diterpenes and polysaccharides.

Actions
1) Diuretic
2) Diaphoretic
3) Anti-inflammatory
4) Antiseptic
5) Carminative
6) Anticatarrhal

Scientific information
S. virgaurea is highly valued in Europe where it is considered to have proved itself over the centuries. It has been approved by *German Commission E* for lower urinary tract diseases and for the treatment and prevention of urinary lithiasis. *S. canadensis* has been in use in Europe for around 700 years.[506]

Neither of the two medicinal *Solidago* spp. has received much scientific attention. Their chemistry though very similar is not identical.

S. virgaurea
In vitro—The whole extract has strong cytotoxicity for tumour cells from prostate, breast, melanoma and small cell lung carcinoma[511]—triterpenes and α-tocopherol-quinone are individually also cytotoxic.[500]

The herb inhibits muscarinic receptor-mediated contraction of bladder tissue.[512]

It has antibacterial activity against a range of organisms[513] and some of the constituents are antifungal against *Candida* and *Cryptococcus* species[514,515] and may also be potential immunostimulants.[502,516]

A combination of *Solidago virgaurea, Fraxinus excelsior* and *Populus tremula* has anti-oxidant, anti-inflammatory and analgesic activities.[517–519]

In vivo—Clinical trials using the above combination found it as effective as NSAIDs in the treatment of mild to moderate osteoarthritis and rheumatoid arthritis and with much fewer side-effects.[520,521]

S. canadensis
In vitro—The lupane triterpenoids inhibit DNA replication giving them a potential in cancer chemotherapy[505] and some of these constituents also have moderate cytotoxicity for several tumour cell lines.[502]

The whole extract is anti-oxidant, the phenolics making a large contribution to this activity.[506,522]

Both *Solidago* species are described as "aquaretic", rather than diuretic, as they increase urine output by increasing renal blood flow and therefore glomerular filtration rate. The increase in urinary output is not accompanied by electrolyte loss.

Solidago spp. are also considered anti-catarrhal with an action in the upper respiratory tract and they may have hypotensive activity.[513] The genus name of *Solidago* is based on the Latin "solidare" to make whole, a reference to the ability of the herb to act as a styptic and to heal wounds. This action is not acknowledged in modern herbalism.

Medicinal uses
Respiratory tract
• catarrh
• allergic rhinitis
• influenza

BHP specific for low grade inflammation of the nasopharynx with persistent catarrh.

Gastro-intestinal tract
As a carminative may be used for:

• flatulent dyspepsia

Urinary tract
• cystitis
• anuria
• oliguria
• urinary tract inflammation
• calculus and gravel

Externally
• throat infection (gargle)
• nasal catarrh and infection (spray)

Pharmacy
Three times daily
Infusion of dried herb   –   0.5–2 g
Tincture 1:5 (45%)   –   0.5–1 ml
Fluid Extract (25%)   –   0.5–2 ml

About a fifth of the available bound flavonoids and tannins are extracted into infusion after steeping the herb for up to 10 minutes.[523] Phenolics (flavonoids and phenolic acids) are best extracted either in water infusions or in tincture using 70% alcohol.[506]

Pharmokinetics
The flavonoids are primarily excreted through the urinary tract.[524]

Precautions and/or safety
For allergic reactions see General Precaution p. 25. *Solidago* is considered to be very safe with no known side-effects.[525]

Historical uses
Internally for bruising and bleeding; ruptures; nausea due to weak digestion; dysmenorrhoea and amenorrhoea; diphtheria. Externally as a styptic and wound healer of great value; to secure loose teeth.

Tanacetum parthenium
[Formerly *Chrysanthemum parthenium*]

Feverfew

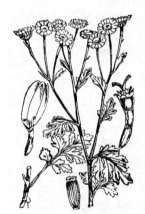

Family Asteraceae, Tribe Anthemideae

Description
Strongly aromatic perennial herb with roots not a rhizome. *Stems* round, erect, 20–60 cm tall, ribbed, sparsely to moderately clothed in short hairs, not much branched from the base. *Basal leaves* petiolate, ovate to ovate-oblong, sparsely to moderately clothed in short hairs and with scattered, pitted glandular hairs, 1-pinnate with leaflets again 1-2-pinnatisect, 3–15 × 2–6 cm; primary leaflets in 3–5 pairs, ovate, all on one plane, shortly petiolate at the base of leaf, ultimate segments ovate to oblong, crenate or serrate. *Cauline leaves* alternate, similar to basal, but above becoming shortly petiolate, smaller and less divided, usually with numerous glandular hairs on the lower surface. *Corymb* with 8–40 loosely packed capitula. *Capitula* 15–30 mm diameter; ray florets 12-numerous; ligules white, disc florets usually numerous, yellow, but few in double forms. *Achenes* c. 1.5 mm long, pale brown, glandular, ribbed; corona lobed, c. 0.2 mm long. Flowers most of the year depending on weather and climate.

Odour—camphorous;   taste—bitter   and camphorous.

Habitat and cultivation
Originally from Europe and temperate Asia feverfew is now a common garden plant. It is a short-lived perennial grown from seed or root division. Prefers light soils and an open sunny situation. Single and double flowered forms are found and one with yellow leaves. Drought and frost resistant.

Parts used
Flowering herb or leaves only.

Active constituents
1) Sesquiterpene lactones, many possessing an α–methylene-γ-lactone structure the predominant one being a germacranolide—parthenolide (0.2–0.9%); also guaianolides including canin and artecanin.[526] Over 45 sesquiterpenes have been characterised so far.[527] Parthenolide content is highest in leaves and flowering tops,[528] is higher in plants harvested in the afternoon and is increased following watering after water-stressing the plant.[529]

Wild *T. parthenium* may naturally have higher parthenolide levels as do the lighter leaf phenotypes[530]

2) Volatile oil including pinene, camphor, limonene, camphene, γ-terpinene, linalool, (E)-β-ocimene and (E)-chrysanthenol[531]
3) Flavonoids including derivatives of kaempferol (tanetin), quercetin, apigenin and luteolin,[532] also santin and centaureidin[533]
4) Polyacetylenes

There is also a small amount of melatonin.[534]

Nutritional constituents
Vitamins: A, B_1, B_2, niacin and C
Minerals: High amounts of iron, manganese, phosphorus, potassium, calcium, chromium and selenium

Actions
1) Anti-inflammatory
2) Stomachic
3) Migraine prophylactic
4) Antipyretic
5) Anthelmintic
6) Antirheumatic

Scientific information
The species name, *parthenium*, is thought to derive from the Greek word *parthenos* meaning a virgin, as the herb was traditionally valued for treating menstrual cramps. It was used in the past for many more applications than it is today, the main recognised use now being that of treating migraines.

Anti-inflammatory
In vitro—Detailed biochemical actions have been explored for the herb and/or its constituents. Both anti-inflammatory and migraine prophylaxis are likely to use at least some of the same biochemical mechanisms. Some of this detail has been elucidated and in summary involves inhibition of the following:-

• arachidonic acid metabolism[535-537] including via both COX-2[538,548] and 5-LOX[548] inhibition

• cytokine expression including that involved in allergic reactions[539-541]
• platelet aggregation and granular secretions from platelets and neutrophils[526,542-545]
• monocyte adherence, a process involved in tissue inflammation[546]
• the synthesis of other mediators of inflammation like nitric oxide production[547]

Whilst parthenolide and the lactones containing the α-methylene-γ-lactone structure have been found to contribute largely to this action, the flavonols, and possibly other constituents are also strongly involved in eicosanoid synthesis inhibition.[548]

In vivo—Given the wide spectrum of anti-inflammatory actions above it is not difficult to understand why feverfew was indicated for rheumatic/arthritic conditions. However there does not appear to have been much clinical investigation into this aspect of the herb. One study has reported no benefit from using the herb in the treatment of rheumatoid arthritis.[549]

Migraine prophylaxis
In vivo—The first clinical studies into the prophylactic effect of *T. parthenium* in migraines were done in the 1980s. Since then a number of studies and/or reviews have appeared assessing benefits of feverfew in both the prevention and treatment of migraines with conflicting results. Some authors have concluded there is no proven benefit of feverfew preparations over placebo,[550-553] others that there is qualified support for the herb reducing migraine frequency and/or some of the related symptoms.[554-560] It has also been reported that the herb may only be effective in people with a migraine frequency in excess of 4 in a 28 day period.[561] A combination of *Salix* and *T. parthenium* also has therapeutic benefits (see *Salix*) and *T. parthenium* combined with *Zingiber officinale*, used sub-lingually in the early phase, helped abort full blown attacks.[560]

More robust testing is still required to satisfy medical criteria of efficacy. However Canada has made a feverfew extract officially available for migraine prophylaxis.[562]

Anticancer
In vitro—Parthenolide has been studied in the context of its anticancer properties. It has:-

- inhibited the growth/increased apoptosis of several cancer cell lines including breast,[563] lymphoma,[564] pancreas,[565] colorectal[566,567] and malignant myeloid leukaemia stem cells which have so far been resistant to pharmaceutical preparations[568]
- helped increase differentiation in human leukaemia cells[569]
- enhanced cell death when used concurrently with chemotherapeutic agents[570,571]
- inhibited mitogen-stimulated proliferation of a number of different cells, an action shared by the whole herb[572]

Parthenolide's action as a cytostatic and apoptotic agent probably involves more than one mechanism.[573] The flavonols, particularly centaureidin, are antimitotic.[533]

Other
In vitro—The whole herb and/or its constituent lactones have antimicrobial activity including against *Leishmania amazonenesis*,[574] *Mycobacterium tuberculosis*,[575] *Staphylococcus aureus, Streptococcus haemolytica, Candida albicans* and *Trichophyton mentagrophytes*.[576] Parthenolide also inhibits the replication of the hepatitis C virus and potentiates the antiviral activity of interferon-α.[577]

The effects of parthenolide on immune cells are numerous and are being explored. Parthenolide inhibits activation-induced cell death of T-cells, a process implicated in severe diseases including auto-immunity.[578]

Medicinal uses
Nervous system
- migraine headaches
- prophylaxis of migraine headaches

Gastro-intestinal tract
As a bitter used for:

- indigestion

Musculoskeletal
- arthritis

Pharmacy
Dried herb in tablet or capsule   – 50–200 mg
Tincture 1:5 (25%)   – 5–20 drops
Ethanol is a slightly better extractive medium than water for the sesquiterpene lactones of *T. parthenium*.[579] For the prophylaxis of migraines the above preparations or fresh leaves (one large or three small taken in a sandwich) once a day, for up to six months. Feverfew preparations may be taken at the start of an attack.

Parthenolide, considered the main active constituent, is often used to standardise the herb and clinical trials using such preparations were based on 0.5 mg parthenolide equivalent a day. However it is likely that there are a number of important active constituents.[580]

The commercial quality has been found to be very variable,[581] preparations showing a 10-fold variation in concentration of herb and an even larger variation in parthenolide content.[582]
CONTRAINDICATIONS—Pregnancy.

Precautions and/or safety
Checks for chromosomal damage from *T. parthenium* used for periods of greater than 11 months continuously found it was safe.[583]

The occasional person develops mouth ulcers from taking the fresh leaf. Other potential side-effects reported include dizziness, indigestion, heartburn, loss of taste, inflammation of mouth and tongue, weight gain[527] and a possible rebound headache may occur on ceasing to use the herb. Many of the above clinical studies checked for adverse reactions and reported a very good safety record for feverfew[551,559,561] even in preparations containing quite high levels of parthenolide.[584]

For allergic reactions—see General Precaution p. 25. A low level of contact dermatitis, up to 4.5%,[585] has been noted through occupational handling of the plant[586] or from airborne exposure, resulting in a type of photosensitive reaction that occurs on sun-exposed skin.[9,587] This may be generalised or may only affect the hands, and/or face.

65% of individuals may have associated blistering of the hands.[9] The sesquiterpene lactones, particularly parthenolide,[588] are considered instrumental in the development of the allergy (predominantly dermatitis),[589] although other phytochemicals may also contribute.[531,590,591]

Interactions

It has been assumed that because the herb can inhibit platelet aggregation it may interact with anticoagulant drugs like warfarin[592] and aspirin,[593] but to date no interactions have been reported *in vivo*. An early study checked the platelet aggregation of long-term feverfew users and found no changes had occurred.[594] Interestingly it is considered possible that NSAIDs may negate the benefit of feverfew in migraine prophylaxis.[595]

Historical uses

Strengthens the womb; helps expel the after-birth; as an emmenagogue, dysmenorrhoea. Pain of the head involving coldness. To lift the spirits; for hysteria and nervousness. For colic; coughs; wheezing; difficulty breathing. Externally to treat freckles; insect bites and as an insect repellent.

Tanacetum vulgare

Tansy

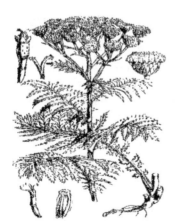

Family Asteraceae, Tribe Anthemideae

Description

A rhizomatous, strongly aromatic perennial which dies back to basal leaves in winter. *Stems* erect,

ribbed and slightly hairy, from 30–200 cm tall, branching above to form the inflorescence. *Basal leaves* petiolate, ovate, obovate or elliptic; pinnate, about 15–25 × 5–10 cm, primary leaflets in 10–15 pairs, lanceolate to narrow ovate, all on one plane, ultimate segments often triangular, serrate. Cauline leaves alternate, similar, but usually glabrous and glandular and becoming sessile and smaller with fewer leaflets higher up the stems. *Flowers* in a corymb with up to 15 or more densely packed capitula. Involucral bracts usually glabrous with a brown margin. Capitula from 6–12 mm across, outer florets female but not or shortly ligulate, disc florets numerous, all yellow. *Achenes* brown, glandular, ribbed, about 1.5 mm long. Flowers midsummer to late autumn.

Habitat and cultivation

Native to Europe and temperate Asia and now naturalised widely in waste and cultivated land. Forms large clumps in most soils and may be grown from root division. Drought and frost resistant.

Parts used

The herb harvested during or just prior to flowering.

Active constituents

T. vulgare exists as different genotypes and 26 different chemoforms having been found in Hungary.[596,597] The constituents and morphology vary according to genotype and geographical location.[597-599]

1) Volatile oil (up to 0.3% in herb, up to 1. 9% in flowers) more than 100 mono- and sesquiterpenes have been identified.[599] Composition depends on chemotype and consists of differing amounts of the main constituents α–thujone (up to 61%), β-thujone (up to 81%), (-)-camphor (most frequently found monoterpene), borneol, 1,8-cineole-bornyl acetate, α-terpineol and/or (E)-chrsysanthenyl acetate (up to 40% or more)[596,598-602]
2) Sesquiterpene lactones including predominantly parthenolide also germacrene D.[603-606] Also some non-volatile sesquiterpenes including davanone,[600,607] tanacetols A and B[608-610]

3) Flavonoids including those based on scutellarein, luteolin, apigenin, quercitin, eupatorin, chrysoeriol and diosmetin[532,611]
4) Terpenoids—artemisia ketone, trans-phytol,[604] pyrethrins, α-amyrin, β-amyrin and taraxasterol[612,613]
5) Sterols including β-sitosterol, stigmasterol and campesterol[612]

Also contains tannins, resin and a pectin polysaccharide (tanacetan).[614,615]

Actions
1) Anthelmintic
2) Emmenagogue
3) Carminative
4) Spasmolytic

Scientific information
In ancient times tansy was used as an embalming agent and insect repellent. It is still known for its repellent properties but is also used in the food flavouring and cosmetics industries.

In spite of the amount of research that has been conducted into the chemical constituents and its variations in make-up, not a great deal has been done into its actions.

In vitro—The essential oil has acaricidal properties tested against the spider mite, *Tetranychus urticae*, β-thujone is considered the main active constituent.[616] The whole herb has partial activity in inhibiting the virus responsible for tick-borne encephalitis.[384]

T. vulgare has anti-oxidant[617] and anti-inflammatory activity.[618] As cited for *T. parthenium* parthenolide also has anti-inflammatory activity but it is present at much lower concentrations in this herb and it is very likely other constituents are contributing to the action.[611]

The polysaccharide fraction has immunomodulatory activity.[619]

Medicinal uses
Gastro-intestinal tract
May be used to improve digestive function, however, it is mainly used as an anthelmintic:

• dyspepsia

• nausea
• nematode infestation[†]

Reproductive tract
As an emmenagogue the herb has been used for:

• amenorrhoea

Externally
• as a lotion for scabies
• as an ointment for pruritus ani
• as an enema for nematode infestation

Pharmacy
Three times daily
Infusion of dried herb   – 1–2 g
Liquid Extract (25%)   – 1–2 ml

As an anthelmintic *T. vulgare* may be combined with other anthelmintic agents and a laxative. The combined herbs are administered once a day, at night or on an empty stomach in the morning, for two weeks. The flowers are stronger than the whole herb.

A scabies lotion may be prepared stronger than that recommended for internal use.

T. vulgare oil is very strong and should be used with great caution. It may be incorporated into an ointment to apply to the anus to kill emerging adults and their eggs.

CONTRAINDICATIONS—Pregnancy.

Precautions and/or safety
Tansy is a strong herb and should not be used continuously for long periods of time. The recommended dosage should not be exceeded. For allergic reactions—see General Precaution p. 25. Photoallergic contact dermatitis has also been observed in patch testing.[620]

The essential oil of tansy may cause convulsions, an activity attributed to the monoterpene ketones.[621]

Historical uses
Hysteria; kidney weakness; fever and ague; gout; epilepsy (essential oil in small doses); joint pains; sciatica. Externally for sprains; swellings;

[†]Includes hookworms, threadworms and pinworms.

rheumatism; mouth and gum sores and loose teeth (gargle); morphew; sunburn; pimples; freckles; eye inflammations. Was used as a strewing herb.

Taraxacum officinale

Dandelion

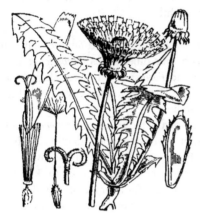

Family Asteraceae, Tribe Lactuceae

Description

Perennial rosette herb with tap root(s). *Leaves* all basal, linear oblanceolate to obovate, runcinate-pinnatifid to not lobed, toothed, glabrous or with sparse short multicellular hairs especially on mid-rib above, 5–30 × 1–10 cm; terminal lobe triangular to deltoid, acute or obtuse, truncate or hastate at base; lateral lobes narrowly to broadly triangular, usually recurved, often toothed, petiole and proximal part of midrib hollow. Scape stout, hollow, glabrous or cobwebby, 3–35 cm tall. *Capitula* 3–5 cm diameter, solitary, terminal. Calyx dull green or reddish, strongly reflexed or recurved at flowering and fruiting. Corolla ligulate, florets golden yellow. *Achene* body cream to greenish brown, ribbed, clavate, 2.5–3.5 mm long. Pappus white, 5–7 mm long. Flowers most of the year with the main season in spring.

Habitat and cultivation

Temperate weed throughout the Northern Hemisphere and naturalised elsewhere in grasslands, lawns and gardens. Self-sows and needs no cultivation but provides better leaves and roots in deep, moist soil. Drought and frost resistant.

Parts used

Leaves gathered throughout the year but before flowering occurs; roots dug from plants two years old or more, in autumn.

Active constituents

Taraxacum is another herb in which polyploidy has been well documented. The herb not only reproduces sexually but can do so asexually, a process called apomixis, this could be a new phenomenon in this species.[622] The normal sexually reproduced plants are diploid but the plant can exist in a polyploid form, mainly triploid and tetraploid,[623] through interaction of the different genetic types. Rural plants can be genetically different from urban ones, the level of pollution apparently making plants less genetically diverse.[624] The constituents of the herb may therefore have some variation depending on genotype.

1) Sesquiterpene lactones, of following types:-
   a) germacranolide including derivatives of taraxinic acid (root and leaf)[625]
   b) guaianolide including a dihydrolactucin, ixerin D and ainslioside (root)[626]
   c) eudesmanolide including tetrahydroridentin B[627] and taraxacolide glucoside (root)
2) Also an ester of γ-butyrolactone glucoside called taraxacoside (root).[628] The sesquiterpene lactones give the herb its bitterness.
3) Flavonoids—glycosides of quercetin[629] (root and leaf); luteolin glucosides[630] (leaf)
4) Phenolic acids including caffeic and p-hydroxyphenylacetic acids and derivatives of caffeoylquinic acid and tartaric acid predominantly cichoric and monocaffeoyltartaric acid, hydroxycinnamic and chlorogenic acids (root and leaf); syringin (root)[626,629,630]
5) Carotenoids including lutein, violaxanthin and β-carotene[631] (leaf)
6) Triterpenoids including pentacylic alcohols taraxasterol, ψ-taraxasterol, taraxerol and β-amyrin (root); β-amyrin (leaf)[632] and

cycloartenol (leaf) and the phytosterols β-sitosterol, stigmasterol (leaf and root) and campesterol (leaf)

7) Coumarins scopoletin, esculetin, cichoriin and aesculin (leaf)[630]

The root has in addition tannins, mucilage, volatile oil and polysaccharides including inulin (up to 40% in autumn), glucans, fructosans and mannans.

The leaf has in addition furan fatty acids,[633] choline and potassium salts (up to 4.25%).

Nutritional constituents
Vitamins: A, B, C, and D in leaf and root; carotenoids in the leaf
Minerals: Potassium, iron, copper in the leaf and root; calcium, sodium, some phosphorous and zinc in the root

Actions
1) Diuretic (leaves)
2) Choleretic
3) Laxative
4) Antirheumatic

Scientific information
Both root and leaf have been used in many traditions over hundreds of years. The root has been an official medicine used as a bitter for atonic dyspepsia and as a laxative.[42] Both herb and root are approved for use by *German Commission E* the former as a diuretic and for prevention of renal gravel the latter as indicated in the pharmacopoeias.

There has been very little modern research into the medicinal use of this herb in humans, early studies using animals forming the basis of the current understanding of its mode of action.

In vitro—The herb is one commonly chosen by Italian herbalists in the treatment of diabetes,[634] one possible explanation may be that it can inhibit α-glucosidase (this is an orthodox approach used to treat type 2 diabetes mellitus).[635]
The root can:-

• stimulate the growth of various bifido-bacteria, an effect likely due to the oligofructans and/or

inulin (see *Cichorium*, inulin is not bio-available in tincture-form)[636]
• inhibit liver cancer cells causing their apoptosis through increased levels of cytokines.[637] (There is an Eastern tradition for using *Taraxacum* spp. to treat breast and uterine cancer.) The root was reported to have antitumour effects[638] and taraxasterol is anti-carcinogenic[639]
• inhibit leukotriene formation in activated neutrophils[625]

In vivo—A clinical trial used *Taraxacum* in combination with four other herbs (*Hypericum*, *Calendula*, *Melissa* and *Foeniculum*) to treat chronic non-specific colitis. The preparation gave a very high level of pain-relief.[640]

Traditionally the action of *Taraxacum* is via stimulation of liver and kidney function. Both parts of the herb are considered to have activities in both areas though the leaves are used for kidney excretion and the root for liver based secretion.

The potassium content of the leaves compensates for loss of this electrolyte which normally occurs with diuretics.

Recent analysis of the flowers has identified flavonoids with good anti-oxidant[641] and anti-inflammatory[642] activity, but this part of the herb is not used in herbal medicine.

Medicinal uses
Cardiovascular system
As a diuretic *Taraxacum folia* (leaves) is indicated where there is oedema:

• hypertension
• ascites

Gastro-intestinal tract
The bitter properties of *Taraxacum radix* (roots) through stimulating digestive secretions make it suitable for treating:

• anorexia
• indigestion
• atonic dyspepsia
• constipation
• cholelithiasis

- jaundice
- cholecystitis

The herb may also be beneficial in hypoglycaemia.

Urinary tract
Taraxacum folia is considered one of the strongest herbal diuretics, comparable in effect to the orthodox drug frusemide. However quite large quantities of the leaves, the juice or fluid extract would be required.

- fluid retention
- kidney lithiasis
- oliguria

Musculoskeletal

- muscular rheumatism

Pharmacy
Three times daily

Leaf

Infusion of dried herb	– 4–10 g
Fluid extract (25%)	– 4–10 ml
Fresh juice	– 10–20 ml

Root

Decoction of dried root	– 2–8 g
Tincture 1:5 (45%)	– 5–10 ml
Fluid Extract (30%)	– 2–8 ml
Juice of fresh root	– 4–8 ml

Dandelion root, roasted, has been used as a coffee substitute.

Precautions and/or safety
The white juice found in the stem has been known to make children, who have ingested it in quantity, nauseous, also causing vomiting, diarrhoea and palpitations. No other toxicity or problems are known for this herb although because of the ability of *Taraxacum* to absorb lead and cadmium from the soil care should be taken when wild-crafting the herb to make medicine.[643]

For allergic reactions—see General Precaution p. 25. There are documented cases of contact dermatitis[644-646] but it is only likely to cause a reaction in those with known contact allergies.[647] A few cases have been reported of children not usually sensitive to the Asteraceae family developing a contact eczema for which *Taraxacum* patch-tested positive.[648,649] The frequency of reaction to dandelion appears to be quite low.[650] There is one recorded case of *Taraxacum* causing *erythema multiforme* after exposure to it whilst gardening.[651]

Historical uses
"Cleanseth imposthumes and inward ulcers in the urinary passages" and to help those with cachexy—meaning a bad habit of the body. Phthisis and skin diseases such as scurvy, scrofula, eczema and eruptive skin conditions generally. The white latex has been used to treat warts.

Tussilago farfara

Coltsfoot, coughwort

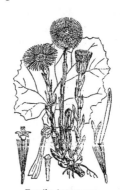

Family Asteraceae,
Tribe Anthemideae

Description
A perennial with creeping rhizomes, and erect flowering stems arising directly from the rhizomes, which lengthen in fruit to 15–35 cm. Flowers in early spring, followed by the appearance of the leaves as flowers fade. *Leaves* all basal, stalked, large 10–30 cm across, orbicular-heartshaped with wide, irregular, shallow lobes. The leaf surface is

deep green but underneath it is covered in soft white hairs. *Flower heads* solitary, bright yellow, 1½–3½ cm consisting of numerous ray florets in many rows. Flower stems are thick with scale-like leaves. Flowers close at night. *Fruits* each have a long white pappus.

Odourless; taste mucilaginous—bitter and astringent.

Habitat and cultivation
Native to all Europe and Britain, *Tussilago* grows in waste places, banks, screes and gravelly places. It is naturalised in parts of USA and considered to be a noxious weed in other places because of its spreading habits. Propagated by division. Frost and drought resistant.

Parts used
Leaves; flowers to a lesser extent.

Active constituents
1) Flavonoids including rutin and hyperoside (flowers); quercetin (leaves)
2) Mucilage (about 8%)
3) Alkaloids of pyrrolizidine type (about 0.015%), including tussilagine,[652] isotussilagine, senkirkine[653] and senecionine[654]
4) Sesquiterpenes including a bisabolene epoxide,[655] farfaratin[656] and tussilagone[657] (flowers)
5) Triterpenoids including arnidiol and fara-diol (flowers), β-amyrin, taraxasterol and the phytosterols sitosterol and stigmasterol (leaves)

Also tannins and inulin.

Nutritional constituents
Vitamins: A, B_{12}, B_6, C, and P
Minerals: Calcium, potassium, zinc, traces of manganese, iron and copper

Actions
1) Expectorant
2) Antitussive
3) Demulcent
4) Anticatarrhal

Scientific information
Tussilago is a widespread herb that has been part of the traditional medicine of many different countries. The botanical name testifies to its well established value across all these countries as a remedy to treat coughs. Both flowers and leaves were at one time official medicines in European pharmacopoeias used to treat chronic and irritable coughs.[42]

There is not a great deal of information available for the herb in the medical literature, most of the scientific interest having centred round its pyrrolizidine alkaloid content (see Precautions).

In vitro—The herb's activity has only been assessed in animal models but includes anti-oxidant and anti-inflammatory activity, via inhibition of arachidonic acid metabolism, inhibition of nitric oxide production and antagonism of PAF.[655]

It had good antimicrobial activity against *Bacillus cereus* and *Staphylococcus aureus*.[658]

In vivo—A decoction of a number of Chinese herbs, including *Tussilago* was effective in clearing up residual airways obstruction in a group of convalescing asthmatics.[659]

Medicinal uses
Respiratory tract
The herb is considered antispasmodic and an aid to mucociliary activity.

- whooping cough
- irritable/spasmodic coughs
- laryngitis
- asthma
- bronchitis
- inflammation of oral/pharynx
- tracheitis

Weiss considers one of *Tussilago's* uses is in the treatment of coughs due to emphysema or silicosis where it would not cure these irreversible conditions but could help to relieve their symptoms. In addition he suggests the bitterness would be an added "tonic" in these debilitating diseases.

Pharmacy
Three times daily

Infusion of dried herb	– 0.6–2 g
Tincture 1:5 (45%)	– 2–8 ml
Fluid extract (25%)	– 0.6–2 ml
Syrup (25%)	– 2–8 ml

Weiss suggests steeping the herb overnight in a thermos (vacuum) flask for use the next morning. It has been used in herbal tobaccos and was formerly used as a smoke inhalation to treat respiratory conditions like asthma.

Precautions and/or safety

The pyrrolizidine alkaloids present in *Tussilago* could theoretically cause hepatotoxicity but in practice the level of these alkaloids are very low. There are no reports to-date of its having done so apart from two cases of veno-occlusive disease initially attributed to *Tussilago* which appear to be cases of incorrect plant identification, the substituted plant being of similar appearance.[660-662]

The alkaloids are also potentially carcinogenic and teratogenic though again no link has yet been found.[663] In fact senkirkine, which is present in very small concentrations in the herb, is not mutagenic to human lymphocytes even at high concentrations.[664]

Coltsfoot is not available in some countries because of the concern over the pyrrolizidine alkaloids, even though it has been used throughout the world over many centuries. Where it is available maximum daily doses, given above, should not be exceeded.

Historical uses

To aid treatment of fevers, scrofulous conditions, calculus. Externally for inflammations or hot swellings; wheals; piles.

BERBERIDACEAE

Berberidaceae are usually shrubs or sub-shrubs which often have spines.

- Leaves are alternate, simple or compound, exstipulate or with minute stipules
- Flowers are nearly always in clusters of three or more, solitary or in fascicles, racemes or panicles
- Sepals and petals are similar in 2 to several whorls, 3 per whorl. Petals are yellow or orange and drop quickly
- Stamens 6, ovary superior with 1 carpel and fruit a 1-few seeded berry

There are 500–600 species mostly from Northern temperate areas and temperate South America.

Berberis vulgaris

Barberry

Description
A glabrous, deciduous, densely branched shrub to 2–3 m high, with angled shoots and three-pronged, needle-like spines to 1.5 cm long on adult shoots.

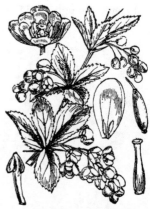

Family Berberidaceae

Wood bright yellow. *Stems* woody, erect, reddish when young, older bark grey. *Leaves* on 1 cm long stalks, lamina dull-green above, alternate, elliptic to obovate, usually serrulate, sometimes entire. *Flowers* in racemes to 6 cm long, with 15–30 flowers, medium yellow, fragrant. *Berries* 9–11 mm long, oblong, scarlet to crimson-scarlet, and shining. Flowers in spring.

Taste—very bitter.

Habitat and cultivation
Originally from Europe, barberry was introduced to other countries to provide stock-proof hedges.

It is hardy, grows from seed, cuttings or layers and produces more berries in poor conditions. Best planted as a hedge and kept trimmed. Frost resistant, drought tender.

Parts used

The root, root bark and stem bark are used in Western Herbal Medicine.

The berries and leaves are also used in various countries, they have medicinal and nutritional value.[1-3]

Active constituents

1) Alkaloids (at least 22 have been identified in all parts of the plant)[4] the most important being the isoquinolones mainly berberine, berbamine, oxyacanthine, jatrorrhizine and palmatine. Also magnoflorine, columbamine, isotetrandine and berberrubine[5-8]
2) Chelidonic acid
3) Tannins

Also contains wax and resin.

Actions

1) Cholagogue
2) Antibacterial
3) Anti-inflammatory
4) Alterative
5) Laxative
6) Anti-emetic
7) Antipyretic
8) Antihaemorrhagic
9) Antiprotozoal
10) Antidiarrhoeal

Scientific information

There are a number of species of *Berberis* used medicinally throughout the world. *B. vulgaris* has been known as a medicine for over 2000 years. The alkaloids are considered central to its actions. Whilst these alkaloids have been well studied, the whole extract as used in herbal medicine has received little attention. Most work has been carried out on berberine and/or its salts,[9] which have been official medicines as bitters.[10]

In vitro—The whole extract has anti-oxidant[11] and antibacterial activity against *Escherichia coli*, *Pseudomonas aeruginosa*, *Staphylococcus aureus*, *Streptococcus mutans* and *S. pyogenes*.[9]

Results of research into the actions of some of the main individual alkaloids are summarised below.

Berberine and/or its salts
In vitro:-

• antibacterial properties for a number of bacteria including *Vibrio cholera*, *Escherichia coli* (it directly reduces their enterotoxins too), *Pseudomonas aeruginosa* and *Bacillus subtilis*[9,12]
• antiprotozoal properties including inhibiting the growth of *Giardia lamblia*, *Entamoeba hystolytica*, *Trichomonas vaginalis*, *Leishamnia donovani* and *Plasmodium falciparum*[13,14]
• antifungal properties against *Candida* spp.,[15] *Trichophyton mentagrophytes* and *Crytpococcus neoformans*[16]
• anti-oxidant[17]
• inhibition of keratinocyte proliferation[18]
• inhibition of HIV-1 reverse transcriptase[19]
• reduction in smooth muscle contraction and intestinal motility[8]
• prevention of ischaemia-induced tachyarrhythmia, increased cardiac contractility and reduced resistance in peripheral blood vessels, lowering blood pressure[8]
• anticancer,[20,21] anticarcinogenic and antimutagenic[22]
• inhibition of inflammatory reactions including COX-2 in colon cancer cells which may have significance for tumour development too.[8,21] (There is a tradition in Eastern Europe of using *Berberis* to treat rheumatic and chronic inflammation, which is attributed to the action of the alkaloids.[23])
• potential as a cholesterol-lowering agent[24]

In vivo:-

• good resolution of eye infections due to *Chlamydia trachomatis*
• antiprotozoal inhibiting the growth of *Giardia lamblia* and *Entamoeba hystolytica*.

Also enhances the effectiveness of the antimalarial, pyrimethamine, in treating chloroquine-resistant malaria[25]

- delays intestinal transit[9]

Berberine has been used in eye drops to treat inflammation, hypersensitivity and allergic conjunctivitis (*Weiss*).

Berbamine
In vitro:-

- inhibits the growth of leukaemia cells including drug-resistant types[26,27] and liver cancer cells[28]
- inhibition of keratinocyte proliferation[18]
- anti-oxidant[29,30]
- antibacterial and antiprotozoal[31]
- anti-arrhythmia, vasodilating and antithrombotic activity[32]
- anti-inflammatory[33] including through inhibition of lipoxygenase[30]

In vivo:-

- increased white blood cells and platelets—used in China to treat leucopenia induced by radiotherapy and chemotherapy

Other alkaloids
In vitro:-

- Palmatine—cytotoxic,[34] antifungal for *Candida*[15] and an inhibitor of HIV-1 reverse transcriptase[19]
- Jatrorrhizine—anti-oxidant[17] and antifungal[35]
- Magnoflorine—anti-oxidant[17]
- Columbamine—anti-oxidant and anti-inflammatory[36]
- Oxyacanthine—anti-oxidant, anti-inflammatory[30] and inhibits keratinocyte proliferation[18]

Medicinal uses
Gastro-intestinal tract
Berberis is a bitter and considered a spleen tonic:

- cholelithiasis
- cholecystitis

- jaundice
- portal hypertension
- dyspepsia

Infectious conditions
- malaria
- leishmaniasis
- dysentery

Pharmacy
Three times daily

Decoction	–	0.5–1 g
Tincture 1:10 (60%)	–	2–4 ml
Fluid Extract (25%)	–	2–3 ml

CONTRAINDICATIONS—Pregnancy.

Historical uses
To cleanse the body of choler and reduce body heat and the manifestations of these problems such as the itch, ringworm and scabs as well as jaundice, bile and agues. For scalds and as a gargle. *Culpeper* also notes that "the berries are as good as the bark and more pleasing". As a yellow dye used to dye leather (Poland) and hair (*Culpeper*). The Indian species *B. aristata* has been used traditionally in wound healing.

Mahonia aquifolium
[Formerly *Berberis aquifolium*]

Oregon grape, mountain grape (because of appearance of clusters of berries)

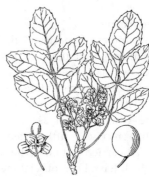

Family Berberidaceae

Description

A many-stemmed and stoloniferous shrub up to 2 m high. Wood yellow. *Leaves* alternate, to about 25 cm long, with a long, dark-red petiole and 3–7 pairs of sessile leaflets and a terminal leaflet, ovate or elliptic-ovate, dark-green and glossy above, prominently veined with undulate and spinose-dentate margins and a spiny apex. *Flowers* yellowish-green, heavily scented, in terminal racemes with brown, 5–10 mm long, membranous scales at the base of the clustered racemes. *Berries* about 10 mm in diameter, globose, blue-black, with a glaucous bloom. Flowers from spring to summer.

Habitat and cultivation

Native from British Columbia to Oregon and grown elsewhere as an ornamental shrub. Grows from seed or cutting and thrives in semi-shade under deciduous trees or along the edge of shrubberies. Frost and drought resistant.

Parts used

The rhizome and root.

Active constituents

1) Alkaloids mainly the isoquinolones berberine and jatrorrhizine. Also oxyacanthine, berbamine, palmatine, columbamine and hydrastine and the aporphine magnoflorine[37–39]
2) Tannins
3) Resin

Also contains a phytosterol[40] and polysaccharides.

Nutritional constituents

Minerals: Manganese, silicon, sodium, copper and zinc

Actions

1) Anticatarrhal
2) Anti-emetic
3) Cholagogue
4) Alterative
5) Laxative
6) Antidiarrhoeal

Scientific information

Mahonia was officially recognised in the USA until 1947 having first come to attention as a medicine in 1877. It was listed as a febrifuge and stomachic. It shares a number of the same alkaloids with *B. vulgaris*. (For their pharmacological activity see the previous herb.)

Antimicrobial

In vitro—The whole extract, as well as some isolated constituents, have antibacterial activity against strains of *Staphylococcus* and *Propionibacterium acnes*[41] and antifungal activity against a range of dermatophytes including *Candida* and *Trichophyton* spp.[31,42,43]

Other

In vitro—*Mahonia* inhibits cytokine induced inflammation, angiogenesis and cancer promotion in stimulated monocytes.[44] It also partially inhibits the production of the cytokines associated with epidermal hyperproliferation and microabscess formation.[45]

The isoquinolone alkaloids, and to a lesser extent the whole root, are immunomodulatory via an anti-complement activity, this may have significance for treatment of auto-immune diseases.[46]

In vivo—Extracts have been beneficial in the topical treatment of psoriasis[47] reducing antibody levels and hyperproliferation of keratinocytes in these lesions.[48]

Mahonia has been considered interchangeable with *B. vulgaris* but may be gentler in its action.

Medicinal uses

Gastro-intestinal tract
- gastritis
- cholecystitis
- cholelithiasis
- jaundice
- portal hypertension
- dyspepsia

Reproductive tract
The anticatarrhal effects are used in this system:

- leucorrhoea

Skin
- psoriasis
- eczema
- dry cutaneous eruptions

Pharmacy
Three times daily
Decoction	– 1–2 g
Tincture 1:10	– 2–5 ml
Fluid Extract (25%)	– 1–2 ml

CONTRAINDICATIONS—Pregnancy.

Historical uses
Psoriasis; pityriasis; syphilis; blood impurities in general; chronic catarrh.

Caulophyllum thalictroides

Blue cohosh

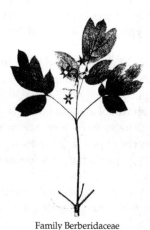

Family Berberidaceae

Description
An erect perennial rhizomatous herb growing to ½–1 m tall with smooth stems covered with a bluish film. *Leaves,* greenish blue divided into 3 or sometimes 5 leaflets. *Flowers,* greenish yellow, each about 1–1½ cm across grow in lax terminal clusters and appear before the leaves. *Fruit* is a 2-seeded drupe with a thin, fleshy blue seed coat. Flowers from April to June and fruits in August in its native environment.

Odour—slight; taste—sweet, bitter and acrid.

Habitat and cultivation
Native to USA growing in moist, rich, shady woods, from New Brunswick to South Carolina and west to Nebraska. Can be cultivated in similar situations either from seed sown when ripe or from root division in autumn.

Parts used
Root and/or rhizome harvested in autumn.

Active constituents
1) Alkaloids (max. 1.1%)[49] of both the aporphine and quinolizidine types including N-methyl-cytisine (caulophylline), batifoline, anagyrine, thalactroidine, magnoflorine and sparteine[50–52]
2) Triterpene saponins based on hederagenin, caulophyllogenin and echinocystic acid[53]

Nutritional constituents
Vitamins: B-complex and E
Minerals: Calcium, magnesium, phosphorus, iron and potassium

Actions
1) Spasmolytic
2) Emmenagogue
3) Uterine tonic
4) Antirheumatic

Scientific information
This herb was an official medicine in the USA until 1950 used for hastening or inducing labour. There is very little scientific information available about it although it has been the subject of some concern in recent years in relation to its use as a partus praeparator.

The alkaloid methylcytisine can bind to nicotinic receptor sites, although weakly, and whilst the effect of this alkaloid and those of the saponin fraction are known in animal models, there are no studies into the physiological effects in humans. (For pharmacological actions of sparteine see *Cytisus*.)

Traditionally *Caulophyllum* was used for a wide variety of complaints but since its introduction to the west it has been mostly used as a female remedy.

Medicinal uses
Reproductive tract
Modern use has focussed on the herb as a uterine tonic and antispasmodic. It may be used to treat:

- dysmenorrhoea
- amenorrhoea
- atony of the uterus

The *BHP* lists threatened miscarriage and false labour pains too. However in the light of recent concerns these uses need careful assessment. See Precautions.

Musculo-skeletal system
- joint pain

Pharmacy
Three times daily
Decoction of dried root/rhizome   – 0.3–1 g
Fluid Extract (70%)   – 0.5–1 ml
    Potter's gives a maximum dosage of 2 g dried or 2 ml fluid extract however the lower maximum given above would seem to be safer.

Precautions and/or safety
There have been several reports in the literature of serious problems occurring in babies born to mothers who were taking *Caulophyllum* as a partus praeparator. Perinatal stroke and heart failure associated with myocardial infarction were attributed to the herb's toxicity.[54-56] As proper identity checks were not carried out at the time it is very difficult to draw firm conclusions as to a causal link. The recommended dosage was also substantially exceeded in one instance.[50] However these cases, even if flawed, do raise questions about the use of the herb during pregnancy. One analysis of how blue cohosh came to achieve the status of a partus praeparator suggests western settlers redefined the indigenous use of the herb for stalled labour into a general labour aid. Furthermore indigenous use involved much lower doses prepared as decoctions, alcohol extraction may change the chemical make-up of the medicine.[57] Given the very vulnerable nature of the population that would be exposed to the herb and the uncertainty surrounding its absolute safety it may be advisable not to use the herb in pregnancy.

    Isolated constituents of the root and rhizome are known toxins in animal models. Large amounts of *Caulophyllum* tincture have been reported to cause tachycardia, diaphoresis, abdominal pain, vomiting and muscle weakness with fasciculations, symptoms akin to nicotinic toxicity.[58]

    Anagyrine has been associated with teratogenicity in animals although there are no reported cases of the whole herb causing human deformities over its long history of use.

Interactions
Some texts advise caution when using this herb with pharmaceuticals used for angina and/or hypertension because methylcytisine has similar physiological effects to nicotine. However this alkaloid is present at low levels in *Caulophyllum* and is estimated to be only 1/40th as strong as nicotine.[59]

Historical uses
Dropsy; epilepsy, hysteria; as an anthelmintic; colic; hiccoughs; asthma; bronchitis; genitourinary complaints.

BETULACEAE

The Betulaceae or birch family consists of 6 genera and over 100 species of deciduous, mostly monoecious trees and shrubs, mainly native to the Northern Hemisphere.

- Leaves alternate, simple
- Male flowers in long, drooping catkins; female flowers in short catkins or clusters; stamens 2–10 in the axils of the bracts
- Fruit a nut or nutlet

Betula alba & Betula pendula

Silver birch

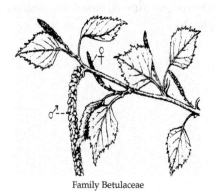

Family Betulaceae

Description

Deciduous tree to 25 m tall. *Bark* black and fissured towards base of trunk, silver-white and peeling above. Branches slender and more or less pendulous. Leaf buds scaly but not sticky. *Leaves* alternate, simple; lamina 3–6 × 1.5–5.5 cm long, ovate to triangular, acuminate, glabrous; margins double toothed. Petiole about 2 cm long. Leaves turn yellow in autumn. *Flowers* monoecious with male and female flowers in different inflorescences—male flowers in drooping catkins 3–6 cm long with 2 stamens; female flowers in erect cylindrical/ovoid catkins up to 3.5 cm long. Wind pollinated. *Fruit* a flattened winged nutlet with persistent styles. Flowers in spring.

Odour—faintly aromatic; taste—somewhat bitter.

Habitat and cultivation

Native to Britain and Europe, *Betula alba* is cultivated elsewhere for its graceful beauty. It grows from seed and is available from garden centres. It can become naturalized. Drought tender, frost resistant.

Parts used

The young leaves and the bark but the sap and leaf buds may also be used. The parts are best harvested in spring.

Active constituents

1) Volatile oil (min. 0.5%) containing over 50 constituents including α-copaene, germacrene D, δ-cadinene and betulenols[1]
2) Flavonoids (approx. 3%) mainly hyperoside and avicularin, also luteolin, quercetrin and myricetin glycosides.[2,3] Flavonoid levels decrease with the age of the leaves[2]
3) Saponins—triterpene and steroidal including betulin (10%–30%),[4] betulinic, papyriferic, pendulic and betuloleanolic acids[5] and betufernanediols A and B.[6] The presence of saponins in *Betula* leaves has been questioned and it has been proposed that dammarane esters, not their glycosides (saponins), are present.[7] Betulin apparently gives the bark its white colour
4) Tannins of the hydrolysable type[8]
5) Resin

Also contains methyl salicylic acid (possibly present only after distillation and as a result of a chemical alteration), fatty acids, sterols,[9] phenolics based on gallic, chlorogenic and coumarolyloquinic acids[10] and lignan glycosides based on secoisolariciresinol[11] The inner bark also contains lignan glycosides, condensed tannins[12] and di- and trisaccharides.[13]

The chemistry of *Betula* can vary with geographic location, age, nutrients, part used and genetic make-up.[11,14] There is a degree of hybridization amongst the species.[15]

Nutritional constituents
Minerals: Potassium, calcium, zinc and phosphorus

Actions
1) Diuretic
2) Antilithic
3) Astringent
4) Cholagogue
5) Bitter

Scientific information
Although *Betula* species have been used for centuries there is little pharmacological information readily available for whole plant extracts. The oil of the related North American black birch, *B. lenta*, is often used to produce "wintergreen oil" because it is chemically very like that of *Gaultheria procumbens*.

Betula has been used in the food industry (it is used to flavour root beer for example) and in cosmetics as the essential oil has a good fragrance. Either the whole extract or the single constituent, betulin, is used.

In vitro:-

• the bark induces interferon production in cell culture in response to infection with the hepatitis C virus[16]
• betulin is anti-oxidant,[17] cytoprotective against alcohol damage in liver cells,[18] antiviral,[19] anti-inflammatory[20] and cytoprotective against cadmium[21,22]
• betulinic acid is anti-inflammatory,[20] antiviral[19] (including derivatives that strongly inhibit HIV),[23] antimalarial[24] and anti-oxidant.[17] It is also showing some promise as an antitumour agent.[25–28] Its concentration in *Betula* is however quiet low[4]

Both betulin and betulinic acid are strong inhibitors of phospholipase A2.[29]

Medicinal uses
Cardiovascular system
• congestive heart failure
• fever

Urinary tract
• cystitis
• lithiasis
• oedema of renal origin

Musculoskeletal
• rheumatism
• arthritis
• gout

Skin
• inflammatory skin conditions

Externally
• arthritis
• neuralgia

Pharmacy
Three times daily
For leaves and bark

Infusion/Decoction of dried herb	–	1–4 g
Tincture 1:5	–	1–5 ml

Other applications
Birch Tar Oil alone, or formulated as a compound, is listed in the *British Pharmaceutical Codex* and has been used externally for the treatment of eczema and psoriasis.

The volatile oil and resin together are known as "empyreumatic oil of birch".

Precautions and/or safety
There are a significant number of people who develop respiratory allergies to the pollen of *Betula* spp.[30,31] There is no indication however that this sensitivity extends to use of the above medicinal preparations.

Historical uses
For sore mouths (as a wash); intermittent fevers (inner bark), analgesic; as a hair conditioner.

BIGNONIACEAE

A dicot family of about 750 species and 110 genera of trees, shrubs and woody vines and rarely herbs mostly of tropical and subtropical regions. There are about 100 species of *Tabebuia* originally from Central and South America and the West Indies. They are among the most common showy flowering trees in tropical regions and yield a good cabinet-making wood.

Tabebuia avellanedae

Lapacho (Spanish), Pau d'arco (Portuguese)

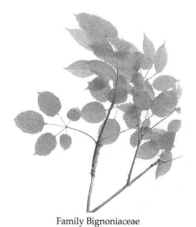

Family Bignoniaceae

Description
An evergreen tree growing up to 20 m. (In cool climates it may become deciduous.) *Leaves*, light green with leaflets 10–15 cm long. *Flowers* many shades of pink or red, trumpet-shaped with golden throats. *Fruit* a smooth pendant capsule, about 30 cm long.

Habitat
Native to Brazil, Paraguay and Argentina, and found also in the Andes in Peru, and Bolivia. *Tabebuia* grows easily in tropical areas such as Florida and Queensland. It is easily propagated from seed or cuttings.

Parts used
The inner bark collected from wild trees throughout the year. The smaller *Tabebuia impetiginosa* from Brazil is also used as a source of bark. The outer bark and wood also contain medicinal constituents in lower concentration.[1,2]

A number of *Tabebuia* species are used traditionally, although *T. avellanedae* is the preferred medicinal species.

Active constituents
1) Quinones[3]
   a) napthoquinones mainly lapachol, β-lapachone, xyloidone, also α-lapachone and furanonaphthoquinones[4,5]
   b) anthraquinones including 2-(hydroxymethyl) anthraquinone and anthraquinone-2 carboxylic acid
2) Flavonoids including quercetin
3) Steroidal saponins
4) Alkaloids including tecomine

Also benzoic acid and benzaldehyde derivatives,[6] iridoid glycosides, phenylethanoids, phenolic glycosides, isocoumarin, lignans, carnosol, indoles and cyclopentene dialdehydes.[7-11] The iridoid, phenylethanoid and lignan glycosides are based on ajugol,[12] osmanthuside H and secoisolariciresinol respectively.[10]

The level of lapachol seems to vary with the quality of material, plant part and method of extraction—the naphthoquinones have poor solubility in water.[5]

Nutritional constituents
Vitamins: Niacin and A (small amount)
Minerals: Iron, calcium, magnesium, potassium, selenium and chromium

Actions
1) Antitumourogenic
2) Antimicrobial
3) Anti-inflammatory

Scientific information
Although this herb has been used extensively by the people of South America for hundreds of years, Western interest began with the scientific study into the herb and its constituents in the late 19th Century. Lapachol was the first constituent to be isolated and identified in 1896 however β-lapachone has probably been more extensively studied.

Antimicrobial
By the mid 1950's lapachol and the other main naphthoquinones were established as being both antibacterial and antifungal.[1] *Tabebuia's* action has been attributed, at least in part, to its ability to inhibit enzyme reactions necessary for mitochondrial respiration.[1]

In vitro—*Tabebuia* and/or its consitituents show good activity against:-

- Bacteria—penicillin G-resistant *Staphylococcus aureus*,[13] methicillin-resistant *S. aureus* (MRSA),[14] *Streptococcus* spp. and *Brucella* spp.,[1] *Helicobacter pylori*[3] and *Clostridium paraputrifactum*.[15] (Intestinal flora, *Bifidobacterium* spp. and *Lactobacillus* spp., are not adversely affected[15])
- Fungi—*Candida albicans* and *Trichophyton* spp.[1,16]
- Viruses—HIV, herpes including HSV-1 and 2, polio and vesicular stomatitis viruses, a number of influenza viruses, retroviruses, Epstein Barr[17,18] and rabies viruses[1]
- Protozoa—*Trypanosoma cruzi*,[1,19-21] *Schistosoma mansoni*[1] *and Plasmodium falciparum*[22]

Anticancer
A number of *Tabebuia's* constituents demonstrate antitumour activity and one of the main ones, lapachol, concentrates preferentially in tumour cells.[1] However no isolated constituent seems to offer a better anticancer effect than that of the whole extract.[1,18] Current interest in the herb has moved in the direction of modifying its active constituents in an effort to enhance their therapeutic applications.[23]

In vitro—The naphthoquinones not only interfere with the energy production of tumour cells they also cause free-radical damage to them and interrupt their nucleic acid synthesis. Constituents inhibit a number of tumour promoting viruses[1] as well as inhibiting the growth of prostatic,[24,25] lung,[26,27] colon[28] and myeloid leukaemia[29] cancer cells (including those resistant to several chemotherapeutic agents), whilst having no adverse effect on normal bone marrow stromal or peripheral blood mononuclear cells.[30]

In vivo—*Tabebuia* was used traditionally for treating cancer. In the 1950's it was widely tested in a Brazilian hospital in the treatment of various types of carcinoma and leukaemia, as well as for impaired immune function and inflammatory conditions.[1,2,5]

The outcomes were promising and the American National Cancer Institute isolated the most active constituent, lapachol, and subjected it to clinical trials. However lapachol alone was not more effective than the whole extract and had the added disadvantage that it increased the likelihood of side-effects. These included nausea and vomiting and an anti-vitamin K activity (an activity that seems to be counteracted in the whole extract by other constituents). Further research was abandoned and there have been no recent clinical trials on the herbal extract.

Other
In vitro—Constituents of *Tabebuia* in addition:-

- inhibit the growth of a keratinocyte line comparable in effect to a standard psoriasis drug, anthralin, suggesting a role in the treatment of this condition[31]
- inhibit nitric oxide production indicating a potential anti-inflammatory role[7]
- show good anti-oxidant activity, comparable with α-tocopherol[6]
- show immunomodulatory activity[5]

Traditional uses of *Tabebuia* are extensive (see Historical uses below) although clinical trials to corroborate them are lacking. Therefore what follows is likely to be a conservative list of the conditions for which the herb may be used.

Medicinal uses
Respiratory tract
Infectious conditions including:

- colds
- influenza
- coughs

Gastro-intestinal tract
- candidiasis
- infections, viral and bacterial
- mucosal inflammation e.g. Colitis

Externally
- fungal infections
- bacterial infections

Research and traditional use of *Tabebuia* suggest it could be used as an adjunct in treating malignant conditions.

Pharmacy
Three times daily (suggested guidelines[1])

Decoction of dried herb	–	0.6–0.9 g
Tincture 1:2 (45%)	–	1.2–1.8 ml

Larger doses may be required to treat malignant conditions.

Precautions and/or safety
Although isolated lapachol is an anti-coagulant at high dose, the whole herb does not have this effect.

Whole extracts are considered safe and there are no reports of toxicity or adverse reactions.

Historical uses
Other actions include cardiotonic, febrifuge, laxative, analgesic, depurative, vulnerary, expectorant and astringent. Used for anaemia (stimulant of red blood cell production), poor circulation; sore throat; polyps, dysentery; cystitis, prostatitis; syphilis; joint inflammation; snakebites; for skin conditions including psoriasis, boils and ulcers. The leaves have been used for treating diabetes.

BORAGINACEAE

The Boraginaceae are a family of annual, biennial or perennial herbs comprising about 2000 species mostly from the Mediterranean and Western Asia.

- Stems and leaves commonly hispid, rarely smooth
- Leaves alternate, simple and without stipules
- Inflorescence often a scorpioid cyme
- Calyx 5-toothed or 5-lobed, corolla 5-lobed, wheel or bell-shaped. Stamens 5
- Fruit usually 2–4 nutlets

Medicinal plants in the Boraginaceae include the genera *Borago, Lithospermum, Pulmonaria* and *Symphytum.*

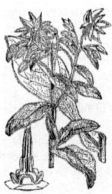

Family Boraginaceae

Borago officinalis

Borage

Description
A sturdy annual beginning as a basal rosette and growing to about 1 × 1 m in flower. Stems and leaves hispid. *Basal leaves* 30 × 20 cm, petiolate, oval-oblong, dark-green, wrinkled, acuminate; base usually rounded. Stem leaves alternate, smaller, becoming sessile. *Flowers*: calyx 10 mm long, becoming longer at fruiting. Corolla about 2.5 cm in diameter with 5 usually bright blue petals (though white and pink flowered forms are known), arranged like a star around the erect, black cone of stamens. *Fruit* 4 nutlets sheltered in the calyx. Flowers from spring to autumn.

Habitat and cultivation
Native to the Mediterranean, *Borago* self-sows freely in any sunny situation and garden soil. Seedlings may be transplanted when small. It is a good bee plant. It is drought and frost resistant.

Parts used
The herb harvested just prior to or at the start of flowering.

Active constituents
1) Saponins
2) Mucilage[1]
3) Tannins
4) Pyrrolizidine alkaloids (PAs) including lycops- amine and intermedine, with smaller amounts of amabiline and supinine. These alkaloids occur in very low concentration, the content being estimated to be of the order of 2–10 ppm (parts per million) or 0.0002% to 0.001% in commercially analysed samples[2]
5) Lipids containing fatty acids, the major one being stearidonic acid (max. 9%)[3] and γ-linoleinc acid (max. 2%).[4] The composition of unsaturated fatty acids is in fact similar to that found in the seed. Their levels have been reported as 4.4% in leaves and 14.6% in stems compared to 25.3% in seeds.[5] The seeds contain oil with omega 3 and 6 essential fatty acids (being particularly rich in γ-linolenic acid)[9] but these are generally in lower levels than found in evening primrose.

Also choline, the polyphenol—rosmarinic acid (around 1.5%),[6] a small amount of dhurrin[7] (a deriv- ative of the cyanogenic glucoside, prunassin) and trace amounts of essential oil. The fresh herb has a very high water content around 94% on average.[8]

Nutritional constituents
Minerals: Potassium, iron[8] and calcium

Actions
1) Diuretic
2) Demulcent
3) Emollient

It is also reportedly expectorant, anti-inflamma- tory, an adrenal tonic and a galactagogue.

Scientific information
Little pharmacological data is available for the herb although some of the constituents have been subject to scientific study.

In vitro—The leaves have very good anti-oxi- dant activity mainly, but not only, attributed to ros- marinic acid.[9]

In vivo—An epidemiological study has found that in areas where *Borago* leaves and stems are boiled and eaten regularly as a vegetable, the incidence of gas- tric cancer is much lower.[5] Therefore there is possibly some protective benefit from its consumption.

There is also a body of clinical and experimen- tal data highlighting the benefits of the particular fatty acids in *Borago* e.g. in the treatment of rheu- matoid arthritis[10] and atopic eczema.[11] The amount of γ-linolenic acid in the herb, after boiling, was around 0.06%.[5]

It was valued traditionally for treating many ailments.

Medicinal uses
Cardiovascular system
• fevers

Respiratory tract
• bronchitis and inflammation of the bronchi

Urinary tract
• urinary tract infections and inflammation

Reproductive tract
• to stimulate milk production

Musculoskeletal
• arthritis

Skin
• herpes simplex
• skin conditions

Externally
• inflammation (as a poultice)

Pharmacy
Three times daily
Infusion of dried herb   – 2–4 g
Fluid Extract   – 2–4 ml

Precautions and/or safety
Because of the presence of unsaturated PAs and their possible hepatotoxicity, *Borago* is deemed

unsafe by some sources. These alkaloids, with the exception of supinine, have shown genotoxicity and carcinogenicity using a standard model.[12] However as stated the alkaloids are present in very low concentration. To date no adverse reactions of any sort have been reported in spite of its long history of human consumption. Apart from in Australia, its use is unrestricted.

Historical uses

The historical use is largely as indicated above. In addition it was used by *Culpeper* to expel venoms and poisons; to raise the spirits in melancholia (adrenal action?); to treat jaundice; with *Fumaria* in the treatment of the itch, ringworm, tetters, sores and scabs. The flowers were also employed in convalescence, depression ("passions of the heart"), as a wash for sore eyes. *Culpeper* does stipulate that the green herb must be used, not the dried. This may account for the diminished use of this herb in modern practice. Borage flowers form part of La tisane de Cinque Fleurs together with flowers of *Calendula officinalis, Cytisus scoparius, Lavandula officinalis* and *Viola tricolour*.

Symphytum spp. [Symphytum officinale, S. asperum and S. x uplandicum]

Comfrey, Russian comfrey

Originally the herb officially consisted of the leaves and/or root of *Symphytum officinale* but in commercial practice at the present time the three species are all used interchangeably.

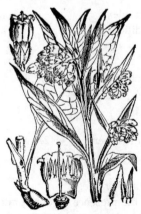

Family Boraginaceae

Description

S. officinale is a perennial herb which dies back in winter. *Stems* grow a metre high in flower. *Roots*, brittle and easily broken, black skinned but white inside, growing very thick with age and forming large clumps. *Basal leaves* very large and long stalked with an ovate or ovate-lanceolate lamina. Densely hispid above and below but not scabrid. *Cauline leaves* smaller, the uppermost sessile with the base continued down the stem to form a narrow wing extending to the node below. *Cymes* densely bristly, calyx 5–8 cm long and lobed nearly to the base. Corolla broadly cylindric, lower part of the tube whitish, expanded upper part and lobes pale pink, occasionally creamy white, often becoming purplish with age and when dried. *Nutlets* 3–6 cm long, but rarely formed. Flowers from spring to autumn.

Habitat and cultivation

Native of Europe and Asia. Propagated by root division, grows almost anywhere but prefers a sunny situation and moist, rich, well-drained soil. Once established it is difficult to eradicate. Dormant from mid-winter to early spring. Drought and frost tender.

Parts used

The leaves and roots are used. The leaves are gathered at the start of or just prior to flowering. The roots are gathered in autumn or spring.

Active constituents

1) Allantoin (around 1.3% in leaves and 0.8% in roots[13] although up to 4.7% has been reported in the latter[14])
2) Mucilage (up to 29%) polysaccharides of fructose and glucose[15] and gum (root)
3) Pyrrolizidine alkaloids (PAs) (0.02–0.18% in dried leaves and 0.25–0.29% in roots[16]) including symphytine, symlandine (these are stereoisomers), cynaglossine, lycopsamine,[17] echinatine and N-oxides of some of the above.[18] The total and individual level of alkaloids seems to be quite variable.[18,19] Echimidine has been reported in the roots of *S. officinale*[20]
4) Tannins (4–6%)

5) Phytosterols—including β-sitosterol and stigmasterol[13]
6) Phenolics including chlorogenic, rosmarinic, lithospermic and caffeic acids[21,22]

Also contains asparagine, resin and triterpenoid saponins (root).[23–25]

Nutritional constituents
Vitamins: A, B_{12} and C
Minerals: Calcium, potassium, phosphorus, iron, magnesium, selenium, sulphur, copper and zinc
Comfrey also contains some protein and eighteen amino acids including lysine.

Actions
1) Vulnerary
2) Demulcent
3) Astringent
4) Anti-inflammatory

Scientific information
The use of comfrey as a medicine dates back thousands of years, both radix and folia were used as tissue healers and soothing agents. The root was listed in the *British Pharmacopoeia* as a medicine to treat wounds and ulcers (both internal and external) the healing action having been attributed to the uric acid metabolite, allantoin.[26] Allantoin is a well established dermatological agent which has been synthesised for use in pharmaceutical preparations to "stimulate tissue formation and hasten wound healing".[26] Comfrey is approved by *German Commission E* for treatment by external application only of bruises, sprains and joint distortions.

Much of the more recent research into the herb has concentrated on the safety issues surrounding the PAs whilst clinical trials have assessed the benefits associated with the external use of the herb.

In vitro—The whole extract is anti-inflammatory, partly due to a strong inhibition of PAF, to which rosmarinic acid and allantoin contribute.[21,27]

The extract and alkaloid fraction also have immunomodulatory activity.[28,29]

In vivo—External preparations of the herb have been effective in the treatment of ankle injuries/sprains (equal to and possibly superior to diclofenac)[30–33] and in promoting the healing of bruises and pain in muscles and joints.[33]

Also in chronic and sub-acute conditions the external use of the herb was able to[34]:

• reduce muscle pain, swelling and overstrain
• effectively treat arthralgia
• effectively treat enthesopathy (pathology occurring at the site of insertion of tendons or ligaments to bones or joint capsules)
• increase mobility in osteoarthritis of the knee[35]

Herbal combinations which included *Symphytum* improved the healing of gum damage due to chronic inflammation and/or dental surgery with no adverse side-effects.[36,37]

Medicinal uses
Gastro-intestinal tract
Used for inflamed and damaged tissue in this tract:

• bleeding gums
• pharyngitis
• oesophagitis
• gastritis
• peptic ulcers
• haematemesis
• ulcerative colitis
• diverticulitis

Externally
An ideal healing agent for all skin and musculoskeletal injuries applied externally over the site of deeper, damaged tissues and around injured skin:

• varicose ulcers
• wounds
• fractures
• hernias
• bruises
• sprains
• mastitis

As an adjunct in the treatment of:

• arthritis
• psoriasis
• eczema

Pharmacy
Three times daily

Infusion of dried herb	–	2–8 g
Tincture 1:5	–	2–5 ml (suggested guidelines)
Fluid Extract (25%)	–	2–8 ml (suggested guidelines)
Ointment or cream	–	10–15% w/w of root or leaves

For open wounds the herb is best applied as a compress or poultice. Although allantoin has poor water solubility[26] it is apparently extracted into cold water macerates[27] and is well absorbed through the skin.

Precautions and/or safety
The external preparations used in the above clinical trials were all very well tolerated.

Since the discovery that livestock that had eaten ragwort which contains PAs developed liver disease scientists have been interested in the potential human health effects of ingestion of these alkaloids. Plants other than comfrey are known to contain them—they are also found in members of the Asteraceae and Fabaceae families—but comfrey has been of particular interest because it has been used extensively both as a medicine and a food.

The scientific evidence against comfrey is largely based on animal experiments which showed a connection between liver abnormalities and the consumption of very large quantities of the herb. PAs have been well researched in the last few decades and it is now known that they are metabolised in the liver, being converted to pyrroles which increases their reactivity and therefore their potential to cause damage.[38] As the liver becomes damaged the alkaloids can go on to damage other tissues e.g. the lungs. Again using animal studies it seems that PAs may persist in the body, being re-released so that they can cause damage long after their initial ingestion.[39]

As far as the PAs in comfrey are concerned their total content varies with:

a) plant part—levels are ten times higher in root than in leaves
b) state of maturation—smaller leaves have higher levels than more mature ones[40]
c) species—content and type of alkaloid may be different[19]

The particular PAs in comfrey are not the toxic ones associated with reported PA poisoning[19] and the toxicity of *Symphytum* in humans needs to be assessed carefully. Firstly the whole herb is likely to behave differently from isolated alkaloids, sulphur-containing amino acids, which occur in quantity in comfrey, for example reduce their toxicity.[19,41] Secondly there is some uncertainty about the presence of the hepatotoxic PAs echimidine and lasiocarpine in *S. officinale*[19,42] and if one or both are present their levels are likely to be very low. The main comfrey PAs are based on retronecine which has low hepatotoxicity and indeed lycopsamine and intermedine have not shown toxicity even at high dose in animal models.[43] Thirdly the hepatotoxicity of *Symphytum* spp. has been based on a rat model and conversion of quantities of herb that would need to be ingested by humans to reach equivalent levels would be very difficult to achieve.[19] (The lowest dose of PAs from comfrey that could cause toxicity according to the World Health Organisation (1989) has been estimated at a very conservative 0.015 mg/kg this equates to 1 mg a day for a 70 kg person or 5 g of dried leaf or 25 ml of 1:5 extract.)

The potential effects of PAs is further complicated by the fact that different animal models have quite different susceptibilities to their toxicity—which animal model is likely to adequately represent human reactions?[19]

Liver function tests on long term comfrey users were normal even though some users had consumed up to 25 g per day of leaf for up to 30 years.[19]

To-date a very small number of human cases have been reported in the medical literature implicating comfrey as a causative factor in hepatic veno-occlusive disease[44] and these appeared in the decade around 1980, nothing has been reported recently. In the cases that have been reported and analysed the link between liver abnormalities and comfrey was not clearly established.[19] A variety of over-the-counter products of leaf and root were shown to contain measurable and variable quantities of hepatotoxic PAs which reflects a need for caution in using these preparations[45]. In countries where the internal use of comfrey is still allowed there is a voluntary restriction on using the root, leaf extracts only are now recommended.

The percutaneous absorption of PAs in toxic form appears to be negligible, again based on animal data.[17]

PAs have also been associated with carcinogenicity and mutagenicity although they have not been associated with human cancers to-date.[39] *In vitro* the isolated alkaloids of *S. officinale* were mutagenic to human lymphocytes at very high concentration only.[46]

Historical uses
Lung and urinary tract problems especially where associated with bleeding. Quinsy; whooping cough and consumption. Joint diseases; wounds and cuts; broken bones and "ruptures". Diarrhoea; dysentery and other "intestinal troubles" including ulcers of stomach and liver. Also used for "defective circulation" and anaemia. Externally to ease the pain of gout. Haemorrhoids; suppurating boils and abscesses; gangrenous ulcers. Historically the root was more highly prized than the leaves.

BRASSICACEAE

[Formerly known as Cruciferae]

The Brassicaceae consist of about 390 genera of annual or perennial plants, rarely small shrubs distributed throughout the world but mainly growing in temperate Northern Hemisphere climates. Some are grown for seed oil e.g. rape, others are used as condiments and some are important vegetables—broccoli, brussels sprouts, cabbage, cauliflower, Chinese cabbages, collards, cress, kale, radish, swedes, turnips, watercress; others are favourite garden flowers—alyssum, honesty, stocks, wallflowers.

- Many members of the family have taproots with a basal rosette of entire or pinnate leaves and one or more erect, leafy, branching stem/s terminating in a raceme
- Leaves are alternate, rarely opposite
- Flowers are bisexual, usually regular in a raceme or corymb
- Calyx is 4 free sepals in 2 whorls
- Corolla is 4 free petals alternating with the sepals, often clawed and forming a cross—hence Cruciferae
- Stamens are usually 6, 2 short and 4 long
- Ovary with 2 united carpels separated by a thin septum with seeds in 1–2 or more rows
- Fruit a pod-like capsule called a silique if long and narrow, and a silicle if broader

Medicinal plants in the Brassicaceae include; *Armoracia rusticana* (horseradish), *Brassica alba* (white mustard), *B. nigra* (black mustard), *Capsella bursa-pastoris* (shepherd's purse).

Members of the family contain mustard oil glycosides, (glucosinolates) which contain sulphur and are responsible for the hot, pungent taste and provide protection from bacteria, insects and fungi.

Armoracia rusticana

Horseradish

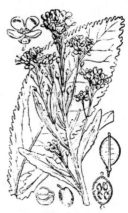

Family Brassicaceae

118

Description

A robust, glabrous perennial, 40–125 cm tall in flower, which dies back to tiny leaves in winter. *Roots*, long white and fleshy. *Basal leaves*, 30–50 cm, oval, toothed, long-stalked, dock-like; lower stem leaves often dissected in linear segments. *Flowers* numerous, white, 8–9 mm across, sweetly scented, borne in panicles on much branched stems. *Seeds* in 2 rows, almost spherical but which do not mature into viable seeds. Flowers in late spring to early summer.

Odour—pungent and irritant; taste—strong, acrid and slightly sweet.

Habitat and cultivation

Native to Asia and Europe, horseradish is grown as a condiment and is naturalized in many countries. Grown from root division, it prefers deep, rich, moist, well drained soil. It is dormant in winter. Once established it is difficult to eradicate. Drought and frost resistant.

Parts used

Root best used fresh, harvested when the plant is dormant in late autumn.

Active constituents

1) Glucosinolates (previously named thioglucosides) including sinigrin (about 83%), glucobrassicin (about 1%) and gluconasturtiin (about 11%).[1] These constituents are rapidly hydrolysed by the enzyme, myrosinase, released when the root is crushed, mainly to isothiocynates.[2] Sinigrin is metabolised to the essential oil allyl isothiocyanate[3] and gluconasturtiin to phenylethyl isothiocyanate. The isothiocyanates give the root its characteristic odour

Also contains asparagine, resin and small amounts of vanillic and gentisic acids.[4] A constituent related to co-enzyme Q and vitamin E, plastoquinone-9, has recently been isolated along with derivatives of β-sitosterol, diacylglycerides and fatty acids.[5]

Nutritional constituents

Vitamins: A, B complex, C (significant amounts) and P

Minerals: Calcium, iron, magnesium, phosphorus, potassium, boron, sulphur and sodium

Actions

1) Circulatory stimulant
2) Diaphoretic
3) Rubefacient
4) Diuretic
5) Antimicrobial
6) Vulnerary

Scientifc information

Although *Armoracia* has a long history of medicinal use there has been very little scientific investigation into the herb itself. It is less popular in modern herbal practice than it once was and it is now used mainly as a condiment.

The glucosinolates are considered to be relatively inert however the isothiocyanates derived from them are well absorbed and biochemically active. Consumption of Brassicas has shown corresponding rises in the level of serum isothiocyanates and it is these that are believed to offer cancer protection.[6,7]

Anti-oxidant and anti-inflammatory

Armoracia has been used both internally and externally for the treatment of musculo-skeletal and nerve inflammation.

In vitro—The main constituents have anti-oxidant activity[8-10] and they, as well as the whole extract, inhibit both COX-1 and COX-2 enzymes.[5]

Anticancer

In vitro—The herb as well as a number of individual constituents are antimutagenic and anticarcinogenic, partly at least, through enzyme modulation of carcinogens.[2,10] The main constituents protect DNA from oxidative damage,[9,11] and based on non-human cell models may decrease the level of spontaneous and irradiation-induced chromosome damage.[12]

Constituents also have a direct effect in inhibiting the growth of some cancer cell lines including colorectal,[5] myeloid leukaemia,[13] lung,[5] breast[11] and ovary.[11] In addition, they or their metabolites, may suppress the promotion of cancer cell development and also block oestrogen receptor sites in oestrogen-dependent cancer cells.[1]

In vivo—Epidemiological evidence suggests that the consumption of Brassicas, which are rich in glucosinolates, are preventative for colorectal cancer.[14]

Other
In vitro—Some of the isothiocynanate constituents have antimicrobial activity.[15]

Medicinal uses
Medicinal use of this herb relies primarily on historical and empirical use. *Armoracia*, like *Capsicum annuum*, was valued as a circulatory and digestive stimulant.

Cardiovascular system
• poor peripheral circulation
• fever

Respiratory tract
• asthma
• bronchial catarrh
• respiratory infections

Gastro-intestinal tract
• anorexia
• poor digestion

Urinary tract
Culpeper regarded this herb as a strong diuretic.

• urinary tract infections
• calculus
• oedema

Nervous system
• neuralgia

Musculo-skeletal system
• arthritis

Endocrine system
Like all glucosinolate containing foods *Armofacia* is goitrogenic, a property that may be used to treat

• hyperthyroidism

Externally
Extensively used for a number of internal and external problems by external application.

• chilblains
• bronchitis
• laryngitis
• pneumonia
• pleurisy
• indolent ulcers
• arthritis
• pericarditis
• sciatica
• rheumatism
• neuritis
• slow-healing wounds

Pharmacy
Three times daily

Infusion of fresh root	– 2–4 g
Fluid extract (50% ethanol)	– 3–5 ml
Syrup	– 5 ml

Syrup made by infusing 4 g fresh root in 30 ml water and adding double weight of sugar.

Externally can be applied as poultice, acetract or syrup. The glucosinolates behave like those found in mustard seed causing counter-irritation, bringing blood to the area of application and increasing the sense of heat. If left on the skin for too long the herb will eventually cause blistering.

CONTRAINDICATIONS—Hypothyroidism—the glucosinolates inhibit the absorption of iodine by the thyroid gland.[15]

Pharmacokinetics
Studies show that isothiocynates are produced in the gut, possibly with the help of gut flora or in uncooked Brassicas by myrosinase activity, and they reach peak plasma levels within 8 hours after ingestion. Some of these are further metabolised to amines, both being excreted via the kidneys some 2–12 hours later.[6,7]

Precautions and/or safety
Large doses can cause vomiting, diarrhoea, Gastro-intestinal-inflammation, cramps, paralysis, coma and death.

Historical uses

Colic; oliguria; scurvy; parasitic worms; paralysis; skin conditions; pertussis; persistent cough from influenza. Externally for "hard swellings" of liver and spleen; freckles. It was applied externally to slow healing wounds where the antimicrobial activity and circulatory stimulation would have been beneficial.

Capsella bursa-pastoris

Shepherd's purse, witches pouches

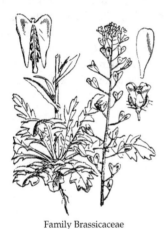

Family Brassicaceae

Description

An annual with an erect, branched stem 15–30 cm tall. *Lower leaves* petiolate, in a rosette, variable in shape from not lobed to runcinate-pinnatifid, 5–15 × 2–5 cm. Upper leaves alternate, clasping stems and sagittate at base, smaller leaves becoming entire. Leaves and stems both hairy. *Flowers* in racemes, 5–20 cm long, pedicels erect in flower and spreading in fruit. Sepals green or pinkish; petals white 2–2.5 × 0.7–1 mm, sometimes reduced or absent. Silicle narrowly or broadly triangular to heart-shaped, 5–10 × 4–7 mm with sharply keeled valves and reticulate veins, greenish brown. *Seeds* pale brown. Flowers and fruits most of the year.

Odour—faint and unpleasant; taste—somewhat acrid and bitter.

Habitat and cultivation

A European weed which is naturalised in other countries, growing in cultivated ground and waste land. It is grown from seed and self-sows freely. It is difficult to cultivate as it goes to seed very quickly.

Parts used

The herb. In Germany the herb, including the seed pods, is an official medicine. *Capsella* can be very variable in its physical appearance.

Active constituents

1) Flavonoids including rutinosides of luteolin and quercitin[16] and diosmin[17]
2) Glucosinolates including sinigrin[18]
3) Polypeptides, not yet characterised[19]

Also contains acids—fumaric[20] and bursic—and bases consisting of choline, acetylcholine, histamine and tyramine,[21] alkaloids possibly yohimbine and ergocristine[17] and volatile oil (approx. 0.02%).[22]

Nutritional constituents

Vitamins: A, C and K
Minerals: Calcium, iron, potassium (significant amounts), sodium, sulphur and zinc

Actions

1) Antihaemorrhagic
2) Urinary antiseptic
3) Antipyretic

Scientific information

Capsella has a centuries-long history of use both as a food and as a medicine. It is used in many cultures including Traditional Chinese and Ayurvedic medicine and was used during World War I as an anti-haemorrhagic (*Grieve*). It is approved by *German Commission E* for the treatment of menorrhagia, metrorrhagia and epistaxis.

As a widespread weed it has attracted interest for reasons other than its pharmacology. Much of the medicinal research was undertaken decades ago, using animal models.

It has been proposed as a bio-monitor for heavy metal pollution particularly for short term changes[23] and this indicates caution is needed in sourcing the herb for medicine making from urban areas.

The medicinal use of the herb relies largely on tradition. The constituents responsible for the accepted use as an antihaemorrhagic have not been identified but it seems unlikely to be due to acetylcholine.[24]

In vitro—*Capsella* is a good antimicrobial, the flavonoid and alkaloid fractions having the strongest and broadest activities.[17]

In Eastern countries the herb had been known as a remedy to treat cancer and research has identified fumaric acid has antitumour properties.[25]

Medicinal uses
Gastro-intestinal tract
• haematemesis
• diarrhoea

Urinary tract
• haematuria
• acute catarrhal cystitis

Reproductive tract
• menorrhagia—uterine haemorrhage (*BHP* specific)

Pharmacy
Three times daily
Infusion of dried herb   – 1–4 g
Fluid Extract (25%)   – 1–4 ml

Historical uses
Inward and outward wounds including haemoptysis; haemorrhoids; uterine cramps; irritation of, and catarrh in, the urinary tract; bound to wrists or feet for jaundice; as a poultice for external inflammations including rheumatic joints, also for bruising; juice used for earache and noises in the ears; inserted into the nose on cotton wool for nose bleeds; as an ointment for all wounds. In China it has been used as an anti-hypertensive.

BURSERACEAE

The Burseraceae or Torchwood family consist of about 600 species of aromatic, deciduous trees or shrubs of tropical and sub-tropical regions mostly North East Africa and Central America. Both frankincense *(Boswellia)*, and myrrh *(Commiphora)*, of the Bible belong to this family.

Commiphora molmol

Myrrh

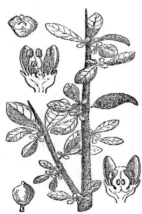

Family Burseraceae

Description

A stunted bush or low tree up to 2.75 m high with a thick trunk bearing numerous irregular knotted branches which divide into stout clustered branchlets each spreading out at right angles and terminating in a sharp thorn. *Leaves* few, trifoliate, obovate-oval, entire and glabrous. Lateral leaflets minute and terminal leaflets 1 cm long. *Flowers* small in terminal panicles.

Odour—harsh and aromatic; taste—bitter and acrid and sticks to teeth.

Habitat

It is a wild plant of Kenya, Ethiopia, Somalia and the Arabian peninsula growing on basaltic soil in very hot areas and is cultivated in east and north Africa.

Parts used

The oleo-resin gum which is discharged through the bark naturally or after cuts are made in it. Commercial myrrh may be derived from other species of *Commiphora*.[1] The resin is yellowish until exposed to the air when it oxidises to a reddish brown colour.

Active constituents[2]

1) Essential oil (7–17%) including:
   a) furanosesquiterpenes which give myrrh its characteristic odour—mainly furanoesudesma-1,3-diene[3] (up to 19%) also furanodiene-6-one,[4] methoxyfuranoguaia-9-ene-8-one,[5] lindesterene,[6] curzerenone; furanogermacranes including isofuranogermacrene
   b) sesquiterpenes including mainly curzerene and germacrone,[7] also β- and γ-elemene and eudesmol derivatives
   c) triterpenes
   d) monoterpenes including isolinalyl acetate
   Numerous constituents have been identified in the essential oil.
2) Gums (55–60%) including proteoglycans based largely on 4-methyl-glucuronogalactone. This fraction is water soluble
3) Bitter ("murr" is Arabic for "bitter")
4) Resin (25–40%) based on triterpenoids including commiphoric acids, commiphorinic acid and commiferin.[8] This fraction is soluble in 90% alcohol.

Some varieties of *Commiphora* notably *C. abyssinica* also contain sterols. Due to the common adulteration of *C. molmol* with other species its chemistry has become rather confused.

Actions

1) Antimicrobial
2) Astringent
3) Anti-inflammatory
4) Carminative
5) Anticatarrhal
6) Vulnerary
7) Antispasmodic
8) Expectorant

Scientific information

Commiphora molmol is regarded as a variety of *C. myrrha* and considered to produce the best quality myrrh. It has been known as a medicine since written records were first kept and has been an official medicine in many countries.[9] Its uses listed in pharmacopoeias include an astringent action on mucous membranes, a gargle/mouthwash for ulcers in mouth or pharynx and internally as a carminative.[9] *German Commission E* has approved its use for external inflammations of oral and pharyngeal mucosa.

A number of *Commiphora* species are used medicinally and it is probable that commercial myrrh is a mixture of these. There is a large body of scientific information based on these other species, which share some chemical similarities, and their pharmacology may prove to be similar, but to-date there is limited information on the species used in western medicine.

Antimicrobial

Modern attention on *C. molmol* has been based on the herb's use as an anti-trematode agent (it was historically used to treat worms). Since 2001 an extract of myrrh, consisting of 8 parts resin and 3.5 parts volatile oil, called *"Mirazid"*, has been marketed for the treatment of schistosomiasis.

In vitro—*Mirazid* was shown to directly affect the integrity of *Schistosoma mansoni* worms which may indicate the *in vivo* action of the extract.[10]

Myrrh has molluscicidal,[11] mosquitocidal,[12] larvicidal[13] and acaricidal[14] activities. The sesquiterpene fraction has antibacterial activity against *Escherichia coli, Staphylococcus aureus, Pseudomonas aeruginosa* and antifungal activity against *Candida albicans*.[15]

In vivo—A number of studies have presented impressive cure rates using *Mirazid* amongst patients infested with the gastro-intestinal parasites from the genera *Fasciola*,[16–19] *Dicrocoelium*,[20] *Schistosoma*[17,21–23] and *Heterophye*.[24] This preparation decreased immunoglobulin E and normalised interleukin levels in the monocytes of patients with fascioliasis.[25] It was effective and also considered safer than the conventional drug praziquantel.

Not all trials have endorsed the anti-parasitic efficacy of *Mirazid*.[26,27] This may be due to differences in dosage level and/or regime used and/or variations in parasitic strains encountered. Further investigation therefore seems to be required to establish the drug's usefulness.[28]

Other

In vitro—Myrrh oil has long been used in perfumery. It is anti-inflammatory through modulation of cytokine and prostaglandin production[29] and has moderate antioxidant activity.[30] The sesquiterpene fraction also has potential local anaesthetic activity.[15]

A reconstruction of an old 18th Century preparation of *Commiphora* spp., *Boswellia* spp., *Aloe* spp. and *Pistacia lentiscus* is anti-inflammatory, antiseptic and anti-oxidant.[31]

In vivo—A product containing myrrh and salt has been marketed as a dentifrice to protect gums.[32] *"Paradontax"* combines fluoride and bicarbonate with extract of myrrh, sage, *Echinacea*, chamomile and rhatany. It has been variously reported as significantly decreasing plaque and gingivitis and having no benefit over standard fluoride toothpaste.[33]

Myrrh is commonly used in Saudi Arabia in the treatment of diabetes.[34]

Medicinal uses
Respiratory tract
- catarrh
- common cold

Externally
The herb is most used as an external agent to counteract infections, reduce inflammation and as an anticatarrhal.

- sinusitis
- pharyngitis
- tonsillitis
- aphthous ulcers
- gingivitis

- fungal infections
- boils
- abrasions/inflammations

Pharmacy
Three times daily
Tincture 1:5   –   0.5–2 ml
The neat tincture can be applied externally.

For sinusitis apply over affected sinuses. As a gargle or mouthwash use 5 ml in a glass of warm water.

Precautions and/or safety
Clinical studies have shown myrrh is safe, it is approved for use as a flavouring by the U.S. *Food and Drug Administration.*

In vitro—The essential oil has very low cytotoxicity.[35] A few cases of allergic dermatitis from topical use have been reported.[36,37]

Interactions
There is one reported interaction between myrrh and warfarin in which the effect of the warfarin was apparently negated.[38]

Historical uses
Extremely long history of medicinal use mainly associated with ability to act as an anti-microbial. Antibiotic for keeping wine (Hebraic texts). To treat wounds and sores; as an embalming agent; for infected teeth; worms; infections of mouth and skin; coughs; chronic catarrh; TB. Was also considered an emmenagogue and therefore used for amenorrhoea. Commonly used in incense.

CANNABACEAE

This is a family of 2 genera, *Cannabis* and *Humulus*, and 4 species from temperate regions of the Northern Hemisphere. The plants are erect or climbing, annual or perennial, dioecious, scabrous and aromatic. They have opposite or alternate leaves which may be simple or palmately divided. The flowers are arranged in axillary inflorescences and are unisexual and apetalous.

Humulus lupulus

Hops

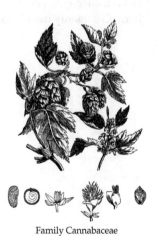

Family Cannabaceae

Description

A dioecious perennial climber with extensive roots, which dies down in winter. *Stems* striate with rough deflexed hairs, twining clockwise to 10 m. *Leaves* opposite, dark green, broadly ovate, either not lobed or 3–5-lobed; lobes acute to acuminate, serrate and sparsely hairy above and below, feeling rough to the touch. Petiole the same length as the lamina. Stipules either 2 per node divided in 2, or 4 per node and entire. *Flowers* without petals. Female flowers sessile, crowded and concentrated in persistent bracts which are triangular and green at first, elongating and turning yellowish to form the strobilus or hop at fruiting. Male flowers in loose axillary panicles, calyx ovate, triangular, green and hairy. Perianth 5-numerous. Achenes ovate-ellipsoid, covered by the glandular calyx. Flowers from late summer and fruits in early autumn.

Habitat and cultivation

Native to Europe, Western and Central Asia, hops are cultivated and naturalised in most countries. Prefers an open sunny situation with rich moist soils. They need extensive support because of their long stems. May be propagated by seed or from root cuttings in spring. Dies back in winter. Frost resistant but drought tender.

Parts used
The female flowers or strobili harvested when present in late summer and autumn.

Active constituents
1) Bitter principle (15–20%), resinous, and containing derivatives of phloroglucinol glucopyranosides—the iso-acids, called α-acids (humulones) and β-acids (lupulones), the former group includes humulone, cohumulone, adhumulone and the latter lupulone.[1-5] The acids degrade to new chemicals on storage, including 2-methyl-3-butene-2-ol,[6] isovaleric acid (3-methylbutanoic acid) and 2-methylpropanoic acid
2) Volatile oil (0.3–1%) mainly mono- and sesquiterpenes[7,8]—myrcene, humulene, caryophyllene, linalool, β-farnesene[9] and 3-methylbut-2-ene-1-al.[10] Improved separation techniques have identified many constituents in this fraction,[11] possibly in excess of 1000[12]
3) Flavonoids up to 0.8%—including a number of prenylflavonoid chalcones[13] predominantly xanthohumol[14] (80–90%)[15] and xanthohumol B[16] and C[17] and prenylflavanones[18] 8-prenylnaringenin[19] and isoxanthohumol.[20] Also kaempferol, quercitin, rutin, isoquercitrin and astragalin[21]
4) Tannin polyphenols (2–4%) including trans-resveratrol and piceid isomers.[22] Procyanidins containing catechin and epicatechin ranging from dimers to octamers have been reported[23,24]

Also phenolic acids (ferulic and chlorogenic), choline, asparagine, tri-methylamine, diphenylmethanol,[25] tribenzylamine,[25] pectin[26] and sitosterol.[20]

The constituents of *Humulus* vary according to the cultivar.[27,28] The genetic make-up, and to some extent the constituents, vary with geographical location[29] and between wild and cultivated plants.[30,31] In addition the plant exhibits polyploidy (diploid, triploid or tetraploid) and aneuploidy (extra or missing chromosomes).[32]

The bitter acids and prenylflavonoids increase in concentration as the flowers mature.[33]

Nutritional constituents
Vitamins: B-complex
Minerals: Magnesium, zinc, copper and traces of iodine, manganese, iron and sodium

Actions
1) Sedative
2) Soporific
3) Spasmolytic
4) Antibacterial (topically)
5) Diuretic
6) Bitter

Scientific information
The medicinal use of hops can be tracked back to the 9th century. It has been used in different cultures across the world mainly as a sedative and bitter, the latter being its official listed use in the *British Pharmacopoeia*.[34] *German Commission E* approved uses are for anxiety, restlessness and as a sedative.

A number of the constituents of *Humulus* have been well studied, chemically and physiologically, due to their importance in the brewing industry. New research has focused on the possible health benefits of *Humulus* extracts in the treatment of female reproductive tract problems and cancers.

Anticancer
In vitro—In the last decade studies have shown hops and/or some of its constituents have a variety of anticancer activities[35] including:-

- cytotoxicity and inhibition of the growth of cancer cell lines including breast, colon, ovary, prostate and leukaemia[36-40]
- chemo-protective and anti-mutagenic activity inhibiting cytochrome activation of food carcinogens[41] and protection of DNA from chemical damage by induction of detoxification enzymes[42,43]
- induced differentiation in cancer cells[35,39]
- anti-oxidant and anti-inflammatory activities (see below)
- inhibition of angiogenesis[44]
- inhibition of invasiveness of cancer cells[45]
- increased cancer cell apoptosis[46]

The phyto-oestrogenic constituents may have raised concern as potential stimulants of hormone-dependent cancers. However they not only inhibit the aromatase production of oestrogen but also decrease breast cancer cell proliferation and induce their apoptosis.[47]

In vivo—To date the only *in vivo* evidence of an anticancer effect is based on epidemiologic studies which have suggested that diets rich in phyto-oestrogens may protect women against breast cancer.[36]

Oestrogenic

It has long been known that *Humulus* had an oestrogen-like activity and one of the strongest phyto-oestrogens has been identified as 8-prenyl-naringenin.[48] Isoxanthohumol can be metabolised to 8-prenylnaringenin by gut flora *in vivo*.[49]

In vitro—*Humulus* and other herbs with phyto-oestrogenic activity are seen as safe alternatives to hormone replacement therapy. The whole extract and 8-prenylnaringenin bind quite strongly to both α- and β-oestrogen receptor sites[50] performing at least as well as phyto-oestrogens from red clover (*Trifolium pratense*).[51] Studies indicate that *Humulus* may have benefit for preventing osteoporosis.[52]

Neither the extract or its constituents have androgenic or progestogenic activity.[53,54]

In vivo—*Humulus* alone or in combination with other herbs was beneficial in the treatment of menopausal symptoms, giving a significant improvement in hot flushes, sleep and mental well being.[55,56]

Anti-inflammatory

In vitro—The whole extract and phloroglucinol fraction have anti-inflammatory activity *via* inhibition of the COX enzymes.[57,58] A high α-acid extract, like ibuprofen, effectively inhibits COX-2 enzyme activity but with less of an inhibitory effect on COX-1 suggesting it would be less likely to have associated gastro-intestinal disturbances whilst still being anti-inflammatory.[58]

In vivo—The reduced α-acids from *Humulus* were used in combination with extracts of *Rosmarinus officinalis* and oleanolic acid to treat patients with osteoarthritis, rheumatoid arthritis or fibromyalgia

giving significant improvement in the former two conditions.[59]

Antimicrobial

Humulus has been traditionally used to treat infectious conditions. With the improved isolation of its constituents scientific studies are verifying activity in a number of fractions.

In vitro—Constituents are:

- effectively antibacterial against *Staphylococcus aureus*, *Streptococcus mutans*, *Bacillus subtilis* and *Mycobacterium fortuitum*
- antiviral against a number of organisims including cytomegalovirus, HSV-1 and 2 and HIV-1 (at non-cytotoxic levels)
- antifungal against *Trichophyton* spp.[60-64]

Constituents of hops, particularly xanthohumol are also active against strains of *Plasmodium falciparum* including those resistant to chloroquine.[62,65]

In addition the polyphenol fraction binds *Vibrio cholerae* and *Escherichia coli* enterotoxins.[66]

Sedative

The better known use for hops involves its effects on the central nervous system.

In vitro—A combination of valerian and hops interacts with melatonin and serotonin receptors.[67] The alpha acids[68] and 2-methyl-3-butene-2-ol are credited with at least some of the sedative properties but the latter may not be present in significant amounts.[69]

In vivo—Hops' effect on the nervous system has been subject to trials as follows:-

- Sleep—*Humulus* and *Melissa* in combination was well-tolerated and effective at improving sleep quality.[70] A hopvalerian combination compared favourably with diphenhydramine in treating mild insomnia and was preferred by participants to the pharmaceutical.[71] It also measured up favourably to benzodiazepines for acute insomnia whilst having none of the withdrawal problems or latent impaired performance associated with this class of drugs[72,73]

- Relaxant—A preparation containing *Humulus* in combination with *Lavandula officinalis* oil, *Melissa officinalis* and *Avena sativa* showed the blend produced changes in brain waves consistent with a state of relaxation and indicating benefits for those coping with mental stress[74]
- Caffeine antidote—Valerian and hops in combination were able to counter caffeine's stimulant effect[75]

Other

In vitro—Constituents, particularly the prenylflavonoids, but also the proanthocyanidins are antioxidant.[39,76-79]

In vivo—*Humulus* in combination with other herbs was effective in the treatment of hyposecretion and chronic inflammation of liver and/or gall bladder.[80]

The bitter α-acid, isohumulone, aids the regulation of fatty acid and carbohydrate metabolism and reduces blood glucose levels in type 2 diabetes.[81] This component is also likely to give the herb its digestive stimulant action.

Medicinal uses

Cardiovascular system
- Palpitations of neurogenic origin

Respiratory tract
- nervous coughs
- irritable coughs (possibly asthma)

Gastro-intestinal tract
- irritable bowel syndrome
- mucous colitis
- nervous dyspepsia
- inflammatory bowel disease
- anorexia

Urinary tract
- irritable bladder

Nervous system
The main use of the herb is due to its ability to influence nervous tension:

- insomnia
- neuralgia

- excitability
- priapism
- restlessness and sleep disorders

Specific indication BHP—restlessness associated with nervous tension headaches and/or indigestion.

Reproductive tract
- dysmenorrhoea
- amenorrhoea
- premature ejaculation
- anaphrodisiac in men

May have a use in the treatment of menopausal symptoms.

Externally
- crural ulcers

Pharmacy

Infusion of dried herb	–	0.5–1 g to aid sleep, or Three times daily
Infusion of dried herb	–	1–2 g
Tincture 1:5 (60%)	–	1–2 ml
Fluid Extract (45%)	–	0.5–1 ml

Fresh dried hops can also be used in a pillow to aid sleep as their scent is carried by the olfactory nerve directly to the limbic system of the brain.

CONTRAINDICATIONS—Depression. There is no science to explain this, however it may be an empirical finding or be based on the herb's depressant effect on the central nervous system.

Pharmacokinetics

In vitro—Studies have found it is possible that levels of 8-prenylnaringenin are increased by intestinal flora[82] and by enzymes present in liver microsomes.[83] Microsomal enzymes also convert 8-prenylnaringenin into metabolites that have oestrogenic potential.[84]

Precautions and/or safety

Symptoms very like those for which *Humulus* is used remedially have sometimes been reported by people who work in contact with them.

Hop farmers show a small incidence of contact dermatitis[85-87] and allergy to the dust[88] however it seems to have lower levels of micro-organisms and endotoxins than that found in other types of farming dust![89] A single case of systemic allergy to wild hops resulting in urticaria, arthralgia and fever has also been reported.[90]

Commercial hops production involves the use of pesticides and these residues have been identified in dried strobili and their extracts.[91,92]

To-date there are no known health problems associated with high phyto-oestrogen diets, and some evidence to suggest they are beneficial, nor are there reports of foetal problems due to their use by pregnant women.[93]

Interactions
The prenylflavonoids can affect the activity of cytochrome P450 notably inhibiting CYP1A1, CYP1B1 and CYP1A2 *in vitro*. Tests so far have established the herb has a positive benefit on cytochrome activity by inhibiting their activation of potential carcinogens.[94] However although to date no drug/herb interactions have been noted drugs metabolised through these particular enzymes may be affected *in vivo*.

Historical uses
To open obstructions of liver and spleen; to "clean" blood; to open bowels; to flush kidney stones. As a depurative for scabs and itch and for sores; tetters and ringworm. As an anthelmintic. In hysteria; delirium and delirium tremens; to soothe inflammation and aid sleep; heart disease; fits; irritable bladder; as a pillow for earache and toothache. Externally for inflammation; neuralgia; rheumatic pains; boils; bruises and gatherings.

CAPRIFOLIACEAE

The Caprifoliaceae or honeysuckle family consists of about 12–15 genera of shrubs or sometimes woody climbers mostly native to temperate regions.

- Leaves opposite, simple or pinnate
- Flowers bisexual, either few and in cymes or many in flat-topped or rounded clusters. Calyx 4–5-toothed, corolla 4–5-lobed, sometimes irregular; stamens 4–5, ovary usually 1–5-celled
- Fruit a berry, drupe, achene or capsule

Lonicera, *Sambucus* and *Viburnum* are medicinal genera in this family.

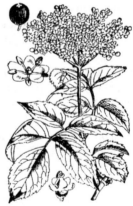

Family Caprifoliaceae

Sambucus nigra

Elder, European elder

Description
Deciduous shrub or small tree to 6 m tall. Bark brownish-grey and cork-like. Vegetative shoots contain pith. *Leaves* pinnate, 3–9 leaflets, ovate, ovate-elliptic or ovate-lanceolate, 2.5–9 cm long. Matt green or green and gold in *S. nigra* "Aurea". *Flowers* regular, in large, flat-topped cymes up to 21 cm in diameter. Calyx very narrow. Corolla 4–4.5 mm, creamy-white, 5 lobed. Anthers cream. *Fruit* a fleshy, globose, black drupe. Flowers in late spring to mid-summer and fruits in late summer to early autumn.

Odour of flowers—faint and characteristic; taste—mucilaginous and sweet. Odour of fruit—characteristic; taste—sweet and sour.

Habitat and cultivation
Native to Europe and Britain, elder grows wild in countries with cooler climates. Easily grown

131

from cuttings or may self-sow. Prefers moist, rich soil and shady situations but will grow in full sun. Drought tender, frost resistant.

Parts used

The flowers are the main medicinal part although in recent time the fruit extracts are also being used. Traditionally, both flowers and fruit, as well as leaves and inner bark have been medicines. Flowers are gathered as they open in early summer. The fruit is harvested when ripe in autumn; the inner bark in early spring before the leaves appear; the leaves in spring.

Active constituents

Flowers[1]

1) Flavonoids (0.8–3%) including rutin,[2] isorhamnetin,[3] hyperoside, isoquercitrin, astragalin[4] and free quercetin and kaempferol
2) Phenolic acids (approx. 3%)—chlorogenic, p-coumaric and caffeic acids
3) Triterpenes (approx. 1%) mainly ursolic and oleanolic acids, also α- and β-amyrin and lupeol[2]
4) Oils:
   a) volatile (up to 0.2%) 76 compounds have been isolated mainly terpenoids[5]
   b) fixed oil rich in free fatty acids, mainly palmitic
5) Sterols (about 0.1%) mainly β-sitosterol, campesterol and stigmasterol[2]

The flowers are rich in minerals (8–9%) especially potassium. They also contain some cyanogenic glycosides,[6] mucilage and tannins.

Leaves[7]

1) Triterpenes similar to those in the flowers
2) Cyanogenic glycosides—sambunigrin
3) Flavonoids—rutin and quercitin

Also fatty acids, lignans, phenolic glycosides and tannins.

Bark

1) Phytohaemagglutinins
2) Enzyme called nigrin-b[8]
3) Tannins
4) Valeric acid[9]

Fruit[10]

1) Flavonoids including quercetin, hyperoside and rutin[11]
2) Anthocyanins (up to 1%)[11–13]
3) Cyanogenic glycosides including sambunigrin[14]

Also contains viburnic acid, a phytohaemagglutinin protein (a lectin),[15,16] vitamin A and rich in vitamin C.[11]

Actions

Flowers

1) Diaphoretic
2) Diuretic
3) Anticatarrhal
4) Anti-inflammatory

Bark was used as a purgative, diuretic and expectorant; leaves as a vulnerary, purgative, expectorant and diuretic; fruit as a sudorific, diuretic, emetic, alterative and laxative.

Scientific information

Records of elder's medicinal use date back over a thousand years. The flowers are listed as a vehicle for skin and eye lotions[17] and their internal use for the treatment of colds has been approved by *German Commision E*.

Modern research has concentrated on examining the properties of the fruit.

Antimicrobial

In vitro—The flowers may have antiviral potential, an extract consisting of *Hypericum, Saponaria officinalis* and *Sambucus* flowers inhibited HSV-1 and some strains of influenza virus.[18]

Fruit—extracts were effective at inhibiting the proliferation of 10 strains of influenza virus types A and B,[19] HIV and HSV-1. The antiviral action seems to be due to the ability of the agglutinin to interact with viral coat-protein thus preventing the virus from entering cells and replicating.[20] In addition cytokine production was increased *ex vivo* suggesting the fruit has a potential immunomodulating activity.[21,22]

The bark is used in Italy as a treatment for HSV-1 and herpes zoster and using feline immunodeficiency virus as a model for HIV it showed susceptibility to this antiviral activity.[23]

In vivo—*Sambucus* has traditionally been used for treating colds. A clinical trial tested the efficacy of elderberry syrup in the treatment of influenza and found it reduced both duration and symptoms effectively.[21,24]

Other

In vitro—Flowers and leaves have potent anti-inflammatory activity[25,26] this has been attributed in part at least to ursolic acid.

Anthocyanins from the fruit demonstrate very strong free-radical scavenging activity[27] protecting endothelial cells from oxidative stress[20] and the whole fruit can inhibit biochemical activities that are associated with initiation and promotion of cancer including COX-2 inhibition.[13]

Nigrin-b is capable of inactivating ribosomes and therefore preventing protein synthesis and may have a future use in cancer chemotherapy particularly as it is non-toxic.[8] The protein agglutinin and nigrin-b are chemically similar.[16]

Diuretic action has been associated more with bark, fruit and leaves and it may be that the high potassium content favours urinary excretion as in *Taraxacum officinale*.

In vivo—The diaphoretic action of the flowers has been demonstrated in healthy subjects by inducing increased sweat gland activity in response to heat.[1] There are no other clinical trials on the therapeutic use of *Sambucus*.

It is still a primary phyto-medicine in central Italy the leaves are used to treat wounds and burns, the flowers for coughs, asthma and externally for eye inflammation.[28] *Weiss* suggests the flowers are useful in increasing non-specific immune function and cooked/heated juice or a puree of elderberries may be a good remedy for long-standing rheumatism, neuralgia and sciatica.

Medicinal uses

Respiratory tract

This is the system in which the herb is mainly used for its ability to help with mucus, fever and inflammation:

- influenza
- lung congestion
- colds (*BHP* specific)
- chronic nasal catarrh with deafness
- dry coughs
- feverish conditions
- sinusitis

Gastro-intestinal tract
- mild laxative effect
- diarrhoea (will regulate extremes of bowel function)

Pharmacy

Three times daily

Infusion of dried flowers	– 3–5 g
Tincture 1:5 (25%)	– 10–25 ml
Fluid Extract (25%)	– 3–5 ml

Also used in syrups or robs for coughs. Commercial *Sambucus* syrup used in above studies contained 38% fruit extract. For diaphoresis best taken as a hot infusion.

Pharmacokinetics

The anthocyanins in the fruit are absorbed intact from the gastro-intestinal tract, are measurable in the blood half an hour after ingestion[29] and excreted in urine within hours.[30] Studies suggest they may have poor bio-availability.[31]

Precautions and/or safety

Unripe fruit can cause diarrhoea, nausea and vomiting. Elder spreads easily and can grow in landfill sites contaminated with cadmium. This may concentrate in the pollen, the fruit has much lower levels[32] and the leaves take up very minimal amounts.[33]

A very small percentage (possibly 0.6%) of allergic individuals show allergy to elder pollen, flowers and berries, this is probably due to the protein (lectin) component.[34]

Historical uses

For phlegm; choler (especially the inner bark). The berries in rheumatism; syphilis; asthma and dropsy and juice used as drops for earache. The root and berries boiled in wine as an emmenagogue. The juice of the leaves sniffed to purge the brain! The distilled water of the flowers used for freckles; morphew; headaches due to a cold cause. A water extract of the flowers or leaves was used for ulcers or sores; for red eyes (as an eyewash); to bathe the hands in palsies. An ointment of the leaves, for bruises; sprains; chilblains; wounds; piles; tumours; swellings. As an insecticide (decoction of the leaves). The flowers for scarlet fever; measles.

Viburnum opulus

Cramp bark, guelder rose

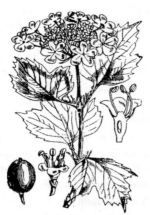

Family Caprifoliaceae

Description
A deciduous shrub to 4 m, with hairless greyish bark. *Leaves* oval, 5–8 cm, usually with three rather deep, irregularly toothed and long-pointed lobes, hairless above. *Flowers* grow in conspicuous flat-topped lax clusters, 5–10 cm across, and are white and of unequal size. The outermost flowers are sterile and some are 1.5–2 cm across—more than twice the size of the innermost flowers. Inner flowers are fertile, about 6 mm across. They are pinkish-white in the bud becoming yellowish-cream as they open. These are followed by glossy, red fruit. Flowers from early to mid-summer, their odour is peppery and sweet. N.B. fresh fruit is POISONOUS.

Habitat and cultivation
Native to all Europe, North Africa and Northern Asia on wet loamy soils in damp woods and hedges. Cultivated and sometimes naturalized elsewhere. Grown from seed or hardwood cuttings. A cultivar *V. opulus* "Roseum", the snowball tree, is common in gardens but has no established medicinal use. Frost resistant but drought tender.

Parts used
The bark of the stem.

Active constituents[10]
1) Bitter—viburnin
2) Valeric acid
3) Salicosides
4) Tannins mainly catechins[35]
5) Hydroquinones including arbutin and methylarbutin
6) Coumarins including scopoletin and scopoline[36]

Also contains resin. Viopudial was identified in 1972 from *Viburnum opulus* but nothing further on its chemistry has appeared since then[37] and it is likely it has been identified as one of the other constituents.

Actions
1) Spasmolytic
2) Sedative
3) Astringent

Nutritional constituents
Minerals: Calcium, potassium, magnesium, phosphorus and iron

Scientific information
V. opulus and *V. prunifolium* were listed in the *United States Pharmacopoeia* of the 19th Century as uterine relaxants and general antispasmodics.[38] *V. opulus* was used by the orthodox profession to treat asthma, hysteria, convulsions, tetanus, palpitations, heart disease and rheumatism. There are almost no studies that have been conducted in recent times. These two *Viburnum's* have been considered interchangeable.

Valeric acid also occurs in the volatile oil fraction of *Valeriana* and is considered sedative (see *Valeriana officinalis*). The salicosides are based on salicylic acid as found in *Filipendula ulmaria* and *Salix* spp. The hydroquinones are like those found in *Arctostaphylos* and should therefore have an antiseptic action in the urinary tract.

In vitro—Older animal-based studies verified that both *Viburnum* species contained at least 4 constituents with an action specific for uterine muscle.[38]

In vivo—The only recent trial involved *V. opulus* in a proprietary capsule with a large number of other herbs which effectively treated hot flushes. It would be very difficult to identify how effective *Viburnum* itself was in this formula.[39]

Medicinal uses

Viburnum opulus has been used primarily as a smooth and skeletal muscle relaxant having been applied to all cases where there is muscular tension.

Cardiovascular system
- hypertension

Respiratory tract
- asthma
- pertussis

Gastro-intestinal tract
- colic
- irritable bowel syndrome
- cholecystalgia
- dysphagia
- nervous dyspepsia

Urinary tract
- urinary spasm (stones)
- enuresis in children

Nervous system
- as a sedative
- migraine

Reproductive tract
- dysmenorrhoea
- threatened miscarriage
- menopausal metrorrhagia

Musculoskeletal
- spasmodic muscular cramps

BHP specific for cramps and pain in ovaries and uterus.

Externally
V. opulus can be applied as an embrocation or lotion as indicated above to treat:

- muscle spasms

Pharmacy
Three times daily

Decoction	– 2–4 g
Tincture 1:5 (45%)	– 5–10 ml
Fluid Extract (25%)	– 2–4 ml

Historical uses
See under Scientific information.

Viburnum prunifolium

Black haw

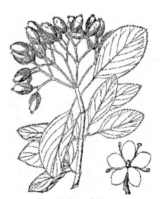

Family Caprifoliaceae

Description
A deciduous shrub or tree up to 6 × 3 m. Trunk erect and branching. *Leaves* opposite, elliptic to ovate, finely toothed, smooth, dull green. *Flowers* small, white, in flat cymes about 10 cm across. *Fruit* blueblack berries, edible after frost. Flowers in spring.

Habitat and cultivation
Native to North America from Connecticut to Florida, Texas to East Kansas in bogs or woodland. Propagated by stratified seed or from cuttings. Frost and drought resistant.

Parts used
The bark of root or stem.

Active constituents[10]
1) Bitter—viburnin
2) Valeric acid
3) Salicin
4) Tannins
5) Triterpenoids including ursolic acid, α- and β-amyrin and oleanolic acid
6) Coumarins including scopoletin[40]

Also contains 1–2 methyl 2,3-dibutyl hemi-melllitate,[41] amentoflavone (a biflavonoid), a trace of volatile oil, resin, arbutin and a number of organic acids.

Actions
1) Uterine sedative
2) Spasmolytic
3) Anti-asthmatic
4) Hypotensive
5) Astringent
6) Antidiarrhoeal

Scientific information
Viburnum prunifolium has been an official preparation (see above). The greater list of constituents probably reflects the greater level of investigation into the herb. It seems to have enjoyed a better reputation than *V. opulus* and a number of papers in the *Lancet* in the late 19th Century attest to its efficacy. There is very little recent research available.

In vitro and *in vivo*—Salicin was not found to inhibit prostaglandin induced uterine muscle contractions.[42]

Amentoflavone has a number of physiological actions—see Appendix III.

This species is mainly used in the female reproductive tract but could be used interchangeably with *V. opulus*.

Medicinal uses
Respiratory tract
As a spasmolytic and anti-asthmatic agent it is used in the treatment of:

• asthma

Reproductive tract
• dysmenorrhoea
• false labour pains
• threatened miscarriage
• metrorrhagia
• post-partum pain
• post-partum haemorrhage

BHP specific is threatened miscarriage with a rise in arterial tension.

Pharmacy
Three times daily
Decoction of dried herb   – 2.5–5 g
Tincture 1:5 (70%)   – 5–10 ml
Fluid Extract (70%)   – 4–8 ml

Historical uses
Disturbance of heart, stomach and nervous system associated with menstruation.

CARYOPHYLLACEAE

The Caryophyllaceae consist of about 70 genera of plants. The stems are often swollen at the nodes. Leaves opposite, simple and entire, with parallel veins. Flowers in terminal cymes or solitary, regular. Herbs in this family include: *Dianthus, Hernaria, Saponaria* and *Stellaria*.

Stellaria media

Chickweed

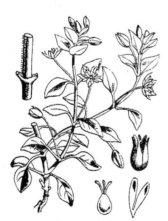

Family Caryophyllaceae

Description
An annual with a fine tap root, forming a loose mat. *Stems* weak, ascending, branching, 15–40 cm long with 1 line of hairs running up the stem and changing sides at each leaf node. *Leaves* opposite, ovate to broadly lanceolate, pointed, with short hairs around the margins, 5–40 × 5–15 mm. Lower leaf stalks about the same length as leaves, but almost absent in upper leaves. *Inflorescence* terminal, cymose and usually lax, with 3–15 flowers. Flower stalks slender with 1 line of hairs. *Sepals* narrow lanceolate, 4–6 mm long, hairy outside. Petals, white, a little smaller or a little larger than sepals. Stamens 3–5. *Capsule*, narrow ovoid about the same size as the calyx. Seeds many, tiny, yellowish brown. Flowers and fruits more or less all year round in both hemispheres, depending on the weather, but specifically from midwinter to mid-summer.

Habitat and cultivation
Native to Europe and naturalized other countries. It grows from seed as a garden weed in cooler weather. It self-sows readily and is frost resistant and drought tender.

Parts used
The herb harvested during or just prior to flowering.

137

Active constituents
1) Saponins
2) Coumarins
3) Flavonoids including isovitexin and apigenin derivatives[1,2]
4) Volatile oil including borneol, menthol, linalool, 1,8-cineole and caryophyllene[3]

Also contains carboxylic acids (triacontanoic acid),[3] triterpenoids (sitosterol),[3] hydrocarbons (hentricontane, pentacosanol)[4] and lipids including γ-linolenic acid and octadecatetraenoic acids.[5]

Nutritional constituents
Vitamins: A (carotenoids),[6] B complex, C (150–350 mg per 100 g) and D
Minerals: Rich in iron, copper, calcium, sodium and some manganese, phosphorus and zinc

Actions
1) Antirheumatic

Externally
2) Antipruritic
3) Vulnerary
4) Emollient

Scientific information
In the past chickweed enjoyed more extensive use than it does in modern practice.

In vitro—It is a strong inhibitor of xanthine oxidase and has moderate anti-oxidant properties, it may be of value in the treatment of hyperuricaemia and gout.[7]

In vivo—The use of the herb is traditional and anecdotal. It is most frequently used in modern practice for external applications but is prized by some herbalists for its nutritional value. *Weiss* did not find *Stellaria* effective in the treatment of rheumatic conditions.

Medicinal uses
Externally
• itches
• eczema
• psoriasis
• abscesses
• indolent ulcers
• boils
• cuts
• bruises
• carbuncles
• wounds

BHP specific for pruritic skin conditions.

Pharmacy
Three times daily

Infusion of dried herb	– 1–5 g
Tincture 1:5 (45%)	– 2–10 ml
Liquid Extract (25%)	– 1–5 ml

Ointment 1:5 in base material.

The herb is used as a cream, poultice or compress. It may be juiced and employed directly, diluted or used as an infusion. Can be eaten fresh in salads.

Precautions and/or safety
A small percentage of individuals tested, including those with no known allergies, showed an allergic or skin irritant reaction to *Stellaria* apparently due to its essential oil.[8,9] A single case of erythema multiforme, in a patient with a previous history of the condition developed after patch testing with the fresh herb.[3]

Historical uses
Externally applied to liver inflammation; cramps; convulsions; palsy; eye inflammations; haemorrhoids; to heal sinews. Internally for hydrophobia (in combination); scurvy; constipation; coughs; hoarseness; obesity.

CLUSIACEAE

This is a family of 40–50 genera of trees, shrubs and herbs often with resinous sap and translucent black or red glands. They mostly come from tropical and subtropical regions except for the mainly temperate genus *Hypericum*.

- The leaves are simple, and without stipules, usually opposite, rarely alternate or whorled
- The flowers are mostly in terminal, cymose panicles and have 2–6 sepals and petals, and numerous stamens
- The fruit is a capsule, berry or drupe

This family has also been known as Guttiferae and sometimes the genus *Hypericum* has been placed with others in a separate family Hypericaceae.

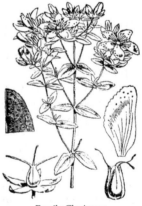

Family Clusiaceae

Hypericum perforatum

St John's wort

Description

A glabrous perennial growing to 1 m high, with slender rhizomes. *Stems* erect, 2-lined and woody at the base, dying back in autumn. *Leaves* opposite, sessile, 10–27 × 1–8 mm, lanceolate to ovate or oblong, dotted with numerous tiny pellucid glands. *Inflorescence* a terminal panicle of dense many-flowered, corymbose cymes with bracts similar to upper leaves. Corolla 8–20 mm in diameter, golden yellow scattered with numerous black glands. Petals obovate, much larger than sepals. Stamens in 3 bundles smaller than or equal to petals, 3 styles. *Capsule* narrow-ovoid, 6–8 mm long, dry. Seeds 0.8–1.3 mm long, rugose. Flowers from mid-summer to autumn.

There is considerable variation in plants of *Hypericum perforatum* but stems should always be

2-lined and leaves should have pellucid, not black, glands.

Odour—aromatic and balsamic; taste—bitter, acrid.

Habitat and cultivation
Originally from Europe, Western Asia and North Africa, St. John's wort is a very common weed in tussock grasslands, pasture, roadsides, riverbeds and waste places. It is declared noxious in some countries because it causes severe photosensitivity in stock that eat it. It is grown from seed and when the flowering stems die back the prostrate, barren reddish leafy shoots remain and form dense mats which may be divided. It prefers an open sunny situation and will die if it becomes overgrown. It is frost resistant but drought tender.

Parts used
The herb gathered during flowering.

Active constituents[1-7]

1) Naphthodianthrones (0.08–0.4%) including hypericin, pseudohypericin, protohypericin and protopseudohypericin. The former two are converted from the latter two in the presence of light.[8] The level of pseudohypercin is twice that of hypericin in the plant[9]
2) Phloroglucinols (up to 4%) including hyperforin and adhyperforin. These are unstable and oxidise to a large extent in the presence of light.[10] Also identified hyperfoliatin[11] and various degradation products of hyperforin[12-14]
3) Flavonoids (2–4%) including hyperoside, rutin, isoquercitrin, quercitrin, avicularin, quercetin[15,16] and the biflavonoids biapigenin,[17] amentoflavone[18] and miquelianin.[19] (Rutin levels appear to be variable and may not always be present).[20]
4) Volatile oil—sesquiterpenes and monoterpenes including caryophyllene, n-alkanes, α- and β-pinene[21]
5) Tannins of catechin type (up to 15%) and procyanidins[22]

Also alkanes, fatty acids, waxy esters,[23] coumarins, caffeic and chlorogenic acids and a number of other phenolic constituents,[24] citric and malic acids, resin and pectin. A diterpene, chromone, phytol, bisanthraquinone glycosides, serotonin and melatonin have also been reported.[25-27]

Hypericin is highest in the flowers and flavonoids are highest in the leaves when the flowers are in full bloom.[28] The time of harvest has the greatest effect on the chemical make-up of the final extract.[29] Plants grown at higher temperatures have a higher concentration of some naphthodianthrones[30] and water availability,[31] geographical area[32] and habitat[29] also alter the levels of major constituents.

Actions
1) Anxiolytic
2) Antidepressant
3) Anti-inflammatory
4) Astringent
5) Antiviral
6) Sedative
Topically:
7) Vulnerary
8) Analgesic
9) Antimicrobial

Nutritional constituents
Vitamins: A and C
Minerals: Iron, calcium, magnesium, zinc, sodium, manganese, copper, chromium and potassium[33,34]

Scientific information
Hypericum was part of traditional Greek medicine and has been used for nervous system disorders since the time of Paracelsus in the 16th century. Depression is amongst the most commonly diagnosed health problems today. As a result *Hypericum* has become one of the best known and studied medicinal herbs as well as one of the most prescribed complementary medicines. There is now a large body of clinical evidence supporting its use in the treatment of depression. In 1998 a standardised *Hypericum* extract was officially approved for use in the treatment of mild to moderate depression in Austria and Germany where it is used extensively to treat this condition in all age groups.[35] *German Commission E* has approved its internal use for

the treatment of psychovegetative disturbances, depressed mood, anxiety and nervous restlessness and the oil for external use on injuries, myalgia and first-degree burns.

Nervous system
In vitro—The mechanism of action of St John's wort as an antidepressant has long been a source of interest with monoamine oxidase (MAO) inhibition initially assumed to account for the effect. However a recent *in vivo* study showed no change in nor-adrenalin or MAO activity but dopamine metabolites were increased.[36] The actions of various constituents or the whole herb are broad and seem to involve modulation/inhibition of binding to the following receptor sites:

- γ-aminobutyric acid (GABA)— amentoflavone,[37] hyperforin[38]
- serotonin—*Hypericum*,[39] amentoflavone,[40] hyperforin[41]
- dopamine—amentoflavone,[40] hypericin,[40] hyperforin[40,41]
- nor-adrenalin or β-adrenergic—*Hypericum*,[39] hypericin,[40] hyperforin[41]
- δ-opiate—amentoflavone[40]
- benzodiazepine—amentoflavone[42]

Additional mechanisms may be via:-

- neuronal and hormonal binding by constituents like biapigenin[43] and adhyperforin[44]
- the reduced breakdown of tryptophan[45] and dopamine[46]
- increased permeability of blood/brain barrier to glucocorticoids[47]
- dis-inhibition of the hypothalmus/pituitary/ adrenal axis[48] leading to increased levels of plasma adrenocorticotrophic hormone (ACTH)[49] and salivary cortisol, (probably mediated through serotonin and dopamine mechanisms).[50–52] More recently it was shown that salivary cortisol is increased at low dose *Hypericum* only, being unaffected by a higher dose.[53] Hypericin and quercetin inhibit the breakdown of cortisol *in vitro*[54]

- inhibition of substance P induced interleukin-6 synthesis. Substance P has been implicated in the development of depression and anxiety and it can increase IL-6 levels which in turn modulates the HPA axis[55,56]
- increased effect of light, a positive outcome of its photosensitizing action[57]

Re-uptake inhibition of dopamine, serotonin, nor-adrenalin and GABA are likely to account for a large part of the herb's antidepressant action.[58,59]

Although it was once considered that the constituents responsible for the activity of the herb were hypericin and pseudohypericin, it is now known that hyperforin, rutin, quercitin and chlorogenic acid are also important. There are still questions surrounding issues of bio-availability of some constituents and their stability.[60] Certainly the level of hyperforin seems relevant to the herb's efficacy, for instance a study found it was effective at the level of 5% but not at 0.5%.[61] The likelihood is that *Hypericum* exerts its action through the synergy of its constituents.[40,62]

In vivo—At least 38 controlled trials have been conducted showing *Hypericum* is both effective and safe with very low rates of adverse reactions and therefore drop-out rates from treatment, for all levels of depression.[63]

Apart from its effectiveness in the treatment of mild to moderate depression (with or without somatic symptoms) in adults[64–77] it has also been beneficial in depressed adolescents[78] and children under 12.[79] It has been used effectively with *Valeriana officinalis* to treat depression with anxiety[80] and alone to treat dysthymia (anecdotal),[81] major depression in youths[82] and somatoform disorder (mental disorder manifesting as physical symptoms).[83–85] The herb seems to accelerate recovery from depression, improving all signs and symptoms of the condition.[86]

In treating mild to moderate depression *Hypericum* was as effective or better than standard antidepressants[87,88] including specifically citalopram,[89] sertraline,[90,91] maprotiline,[92] fluoxetine[93–96] and imipramine[97–99] with considerably fewer side-effects and with the added advantage of improving associated somatic symptoms[100] including anxiety.[97]

In the treatment of moderate to severe/major depression it gave significant improvement[101,102] and was superior or equal to fluoxetine,[103–106] paroxetine,[107] amitriptyline,[108] imipramine[109] and sertraline.[90]

However *Hypericum* did not help ameliorate social phobia.[110]

Some studies have disputed the herb's value in treating major depression[111–113] and critics suggest that skewing of the data has produced positive outcomes.[114–116] On the other hand in trials where no significant improvement occurred the variable quality of extracts used[117,118] or compliance problems[119] have been cited as possible factors for negative outcomes.

It seems that an early response to *Hypericum* treatment (in the first 2 weeks of use) is a good indicator of its likely long-term success.[104,120]

An interesting side study undertaken into the cardiac electrical conductivity in patients using either imipramine or high dose *Hypericum* to treat depression showed that at the end of the trial period whilst the imipramine group showed a significant increase in cardiac conduction abnormalities there was actually a reduction of these in the *Hypericum* group.[121]

The use of *Hypericum* in the nervous system has become more extensive than just the treatment of depression. Other clinical trials with the herb show:-

- a possible shielding effect on the central nervous system indicated by increased output of baseline values in electrical brain activity[122]
- benefit for the treatment of psychological aspects of menopausal problems[123,124]
- some improvement in treating premenstrual problems[125] associated with dysphoria (PMDD),[126] not corroborated[127]
- positive results treating obsessive-compulsive disorder within one week of treatment,[128] not corroborated[129]
- a possible benefit in treating schizophrenia[130]
- benefit for seasonal affective disorder (SAD)[131]
- improvement in sleep patterns[132,133] and increased nocturnal levels of melatonin,[1] not corroborated[53]

- good supportive effect in the treatment of depression in alcoholics[134]
- good results in the topical treatment of otalgia (combined herbal preparation) as effective as anaesthetic ear drops[135]

Hypericum does not adversely affect cardiovascular or cognitive function[136] and may improve the latter.[137,138]

It did not help painful polyneuropathies,[139] the cessation of smoking[140] or improve memory.[141]

Cancer
In vitro—Studies have been conducted into the potential of *Hypericum* as an anticancer agent. It effectively inhibits both high and low grade bladder cancer,[142,143] prostatic cancer[144] and leukaemia cells.[145,146] Light exposure enhances the anti-proliferative effects of fresh and dried *Hypericum* extracts on leukaemia and glioblastoma cells.[147] It also improves the repair mechanism of DNA which may help prevent mutations.[148]

Of the individual constituents, hyperforin is active against a number of cancer cell lines[149] including fibrosarcoma[150] and B-cell chronic lymphocytic leukaemia cells whilst having no deleterious effect on normal lymphocytes.[151] It also inhibits angiogenesis.[152] Hypericin and pseudohypericin are activated by light to become cytotoxic[9] and hypericin strongly inhibits protein kinase C which is involved in tumour development and angiogenesis.[153]

All the main constituents strongly inhibit CYP enzyme conversion of pro-carcinogens into their active forms (see below).[154,155] They may therefore have a role in cancer prophylaxis.

Again no one constituent is likely to be responsible for observed anti-proliferative effects[156] and synergism probably underlies this action.[157]

Detoxification
In vitro—The main constituents induce pathways involved in detoxification by activating the nuclear receptor group pregnane X.[158] This receptor helps detect and detoxify lipophilic toxins. Bile acids can be toxic to liver cells and *Hypericum*, through activation of pregnane X, may be protective in disease

conditions like biliary cholestasis.[159] This mechanism is also involved in herb/drug interactions (see below).

Anti-oxidant

In vitro—*Hypericum* and some of its constituents are strong anti-oxidants[160–165] including against oxidation from UV irradiation and topical use may protect skin from sun damage.[166]

Anti-inflammatory

In vitro—The herb inhibits COX-2 whilst hyperforin strongly inhibits 5-LOX and COX-1,[167] both inhibit other inflammatory mediators[1,168–170] and are also immunomodulatory.[171,172] All these actions may help explain the observed anti-inflammatory activity.

In vivo—*Hypericum* was found to be an effective topical treatment for atopic eczema.[173]

Antimicrobial[1]

In vitro—The herb and/or its constituents have a range of antimicrobial activity including:

- antiviral against a bovine virus similar in structure to hepatitis C virus. Also the following viruses—hepatitis B, human cytomegalovirus, parainfluenza virus type 3, vesicular stomatitis, Sindbis, vaccinia, HSV-1 and 2 and the retroviruses, of which HIV is a member[174,175]
- antibacterial against a number of Gram-positive bacteria[161,176] including *Staphylococcus* spp.[177] and specifically MRSA, *Helicobacter pylori*,[178] *Escherichia coli*, *Proteus vulgaris*, *Streptococcus sanguis* and *S. mutans*, *Shigella* spp.[179,180]

In vivo—Small clinical trials conducted using hypericin have so far failed to improve either chronic hepatitis C[181] or HIV[182] infection. However, some studies had indicated that HIV patients were achieving improvements using the whole herb[183] but no confirmation has emerged. Caution is necessary in using *Hypericum* in patients on protease inhibitors for AIDS as it has been reported to reduce drug serum levels (see Interactions).

Other

The photosensitizing activity of *Hypericum* is related to the naphodianthrone fraction and presents possibilities for future treatment of conditions like psoriasis.[184]

Medicinal uses
Nervous system
- depression
- anxiety
- depression associated with menopause (*BHP* specific)
- sciatica
- excitability
- neuroses
- neuralgia including shingles

Musculoskeletal
- fibrositis

Externally
Topical actions suit *Hypericum* to the treatment of:

- wounds
- burns
- contusions

Pharmacy
Three times daily
Infusion of dried herb   – 2–4 g
Tincture 1:10 (45%)   – 2–4 ml
Fluid Extract (25%)   – 2–4 ml

The clinical trials on depression were based on standardized extracts with daily doses ranging from 300–1200 mg *Hypericum*, the majority used 900 mg daily. Trials were conducted over a minimum of 4 weeks, but usually carried out over 6–12 weeks. The standardization of extracts is complicated by the number of known active constituents and probable synergism. Standardization of a few marker constituents does not ensure that products are chemically or pharmacologically the same.[185,186] In addition high hypericin preparations have been noted to induce side-effects like hypersensitivity.[182,187]

The quality of extracts can be assessed visually, they should have a red hue. The phloroglucinols seem to be better extracted in alcohol than the napthadianthrones. Light-exposure of alcohol extracts, even of short duration, can cause the significant loss of active constituents—especially hyperforins—so storage of preparations is important.[188,189]

Commercial products appear to differ quite markedly in their actual level of active constituents compared to that claimed on the label[190-192] and they may deteriorate anyway, over months.[193] (Variability of quality is apparently worse in teas and functional foods[194]). Constituents are more bio-available from soft gelatine capsules than from hard ones.[195]

Hypericum oil is made by macerating the flower heads only, in vegetable oil and exposing the macerate to sunlight for six weeks. The oil should be bright red by this time, the colour is believed to be due to the presence of hyperforins (although these are unstable in normal conditions) and breakdown products of hypericin. It will also contain flavonoids which increase on exposure to light.[196]

Pharmacokinetics
Studies show maximum plasma levels of the main constituents after tablet ingestion occurs within 8 hours and their halflife is not more than 19 hours, the flavonoids reach maximum concentration in about half that time and have a much shorter half-life (maximum of 6 hours).[197] Hypericin and hyperforin were detectable in plasma 7 days after discontinuation of therapeutic doses.[198] It takes 4 days to reach a steady-state of plasma levels of naphadianthrones.[199] Repeated dosing of *Hypericum* does not lead to the accumulation of hyperforin.[200]

Precautions and/or safety
In vivo Hypericum oil has been declared safe for topical use.[201] Apart from the potential to interact with other medications, the good safety and tolerability of *Hypericum* in various dosage forms emerges from all the trials that have been conducted to-date[83,202] with much lower drop-out rates and side-effects than that recorded for pharmaceutical antidepressants.[75,203-205] In healthy volunteers the herb does not affect blood vessel tone, skin conductance,[206] cognitive or psychomotor function.[207]

Minor side-effects are estimated to occur at the rate of 1–3%, which is ten times less than with pharmaceutical antidepressants,[208] and at the same rate as for placebo.[209] These include nausea, rash and itch, fatigue, restlessness, photosensitivity, acute neuropathy, dizziness and constipation.[210-212] The phototoxic rash associated with *Hypericum* which causes erythema, itch and heightened sensory nerve sensation has been well documented and is referred to as "hypericism". It is considered to have a very low incidence though[209] and studies on volunteers taking *Hypericum* with subsequent exposure to light at various wavelengths showed no detectable increase in erythema or melanin.[213] Even at high doses of hypericin UVA light failed to cause significant erythema *in vivo*.[214] *In vitro* keratinocyte reaction was shown to occur on exposure to UVA and white light however the level of hypericin required to cause this reaction would not be expected to be reached in the course of antidepressant therapy.[215] However in HIV patients hypercin treatment did result in a majority experiencing a phototoxic reaction.[216]

It may be prudent to advise patients using the herb to stay out of the sun. Caution may also be necessary if the patient is receiving ultraviolet A (UVA) therapy.[217]

The phototoxicity of hypericin and data from *in vitro* studies has raised concern about possible damage to retinal[218] and lens[219] cells. It may be advisable to also protect eyes from intense light when taking the herb.

Adverse events of a more serious nature have appeared in the literature. These are listed below with the number of cases reported in brackets:-

- impotence (1)—this may be linked to the muscle relaxant effect reported in isolated *vas deferens*[220]
- psychosis (17), mainly mania[221-224] and hypomania[225,226]
- fatal bone marrow necrosis (1)[227]
- suicidal and aggressive thoughts (1)[228]
- bigeminy/digoxin poisoning upon cessation of *Hypericum* (1)[229]

- severe phototoxic reaction with laser treatment (1)[230] reversible erythema after UVB light exposure (1)[231]
- serotonin syndrome† when used with SSRIs (5)[232]

A retrospective study has suggested *Hypericum* may increase levels of thyroid stimulating hormone.[233]

No toxicity was found on animal foetal development[234] and *in vitro* genotoxicity with hypericin and exposure to UVA light appears to be low.[235] Mutagenicity tests have been negative in mammalian models.[236]

There are no reports of problems with use of the herb in pregnancy or breast-feeding—*Hypericum* is frequently used to treat post-natal depression.[237,238] One analysis showed that no hypericin and very little hyperforin, are secreted in breast milk and they are undetectable in the baby's plasma.[239]

Interactions
In vitro—*Hypericum* has been shown to affect drug metabolism in two ways, both probably occurring through induction of nuclear receptor pregnane X. The first is through the cytochrome P450 isozymes, enzymes that alter drug metabolism and the second through P-glycoprotein a membrane protein that affects drug absorption[240] and efflux. These systems are used by the body to process or breakdown foreign chemicals as well as the natural metabolites of cell function. *Hypericum* particularly induces CYP3A4[241] which metabolises 60% of clinically relevant drugs, an effect that seems to correlate to the level of hyperforin.[242] *In vivo* CYP3A4 and CYP2E1 were also induced by long term exposure to *Hypericum*.[243,244] Other Cytochrome P isozymes have been induced *in vitro* and/or *in vivo* by *Hypericum* and/or its constituents and although results

have been inconsistent, hyperforin does seem to be implicated.[245-249] P-glycoprotein has also been induced *in vitro* and *in vivo*, by the whole extract[250] and by quercetin and hyperforin,[251] the latter again correlating strongly to the level of induction.[252]

Because these two pathways are inducible by *Hypericum*, it may cause variable effects for any particular drug/herb interaction and the level of interaction will likely depend on the type of preparation used, dosing regime, route of administration[253] and the length of exposure to the herb (see below). Another possible problem in assessing potential interactions is exemplified by the physical interaction that occurs when *Hypericum* and warfarin are mixed *in vitro* forming a precipitate that reduces the apparent level of warfarin.[254] Immunoassays are more reliable to measure serum drug levels as they are unaffected by the presence of hypericin or hyperforin.[255]

In vitro—ritonavir and erythromycin levels were increased by short term exposure to *Hypericum*[253] and studies have predicted interactions may occur with docetaxel,[256] paclitaxel,[257] ritonavir[54] and etoposide amsacrine.[258]

In vivo—*Hypericum* has been implicated in the majority of interactions between pharmaceuticals and herbs.[259] Based on the cytochrome pathway for their metabolism, it would be expected that the anti-retrovirals—amprenavir, lopinavir, saquinavir, atazanavir[260]—would be affected by their co-administration. Predictions of this sort however are not necessarily accurate as there are many variables involved[261] (for example there is a sex-related difference in the levels of induced CYP3A4[262]—higher in women, and *in vivo* studies will be needed to confirm them).[263] An *in vivo* study showed androgen levels were effectively unchanged after using St. John's wort even though these sterols are also metabolised by CYP3A4.[264]

It should be noted that the level of hyperforin could be critical to producing drug/herb interactions as low- hyperforin *Hypericum* appears not to interact significantly with other drugs.[252]

Of the clinical studies that have confirmed drug interactions co-medication of *Hypericum* with pharmaceuticals found in the main the latter's bioavailability had decreased.[265]

---

†The possible symptoms are: euphoria, drowsiness, sustained rapid eye movement, overreaction of the reflexes, rapid muscle contraction and relaxation in the ankle causing abnormal movements of the foot, clumsiness, restlessness, feeling drunk and dizzy, muscle contraction and relaxation in the jaw, sweating, muscle twitching, rigidity, high body temperature, mental status changes (including confusion and hypomania—a "happy drunk" state), shivering, diarrhoea, loss of consciousness and death.

No relevant interaction occurred with digoxin, alprazolam, caffeine or tolbutamide with low-hyperforin *Hypericum*[266] and the standardised herb was not found to alter the pharmacokinetics of carbamazepine,[267] dextromethorphan, mycophenolic acid or pravastatin.[279]

In vivo reports of interaction do exist for the following pharmaceuticals:-

- Anti-fungal: **voriconazole** (initially the level rose but long term it decreased)[268]
- Cancer medicines: **imatinib**,[269,270] **irinotecan**[271]
- Cardiovascular medicines: **digoxin**,[272,273] **warfarin**,[274] **phenprocoumon, simvastin**,[275,276] **verapamil**[277]
- Gastro-intestinal medicines: **omeprazole**[278]
- HIV medicines: **indinavir**,[279] **nevirapine**[280]
- Hormone: **contraceptive pill**[281,282] note *Hypericum* did not alter hormone levels or seem to cause ovulation when used with low dose "pill" but it did cause break-through bleeding.[283] There have been 5 cases of failed contraception reported[284]

- Immunosuppressants: **cyclosporin**,[285–289] **tacrolimus**[290,291]
- Psycho-actives: **amitriptyline**,[292] **quazepam**,[293] **methadone**,[294] **alprazolam**[295] (this was not corroborated by another study where no significant interaction occurred with normal doses),[296] Selective Serotonin Re-uptake Inhibitors (SSRIs)-e.g. **sertraline, paroxetine**[232]
- Respiratory medicines: **theophylline**[266] (has been contradicted);[297] **fexofenadine**, the level was raised after a single dose but decreased long-term[298,299]

Historical uses

Externally to dissolve swellings; hard tumours; caked breasts; ecchymosis (bruises) and to open up obstructions. Culpeper mainly used the seeds. Used in a broad range of pulmonary and urinary problems including suppression of urine. Also used for haemoptysis; dysentery; worms; haemorrhages; jaundice. Enuresis as a tea at night.

CUPRESSACEAE

The Cupressaceae or Cypress family are gymnosperms and consist of about 21 genera of widely distributed resinous, coniferous, usually evergreen, monoecious or dioecious trees and shrubs. They are distinguished from pine and yew families by having opposite or whorled leaves, usually flattened and scale-like, or sometimes needle-shaped as in *Juniperus*.

- Their cones are woody, leathery or berrylike with few cone scales
- Seedlings usually have 2 cotyledons

Medicinal plants of this family include *Juniperus* and *Thuja*.

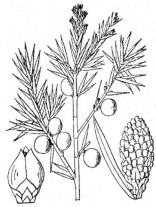

Family Cupressaceae

Juniperus communis

Juniper, genevre

Description
An erect or prostrate evergreen shrub or small tree to 12 m. *Leaves* ternate, all linear, spreading and sharp-pointed, with a single, white, longitudinal band above, weakly keeled below. *Flowers*, tiny, appear in late summer. Female berry-like green *cones* ripen to blue or black in two years and are glaucous, 0.25–0.5 cm in diameter, mostly three-seeded. A very variable species.

Odour—characteristically spicy; taste—sweet and aromatic.

Habitat and cultivation
Originally from Eurasia and North America, many ornamental cultivars of *Juniperus communis* are common, but the true species is hard to find in the Southern hemisphere. It may be grown from seed or cuttings and is tolerant of most soils and situations.

147

Parts used
The berries gathered from the second autumn onwards. Only the ripe blue-black berries are used medicinally and it may take three years for them to fully mature.

Active constituents[1,2]
1) Volatile oil (0.5–3.4%)[4] including predominantly
   a) α- and β-pinene, sabinene, limonene and myrcene,[3] p-cymene and also terpinen-4-ol, 1,4-cineole, camphene and codenine
   b) sesquiterpenes[4]—caryophyllene, cadinene and elemene
2) Flavonoids
3) Resin (up to 10%)
4) Bitter glycoside—juniperin
5) Tannins (condensed type)

Also contains diterpenes (including isocupressic acid)[5] and up to 30% sugars. Over 200 constituents have been isolated.[4]

The composition of the oil is variable, geographical location, maturity of berries,[6] environment and method of extraction being important factors.[4,7,8] As unripe berries are present alongside the ripe ones they may be harvested together. These immature berries or other aerial parts may contribute to chemical differences.

Nutritional constituents
Vitamins: C
Minerals: Potassium, selenium, calcium, magnesium and iron

Actions
1) Diuretic
2) Urinary antiseptic
3) Antirheumatic
4) Carminative
5) Stomachic

Scientific information
Juniper and its oil have been official preparations in a number of pharmacopoeias, listed as carminative, they were used to treat colic and flatulence.[9] *German Commission E* has approved its use for dyspepsia and as a supportive herb in the treatment of urinary tract problems. *Culpeper* regarded it as a powerful diuretic.

Actions attributed to the herb have been derived using animal models, there are no studies reported on its pharmacological action in humans. The volatile oil is considered central to its actions.

Antimicrobial
In vitro—The berries and their essential oil have enjoyed a reputation as antimicrobials an action confirmed by modern research. They are active against a range of bacteria including *Propionibacterium acnes, Staphylococcus aureus, Enterococcus faecalis, Salmonella enteriditis, Yersinia enterocolitica,* have moderate activity against various strains of *Helicobacter pylori* and are antimycobacterial with activity against the organism responsible for tuberculosis.[2–12] The oil also has strong antifungal activity including against *Candida* spp., *Cryptococcus neoformans* and *Trichophyton* spp.[2] The antimicrobial activity has proven to be variable, possibly dependent on the composition of the oil which is apparently more effective when levels of α-pinene, β-pinene and p-cymene are relatively high.[2,13]

In vivo—A combination of herbs, which included *Juniperus*, was used as a mouthwash in the treatment of gingivitis but had no benefit in inhibiting plaque growth or improving gingival health.[14]

Other
In vitro—Juniper has potential anticancer activity[15] and inhibits COX and PAF-mediated inflammation.[16]

The oil protects brain astrocytes from induced apoptosis.[17] Terpinen-4-ol inhibits antigen-induced inflammation[18] and is also credited with being the major contributor to the diuretic/aquaretic property of *Juniperus*.

Medicinal uses
Gastro-intestinal tract
• flatulent colic
• dyspepsia

Urinary tract
• cystitis, acute and chronic
• urethritis
• lithiasis

Musculoskeletal
- arthritis
- rheumatism
- gout

Externally
- arthritis
- myalgia
- neuralgia

Pharmacy
Three times daily

Infusion	– 100 ml of 1:20 extract of bruised berries
Tincture 1:5 (45%)	– 1–2 ml
Fluid Extract (25%)	– 2–4 ml

CONTRAINDICATIONS—Pregnancy. The volatile oil can stimulate uterine muscle and therefore act as an emmenagogue. (Animals have suffered abortions from eating plants containing isocupressic acid.)

Precautions and/or safety
In modern texts, including *German Commission E, Juniperus* has been contra-indicated in renal disease due to the irritant effect of the volatile oil on kidneys. It is also stated that it should not be used for longer than six weeks continuously for this reason. Older texts do not appear to have limitations imposed on the herb's use. Problems of safety may have arisen after dosing experimental animals with relatively large amounts of oil. Also oil high in α- and β-pinene, if prepared from unripe berries, needles and branches, would increase its potential to cause toxicity or irritation. Recent animal experiments using the characterised oil found no renal changes indicative of toxicity even after 4 weeks administration of large doses[19] thus challenging earlier findings. Normal use is not based on ingestion of the volatile oil.

Interactions
A review has suggested that there is a variable amount of vitamin K in *Juniperus* and that it may reduce the effectiveness of anti-coagulant therapy.[20] No interactions have been reported.

Historical uses
Pestilence; to counter poison; baldness—essential oil or infused oil used as a scalp rub. Cough; dyspnoea; consumption; ruptures; cramps; convulsions, epilepsy; sciatica; agues; to expedite labour; strengthen brain, optic nerves and memory; piles; worms in children.

Thuja occidentalis

Thuja, arbor-vitae, white cedar

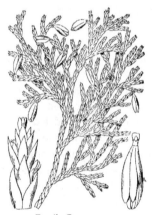

Family Cupressaceae

Description
A spreading evergreen monoecious tree to 20 m with branchlets flattened, in a horizontal plane. Trunk strongly buttressed, dividing near the ground into several trunks. *Leaves* scalelike, 4-ranked, dimorphic, dark green above, yellowish green beneath, glandular and aromatic. *Female cones* erect, ovoid-oblong, about 1 cm long, scales in 4–5 pairs; the middle pairs bearing 2–3 small 2-winged seeds.

Odour—camphoraceous; taste—bitter.

Habitat and cultivation
Native to North America from Nova Scotia to North Carolina and Illinois and may be grown in other countries from seeds or cuttings taken with a heel in spring, kept moist in summer to root in autumn. The true species is hard to find and very slow growing. New estimates suggest slow growing trees could be older than one and a half thousand years.[21]

Parts used
Leaves and twigs.

Active constituents[1,22]
1) Volatile oil (up to 4%) including:
   a) monoterpenes mainly thujone (65%)—a mixture of α and β isomers also fenchone, sabinene, α-pinene and smaller amounts of borneol, camphor and myrcene
   b) diterpenes based on isopimaric acid[23]
2) Flavonoids including thujin (a conjugate of quercetin), kaempferol and quercetin
3) Mucilage
4) Tannins

Also contains β-sitosterol, polysaccharides, proteins and a number of lignans including deoxypodophyllotoxin[25] and secoisolariciresinol.[24]

Thujone content in the volatile oil has been estimated at around 0.76% of dried twigs predominantly in the form of α-thujone. Its level can vary significantly with the method of extraction, being much lower in water extracts and increasing as the content of alcohol in the extracting medium rises.[22]

Nutritional constituents
Vitamins: C

Actions
1) Stimulant[†]
2) Expectorant
3) Astringent
4) Diuretic
5) Counter-irritant
6) Anthelmintic

Scientific information
The name Arbor-vitae—tree of life—derives from the use of the leaves of *Thuja* to treat scurvy, a practice introduced to European explorers by Native Americans. The herb was an official preparation in the United States until 1936.[25]

In vitro—The polysaccharides have received the most scientific attention. They inhibit HIV-1

and are immunomodulatory, stimulating T-cell activity[26] and cytokine production.[22] It has been postulated that although the polysaccharides are unlikely to be bio-available systemically when the whole extract is taken orally, they may still modulate mucosal immune activity through contact with lymphatic tissue in the gut such as Peyer's patches.[22]

In vitro—A constituent, B-thujaplicinol isolated from the heartwood of the tree has shown promise as an AIDS treatment,[27] inhibiting HIV-1.[28]

In vivo—*Thuja* in combination with *Echinacea* and *Baptisia* was effective in treating the common cold, reducing the duration and severity of symptoms.[22,29] This same combination used in conjunction with antibiotic therapy to treat acute bronchitis improved the recovery rate compared to antibiotics used alone.[30]

Thuja is an effective agent against naked viruses and in a preliminary study a tincture applied to verruca pedis was a very effective treatment.[31] (*Weiss* states it is effective on small warts but not on large, solid ones.)

For physiological effects of thujone see Appendix III.

Medicinal uses
Respiratory tract
• bronchial catarrh (*BHP* specific with associated circulatory weakness)

Urinary tract
As an antiseptic and to improve the tone of the bladder.

• cystitis
• enuresis
• incontinence (including that due to prostatic enlargement)
• irritable bladder

Reproductive tract
• prostatitis
• amenorrhoea
• spermatorrhoea
• impotence
• possible use in uterine cancer

[†]Nerve, uterus, circulation and immune system.

Musculoskeletal
• rheumatism

Skin
• psoriasis
• warts

Externally
• fungal infections
• warts, particularly genital and anal

Pharmacy
Three times daily
Infusion of dried herb   – 1–2 g
Tincture 1:10 in 60% alcohol   – 1–2 ml
Fluid Extract in 50% alcohol   – 2–4 ml
    Tincture can be applied externally to warts and fungal infections. In the clinical trial in which verrucae were treated, the tincture was applied weekly for three weeks. They took 4 to 8 weeks to disappear and in all cases were gone within 3 months.
    CONTRAINDICATIONS—Pregnancy.

Precautions and/or safety
Thujone is toxic in large doses. The fresh herb in high enough doses can cause vomiting, stomach ache, diarrhoea, gastroenteritis and possibly more severe symptoms including convulsions and renal or hepatic toxicity, effects attributable to thujone.[22]

Historical uses
Used in intermittent fevers; dropsy; coughs; scurvy. The essential oil was used for parasites (very toxic).

DIOSCOREACEAE

The Dioscoreaceae or Yam family consists of 9–10 genera of monocotyledons of tropical or warm temperate regions, twining, leafy, sometimes woody vines, with rhizomes or tuberous roots. The most important genus is *Dioscorea*, several species of which are cultivated for their edible tubers. The inedible tubers of several Mexican species contain saponins and are gathered wild for the production of drug hormones.

Dioscorea villosa

Wild yam

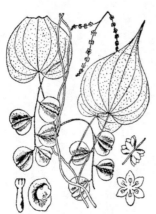

Family Dioscoreaceae

Description
A herbaceous twiner from 1.5–5 m long, growing over bushes or fences. *Root* horizontal, 1.5 cm in diameter, oval, flattened, seldom branched but marked on the upper surface with scars of previous years' stems. *Stems* slender and twining. *Leaves* arranged differently according to their position—basal leaves sometimes in fours, middle section leaves nearly opposite and upper leaves alternate. *Leaf blades* ovate with 7–11 ribs, downy and greyish beneath; base cordate, margin entire or wavy, apex pointed. Petioles nearly as long as the blade and dilated at the base. *Inflorescence* in drooping axillary racemes and panicles. Flowers very small, dioecious, greenish yellow. Male flowers grow in elongated panicles, have 6 stamens and a minute, abortive ovary. Female flowers grow in racemes, with 6 abortive stamens and an oblong, sharply triangular 3-celled ovary. *Fruit* an oval, 3-celled, 3-winged membranaceous pod. Seeds winged, 2 in each cell.

Habitat
Indigenous to North America, in wet woods and swampy ground, from Canada and New England to Wisconsin and southward but is common only in the south. It is collected in the wild.

Parts used

The fresh root and rhizome collected in autumn. *Grieve* states that the herb must be harvested in the first year to prevent loss of its therapeutic value.

Active constituents[1]

1) Phytosterols including β-sitosterol, campesterol and stigmasterol[2]
2) Steroidal saponins (up to 0.4%) including diosgenin (glycoside = dioscin) (up to 3.5%) and protodioscin[3]
3) Alkaloids
4) Flavonoids based on flavan-3-ol[3]

Also contains tannins, mucilage and starch.

Nutritional constituents

Vitamins: C and A
Minerals: Calcium, chromium, magnesium, phosphorus, potassium and sodium

Actions

1) Anti-inflammatory
2) Spasmolytic
3) Cholagogue
4) Mild diaphoretic
5) Antirheumatic

Scientific information

The steroidal saponin, diosgenin, from *Dioscorea* spp. had become a predominant source of starting material for the manufacture of steroidal drugs including corticosteroids and sex-hormones.[4] Initially Mexican yam was the main plant used, to the extent that it was nationalised by the Mexican government, its harvesting and processing leading to substantial changes in the lives and economy of people in that country.[5] The price of Mexican yam escalated and alternate species were sought in other countries. *Trigonella foenum-graecum* is a more recently established source of diosgenin.[6]

Dioscorea spp. are found in the nutritional and medicinal tradition of many countries and their uses bear many similarities. Research has been conducted on a number of different species and on diosgenin but not a great deal has been published on the whole extract of *D. villosa*.

Hormonal

In vitro—The herb has an anti-oestrogenic activity[7] but failed to have much effect on the hormone receptor sites in breast cancer cells.[8]

In vivo—A cream containing *Dioscorea* was used to treat menopausal symptoms in otherwise healthy women and found to have no effect on hormone or lipid levels, blood pressure and weight and no significant reduction of menopausal flushing or sweating.[9] It has been suggested that extracts with a diosgenin content of less than 3.5% have no oestrogenic activity.[1]

A supplement containing *Dioscorea* was given to a group of older people and the effects on levels of dehydroepiandrosterone (DHEA) metabolites and lipid levels were monitored. Whilst DHEA levels were unchanged there was a favourable shift in serum lipids to reduce triglyceride and raise HDL levels.[10]

Other

In vitro—One of the flavan-3-ol glycosides has antifungal activity against *Candida* spp. including *C. albicans*.[3]

Disogenin

A good deal more research has been carried out on this constituent. *In vitro* studies show that it:-

- inhibits tumour cell growth of a number of different cell lines[11–13] including leukaemia,[14–17] breast cancer,[18] colon cancer[19] and osteosarcoma cells[20]
- inhibits the invasive ability of tumours[21]
- induces differentiation in a leukaemia cell line[22]
- affects neuronal activity through altered membrane conductance[23]
- protects neurones from oxidative stress and toxicity including that from HIV infection[24,25]
- inhibits inflammation,[26] including through inhibition of 12-LOX[27] and by interfering with the process behind the chronic destructive inflammation of rheumatoid arthritis involving the up-regulation of COX-2[28]
- inhibits osteoclastogenesis[21]

It seems that diosgenin may be poorly absorbed however as serum levels of unmodified diosgenin were low after large doses were taken orally over a month.[29]

Medicinal uses
Cardiovascular system
• intermittent claudication

Gastro-intestinal tract
• intestinal colic
• bilious colic
• cholecystitis
• diverticulitis
• cramps

Reproductive tract
• dysmenorrhoea
• ovarian and/or uterine pain
• nausea in pregnancy

Musculoskeletal
• muscular rheumatism
• gout
• cramps
• rheumatoid arthritis (acute)

Pharmacy
Three times daily
Decoction of dried root   – 2–4 g
Tincture 1:5 (45%)   – 2–10 ml
Fluid Extract (45%)   – 2–4 ml

Precautions and/or safety
A report into the safety of the herb found it was not genotoxic in standard tests.[1]

DROSERACEAE

The sundew family consists of 85 species of perennial herbaceous plants often growing as a rosette. The upper surface of the leaves is covered with long, glistening, glandular hairs which attract and trap insects. The flowers are regular, often in branching clusters, commonly in parts of 5. The fruit is a capsule. Sundews get their name from the sparkling, sticky hair drops which do not dry out in the sun.

Drosera rotundifolia

Sundew, common sundew

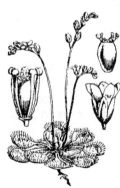

Family Droseraceae

Description
A small insectivorous perennial. *Leaves* reddish, circular-bladed, covered with glistening, glandular hairs on the upper surface and growing in flattened rosettes. Leaf stalks hairy. *Flower* stems slender, leafless, 6–8 cm, bearing a few short-stalked flowers each 0.5 cm across with 6 white petals. Flowers from June to September in Europe and North America.

Habitat and cultivation
This *Drosera* is native to Europe growing in poor peaty bogs and damp heaths, often in sphagnum moss. It also grows in North America from Newfoundland to Florida, in Illinois and Minnesota. It is generally collected wild but may be grown from seed or by division of the stolons if its natural growing conditions can be provided. It is drought and frost tender.

Parts used
The herb gathered during flowering in the summer or early autumn.

Active constituents
1) Naphthoquinones—1,4-naphthoquinones including plumbagin (2-methyl-5-hydroxy-1,4- naphthoquinone),[1] 7-methyljuglone

155

(5-hydroxy-7-methyl-1,4-naphthoquinone)[2] and its derivative rossoliside.[3] (A methylnaphthazarin derivative has been identified as an extraction artefact of rossoliside.)[4]

2) Flavonoids including hyperoside, quercetin, isoquercitrin[5], droserone and droserin
3) Tannins including ellagic acid[5]

Also contains citric and malic acids, resin and a red pigment.

Levels of 7-methyjuglone show relatively small variations according to location but annual conditions are significant in determining its concentration.[2] It has been reported that cultivated samples of the herb do not contain plumbagin and it may not occur in all wild specimens either.[2,3]

Actions
1) Antispasmodic
2) Demulcent
3) Expectorant
4) Bronchial muscle relaxant
5) Antitussive
6) Anti-asthmatic

Scientific information
Drosera was an official medicine in a number of different countries having been used for chronic bronchitis, pertussis and asthma.[6] Other species were acceptable substitutes in the past and current pressure on *D. rotundifolia* supplies has led not only to its cultivation but also to the other species being used in its place.[7]

D. rotundifolia is not well characterised or studied and its use is dictated by folklore.

In vitro—*Drosera* is strongly anti-inflammatory, an effect attributed to the flavonoids.[5,7] Indeed their level is high whilst that of the naphthoquinones is relatively low.[7]

Other members of this species have a broad spectrum of antimicrobial activity.[8,9]

Plumbagin is:-

- antibacterial*[,10,11]
- antifungal**
- antimycobacterial[12]
- anti-oxidant[13]
- an inhibitor of platelet aggregation[14]
- antiparasitic***
- antiviral[15]
- antiproliferative[16]
- cytotoxic[17]

In vivo—*D. peltata* (a common substitute for *D. rotundifolia*) used in a herbal combination improved the symptoms of patients with chronic obstructive pulmonary disease (COPD) comparable to or better than using the combined conventional medicines salbutamol, theophylline and bromhexine.[20]

Medicinal uses
Respiratory tract
- asthma
- bronchitis
- pertussis
- tracheitis
- coughs, dry and painful

BHP specific for asthma and/or chronic bronchitis with gastric ulceration or gastritis.

Gastro-intestinal tract
- gastric ulcers
- gastritis

Pharmacy
Infusion of dried herb – 1–2 g
Tincture 1:5 (60%) – 0.5–1 ml
Fluid extract (25%) – 0.5–2 ml

Historical uses
The juice was supposed to be effective in the treatment of corns and warts. In America as a cure for arteriosclerosis and old age! Mental disorders. Impotence; frigidity; amenorrhoea.

*Including against *Staphylococcus* spp. (*S. aureus*),[18] *Streptococcus* and *Pneumococcus* spp.[20]
**Including against *Candida albicans*.
***Including against *Leishmania* spp.[19]

EPHEDRACEAE

The Ephedraceae consists of just one dioecious genus. The species comprise much-branched straggly shrubs of slender green stems, native to dry and desert regions of the Northern Hemisphere and South America. The leaves are dry and scale-like and grow in groups of 2–3 at each node. Flowers consist of male cones, also at the nodes, which have several stamen-like structures and female cones on different plants, have a terminal ovule. Seeds have a fleshy red coat.

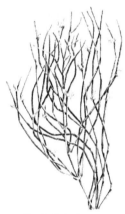

Family Ephedraceae

Ephedra sinica [Restricted Herb]

Ma Huang

Description
An evergreen shrub growing to about 50 cm. *Stems* long, narrow and spreading, leaves tiny and scale-like. Male and female cones grow on separate plants.

Habitat and cultivation
Native to usually semi-arid rocky hills in Northern China and Inner Mongolia. Plants propagated from seed sown in autumn or root division in autumn or spring. Needs well-drained soil to grow.

Parts used
Young dried stems. *E. equisetina* and *E. gerardiana* may also be used.[1]

Active constituents
1) Alkaloids (around 2%), including mostly (−)-ephedrine and (+)-pseudoephedrine. Also norephedrine, norpseudoephedrine, methyl-ephedrine and methylpseudoephedrine.[2]

157

Also contains flavonoids, proanthocyanidins and tannins, volatile oil and organic acids

Actions
1) Bronchodilator
2) Anti-asthmatic
3) Hypertensive
4) Stimulant

Scientific information
Ephedra has been in use in Chinese medicine for thousands of years. It has been, and still is, an official medicine in a number of countries and is approved for use in mild bronchospasm by *German Commission E*. It is used mainly as a source of ephedrine in the west. **This is a restricted herb and it is not available for use by herbalists in most countries.**

Its alkaloids are adrenergic, stimulating the sympathetic nervous system. Both of the major alkaloids are strongly sympathomimetic, causing bronchodilation, vasoconstriction and stimulating the heart and the central nervous system.

Medicinal uses
• allergic conditions[†]
• enuresis

_____

[†]Including asthma, hayfever, urticaria and sinusitis.

• chronic postural hypotension
• myasthenia gravis
• narcolepsy

CONTRAINDICATIONS—Glaucoma, phaeochromocytoma, prostatic enlargement, hyperthyroidism, coronary thrombosis and severe hypertension.

Precautions and/or safety
The action of *Ephedra's* alkaloids can cause a rise in blood pressure, although this should not occur with a properly identified whole extract. The level of active alkaloids is clearly much lower in herbal extracts compared to pure drugs, like ephedrine, used within the pharmaceutical industry.

Overdose of the herb can cause palpitations, tremor, insomnia, hypertension, anorexia and nausea.

Interactions
Should not be used with monoamine oxidase inhibitors, cardiac glycosides, halothane, guanethidine, ergot alkaloid derivatives or oxytocin.

EQUISETACEAE

The Equisetaceae or horsetail family are Fern Allies and are a very ancient and primitive form of plant life.

- Stems are jointed, longitudinally grooved and siliceous
- Leaves each have 1 unbranched vein and are united into whorls sheathing the stems at the nodes
- The spores are in sacs arranged like small cones at the top of fertile stems

Description
A creeping perennial with hairy rhizomes and both sterile and fertile hollow, jointed stems, longitudinally grooved and impregnated with silica. *Fertile stems* brown, appearing first, shorter than sterile stems, unbranched, which die after spore dispersal. Their 4–6 sheaths are also brown with dark brown teeth. Cones 10–40 mm long. *Sterile stems* green, 10–80 cm × 1–5 mm, branched, erect or decumbent, rough, with 6–19-toothed green sheaths. Branches are numerous, spreading, and arranged in whorls. Dies back in winter.

Equisetum arvense

Horsetail

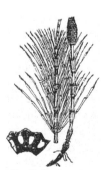

Family Equisetaceae

Equisetum hymale

Horsetail

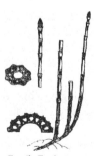

Family Equisetaceae

Description
Evergreen, creeping, slender, rhizomatous perennial similar to *E. arvense* but sterile stems green, taller, 30–100 cm with very few branches and those growing upright from the nodes rather than spreading. *Stems* hollow, jointed, each joint with a broad white band with a narrower black band top and bottom and 10–30 narrow blunt teeth; furrowed, with 14–40 ridges. *Fertile stems* also green, topped with a shorter, rounder cone. Does not die back in winter. *E. hymale* is the species used in Traditional Chinese Medicine.

Habitat and cultivation
Equisetums are cosmopolitan weeds in damp, wet areas of temperate regions of the Northern Hemisphere. They are considered noxious because they spread and their high silica content destroys the teeth of stock that eat them. Grown from spores or root division. Frost resistant and drought tender.

Parts used
The sterile stems of the herb harvested mid to late summer.

Active constituents[1,2]
1) Flavonoids[3-5] (up to 1%) including apigenin, kaempferol, luteolin and quercetin glycosides. There are two chemotypes of this herb, one found in Asia and North America and the other in Europe, they vary in their specific flavonoids[4]
2) Phytosterols including β-sitosterol (around 60%), campesterol (around 33%), isofucosterol (around 6%) and trace amounts of cholesterol[6]
3) Silica in various forms including as elemental silica,[7] silicic acid[8] (5–8%) a small proportion of which is in a soluble form (*E. hymale* is richer in silica. The horsetail family is known to have the highest concentration of silica in the plant world[7])
4) Volatile oil including hexahydrofarnesyl acetone, cis-geranyl acetone, thymol and trans-phytol[9]
5) Phenolics including pterosins (onitin and its glucoside)[10] and caffeic acid derivatives[11-13]

6) Saponins—equisetonin
7) Alkaloids at very low levels, including nicotine, palustrine and palustrinine[14]

Also contains tannins, a bitter, aconitic acid and lectins.[15]

Nutritional constituents
Vitamins: Pantothenic acid, C and E[16]
Minerals: Silica, selenium, copper, zinc, manganese, magnesium, sodium, iron, iodine, potassium and calcium

Actions
1) Astringent especially for genitourinary tract
2) Antihaemorrhagic
3) Diuretic
4) Antilithic Locally
5) Styptic
6) Vulnerary

Scientific information
This herb has been used medicinally since ancient Greek and Roman times but was also used in traditional medicine in Asia and North America. It was listed as an official preparation in a number of European pharmacopoeias until fairly recently as a mild diuretic.[17] *German Commission E* has approved the herb for internal use to treat bacterial infections and inflammation of the lower urinary tract and renal gravel and externally to aid poor healing wounds. Its diuretic effect is considered to be due to saponins and flavonoids. The Chinese have used it for conjunctivitis and dysentery and the Germans for bleeding in the gastrointestinal tract.

In vitro—In contrast to earlier reports[18,19] the whole extract has very good anti-oxidant activity comparable with ascorbic acid, and likely due to the high vitamin C and E, copper and zinc levels.[16]

Equisetum inhibits platelet aggregation, an action that may be attributable to the phenolic fraction[20] and also, according to the *BHP*, causes a mild increase in leucocytosis.

The volatile oil has very good antimicrobial activity against a number of organisms including *Staphylococcus aureus, Escherichia coli, Klebsiella pneumoniae, Pseudomonas aeroginosa, Salmonella enteritidis, Aspergillus niger* and *Candida albicans*.[9]

Onitin and luteolin are protective of hepatic cells[10]—the herb is used in the East for treating hepatitis.

In vivo—*Equisetum* in a topical combination with fatty acids and *Hypericum perforatum* was effective in treating and preventing pressure ulcers,[21] this supports the traditional use of the herb as a vulnerary.

Although animal testing has confirmed some of the traditional uses of horsetail, there are very few human based studies and the long tradition of medicinal use is the best guide to its applications.

Medicinal uses
Respiratory tract
To heal and strengthen lung tissue has been applied to:

- haemoptysis

Urinary tract
The astringency may help to improve bladder tone and reduce prostate enlargement. Silica aids tissue healing.

- cystitis
- enuresis
- urethritis
- incontinence
- oedema associated with menopause or arthritis
- lithiasis
- haematuria
- prostatitis
- prostatic enlargement

BHP specific for prostatitis, prostate enlargement, incontinence and enuresis in children.

Externally
The herb is considered an aid to strengthening connective tissue due to its silica content. Used for:

- bleeding
- haemorrhoids (ointment)
- slow healing wounds

Can be used as a wash for nose, eyes, mouth and vagina.

Pharmacy
Three times daily
Infusion of dried herb   – 1–4 g
Fluid extract (25%)   – 1–4 ml

For infusion/decoction pour 150 ml boiling water over 2–4 g *Equisetum* in a pan. Boil for 5 minutes and infuse for 10–15 minutes. (According to *German Commission E* monograph 34% of its flavonoids are available after 5 minutes of infusion and 40% after 10 minutes.)

Pharmacokinetics
In vivo—Studies have been conducted into the metabolism of the flavonoid quercetin from a standardised extract of horsetail. It is predominantly metabolised to benzoic acid derivatives and excreted in urine as hippuric acid.[22]

Precautions and/or safety
The herb is apparently toxic to cattle in large quantities but is not known to cause a problem in normal therapeutic doses in humans.

There is a reported case involving the use of herbal mixtures to aid smoking cessation consisting of both tablets and liquids (only the latter contained *Equisetum*) which resulted in transient but complete atrioventricular block in an otherwise healthy man.[23] Seborrhoeic dermatitis attributed to the nicotine in horsetails has also been reported.[24]

Historical uses
To ease bowels; for "coughs that come, by distillation, from the head" (*Culpeper*); chilblains, rheumatic, arthritic and skin problems; dropsy; a strong infusion as an emmenagogue.

ERICACEAE

Ericaceae usually consist of shrubs, often low and creeping, or sometimes small trees. Widely distributed on acid soils mainly in temperate areas of the world.

- Leaves are generally entire or toothed and undivided
- Flowers usually drooping, either solitary or in small clusters or racemes in the axils of the leaves, or forming short, terminal, leafy racemes
- Calyx of 4 or 5 divisions, either free or with a tube adhering to the ovary
- Corolla inferior or superior, usually ovoid or globular, sometimes small and campanulate, with 4 or 5 lobes
- Stamens twice as many, or rarely the same number, as the lobes of the corolla
- Ovary usually the same number of cells as the lobes of the corolla
- Fruit a capsule or berry with one or several small seeds, with a fleshy albumen in each cell

Arctostaphylos uva-ursi, Vaccinium myrtillus and *Gaultheria procumbens* are medicinal herbs belonging to this family.

Arctostaphylos uva-ursi

Bearberry, uva-ursi

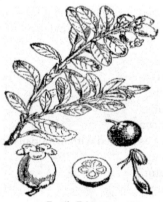

Family Ericaceae

Description

A prostrate, evergreen shrub with semi-trailing, pale brown, smooth, woody stems and numerous branches with small, (about 2 cm long), obovate or oblong entire leaves, leathery, glossy dark green above, paler and veined beneath. *Flowers* grow in compact, drooping terminal racemes of 4–6 and are white with a red tip, waxy and urn-shaped. They bloom between November and December.

162

The ovary and fruit are free, the sepals being at the base of the berry, not crowning it. *Fruit* is a thick-skinned, glossy, bright red berry with 5 or fewer seeds, ripening in autumn.

Odour—slightly aromatic; taste—astringent and bitter.

Habitat and cultivation
Bearberry is native to the whole Arctic and temperate zone of the Northern Hemisphere south to the Mediterranean and California. Grows in dry, heathy, mountainous places on moors and banks. Grown from seed, cuttings or layers in cooler, open places. Drought and frost resistant.

Parts used
The green leaves harvested in early autumn.

Active constituents
1) Hydroquinone derivatives including arbutin (6–9%)[1] and methylarbutin, also free hydroquinone. The arbutin level varies with geographical location and time of year, being highest in autumn.[1]
2) Polyphenols (tannins)—(10–15%) mainly gallotannins, also catechin and corilagin.[2] A tannin level of 6–7% is generally quoted (*BPC*), although the range can be anywhere between 10%–20%, this higher level may reflect total polyphenols rather than just tannins. However a study of commercial bearberry teas found a tannin content of between 17% and 22%[3]
3) Phenolic acids including mainly gallic acid and also p-coumaric and syringic acids[4]
4) Flavonoids, mainly quercetin and myricetin glycosides
5) Iridoids including monotropein[5]

Also a phenolic glucoside (piceoside)[6] and triterpenes including ursolic acid. Ericolin is not widely cited as a constituent of this herb in modern literature.

The total phenolic content is around 30%.[7]

Nutritional constituents
Vitamins: C and A
Minerals: Calcium, iron, magnesium and potassium

Actions
1) Urinary antiseptic
2) Astringent

Scientific information
The herb has a long history of medicinal use mainly as an astringent and haemostatic, but modern uses date back only to the 18th Century. *Arctostaphylos* has been an official preparation in a number of pharmacopoeias[8] and it is approved by *German Commission E* for the treatment of inflammatory conditions of the lower urinary tract and for catarrh of the bladder and renal pelvis.

Although bearberry had been considered a diuretic pharmacological studies do not bear this out. Instead it is a urinary antiseptic in which arbutin is likely to contribute significantly.[9] The herb also has a very high tannin content and is therefore an effective astringent.

The leaves have been used by the Carrier people from northcentral British Columbia as a poultice on wounds and for high blood pressure, menstrual cramps and as a mood enhancer in menopause.[10]

Antimicrobial
In vitro—*Arctostaphylos* is a very good bacteriostatic agent against a number of *Helicobacter pylori* strains, an action ascribed to the tannins.[11] The herb and/or arbutin also show growth inhibition of a number of infective organisms including *Streptococcus, Enterobacter, Klebsiella* and *Shigella* spp., *Bacillus subtilis, Pseudomonas aeruginosa, Salmonella typhimurium, Proteus mirabilis, Escherichia coli, Ureaplasma urealyticum* and *Mycoplasma hominis*.[12-15] Corilagin is antibacterial and increases the effectiveness of β-lactam antibiotics, e.g. oxacillin (a penicillin), against MRSA.[2]

Ex vivo—Urine from volunteers who had consumed arbutin or whole *Arctostaphylos* extract showed an impressive range of antibacterial activity when tested at an alkaline pH.[15]

Antiviral activity against HSV-2, influenza virus A2 and vaccinia virus by aqueous extracts has also been reported.[15]

In vivo—A preparation containing *Arctostaphylos* and *Taraxacum officinale* (root and herb) was taken over the course of a month and found to be very effective in preventing the development of cystitis in the following 12-month period in a group of women who had had recurrent bladder infections.[16]

The antibacterial effects of the herb are due largely to the conversion in the kidney tubule of arbutin to hydroquinone and hydroquinone esters (see Pharmacokinetics).

Anti-oxidant

In vitro—*Arctostaphylos* is a very strong anti-oxidant, an action likely due to the phenol fraction.[7] (The total phenolic content of this herb is comparable with that of green tea.[7])

Hydroquinone is also an anti-oxidant, inhibiting lipid peroxidation, and may have an inhibitory effect on protein glycation.[17]

Other

In vitro—The herb, and arbutin in particular, strongly inhibit the enzyme tyrosinase[18-20] which is responsible for melanin production and this may represent a treatment option in conditions where melanin production is undesirable e.g. to lighten dark blemishes.[15]

Medicinal uses

Gastro-intestinal tract

The astringency of the tannins is effective in the digestive tract:

- diarrhoea
- haemorrhage

Urinary tract
- pyelitis
- urethritis
- dysuria
- prostatitis
- cystitis (*BHP* specific)

Externally
- leucorrhoea (douche)
- haemorrhage

Pharmacy

Three times daily

Infusion	– 1.5–2.5 g
Tincture 1:5 (25%)	– 2–4 ml (suggested guidelines)
Fluid Extract (25%)	– 1.5–2.5 ml

According to *Weiss* arbutin is difficult to extract from the tough leaf and therefore is best prepared as a decoction. It should be boiled, covered and steeped for half an hour, however this process would increase the tannins extracted too (see below).

Arbutin is slightly better and more quickly absorbed from aqueous extracts of *Arctostaphylos* than from coated tablets.[21]

CONTRAINDICATIONS—Pregnancy (*BHC* and *German Commission E*).

Pharmacokinetics

The enzyme responsible for converting arbutin to hydroquinone is not found in mammalian tissues and hydroquinone produced in any quantity is therefore presumed to be the result of gut flora or infecting microbes.[22] Hydroquinone absorbed from the gut is converted in the liver to hydroquinone esters for renal excretion, being released again in its free form in the kidneys, particularly if urine is alkaline. It has also been shown that *E. coli* organisms absorb arbutin metabolites and convert them to hydroquinone within their own cells without the requirement of an alkaline pH.[23] Hydroquinone and its esters' antibacterial activity is maximal 3–4 hours after dosing.[15] Although bearberry itself is only weakly bactericidal, its action in inhibiting *E. coli* strains from adhering to host cells walls is strong and this would add to any direct antimicrobial effect.[24] *In vivo* oral dosing with an infusion resulted in over 50% of arbutin being excreted within 4 hours, mainly as hydroquinone glucuronide and hydroquinone sulphate,[25] and 75% being excreted within 24 hours. Free hydroquinone is excreted in insignificant quantities.[26]

Precautions and/or safety

The high tannin content of this herb can lead to gastric irritation and large doses may cause nausea and vomiting. Tannin levels may be reduced by preparing a cold infusion and/or gastric irritation may be counteracted by first giving a demulcent.

A case of bull's-eye maculopathy has been reported after the herb was used for 3 years, the speculated cause being the herb's inhibition of tyrosinase.[27]

It is recommended in the *BHC* that this herb should only be used short term—maximum 7 days. However the *Commission E monograph* (1984) does not note this restriction but advises that long term use should not be undertaken without consulting a practitioner.

Hydroquinone has no reported carcinogenic effects in humans but can produce gene mutations in high enough concentrations. Arbutin and *Arctostaphylos* itself appear to be devoid of genotoxicity even at relatively high doses.[22] The hydroquinone content of bearberry generated by human metabolism is low and the herb is considered safe when used as recommended.

Historical uses
Bladder and kidney disease; tonic to urinary tract; with tobacco as a smoking mix.

Gaultheria procumbens

Wintergreen, checkerberry

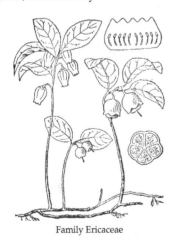

Family Ericaceae

Description
Dwarf evergreen shrub, 10–15 cm, with thin creeping rootstock from which grow erect hairy stems topped with a few leaves. *Leaves* 2–4 cm long, pointed elliptic, stiff, leathery with toothed margins; glossy dark green above and paler beneath. *Flowers* white, 7.5 mm long, solitary, drooping, growing on paired stalks from base of leaf axils. Blooms mid to late summer. *Fruit* scarlet 7 mm berries.

Habitat and cultivation
Native to North America from Newfoundland to Georgia and also to most of Europe and the north of Britain growing in open woods, thickets, rocky moors and mountainous regions. It grows on poor sandy soils. Cultivated in similar conditions elsewhere. Drought and frost resistant.

Parts used
Leaves and stems.

Active constituents
1) Phenolic compounds including gaultherin and salicylic, p-hydroxy benzoic, gentisic, vanillic and caffeic acids[28]
2) Volatile oil (up to 1%) containing mostly (98%) methyl salicylate (min. 85 µg/g)[29] produced through hydrolysis (either by enzyme action or steam distillation) of gaultherin, which consists of the disaccharide primeverose bound to methyl salicylate. *Gaultheria* is the richest plant source of total and free salicylic acid, the level being especially high in the cultivated herb.[28]

Actions
1) Anti-inflammatory
2) Antirheumatic
3) Diuretic
4) Mild analgesic

Scientific information
By 1843 wintergreen was a recognised source of salicylates, these were being used commercially in both the pharmaceutical and food industries (methyl salicylate formed the base of many synthetic flavours). Through excessive harvesting *Gaultheria* in the wild became seriously depleted. *Betula lenta*, a North American variety of birch was the main natural alternative source of methyl salicylate but it was

and still is also chemically synthesised. Methyl salicylate is usually sold as wintergreen oil[8] however it is possible to distinguish between the naturally derived and synthetic chemical.[30]

The pharmacology of the whole extract is not well studied or much used in modern phytotherapy, and it is the isolated oil, widely sold as wintergreen oil, that is well known. The synthetic version of salicylic acid—acetyl salicylate or aspirin—is by contrast one of the best studied pharmaceuticals. The natural salicylates whilst sharing some of the pharmacological effects of their synthetic counterparts do not have their range of activity. Indeed due to the irritant potential of salicylic acid and aspirin, alternative chemical derivatives have been sought to use as anti-inflammatory medications and gaultherin has been tested in this context as the presence of the disaccharide renders the salicylate non-irritant.[29]

In vitro—*Gaultheria* has antifungal activity against some species including *Microsporum gypseum* and *Trichophyton mentagrophytes*.[31]

However it is mainly as an external application of the essential oil that *Gaultheria* is used today.

Medicinal uses
Musculoskeletal
The herb is used internally in the treatment of:

* rheumatoid arthritis
* rheumatism

Externally
As a liniment the essential oil (mainly) is used for:

* neuralgia
* myalgia
* sprains
* sciatica

Pharmacy
Three times daily
Infusion of dried herb　　–　0.5–1 g
Fluid Extract (25%)　　　–　0.5–1 ml
　It is easily absorbed from the skin but may cause reactions.

Precautions and/or safety
The essential oil must not be taken internally.

Salicylate poisoning can occur with very large doses of herb or ingestion of the essential oil[32] leading within 2 hours to symptoms including nausea, vomiting, pulmonary oedema, convulsions and tinnitus. One teaspoon of wintergreen oil has been calculated as equivalent to about 21 adult aspirin tablets.[33] 6 ml of oil may be a lethal dose for a child and 30 ml for an adult. A case of an infant being poisoned by accidentally swallowing the oil and developing laryngeal oedema[34] has been reported.

Although topical applications of salicylate-containing herbs rarely cause problems, there are cases of patients with skin diseases who, having been exposed to extensive amounts of these preparations, developed signs of toxicity.[35] This is an uncommon event.[36]

The FDA estimates the incidence of sensitivity to salicylates could be as high as 5% of the population[37] and in susceptible individuals this may precipitate asthma,[38] eczema,[39] urticaria,[40] gastrointestinal problems,[41] headaches, recurrent mouth ulcers, irritability and at worst anaphylaxis.[8]

Some sources warn that salicylates in plants could have antiplatelet activity, there are no reported cases to date[42] (see *Salix*).

Historical uses
Emmenagogue; chronic mucus discharges; galactagogue. Externally as an insect repellent.

Vaccinium myrtillus

Bilberry, blueberry

Description
A shrubby perennial with creeping rootstock 0.6 × 1 m. *Stems* green, erect, wiry, branched. *Leaves* oval, 1–2 cm long, leathery with conspicuous veins and finely serrate margins, bright green. *Flowers* reddish pink or red and white, solitary and bell-shaped, blooming in spring. *Fruit* blue-black, sweet-tasting, globular berries.

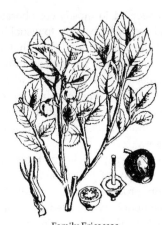

Family Ericaceae

Leaf odour and taste faintly bitter and astringent. Fruit odour—faintly spicy; taste—slightly bitter and pungent.

Habitat and cultivation
Native to woods and forest meadows of Northern Britain, Europe and North America, bilberries prefer a moist, acid soil and semi-shade. They are propagated by cuttings and division in autumn and are frost resistant but drought tender. *V. corymbosum* is grown as a commercial fruit and is also known as blueberry. It is not the medicinal blueberry.

Parts used
The ripe fruit harvested in the autumn. Historically the leaves have also been used.

Active constituents
1) Flavonoids including at least 15 different anthocyanins comprising 0.1–0.25% of the whole extract.[43–50] Also (–)-epicatechin, (+)-catechin, procyanidins (mainly trimers)[51] and the flavonols quercetin[52,56] and myricetin.[53] The flavonoid level is generally higher in sun-exposed leaves and fruit.[54] During maturation of the fruit anthocyanin levels rise and procyanidin and quercetin levels fall[55]
2) Phenolics—the total phenolic content of most berries is high but *Vaccinium* berries is amongst the highest[73]
   a) phenolic acids—derivatives of hydroxycinnamic acid including predominantly ferulic but also p-coumaric, caffeic and chlorogenic acids[56]
   b) polyphenols including trans-resveratrol,[57,58] the content of which varies with geographical location and is reduced by cooking[58]
3) Alkaloid of the quinolizidine type including myrtine and epimyrtine[59]
4) Volatile oil including methyl salicylate, farnesol, vanillin, myristicin and citronellol[60]
5) Tannins in fruit and leaves[61]
6) Iridoid glucosides—monotropein[62]

Also contains fruit acids and sugars, pectin, hydroxy-fatty acids,[63] arbutin and proteins.[64] Carotenoids and sterols have been isolated from the fruit.[65]

N.B. *Potter's* states that *V. myrtillus* does not in fact contain arbutin or any other hydroquinone derivatives that occur in other species of the genus. Very low levels of hydroquinones have been reported more recently in the leaf.[66]

Nutritional constituents
Vitamins: C and E
Minerals: Phosphorus, iron, zinc, magnesium, potassium, sulphur, selenium and smaller amounts of boron, calcium, copper, manganese, sodium and silica[67,68]

Actions
1) Astringent
2) Urinary antiseptic
3) Anti-oxidant
4) Collagen stabiliser
5) Nutritive

Scientific information
Vaccinium has been in use as a medicine for over 1000 years, has been an official medicine in a number of European countries[8] and is approved by *German Commission E* for the treatment of acute non-specific diarrhoea and for local use in mild mucosal inflammation of throat and mouth.

Much of the recent work on the pharmacology of this herb has centred round the *in vitro* effects of the anthocyanins or anthocyanosides and their aglycones, called anthocyanidins. The anthocyanins appear to be more physiologically active although their intestinal absorption was at one time in doubt. Studies now indicate they are absorbed and excreted in this glycosidic form.[69,70] One of the main reasons for the interest in these phytochemicals is that they are very water-soluble and occur in high enough levels in plants to have the potential of reaching effective levels *in vivo*.

Anti-oxidant

In vitro—*Vaccinium*, its anthocyanins[71] and also the catechin and procyanidin fractions are all strong anti-oxidants.[43,51,72-74] The anti-oxidant strength of the herb is directly correlated with its total phenolic content.[56] *Vaccinium* is a potent preventative of low density lipoprotein oxidation and if this action extends to *in vivo* the herb may offer protection against atherogenesis.[75]

In vivo—Serum anti-oxidant potential increased with the consumption of the herb[70] and the serum levels of quercetin was found to be higher in people who consumed bilberries (and other berries) than those on a normal diet.[76]

Anticancer

In vitro—*Vaccinium*, individual anthocyanins and anthocyanidins inhibit a number of different cancer cell lines.[74,77-79] In addition the herb and/or its constituents are:-

- anti-oxidant
- able to inhibit angiogenesis and therefore tumour growth[73,80]
- able to promote enzyme detoxification, protecting against chemically induced tumour formation[81]

In vivo—Epidemiological studies suggest eating berries like *Vaccinium* may be protective against cancer development.[82]

Vision

The effects of bilberry on vision were established in more recent times. It was said that night vision of pilots in World War II was improved through eating bilberry jam and this prompted research into a possible connection. Studies were conducted in the 1970's and seemed to mostly corroborate both *in vivo*[83-87] and *in vitro*[88,89] benefits to visual function.

In vitro—Recent studies found that *Vaccinium* as well as a number of the anthocyanins and resveratrol protect retinal pigment[90] and retinal cell membranes[91] from damage due to oxidation. Oxidation damage is implicated in age-related vision deterioration, retinal disorders and macular degeneration.

In vivo—A survey of clinical trials purporting to test the benefits of *Vaccinium* anthocyanins for night vision produced mixed results.[92] Possible flaws in methodology are cited as accounting for some of the lack of consistency, in particular, many studies used subjects who were not suffering from impaired night vision to begin with and therefore there was no measurable benefit from using the herb.[93]

Clinical trials into other benefits on visual function showed that the anthocyanins were protective in a number of disorders including diabetic retinopathy, retinitis pigmentosa, macular degeneration, anticoagulant-induced haemorrhagic retinopathy,[94] cataracts[95] and glaucoma.[96] The anthocyanins also normalise connective tissue production in diabetic retinopathy, a process that is disordered by the disease, and can lead to loss of vision.[97]

Antimicrobial

In vitro—*Vaccinium*'s phenolic component has antibacterial activity against strains of Gram-negative organisms including *Salmonella*, *Staphylococcus*, *Bacillus* and *Helicobacter* (including *H. pylori*[98]). Some of this activity seems related to disruption of the bacterial cell wall but there is also direct immobilisation of pathogens.[99] The leaf extract also has antibacterial activity.[100]

Whole extracts were antiviral to tick-borne encephalitis virus.[101]

Other

In vitro—The herb has low to moderate anti-inflammatory activity[102,103] but the anthocyanidin, cyanidin, has very strong activity.[104]

Ex vivo—Blood from healthy individuals who had consumed bilberries strongly inhibited platelet aggregation.[105]

In vivo—Much early work into the benefits of *Vaccinium*'s anthocyanins for strengthening and protecting blood vessels is no longer easily accessible nor have they been subjected to recent clinical studies. The herb had been tested in the treatment of a variety of circulatory disorders, including venous and vascular permeability problems, apparently with positive results.[106-110]

Most studies on the herb's effect on inflammation and connective tissue support was carried out using animals and may suggest mechanisms of action as well as applications for clinical use. These showed the herb promoted synthesis and stabilisation of collagen and enhanced cross-linkages of fibres. It also inhibited the release of enzymes that lyse collagen and decreased release of inflammatory prostaglandins, leukotrienes and histamine.

Cyanidin is protective against aspirin-induced ulceration.[74,111]

Medicinal uses
Cardiovascular system
Due to the beneficial effects in strengthening blood vessels, the herb may be used to treat:

- varicose veins
- venous insufficiency
- phlebitis
- oedema
- blood purpura
- fragile capillaries

Gastro-intestinal tract
The fruit acids and pectin act as soluble fibre and make the herb a bulk laxative but it is also astringent:

- constipation—raw berries
- diarrhoea—dried berries
- dysentery
- dyspepsia

Weiss claims a "marked anti-emetic" effect.

Urinary tract
Vaccinium was traditionally used for the treatment of problems in this system. The anthocyanosides are excreted via kidneys. The herb's astringency, antimicrobial and diuretic[8] activities suggests it may be useful in conditions like:

- haematuria

Nervous system
- poor night vision
- hemeralopia (day blindness)
- glaucoma
- diabetic retinopathy
- retinal degeneration
- cataracts

It is possible that by reducing permeability of the blood/brain barrier, *Vaccinium* may be useful in psychotic conditions like schizophrenia.[60]

Reproductive tract
- vaginal discharge

Grieve lists *Vaccinium* as anti-galactogogue, an action not mentioned elsewhere.

Musculoskeletal
It may help improve excretion of uric acid. As an agent that strengthens connective tissue and prevents inflammatory damage the herb is used in the treatment of:

- rheumatoid arthritis
- osteoarthritis
- gout
- periodontal disease

Externally
With the high tannin content it may be used externally to treat:

- wounds
- ulcers
- infections

Pharmacy
Three times daily
Decoction dried herb   –   2–4 g
Fluid Extract (25%)   –   2–4 ml

Scientific investigations used extracts standardised to contain 25% anthocyanins.

Pharmacokinetics
The anthocyandins reached maximum levels in urine 3–4 hours after ingestion.[74]

Precautions and/or safety
It has been recommended by some surgeons that *Vaccinium* supplements be discontinued 2 weeks prior to surgery due to potential antiplatelet effects.[112]

The leaves have been reported to be toxic in animals due to the presence of hydroquinones. It is possible that the inconsistent levels of this constituent have arisen from contamination of the leaves with other species of this genus.[66] The anthocyanidins are non-toxic.[60,74]

Interactions
Due to its antiplatelet activity bilberry could interact with antithrombotics but there are no reports of interactions to-date.[113]

In vitro—*Vaccinium* inhibited organic anion-transporting polypeptide-B found in intestinal epithelial cells and this may affect the absorption of drugs which use this mechanism if the two are consumed concomitantly.[114]

Historical uses
Scurvy; agues; vomiting; old coughs; menorrhagia; haemoptysis; ulcer in the lung; discharges or bleeding generally whether internal or external; dropsy; gravel. Leaf extracts for diabetes mellitus type 2.

EUPHORBIACEAE

The Euphorbiaceae or spurge family consists of 283 genera and 7,300 species of monoecious and dioecious herbs, shrubs, trees and even some spiny succulents, often with milky juice. They grow worldwide but mostly in the tropics. Among the medicinal plants of this family are the *Chamaesyce, Euphorbia, Phyllanthus, Ricinus* and *Stillingia* genera.

Chamaesyce hirta
[Formerly *Euphorbia pilulifera*]

Asthma plant, pill-bearing spurge

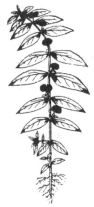

Family Euphorbiaceae

Description

Annual, erect or spreading with several radiating, reddish stems 10–30 cm long, moderately to densely hairy. *Leaves* opposite, moderately hairy above, densely hairy below, oval to elliptic, 2–4 cm long, serrate, dull reddish green, often with a purple spot about mid vein. *Flowers* reduced and clustered in a cup-shaped involucre to form a flower-like cyathium, in small axillary or terminal leafless clusters. *Seed* capsule smooth. Seeds rugose, reddish brown.

All parts of the plant exude a copious amount of white latex if broken.

Habitat and cultivation

Native to several tropical countries e.g. India and Northern Australia, it is a widespread and troublesome weed of crop lands and any open disturbed wasteland. Grows from seed, self-sows freely.

Parts used

The herb harvested during flowering.

Active constituents[1,2]

1) Flavonoids including quercitin, quercetrin, myricitrin and cyanidin[3,4]
2) Triterpenes including taraxerol, α- and β-amyrin, friedelin[5]

171

3) Sterols including β-sitosterol, campesterol and jambulol
4) Polyphenols
   a) tannins including ellagitannins (euphorbin A and B)[6]
   b) phenolic acids including gallic acid and its derivatives

Also contains shikimic, hentriacontane and melissic (myricyl) alcohol and acid; choline and a small quantity of alkaloids.

Nutritional constituents
Vitamins: C[1]
Minerals: Calcium, copper and iron[7]

Actions
1) Anti-asthmatic
2) Expectorant
3) Spasmolytic
4) Antiprotozoal

Scientific information
Euphorbia has been a recognised medicinal herb in many different parts of the world, used to treat a variety of conditions (see Historical uses).[8–11] It was an official preparation in the *British Pharmaceutical Codex* indicated for the treatment of coughs and asthma, which is its main use in modern phytotherapy, and with an acknowledged application in the treatment of amoebiasis.[12]

In vitro—Recent studies have been concerned with the antimicrobial activity of *Euphorbia* as so many traditions have used it for treating general infections. Extracts have a broad spectrum of antibacterial activity, especially against *Escherichia coli*, *Proteus vulgaris*, *Pseudomonas aeruginosa*, *Staphylococcus aureus*,[13–15] *Bacillus cereus*,[9] *Vibrio cholerae* and *Shigella* spp.[16] (including *S. flexneri*[17]). A low activity against *Helicobacter pylori*[8] has also been reported as well as some antifungal activity against *Candida albicans*.[9,18]

The herb has been used traditionally in the treatment of protozoan parasites and it has been tested against *Plasmodium falciparum* and reported to have a range of activity from weak[10] to very good,[19] achieving over 80% inhibition in one study.[20]

It was also strongly anti-amoebic to *Entamoeba hystolytica*[21] and with its apparent spasmolytic and antibacterial actions, attributed to the polyphenols,[22] this could explain its widespread traditional use in treating diarrhoea and dysentery.[23] Anti-amoebic activity demonstrated in fresh plant aqueous extracts was much reduced in extracts made from dried herb.[24]

In vivo—The herb effectively treated intestinal amoebiasis particularly acute cases of short duration.[25]

Choline and shikimic acid are active in relaxing smooth muscle but a detailed pharmacology for the herb itself is lacking.

Euphorbia has also been used in:

- Asia for worms and viral fever[26]
- Africa as a diuretic[27] and to treat asthma,[13,28] peptic ulcers, dysentery and diarrhoea[29]
- Australia for coughs, chronic bronchitis and pulmonary disorders.[29]

Medicinal uses
Respiratory tract
- asthma
- bronchitis
- upper respiratory catarrh
- laryngeal spasms

BHP specific for bronchitic asthma.

Gastrointestinal tract
- amoebiasis

Pharmacy
Three times daily
Infusion of dried herb   – 120–300 mg
Tincture 1:5 (60%)   – 0.6–2.0 ml
Fluid extract (45%)   – 0.12–0.30 ml

Precautions and/or safety
The herb has a very low toxicity *in vitro*.[10,16]

Historical uses
Emphysema; hayfever and coryza; as a sedative;[30] to treat snake bites.[5]

FABACEAE

Fabaceae—the pea family, formerly Leguminosae. This is the third largest plant family in the world with over 650 genera. The Fabaceae is a cosmopolitan family of trees, shrubs, lianes, water plants and herbaceous plants and most have root nodules containing nitrogen-fixing bacteria which make atmospheric nitrogen available to the plant.

Economically the Fabaceae family is important because many genera produce edible seeds e.g. peanuts, carob, chick peas, soya beans, lentils, peas and beans. Melilot, clovers and lucerne are important fodder crops.

Characteristics
- The flowers are grouped into racemes, spikes, panicles or heads
- The calyx is tubular usually with 5 sepals more or less united
- The corolla usually has 5 petals and is butterfly-shaped—the uppermost petal is large and showy and called the *standard*; the two side petals form the *wings* and the two lowest, more or less united, form the *keel*
- Inside the keel there are usually 10 stamens with their filaments fused into a tube. Sometimes 1 stamen remains separate, and occasionally all the filaments are separate
- The pistil is simple with 1 carpel which contains a number of ovaries
- The fruit is a pod which splits into 2 separate halves. In a few species the pods break up into sections instead of splitting
- The leaves are usually compound and alternate. There are stipules present sometimes in the form of spines. Often some leaflets are changed into tendrils used for climbing

Fabaceae is sometimes treated as 3 families: Caesalpinioideae, Mimosoideae, and Papilionoideae.

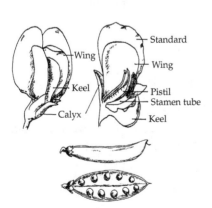

173

Baptisia tinctoria

Wild indigo

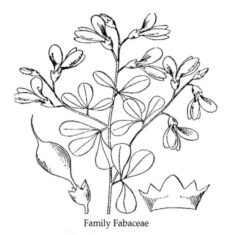

Family Fabaceae

Description
A slender, glaucous, bushy-branching perennial herb which grows 30–60 cm tall. *Root* large, irregular, ligneous, light yellowish-brown inside, black externally. Numerous rootlets. *Leaves* trifoliate, mostly sessile, dark blue-green with a light green stripe on the midrib, leaflets rounded or cuneate-obovate. *Stem* smooth, glabrous, round, branching. *Inflorescence* short, loose, few-flowered in terminal racemes. Flowers canary yellow, about as long as leaflets, calyx cup-shaped. *Fruit* an oval, centrally inflated legume stalked in the persistent cup of the calyx. *Seeds* many, ovoid and cinnamon brown.

Habitat and cultivation
Indigenous to Canada and USA in open, sunny areas of well-drained sandy soils. Grows in some other countries. Grown from seed sown in winter/spring. Frost resistant, drought tender.

Parts used
The roots gathered in the spring or autumn of the second year onwards. The fresh root was preferred by the Eclectics.

Active constituents
1) Alkaloids including cytisine[1] (probably identical to baptitoxin)[2]
2) Polysaccharides including arabinogalactan-proteins (glycoproteins)[3] and heteroglycans[4]
3) Flavonoids including isoflavones (genistein)
4) Oleo-resin
5) Coumarins

Actions
1) Antimicrobial
2) Immunostimulant
3) Laxative
4) Antipyretic
5) Mild cardioactive

Scientific information
Baptisia was a valued medicine for indigenous North Americans. It was introduced to European settlers in the late 18th Century and they found it effective for treating infectious diseases. In recent times it has suffered from over-harvesting.

In vitro—The arabinogalactan-proteins in *Baptisia* may have similar physiological properties, but are not structurally the same, as those found in *Echinacea* spp.[5]

The water-soluble polysaccharide or heteroglycan fraction is immunostimulating.[4,6]

In vivo—Recent studies have mainly been carried out on *Baptisia*, in combination with other herbs, to treat upper respiratory infections. They were significantly better than placebo in reducing these infections.[7-9] The mode of action is likely to be antiviral as well as stimulation of non-specific immune function (increased macrophage activity)[9,10] and/or immuno-balancing.[8]

Isoflavones are oestrogenic.

Medicinal uses
Cardiovascular system
• fevers
• lymphadenitis

Respiratory tract
The specific application of *Baptisia* is for infections in the upper respiratory tract:

• tonsillitis
• pharyngitis
• acute catarrhal infections

Gastro-intestinal tract
- aphthous ulcers
- stomatitis
- gingivitis

Skin
- boils

Externally
- indolent ulcers
- sore nipples
- leucorrhoea (as a douche)

Pharmacy
Three times daily

Decoction	–	0.3–1 g
Tincture BPC (1934)	–	2–5 ml
Fluid Extract (60%)	–	0.3–1.3 ml

The recommended ratio in the *BHP* for the ointment is 1 part fluid extract to 8 parts of base.

To date *Baptisia* has been found to be non-toxic,[7,9] although cytisine itself, being similar to nicotine, is toxic.[1]

Historical uses
Liver problems, venereal disease, pains of varied nature, sepsis, intermittent fevers including typhus and scarlatina.

Cassia acutifolia and *Cassia angustifolia*
[Formerly listed as *Cassia senna*]

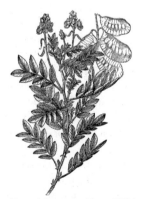

Alexandrian senna (*C. acutifolia*)

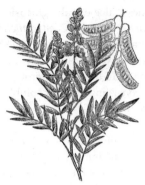

Family Fabaceae
Tinnevelly senna (*C. angustifolia*)

Description
C. acutifolia is a small shrub to about 60 cm high. The *stems* are erect, smooth and pale green, with long spreading branches with leaflets arranged in 4–5 pairs. They have an asymetric base and a thin stiff, brittle, light green lamina, often marked with transverse/oblique lines. They have a faint peculiar odour and a mucilaginous, sweetish taste (*Grieve*). *Flowers* are small and yellow and fruit is a pod 5 cm × 20–25 mm containing 5–7 seeds. *C. angustifolia* is an annual growing in the Middle East and India. It differs from *C. acutifolia* in the pod size which is 5 cm × 15–18 mm containing 7–10 seeds. These pods taste more bitter and harsh.

Odour—characteristic; taste—mucilaginous then slightly bitter.[11]

Habitat
Alexandrian senna is native to Egypt, Sudan and Nigeria. Tinnevelly senna is cultivated in India.

Parts used
The leaves and the fruit pods.

Active constituents[11]
1) Hydroxyanthracene glycosides (min. 3%) mainly the dianthrones—sennosides A (41%) and B (44%),[12] also C and D[13,14,†] and small amounts of free anthroquinones rhein, aloe-emodin and crysophanol. Also rhein

---

†The constituents of the two varieties of *Cassia* only differ in their quantity of these constituents. *C. acutifolia* pods contain 2.5–4.5% and *C. angustifolia* 1.2–2.5% hydroxyanthracene glycosides (calculated as sennoside B) whilst leaf content for both is a minimum of 2.5%.

8-glucosides,[15] aloe-emodin glucosides,[16–18] tinnevellin 8-glucoside (*C. angustifolia*)[19] and 6-hydroxymusicin glucoside (*C. acutifolia*)[20]

2) Naphthalene glycosides
3) Flavonoids including kaempferol
4) Mucilage consisting of water soluble acidic polysaccharides[21]

Also contains pinitol, sugars and a gum isolated from the seeds containing galactomannans.[22]

The powder, on storage, may degrade to sennidin glucosides and sennosides oxidise at high temperatures to rhein 8-O-glucoside.[23]

Nutritional constituents
Minerals: Low levels of calcium, copper, magnesium, manganese and zinc[24]

Actions
1) Laxative

Scientific information
Senna was introduced to the west by the Arabs in the 9th Century although its recorded use dates back as far as 1550 BC.[25] It has been a recognised medicine ever since and is still an official medicine in modern allopathic medicine, used to treat constipation.[1] As a result its constituents are relatively well studied. The trend in laxative use is apparently declining. It had been a regular self-administered treatment, persisting more in the older age groups.[26] Senna is however still one of the more popular over-the-counter products for constipation[27] and it is used in hospitals.

Laxative
Sennosides A and B are considered the main active constituents.[15] The strength of cathartic activity within this species is directly related to the level of sennosides.[28] They pass to the large colon intact where gut flora metabolise them to produce active rhein anthrone which on absorption into the lumen wall stimulates the colon, through nerve and the immune cell stimulation, causing evacuation.[29–31] Sennoside administration has been shown to increase peristalsis or propulsive activity in the ascending and descending colon, thereby reducing bowel transit time,[32–35] and to increase the calibre of the lumen of all parts of the colon.[36] By reducing transit time fluid re-absorption is reduced but there is also an increase in secretion of fluid into the colon, thus making stools more "fluid".

In vivo—Many clinical trials have been conducted using pharmaceutical senna preparations with standardised sennoside levels, to stimulate bowel function. They were found effective:-

- after opiod therapy[37–39] (as effective as lactulose)[40]
- as a bowel cleanse preparatory to colonoscopy[41]
- in children[42] although the benefits in chronic functional constipation were limited[43]
- in pregnancy[44] and postpartum[45]
- after abdominal[46] and anorectal[47] surgery
- in the constipation phase of irritable bowel syndrome[11]
- in elderly patients used alone[48] or in combination with other laxative aids[49–51]

In prescribed doses sennosides do not disrupt the normal pattern of bowel emptying,[11] alter gastric emptying or small intestine transit time.[52] Senna's effect on bowel function does not persist on cessation of its use.[53,54]

A combination of senna and psyllium has been very effective in treating constipation,[55] improving bowel function more than either agent alone.[56]

Other
In vitro—*Cassia angustifolia* has:

- limited anti-hepatoma activity[57]
- inhibits the generation of mutagens and has anti-mutagenic activity[58]
- virucidal activity against HSV-1 an activity isolated to the anthraquinone fraction. (Aloe-emodin has a much wider antiviral action against a range of enveloped viruses.)[59]

In Asian countries *Cassia* has been used traditionally as a topical agent to treat inflammation and *in vitro* studies have lent some support to this use.[60]

In vivo—Serum oestrogen levels in pre-menopausal women fell when senna was used throughout the cycle as the opportunity for hormone re-absorption from the colon was reduced.[61] However the decreased transit time did not alter oxidative status or the level of plasma cholesterol or triglycerides.[62]

Medicinal uses
Gastro-intestinal tract
- constipation
- haemorrhoids (which require soft stools)
- anal fissures (which require soft stools)

Pharmacy
Once daily
Infusion
Dried pods   – 3–6 (*C. acutifolia*)
              – 4–12 (*C. angustifolia*-steeped in 150 ml of warm water for 6–12 hours)
Dried leaf   – 0.5–2 g in a cup of water
Fluid Extract:
Pods BPC (1973) – 0.5–2 ml
Leaves (25%)   – 0.5–2 ml

The herb takes 8 to 14 hours to act and is best taken at bedtime or perhaps as a split dose, one at bedtime and the other in the morning.

It has been suggested that a hot infusion should be used to minimise possible microbial contamination.[63]

CONTRAINDICATIONS—Intestinal obstructions, inflammatory bowel disease, appendicitis, abdominal pain of unknown origin.

Pharmacokinetics
Rhein anthrone is taken up in small amounts from the colon and is metabolised to glucuronide and sulphate derivatives which can be found in urine and bile.[31] The serum half life of rhein anthrone is between 4 and 12 hours[31] and it is detectable in urine for 24 hours.[64] Plasma levels of rhein show two peaks, one after 3–5 hours, presumed to be free rhein and the other after 10–11 hours relating to the bacterial release of rhein from the sennosides, aloe-emodin is below detection level.[65]

Precautions and/or safety
Clinical trials have reported the herb is safe when used at recommended doses.[48,66,67] Used in preparation for colonoscopy in patients with ulcerative colitis it did not cause relapse from the remission phase of the disease.[68]

Senna in all its forms is not genotoxic, *in vitro*[69] in particular the anthraquinone glycosides appear to be safe.[70] *In vivo* assessment supports this finding too at prescribed doses.[71]

These preparations have also been declared safe for use in pregnancy and lactation,[72–74] although *German Commission E* contraindicates such use.

The herb can cause griping and should therefore be administered with a carminative. Clinical studies comparing various laxatives have found that senna tends to be associated with more side-effects.[75–77] It should not be used for longer than 10 days at a time. Overdosing can lead to fluid and electrolyte loss through diarrhoea and chronic use may lead to dependence and the need for higher doses.[11]

Because of the decreased colon transit time senna reduces the potential to absorb deoxycholic acid, the increased levels of which have been associated with cholesterol saturation of bile and gall stone development.[78]

There are a number of anecdotal reports of problems caused through the overuse/abuse of *Cassia*. These include reversible acute hepatic failure with renal impairment,[79] hepatitis,[80,81] hypogammaglobulinaemia,[82] finger-clubbing[83] and hypertrophic osteoarthropathy.[84] In children under 6 years of age *Cassia* intake has resulted in severe nappy rash, blistering and skin sloughing.[85]

Rhein increases apoptosis of colon cells *in vitro* and stimulates leucocyte activity.[86] *In vivo* a highly purified extract of sennosides affected the cell growth of the colon epithelium quite dramatically when administered as a once only enema causing widespread apoptosis and consequent replacement by cell proliferation.[87] There is concern that chronic use of *Cassia* can lead to cancer and this may be a possible mechanism. Chronic use has certainly been linked to the development of *pseudomelanosis coli*. This is due to the deposition of a greater number of apoptic bodies in the colon mucosa that contain a melanin-like pigment derived from the anthroquinones and/or cell death.[88] It has been suggested this condition may lead to bowel inflammation and possibly bowel cancer although no link has been found to date[11] and there are no epidemiologic data actually linking senna use to increased colon cancer.[89] Furthermore there was no evidence of inflammation or increased incidence of cancer even when used by people at high-risk for developing colorectal cancer.[90,91] At present *pseudomelanosis coli* is considered harmless and reversible.[11,92] A retrospective study of patients with urinary tract cancers has deduced that senna may be causally linked.[93]

Alteration to the bowel structure from laxatives has been described but is another controversial aspect of senna use.[11,89] The colon in stimulant laxative users may lose its structure, namely the haustral folds, and this could indicate either neuron or muscle damage may have occurred.[94]

Interactions

Because of the decreased transit time through the colon it is possible that senna may interact with drugs with which it is co-administered and which are absorbed from this area. *In vivo* concomitant administration of senna and oestrodiol resulted in reduced serum hormone levels although the effect was not significant.[95]

Chronic use or abuse of *Cassia* may lead to hypokalaemia which could potentiate the effect of cardiac glycoside drugs like digitalis or anti-arrhythmics or exacerbate potassium deficiency induced by thiazide diuretics or adrenocorticosteroids.[11]

Historical uses

As for modern uses.

Cytisus scoparius
[Formerly *Sarothamnus scoparius*]

Broom, Scotch broom

Description

Much branched deciduous shrub to 3 × 2 m, with slender, erect, arching stems and green, more or

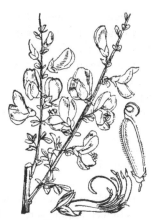

Family Fabaceae

less 5-angled twigs. *Leaves* trifoliate and petiolate when mature, younger leaves sub- sessile and 1–2-foliate, soft green. Leaflets elliptic to obovate 4–16 mm long, terminal leaflet longer than lateral leaflets. *Flowers* pea-shaped, usually solitary, rarely paired, in leaf axils. Calyx glabrous, bilabiate, about ¼ length of corolla. Corolla golden yellow, 16–25 mm long. *Pods* black, many-seeded, oblong, 15–60 mm long with hairy margins. *Seeds* ellipsoid, brown or greenish brown, about 3 mm long. Flowers late spring to mid-summer.

Habitat and cultivation

Native to Britain, Europe and Asia, grows in light to medium acid soils in sunny situations. *Cytisus* is naturalised elsewhere and is often a troublesome weed. It grows from seed or cuttings and is drought and frost resistant.

Parts used

The flowering tops harvested in early spring.

Active constituents

1) Quinolizidine alkaloids (0.10% of fresh plant) mainly (−)-sparteine, (−)17-oxosparteine, (+)-lupanine and derivatives of lupanine. Alkaloid levels are highest in the leaves, much lower in flowers[96,97]
2) Flavonoids including the isoflavonoids genistein and scoparin, also flavonols including quercitin and isoquercitin[98,99]

3) Phenethylamines including tyramine and hydroxytyramine, levels much higher in flowers[96,100]

4) Volatile oil including eugenol, isovaleric and benzoic acids

Also contains tannins, caffeic and p-coumaric acids. The seeds contain lectins.[101]

Actions
1) Peripheral vasoconstrictor
2) Antihaemorrhagic
3) Diuretic

Scientific information
Broom was used medicinally by the Anglo-Saxons and was at one time an official preparation.

There are very few studies of this herb in recent times and most knowledge comes from traditional use and the observed actions of its best known constituent, sparteine, which has been used in orthodox medicine.

In vitro—The herb has good antioxidant properties.[102]

Cytisus is a herb with cardiac activity however this activity is not based on glycosides, as in the case of *Digitalis* and *Convallaria*, but is due to the alkaloids, mainly sparteine.

Sparteine has been subjected to pharmacological study.[1] It reduces the irritability and conductivity of the heart. Its action occurs via the autonomic ganglia, small doses stimulate and large doses paralyse them. It potentiates the effect of adrenaline in raising blood pressure. It also depresses respiration and is a stimulant of uterine contractions (though *Potter's* suggest this action is unpredictable in inducing labour, *Weiss* states it is used instead of quinine in obstetric practice and there are many reports of its use as an oxytocic agent[1]).

The phenethylamines have vasoconstrictor activity.

Medicinal uses
Cardiovascular system
The effect of *Cytisus* is to reduce overactivity of the heart and so produce a regular, effective heart stroke. The peripheral constriction produces a rise in pressure. Overall venous return and cardiac output benefit:

• arrhythmias
• palpitations
• myocardial weakness
• tachycardia
• cardiac oedema
• hypotension
• post-infectious myocarditis

BHP specific is for functional palpitations with lowered blood pressure.

N.B. *Weiss* states the herb will not adequately treat absolute arrhythmia or paroxysmal tachycardia.

Reproductive tract
As a vasoconstrictor and anti-haemorrhagic, the herb may find use in the treatment of:

• menorrhagia

Pharmacy
Three times daily
Infusion of dried herb   – 1–2 g
Tincture 1:5 (45%)   – 0.5–2 ml
Fluid Extract (25%)   – 1–2 ml
CONTRAINDICATIONS—Pregnancy, hypertension.

Historical uses
Cytisus was considered a cathartic and emetic agent. Used in gout; joint pains in general; liver obstructions; sciatica; tumours. Also for ague; bladder and kidney problems including stones. The oil used for toothache. As an ointment for stitches in the side or spleen pain; for lice.

Galega officinalis

Goat's rue

Description
An erect, leafy, hairless perennial herb growing from 0.5–1 m high in flower. *Stems* rounded,

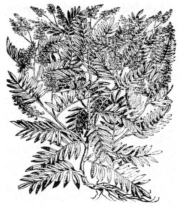

Family Fabaceae

ribbed, hollow and more or less glabrous. *Leaves* pinnate with oblong, fine- pointed or notched leaflets 20–50 mm long, in 4–9 opposite pairs; pinnately veined; stipules ovate-lanceolate with 1–3 basal lobes. *Flowers* in erect axillary or terminal racemes. They are short-stalked and 8–15 mm long. Calyx campanulate with 5 sub-equal teeth, glabrous or with scattered short hairs at the base of the tube and teeth, slightly swollen at the side. Corolla white or pale lilac, 10–13 mm long. *Seed* pods glabrous, more or less cylindric, 2–3 cm × 4 mm, with thickened parallel veins, containing 2–8 smooth, oblong seeds. Flowers in summer through to autumn.

Habitat and cultivation
Native to Europe and Asia Minor and cultivated elsewhere. Grown from seed and self-sows. Prefers an open sunny situation and rich, moist soils. Dies back in winter. Drought and frost tender.

Parts used
The herb harvested just prior to or during flowering.

Active constituents
1) Alkaloids including galegine[103] and peganine[104]
2) Saponins of triterpenoid type and β-sitosterol[105]
3) Flavonoids based on kaempferol and quercitin[106]

Also contains a bitter compound and tannins.

Actions
1) Hypoglycaemic
2) Galactagogue
3) Diuretic (mild)

Scientific information
Galega has been associated with treating diabetes since the Middle Ages and was used in Europe and other parts of the world.[107,108] It was from this herb that metformin, a current drug commonly used to treat type-2 diabetes, was developed.[109]

In vitro—The herb has significant antibacterial activity to both Gram-positive and Gram-negative organisms.[110] A water-soluble fraction inhibits platelet aggregation (it consists of a polysaccharide and protein).[111,112]

Goat's rue does not contain any known phyto-oestrogenic constituents.[113]

Galegine is a glucokinin derived from the purine guanidine. It has been identified as a poison to some live-stock if eaten in excess which has led to *Galega* being listed as a poisonous plant in some countries.[114] It is active as a hypoglycaemic agent.[115]

The name *Galega* derives from gale-"milk" and *ega*- "to bring on" a clear acknowledgement of the herb's galactagogic properties. There are no current *in vivo* evaluations of the herb as an anti-diabetic agent or as a galactagogue but earlier clinical studies had examined these actions.[116,117]

Medicinal uses
Reproductive tract
• to increase lactation/milk flow

Endocrine system
• diabetes

Pharmacy
Three times daily
Infusion of dried herb   – 1–2 g
Tincture 1:10 (45%)   – 2–4 ml
Fluid Extract (25%)   – 1–2 ml

Galega is particularly used for type 2 or late onset diabetes. The *BHP* states that its effect is gradual and if the patient is using insulin then this needs to be continued. The treatment regime can be adjusted as the blood and/or urine glucose levels improve.

Precautions and/or safety
Careful monitoring of glucose levels is necessary when treating diabetes.

Historical uses
Used as a footbath for tired feet. The American *G. virginiana* is also diaphoretic and anthelmintic. This was an official medicine in the *United States Pharmacopoeia. Weiss* mentions the seeds of *G. officinalis* as the part used in the treatment of diabetes but does not apparently hold them in very high regard.

Glycyrrhiza glabra

Liquorice, licorice

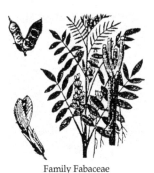

Family Fabaceae

Description
A robust erect, hairless perennial to 1.5 m, which dies down in winter. *Leaves*, mat green, pinnate with 9–17 elliptic to oblong leaflets, 2.5–5 cm, and a terminal leaflet, sticky beneath; stipules minute or absent. *Flowers* numerous, growing in axillary, long stalked, spike-like clusters. Each flower is bluish or violet, about 1 cm, with a glandular-hairy calyx and an erect standard much longer than the wings or keel. *Fruit* 1.5–2 cm, oblong, much flattened and hairless. Flowers in summer.

Odour—faint and characteristic; taste—very sweet and mildly aromatic.

Habitat and cultivation
Native to south east Europe, central and south west Asia growing in stony places, dry woods and ditches. Grows easilty from seed. Cultivated commercially in well- drained, rich moist soil. Does best in cold winter climates. May be divided and replanted in autumn. Dies back in winter and does not appear until late spring.

Frost resistant, drought tender.

Parts used
Root and stolons harvested from autumn of the fourth year onwards (preferably). Outer cortex may be stripped or left.

Active constituents[118]
1) Triterpene saponins predominantly glycyrrhizin (2–25%) which is a mixture of calcium and potassium salts of glycyrrhizic acid, also called glycyrrhizinic acid. Its aglycone 18-β-glycyrrhetic acid (glycyrrhetic acid) also called glycyrrhetinic acid or enoxolone, is present in small quantities and produced on hydrolysis of glycyrrhizin. Other terpenoids have been isolated[119–123]
2) Flavonoids (approximately 1%) including:
   a) flavonones—liquiritigenin, isoliquiritigenin, liquiritin and its apioside, isoliquiritin and licochalcone A
   b) isoflavonoids—including glabridin (about 0.2%), glabrene and fomononetin[124–131]
3) Bitter (glycymarin)
4) Polysaccharides based on a backbone of galactose residues[132–134]

Also contains up to 45 other phenolic constituents including salicylicates,[135,136] a trace of volatile oil, sterols (β-sitosterol[137]), asparagine, coumarins[138] including umbelliferone,[139] a trace of tannins and a ketone based on propanone.[140]

Glycyrrhizin is the predominant constituent of all *Glycyrrhiza* species, although its content varies widely with geographical location[127,141] being up to 4% in European root but much higher in Chinese grown liquorice. Content is also influenced by extraction method for example it is better extracted using 70% ethanol than 50% ethanol.[126] Glabridin is a distinctive flavonoid found in *G. glabra* and helps

to distinguish it from the other medicinal varieties, *G. uralensis* and *G. inflata*, although all three are
closely related. In central Asia where both *G. glabra*
and *G. uralensis* grow together a hybrid is produced
but it lacks glabridin.[141]

Nutritional constituents
Vitamins: E and B complex, biotin, niacin and pantothenic acid
Minerals: Phosphorus, manganese, iodine, chromium and zinc
    Also contains lecithin.

Actions
1) Expectorant
2) Adrenocorticotropic
3) Demulcent
4) Anti-inflammatory
5) Spasmolytic
6) Mild laxative

Scientific information
Glycyrrhiza has been named from the Greek *glykos* =
sweet and *rhiza* = root. Its medicinal use has a long
history, over 4000 years, and is widespread being
found in all the major ancient cultures. It has been
an official medicine in very many countries as a
demulcent and expectorant,[1] actions attributed to
glycyrrhizin,[118] and is approved by *German Commission E* for the treatment of upper respiratory
catarrh and for gastric and duodenal ulcers.
    Glycyrrhizin is around 170 times sweeter than
sucrose[142,143] (a value of 50 times sweeter has been
reported elsewhere[118]). It is widely used in com-
merce as a flavouring agent (in the tobacco industry, for beverages, as a foaming agent in beer and
also in confectionery) apart from being one of the
most frequently used herbs worldwide.
    There is a vast volume of new research into the
herb and its constituents as they appear to have a
broad spectrum of activity and may provide the
basis for developing new medicines.

Endocrine effects
The adrenal-like effects of *Glycyrrhiza* have been
appreciated for a long time and many studies have
helped to elucidate its mode of action.

In vitro—The mechanism of action and the effect
of liquorice's constituents, mainly glycyrrhetic acid,
on adrenocortical function is seen as two-fold:-

- inhibition of the enzyme 11β-hydroxysteroid
  dehydrogenase which converts active cortisol
  to the inactive cortisone, so that it raises levels
  of free cortisol.[144] Cortisol is also capable of
  binding to mineralocorticoid receptor sites[145]
  and behaving like aldosterone, the enzyme's
  inactivation of cortisol prevents it from doing
  so. By inhibiting enzyme inactivation of cortisol an apparent mineralocorticoid excess
  occurs. Glycyrrhetic acid and at least one
  of its metabolites[146] are much more potent
  inhibitors of this enzyme than glycyrrhizic
  acid[147]
- interaction with the mineralocorticoid and
  gluco-corticoid receptors directly although this
  binding is very weak, glycyrrhetic acid's affinity being four orders of magnitude lower than
  aldosterone[148] and five orders of magnitude
  lower than dexamethasone[149]

The inhibition of 11β-hydroxysteroid dehydrogenase has further ramifications as the enzyme may
be partly responsible for the differentiation of precursor fat cells to adipose cells a process that has
been prevented by carbenoxolone, a derivative of
glycyrrhizin.[150] *In vivo* liquorice was indeed shown
to reduce body fat.[151]
    The isoflavonoids glabridin and glabrene also
have endocrine effects and have shown similar
benefits to that of HRT in osteoblasts and endothelial cells from post-menopausal women.[152,153]
In vivo—The measured effects of *Glycyrrhiza*
in normal healthy people, presumed to be due to
inhibiting 11β-hydroxysteroid dehydrogenase, are:-

- raised levels of renal and urinary cortisol and
  sodium[154]
- raised blood pressure (as little as 50 g of
  liquorice daily was reported to cause a rise and
  studies using 50–200 g daily recorded a range
  of increase from 3.1–19.0 mm Hg in systolic
  pressure, diastolic pressure showed smaller
  rises)[155,156,299]

- decreased levels of potassium, aldosterone (more marked in men than in women), anti-diuretic hormone, plasma rennin activity and urinary cortisone.[156,157]

It does not change plasma cortisol and ACTH levels.[158] Metabolic changes caused by liquorice or its constituents persist for a short time after ceasing their use.[159]

The effects of *Glycyrrhiza* on adrenal function has lead to it, or glycyrrhizic acid, being used as a supportive therapy for conditions of adrenal insufficiency like Addison's disease.[118] In fact a case of primary adrenocortical insufficiency was masked due to the patient's excessive consumption of liquorice.[160] It may also be useful in treating hyperkalaemia associated with diabetes mellitus.[161]

Liquorice given to normal pre-menopausal women resulted in:-

- lowered testosterone levels whilst using the extract, probably due to inhibition of 11β-hydroxysteroid dehydrogenase which catalyses the conversion of androstenedione to testosterone[162] (may be supportive in treatment of hirsutism and polycystic ovary disease)
- lowered plasma renin and aldosterone levels[163]
- unaltered cortisol and luteal hormones[164]
- unaltered blood pressure[163,164]
- increased parathyroid hormone, 25-hydroxycholecalciferol and urinary calcium[164]

The effect of liquorice on male serum testosterone levels is somewhat controversial. Some studies have reported reductions in levels[165,166] whilst others found no significant changes.[162,167] The latter researchers concluded that moderate *Glycyrrhiza* intake mainly induces changes in cortisol levels with marginal effects on androgen hormones.

In both men and women, over a range of ages, regular liquorice intake was linked to reduced prolactin levels and a lower response of prolactin production to thyrotropic releasing hormone (TRH).[168]

Anticancer and Immune modulation
In vitro—*Glycyrrhiza* and a number of its constituents have been identified as possible anticancer

agents[169,170] by directly inhibiting the growth of myelogenous and monoblastic leukaemia cells,[171–173] prostate,[174–178] breast,[173,179,180] hepatoma,[181] gastric,[182] colon[183] and lung[184] cancer cells.

Constituents in the herb are phyto-oestrogenic[185] and can bind to oestrogen receptor sites. They are also able to bind more weakly to progesterone receptor sites[186] and this may affect hormone-dependent cancer cells. The flavonoids glabridin, isoliquiritigenin and glabrene in isolation have a biphasic effect on breast cancer cells i.e. they are stimulatory at low dose but cytotoxic at high dose, the latter effect being irrespective of the hormone-dependent status of the cells.[187–189] The whole extract does not cause increased proliferation of oestrogen-dependent breast cancer cells[190] and binds only weakly to oestrogen receptors.[191]

Indirectly too the herb may be protective against cancer as constituents are:-

- anti-mutagenic—standard tests found some of the herb's flavonoids were able to protect against damage by a range of potential carcinogens
- desmutagenic i.e. they deactivate potential carcinogens[192–196]
- anti-angiogenic[197]

In addition higher levels of glucocorticosteroids have been found to decrease cancer cell proliferation and *Glycyrrhiza* increases cortisol levels.[198]

The herb may have some general support for the immune system too. *Glycyrrhiza* used with *Echinacea in vitro* increased phagocytosis, the effect of the two herbs being greater than that induced by either one alone.[199] Licochalcone-A alters cytokine production and may be immunomodulatory[200] and glycyrrhizin increases interferon production.[201]

In vivo—No trials have specifically used *Glycyrrhiza* or its constituents to treat cancer but a proprietary preparation, PC-SPES, containing liquorice was hailed for some time as very beneficial for treating prostate cancer. It has since been shown that the preparation was adulterated with pharmaceuticals including an oestrogen analogue and interpretation of the benefits due to the herbs themselves is not possible.[202]

Liquorice improved immune function by enhanced T-cell production within 24 hours of its having been taken, the effect persisting for days afterwards.[203] Used in combination with other herbs it improved the symptoms associated with allergic asthma[204] and Familial Mediterranean Fever.[205]

Gastro-intestinal system

In vitro—Isoliquiritigenin is an antagonist of acid-producing parietal cells in the stomach.[206]

In vivo—Liquorice was used as a watery paste to treat gastric ulcers in the mid 20th Century. This preparation reduced symptoms, healed ulcers and protected against their future development. The potential for unwanted effects like pseudoaldosteronism (see under Precautions) prompted the development of new compounds from its constituents including carbenoxelone and deglycyrrinized liquorice. The former although effective still had side-effects,[207] the latter was useful in the treatment of erosive gastritis, duodenitis and/or ulcers[208–212] but newer pharmaceuticals have largely displaced both preparations.

Glycyrrhiza and/or its synthetic derivatives:-

- stimulated the release of secretin and therefore pancreatic bicarbonate production via raised prostaglandin levels in the gastric mucosa.[213] This is probably part of the mechanism by which the herb protects the mucosal lining from ulceration[214]
- decreased gastrin secretion thereby reducing acid secretion postprandially[215]
- reduced aspirin-induced faecal blood loss[216]
- were as effective as antacids and cimetidine in treating chronic duodenal ulcers[217]

Glycyrrhiza has been used, in combination with other herbs, to successfully treat infantile colic (tea)[218] and functional dyspepsia.[219,220]

Hepato-protective

In vitro—Constituents of the herb:-

- stimulate the proliferation of healthy, function-ing hepatocytes (isoliquiritigenin)[221]

- directly protect hepatocytes from chemical damage by enhancing the cell's detoxification enzyme activity (glycyrrhizic acid)[222–224]
- protect hepatocytes from damage caused by cholestasis (glycyrrhizin and glycyrrhetic acid).[225]

In vivo—Japan and Russia have used a preparation containing glycyrrhizic acid for decades to treat:-

- chronic hepatitis (from hepatitis B and C infections)[226–228] results being equal to, or better than, interferon therapy[229,230]
- all types of hepatitis[228]
- sub-acute liver failure due to viral hepatitis—endogenous-interferon production and sur-vival rate improved[231]

A recent review of the use of glycyrrizin in trials to treat chronic hepatitis C indicated it had a limited effect, improved liver function was not sustained on cessation of therapy and there was no reduction in viral load.[232]

Intravenous administration of glycyrrhizin was used to treat oral lichen planus in hepatitis C patients with some success.[233]

Antimicrobial

In vitro—The whole extract as well as the main saponins and flavonoids[135] are very effective and safe antimicrobials against:-

- bacteria—a large number of *Helicobacter pylori* strains, including some that are antibiotic-resistant,[234–236] *Streptococcus mutans*,[237] *Propi-onibacterium acnes*,[238] *Staphylococcus aureus*, including Methicillin-resistant strains (restor-ing their sensitivity to oxacillin),[239–241] *Enterococ-cus faecalis, Bacillus subtilis*[240] and *Micrococcus luteus*[240]
- fungi—*Trichophyton mentagrophytes*[127] and *Candida albicans*[242]
- viruses—Epstein Barr,[243] several DNA and RNA viruses including HSV,[244] corona virus associated with SARS,[245] HIV,[246,247] Japanese encephalitis virus strains, latent Karposi sarcoma-associated herpes (has been very diffi-cult to treat to date)[248] and hepatitis B virus[249–251]

Licochalcone A has in addition antimycobacterial activity against *Mycobacterium tuberculosis*, some *Legionella* species[252] and strong activity against *Leishmania* spp.[253]

Glycyrrhizin inhibits dental plaque formation[254] and enamel dissolution.[255]

In vivo—Tests using liquorice or its constituents as an antimicrobial in dentifrice have not been clear—with both negative[256,257] and positive[258] results having been reported.

Anti-oxidant

In vitro—*Glycyrrhiza* has good anti-oxidant activity.[259–261] Seven individual flavonoids, including glabridin, the most abundant and most potent, also have good activity.[262–265] Glycyrrhetic acid has both anti-oxidant and pro-oxidant activity, the latter action has been suggested as a mechanism for apoptosis of tumour cells through increased membrane permeability.[266]

Ex vivo—LDL was protected from oxidation by prior dosing with *Glycyrrhiza*.[267]

In vivo—Oxidation of LDL is considered a crucial step toward the development of atherosclerotic lesions. Liquorice given to patients with hypercholesterolaemia was anti-oxidant, increased LDL resistance to atherogenic changes and lowered LDL-cholesterol (5%), triglyceride levels (14%) and systolic blood pressure (10%).[268] This latter finding is in contrast to systolic rises in normal, healthy people. The herb may therefore prove beneficial in the treatment of cardiovascular disease. *Glycyrrhiza* (and glabridin) also reduced LDL oxidation in people with normal lipid levels.[267]

Anti-inflammatory

In vitro—*Glycyrrhiza* has a reputation as an anti-inflammatory. Apart from effectively increasing levels of cortisol, the herb has demonstrated inhibition of both 5-LOX and COX-2,[269] platelet aggregation[270] and some activity against fibroblasts derived from rheumatoid arthritis cells.[271]

Various of the herb's constituents also inhibit platelet aggregation[272], inflammatory cytokines[273] and serum complement factors which are commonly involved in chronic inflammation e.g. in autoimmune and allergic reactions.[274–277]

Topical

In vitro—*Glycyrrhiza* and/or glycyrrhizin added to a topical preparation increases its free radical scavenging activity and enhances skin protection from oxidative[278] and UVB radiation[279] damage.

Various flavonoids in *Glycyrrhiza* inhibit tyrosinase[280,281] and in fact liquorice extracts have been used in hyperpigmentation disorders.[282]

Topical preparations themselves benefit from the herb's anti-oxidant activity as it helps to stabilise them.[283]

In vivo—Some of *Glycyrrhiza*'s constituents have been tested topically. A gylcyrrhizic acid preparation safely reduced fat deposition (through its inhibition of 11β-hydroxysteroid dehydrogenase[284]) glycyrrhizin was effective in controlling the symptoms of atopic eczema[285] and a mouthwash containing deglycyrrhized liquorice was effective in resolving aphthous ulcers.[286]

Other

In vitro—Some of the flavonoid constituents of *Glycyrrhiza* inhibit the enzymes xanthine oxidase (associated with gout) and monoamine oxidase (associated with neuron function)[138,287] and inhibit the re-uptake of serotonin.[288] The latter two observations may give the herb benefits for use in depression.

The polysaccharide fraction is immunostimulatory.

In vivo—The mineralocorticoid properties of liquorice derivatives have been used for treating hypotension.[289]

Liquorice was used with the antibiotic, nitrofurantoin, in the treatment of urinary tract infections where it increased urinary elimination of the antibiotic, reducing its side effects.[290]

The herb is considered a tonic and has wide applicability. It is also a suitable addition to children's prescriptions to improve the taste.

Medicinal uses
Respiratory tract
- bronchitis
- bronchial catarrh
- asthma
- coughs
- irritation of the respiratory mucosa

Gastro-intestinal tract
• peptic ulcers
• chronic gastritis
• colic
• ulcers anywhere in this tract

Musculoskeletal
• arthritis
• rheumatism

Skin
• chronic skin disease

Endocrine system
Glycyrrhiza's support of adrenal function through decreasing hormone catabolism, supports its anti-inflammatory effect, and gives it a use in:

• Addison's disease/adrenocortical insufficiency
• auto-immune diseases
• aid to withdrawal of steroid therapy

Pharmacy
Three times daily
Decoction   – 1–4 g
Fluid Extract (20%)   – 2–5 ml

At recommended doses *Glycyrrhiza* is considered a safe herb and has no teratogenic or mutagenic activity. The safe level of glycyrrhizic acid is set at 0.2 mg/kg per day e.g. 12 mg for a 60 kg person equating to 6 g of liquorice a day based on a glycyrrhizin content of 0.2%.[291] Most authorities have set maximum safety limits much higher for instance the *Dutch Nutrition Council* level is 200 mg glycyrrhizic acid a day[291] and *German Commission E* has specified 100 mg glycyrrhizin a day. Individual differences in absorption, sensitivity and metabolic rate would also affect these limits.

CONTRAINDICATIONS—Hypertension, pregnancy, hypokalaemia, cirrhosis of the liver. Large doses of liquorice should not be used for more than 6 weeks.

Pharmacokinetics
Glcyrrhizin, which is considered the main active constituent in liquorice, seems to have poor bioavailability from the whole extract.[292] After ingestion it is hydrolysed to glycyrrhetic acid in a two-step process by gut flora in the colon and for each person this process will vary according to their flora. Glycyrrhetic acid is well absorbed and its level rises in plasma soon after liquorice ingestion, taking 12 hours to reach a maximum. It is transported to the liver by a protein carrier where it is conjugated before being secreted into bile. On reaching the colon a second time re-absorption occurs after the flora have once again hydrolysed the conjugates and so glycyrrhetic acid is recycled,[293] a process called enterohepatic cycling, and this gives rise to a second plasma peak of glycyrrhetic acid some time later. This process could cause a cumulative effect in plasma levels.[294] It is likely that transit time in the bowel also alters the level of re-absorption, a slow transit tending to raise plasma levels.[147]

A small amount of glycyrrhizin is absorbed intact and excreted in urine within 24 hours, the main urinary metabolite being glcyrrhetic acid, however, only about 1–2% is excreted by this route.[295,296] The urinary metabolite is detectable for some time after liquorice intake is stopped (5 days for chronic intake and up to 51 hours after a single large dose).[297]

The study of the flavonoids *in vitro* suggests liquiritin is poorly absorbed but it too appears to undergo changes by gut flora into liquiritigenin and davidigenin which are well absorbed.[298]

Precautions and/or safety
Blood pressure rises due to *Glycyrrhiza* may be significantly higher in people with essential hypertension (one study found the average rise was 15.3 mm Hg systolic and 9.3 mm Hg diastolic pressure but the individual range is wide), gender is not a factor in this increase.[155,299] A high salt intake exacerbates liquorice-induced hypertension.[300]

In high enough doses or with chronic use the adrenocortical effects can lead to an excessive increase in potassium loss and sodium and water retention a condition called pseudoaldosteronism. It results in hypokalaemic myopathy, oedema, hypertension and metabolic alkalosis.[301–308]

Pseudoaldosteronism can occur with no attendant hypertension.[309]

Various forms of liquorice use can cause hypokalaemic myopathy but symptoms disappear in most cases by refraining from further use.[310] Most adverse event reports have occurred from the consumption of excessive or chronic liquorice confectionery or in people who already had existing health problems when they used reasonable amounts of the herb.[311–314] However pseudoaldosteronism has been recorded in healthy people taking as little as 7 g of liquorice, equating to 500 mg of glycyrrhizic acid, daily for a week[315] and symptoms have been reported from just using a liquorice mouthwash or chewing gum.[316,317] Interestingly, aqueous extracts are associated with fewer and less severe side effects than reported for the equivalent amount of herb in confectionery form.[318]

More serious side-effects attributed to liquorice use include:-

- rhabdomylosis which can result from severe hypokalaemia (to date 77 cases have been reported)[319–321]
- severe hypokalaemic paralysis which is life threatening.[322–324] A case of paralysis occurred with ingestion of small amounts of liquorice contained in a laxative[325]
- encephalopathy[326,327]
- transient visual loss possibly associated with smooth muscle vasoconstriction in retinal or occipital vessels, similar to migraine[328,329]
- arrhythmia,[330] severe tachycardia[331] and hypertensive crisis[332]

There appears to be a range of sensitivities to *Glycyrrhiza* and/or its constituents.

As 11β-hydroxysteroid dehydrogenase can act as a detoxifying enzyme for external chemicals liquorice by its inhibition of this enzyme may counter this protective effect.[333]

Reported reduction in men's testosterone levels occurred with doses of 7 g liquorice daily (0.5 g glycyrrhizic acid).[165]

In pregnancy—a retrospective study associated a shorter gestation and increased pre-term deliveries (less than 37 weeks gestation) in women consuming large amounts of liquorice confectionery (estimated to be more than 500 mg glycyrrhizin per week).[334,335] Birth weight and maternal blood pressure were not affected but fluid retention could be relevant to maternal hypertension.

Although there have been a few fatalities linked to the herb's use, in the majority of cases side-effects that have been recorded, whether serious or not, have been reversible. It may take anywhere from weeks to months for disturbed biochemistry to return to normal.

Interactions

In vitro—*Glycyrrhiza* and some of its constituents (not glycyrrhizin) inhibit CYP3A4.[336–338] Glabridin also inhibits isozymes CYP2B6 and CYP2C9.[339] There is the potential for drug/herb interactions based on these effects.

In vivo—Other possible and/or reported interactions are:-

- **diuretics**—further reductions of already low potassium levels—reported interaction led to hypertension, oedema, rhabdomylosis, respiratory and kidney failure[340]
- **cardiac glycosides**—hypokalaemia can affect heart muscle function—reported interaction led to digitalis toxicity[341]
- **corticosteroids**—raised levels of corticoids—steroidal nasal spray and/or diuretic led to severe hypokalaemia and hypertension[342]

In vitro Glycyrrhizic acid complexes with lappaconitine, an antiarrhythmic agent, although no *in vivo* problems have so far been reported.[343]

Historical uses
Dropsy; to prevent thirst (diabetes?); "all diseases of breast and lungs"; tuberculosis; dry cough, hoarseness; mild laxative; kidney pain; ulcerated kidneys and bladder; strangury; heat of urine. Externally used in eyes for "rheumatic distillations" (powder).

Melilotus officinalis

Melilot, sweet clover

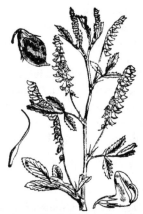

Family Fabaceae

Description

A biennial herb with a woody tap root. *Stems* more or less glabrous below, sparsely hairy above, decumbent or erect to 1.5 m high in flower. *Leaves* pinnately trifoliate, sparsely hairy when young otherwise glabrous, petioles 5–25 mm long, leaflets narrowly elliptic or obovate, serrate, 10–25 mm long. *Flowers* numerous, yellow, in lax and slender racemes. Corolla 4–6 mm long, wings greater than keel. *Pod* glabrous, about 3 mm long, 1–2 seeded, transversely rugose, seeds light brown, 2–3 mm long. Flowers from spring to summer. It may be distinguished from the very similar *M. albus* by the latter's white flowers and reticulately veined seed pods.

Odour—of coumarin, sweetish; taste—bitter, somewhat salty and pungent.

Habitat and cultivation

Native to Europe and Asia, melilot grows wild in many countries, in dry waste places and near the coast. It is grown from seed and self-sows. Drought and frost resistant.

Parts used

The herb, harvested during flowering and dried carefully.

Active constituents

1) Coumarins (up to 1.4%) including free coumarin, o-coumaric acid, dihydroxycoumarin, melilotin, melilotic acid and melilotol.[344] These develop on drying
2) Flavonoids (about 0.1%)[345] including robinin
3) Tannins

Phenolics other than the flavonoids[345] and saponins have also been isolated from *Melilotus*.[346]

Actions

1) Spasmolytic
2) Carminative

Scientific information

Melilotus was known to and used by the 2nd century physician Galen. It was at one time an official medicine. In the 1920's attention was drawn to the herb when cattle grazing it developed haemorrhages. Studies isolated the causative factor, dicoumarol, and from this was developed the antithrombotic warfarin.[347] *Melilotus* develops dicoumarol through fermentation as it decomposes and it is not actually a component of the properly prepared herb.[348]

In vitro—*Melilotus* has some limited anti-oxidant and anti-inflammatory activity due to its phenolic content.[345,349]

The coumarins are important to the activity of the herb and they had been shown to be anti-oedematous and antiinflammatory, increasing blood and lymph flow and helping to repair damaged blood vessel walls.[350] *Ex vivo* and *in vivo* the coumarins are absorbed through the skin and may act on the local circulation.

In vivo—*Melilotus* has been used with other herbs to treat chronic venous insufficiency with both subjective and objective measures being significantly improved by topical application[351] and with internal treatment.[352]

Preparations containing the coumarins and/or the whole herb were able to reduce lymphoedema caused by node removal in the treatment of metastatic cancer.[353,354] The reduced oedema though modest (5%) was significant.

An internal preparation containing the herb was developed in Italy and marketed as *Cellasene* for reducing cellulite. The action of *Melilotus* in the product was intended as a circulatory stimulant to reduce oedema.[355] Reported trials of the product have given contradictory outcomes with a few claiming efficacy whilst at least one found it failed.[356]

The herb is used in other traditions as a sedative.[357]

Medicinal uses
Cardiovascular system
• haemorrhoids
• varicose veins
• varicose ulcers
• post-traumatic oedema
• lymphoedema
• thrombosis
• thrombophlebitis

Pharmacy
Infusion dried herb – 1–2 teaspoons per cup boiling water (dose 3–4 cups a day—*Weiss*)
Tincture 1:5 (45%) – 1–5 ml[+]
Fluid Extract (25%) – 0.6–2 ml

Precautions and/or safety
In vivo—Studies reported only minor side effects like transitory gastro-intestinal problems.[354]

Coumarin (benzo-α–pyrone), which has been used as a food additive, itself has no anti-coagulant activity and adverse effects in humans occur rarely and with high doses only. The *European Commission* safety limit has been set at 0.1 mg/kg/day, probably a very conservative level given that much larger doses have been used for months at a time without problems. Doses of coumarin of up to 7000 mg/day in humans have been well tolerated and where liver enzymes have risen in patients subjected to very high doses, these are reduced on cessation of the drug. Topical application results in very much lower systemic levels.[358] Coumarin

is considered to be non-genotoxic and although hepatotoxicity has been reported in rodents this appears to be a peculiarity of their metabolism.

There are suggestions that the herb may increase bleeding time and should not be used prior to surgery but this is speculative, there are no reports of this having occurred in the literature.[359]

Interactions
The herb could potentially interact with blood thinning agents like warfarin[360,361] but to date this has not been reported and as the herb contains coumarins with no significant anti-coagulant activity the interaction would seem very unlikely.

Historical uses
In combination with other herbs as an ointment or poultice to soften all swellings; the juice as eye drops to clear sight. Also used externally for abdominal and rheumatic pain, loss of senses and apoplexy. As an analgesic for head and ear aches. For flatulence.

Piscidia piscipula
[Formerly *P. erythrina*]

Jamaican dogwood, fish poison tree

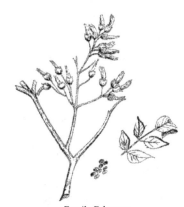

Family Fabaceae

Description
Evergreen shrub 5 × 2.5 m. *Bark* yellowish or greyish brown. *Stems* erect, slender. *Leaves* divided into 3–4 pairs of leaflets, ovate to obovate, up to 10 cm

---

[+]Suggested dosage based on *German Commision E* recommendation. Alcohol strength based on that used for coumarin-containing *Trifolium pratense*.

long, undulate or slightly toothed. *Flowers* small, pea-shaped, white, striped red. *Fruit* a pod to 10 cm long with longitudinal wings.

Habitat and cultivation
Originally from the West Indies and southern Florida *Piscidia* grows in moist, well-drained soil and sunny sheltered situations. It is drought and frost tender. It is propagated from stratified seed.

Parts used
The root bark.

Active constituents
1) Isoflavonoids over 20 have been identified some being complex, called coumarono-chromones, and others containing amino groups.[362] The main isoflavonoids are eryth-bigenin, piscidone, ichthynone, jamaicin, genistein, lisetin and rotenone[363–370]
2) Organic acids including piscidic, fukiic and methylfukiic acids

Also contains tannins and β-sitosterol.
    Some variability in the constituents occurs with the geographical area in which the plant grows.

Actions
1) Sedative
2) Antitussive
3) Spasmolytic
4) Anti-inflammatory
5) Anodyne

Scientific information
Western interest in this herb appears to date back to the 1840s. Whilst the actions of *Piscidia* are utilised by herbalists, little detail of the pharmacology is available.
    In vitro—*Piscidia* is used in Guatemala to treat fungal infections and this use has been verified.[371]
    Rotenone, an insecticide whose activity is based on its ability to interfere with oxygen metabolism via mitochondria, is a neurotoxin.[372] There is current concern that it may contribute to the development of Parkinson's disease based on animal and *in vitro* studies.[373]

In vivo—There are no human trials available but animal studies have indicated the herb has spasmolytic activity, is hypotensive and depressant to the myocardium.
    Piscidia used as a fish poison, was thrown into the water, causing fish to float to the surface where they were easily caught. The active constituent in this process is considered to be piscidic acid.

Medicinal uses
Nervous system
Primarily active on nerve tissue making it useful for:

• insomnia
• neuralgia
• migraine

BHP specific for insomnia due to neuralgia and nervous tension.

Reproductive tract
• dysmenorrhoea

Pharmacy
Three times daily
Decoction of dried herb   – 2–4 g
Tincture 1:5 (45%)   – 5–15 ml
Fluid Extract (60%)   – 2–8 ml
    CONTRAINDICATIONS—Pregnancy, brady-cardia, cardiac insufficiency.

Historical uses
Asthma; whooping cough; toothache.

Trifolium pratense

Red clover

Description
Erect or decumbent perennial not rooting at the nodes, with stems sparsely hairy below and moderately or densely hairy in the upper parts. *Leaves* alternate, trifoliate, usually moderately hairy on petioles and under surface of leaflets, and more or less glabrous on upper surface. *Petioles* up to 200 mm long; leaflets ovate, elliptic or obovate,

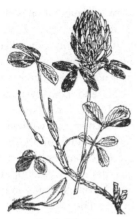

Family Fabaceae

usually more or less entire with a crescentic spot towards base, about 15–40 mm long. *Inflorescence* terminal, spicate, globose to ovoid, usually sessile and with 2 leaves immediately below it. *Flowers* numerous, sessile, corolla pink or purple-pink, 10–16 mm long. *Pod* glabrous and straight, 2–3 mm long 1-seeded. Flowers from spring to autumn.

Habitat and cultivation
Native to Europe, West Asia and North Africa, red clover is common throughout the world, both cultivated and naturalised in pasture, waste places and gardens.

It is grown from seed and self-sows in light, well-drained soils, in open sunny situations. It is grown instead of lucerne in areas with a cool spring climate, but will grow in any ordinary garden soil as long as it does not get too dry in summer. Commonly grown as fodder. Frost and drought resistant.

Parts used
The flower heads. Most commercial products also contain some of the small leaflets.

Active constituents[374]
1) Flavonoids
   a) mainly isoflavones (up to 0.6%) over 20 have been identified including formononetin and biochanin-A with lower levels of daidzein, genistein and pratensein[375-379]
   b) flavones[380]

2) Phenolic acids including salicylic, coumaric and caffeic acids
3) Procyanidins—polymers based on epicatechin and catechin[381]
4) Volatile oil containing more than 40 compounds

Also contains sitosterol, fatty acids and long chain hydrocarbons and alcohols.

The levels of isoflavone may vary over the season, daidzein and genistein levels are higher in mid-summer whilst formononetin and biochanin-A peak in autumn.[382] Higher ambient levels of UV-B radiation increase the content of the latter isoflavones and caffeic acid also.[383] Leaves have the highest content of isoflavones and contain some not found in the flowers.[375] Flowers have the lowest isoflavone levels of all the aerial parts of the plant.[384] Many cultivars of *Trifolium* exist which may differ in their isoflavone concentrations but site and plant age, plant-part, growing conditions and maturity at harvest all contribute to a variable chemical make-up.

Nutritional constituents
Vitamins: A, B-complex, C, F and P
Minerals: Rich in magnesium, calcium, potassium and copper also some selenium, manganese, sodium and zinc

Actions
1) Dermatological agent
2) Mild antispasmodic
3) Expectorant
4) Alterative

Scientific information
Red clover is of interest to the agricultural sector as a food crop for livestock and for its value in soil improvement. Recent interest in the medicinal value of the herb is due to its good phyto-oestrogenic potential, the isoflavones being structurally similar to 17β-oestradiol, and it is being trialled as a safer treatment for menopausal symptoms than HRT. The leaves have a much higher level of hormone-like constituents and they have been used in the main for commercial extracts, being further

processed to enhance the isoflavone levels so that they represent 30% or more of the total.[376] Traditionally this part of the herb was not used, neither was *Trifolium* used for its hormone-like properties. Very little recent research has in fact been carried out into its traditional uses.

Hormonal

In vitro—The flowers do have significant phyto-oestrogenic activity[385] although most studies have used isoflavone-enriched extracts. The extracts bind to both α- and β-oestrogen receptor sites[386] (and also to those for progesterone and androgen)[375,387] and are deemed to have a high enough hormone activity to act like synthetic oestrogens (HRT).[388] Of the isolated isoflavones genistein has the strongest oestrogenic activity.[389]

In vivo—Trials using isoflavone-rich *Trifolium*, with or without the isoflavones from other plant sources, have reported benefits for post-menopausal women in:-

- the relief of menopausal symptoms[390,399]
- vaginal tissue structure[399]
- reduced risk factors for breast cancer[390]
- bone density[391,392]
- blood pressure and endothelial function in type 2 diabetes[393]

Some studies failed to corroborate improvements in menopausal symptoms.[394,395] Extracts did not improve short term cognitive function in post-menopausal women.[396]

Cardio-vascular

Epidemiological studies have suggested isoflavone rich diets, particularly soy-based ones, are preventative for cardiovascular disease.

In vitro—The herb increases nitric oxide synthesis in endothelial cells suggesting a possible benefit for blood vessel tone and reduced atheroma formation.[397]

Ex vivo—Blood vessel walls benefited from isoflavone supplementation.[398]

In vivo—Trials to determine hormonal benefits also analysed effects of isoflavones derived from *Trifolium* alone or in combination with other isoflavone sources, for cardiovascular health.

Isoflavone supplements have been given to woman at different stages in their reproductive life. They improved lipid (triglyceride,[399] HDL cholesterol[390,392,400]) and homocysteine[390] levels in post-menopausal women with little, or no, benefit for pre-and peri-menopausal women.[400-402]

A number of reviews of the above clinical trials have commented on discrepant results for cardiovascular and menopausal symptom relief.[403-406] Inconsistencies may be due to variability in the chemistry and/or quality[407] of different extracts used or their method of processing.[375] There has been better consistency across studies examining *Trifolium* extracts in maintaining bone and arterial health in post-menopausal women.[408]

A quite different *Trifolium* isoflavone preparation, one rich in formononetin, reduced arterial stiffness in both genders without affecting blood pressure levels[409] whilst the isolated isoflavone, biochanin-A, lowered low-density lipoprotein in men but not in women.[410]

Anticancer

Traditionally *Trifolium* has been used in treating cancers and this is supported by epidemiological studies showing cultures with isoflavone-rich diets have a lower incidence of prostate cancer, and also of benign prostatic hyperplasia.[411]

In vitro—The isoflavones stimulate differentiation of cancer cells,[412] may reduce the risk of oestrogen-related carcinogenesis[413] and inhibit COX activity which has been linked with, among other things, cancer development.[414] Biochanin-A protects cells from external chemical carcinogens.[378,415]

In vivo—There is evidence to suggest that red clover isoflavones are beneficial in treating prostatic cancer.[411,416]

Other

Red clover is anti-oxidant *in vitro*,[315,387,417] an action attributed to the isoflavones and phenols[418] however *in vivo* isoflavones did not improve the anti-oxidant status in women.[400]

Medicinal uses

Respiratory tract
- whooping cough
- coughs
- bronchitis

Skin
Used in the treatment of skin problems where it may act as an alterative for:

- psoriasis
- eczema (*BHP* specific)
- chronic skin diseases (*BHP* specific)

Externally
It can be used topically too for the treatment of the above skin problems.

Pharmacy
Three times daily

Infusion	–	2–4 g
Tincture 1:10 (45%)	–	1–2 ml
Fluid Extract (25%)	–	2–4 ml

For external use an infusion or the fluid extract can be used directly or added to an ointment base to give a 10–15% concentration of herb—volume to weight.

Pharmacokinetics
Liver microsomes convert biochanin-A and for-mononetin into genistein and daidzein respectively[413] and serum levels of isoflavones appear to have a relatively long half-life.[419] *In vivo* the isoflavonoids are mainly conjugated in the liver, undergo enterohepatic cycling and are excreted in bile and urine.[420,422]

Precautions and/or safety
The isoflavone-rich extracts used in these trials, in some cases amounting to a daily intake of between 80–160 mg of red clover derived isoflavones, were without side-effects. Red clover is considered safe.[421,422]

In vitro—Breast cancer cells were induced to proliferate when exposed to a commercial preparation of *Trifolium* creating concern over their suitability for use in women with hormone-dependent breast cancer.[423] On the other hand the isoflavones inhibited the production of mutagenic metabolites from endogenous hormones which could give them a protective role against increased cancer risk.[413]

In vivo—Checks on hormone levels and breast density changes in women at risk for the disease found isoflavones did not alter these parameters and they are not therefore considered to increase the risk of breast cancer.[394]

Interactions
In vitro—*Trifolium* inhibits CYP3A4.[424]

Some sources caution against using the herb with anticoagulant therapy because of its coumarins (see *Melilotus*). However the coumarin content is low and dicoumarol has not been identified in it. There are no reported interactions of *Trifolium* with any medicines.

Historical uses
The herb has a folklore tradition of being used in the treatment of cancerous growths.

Trigonella foenum-graecum

Fenugreek

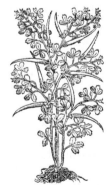

Family Fabaceae

Description
An erect almost hairless annual, 15–50 cm tall. *Leaves* alternate, trifoliate, oblong to ovate, toothed near the apex. *Flowers* whitish-yellow, stalkless,

solitary or paired in the axils of the upper leaves. Each flower 1–1.5 cm, in a hairy calyx with equal, linear, lance-shaped teeth. *Fruit* is a small, erect, linear, hairless pod, 7–10 cm, progressively narrowing to a slender beak, 3–5 cm.

Odour—spicy, characteristically of curry; taste—somewhat bitter and seeds are mucilaginous when chewed.

Habitat and cultivation
Native to Asia and introduced, and sometimes naturalised, in much of Southern Europe. Always grown from seed which germinates easily. Grows in any ordinary garden soil, like a dwarf pea. Sometimes grown as a fodder crop and is used in veterinary treatments. Drought and frost tender.

Parts used
The dried mature seed.

Active constituents
1) Steroidal saponins including diosgenin (up to 0.9%),[425] yamogenin, methyl-protodioscin, methyl-protodeltonin[426,427] and a number of other furostanol saponins[428,429]
2) Alkaloids including trigonelline (up to 0.36%)
3) Mucilage (up to 30%)
4) Volatile oil
5) Flavonoids including vitexin, quercetin, luteolin and naringenin[430]

Also contains a high level of protein[431] including the unusual amino acid 4-hydroxyisoleucine[432] and seven essential amino acids,[433] a number of fatty acids, a derivative of β-sitosterol,[434] phytate[435] and dietary fibre (up to 51%) containing galactomannan, some of which is comprised of mucilaginous fibre and the rest is neutral fibre.[436]

The total phenolic content of *Trigonella* is around 5% of its dry weight.[437]

Nutritional constituents
Vitamins: A, C and D as well as B1, B2 and niacin
Minerals: Calcium, phosphorus and iron
Also contains choline, lecithin and an oil resembling cod liver oil.

Actions
1) Hypoglycaemic
2) Laxative
3) Demulcent
4) Expectorant
5) Galactagogue
6) Nutritive
7) Antipyretic
8) Orexigenic Topically
9) Emollient
10) Vulnerary

Scientific information
Trigonella was used by the ancient Egyptian, early Greek and Roman civilisations as a medicinal and culinary herb—the name *foenum graecum* means "Greek hay"—and has long traditional use in many countries both as a medicine and as a spice. The herb has been an official medicine and is approved by *German Commission E* to stimulate appetite and as a topical anti-inflammatory.

Apart from its hypoglycaemic properties, which are the focus of current interest, it is also seen as a replacement source of the steroidal saponin, diosgenin, as yams have become too expensive.[438] Other parts of the plant are also used as a food, the aerial parts are in fact a richer source of phenols (anti-oxidants).[439] Traditionally the herb was used to aid convalescence, possibly because of its rich nutritional content.

Hypoglycaemic
The seeds have been used in Eastern cultures to treat diabetes and hypercholesterolaemia and it is this aspect of *Trigonella* that has been most studied in recent times.

The alkaloid trigonelline was believed to be the active constituent in glucose control but more recent studies point to the fibre (combined mucilaginous and neutral fibre) and gum as possibly stronger hypoglycaemic agents. The proposed mechanism of action, based on animal experiments, is through delayed gastric emptying with direct interference of intestinal glucose absorption,[440] the fibre content slowing down glucose uptake, and possibly also through activation of insulin signalling in adipocytes and liver cells.[441]

In vitro—4-hydroxyisoleucine increases glucose-induced insulin release from β-cells of Islets of Langerhans[442] and it too may make a contribution to improved glucose metabolism.

In vivo—*Trigonella* used to treat non-insulin dependent (type 2) diabetes improved glucose control, both fasting and postprandial levels, and reduced glycosuria, glycated haemoglobin and insulin levels.[443-448] The results of using *Trigonella* were comparable to dietary control and exercise but with the added advantage of decreased insulin resistance.[445,449] However, blood sugar levels in severe type-2 diabetes were more resistant to change.[457]

Trigonella was also beneficial in the management of type 1 or insulin dependent diabetes giving improved glucose tolerance as well as reduced fasting blood glucose levels and glycosuria.[450]

The whole seeds appear to have the strongest hypoglycaemic effect compared to their isolated constituents or the leaves and even after being cooked they still retain some activity.[444,447] There are a number of reviews of the clinical trials to-date on *Trigonella* in the treatment of diabetes that conclude in the main the herb shows good potential.[436,451-453]

4-hydroxyisoleucine improved the rate of glycogen re-synthesis post-exercise in trained athletes without increasing insulin levels.[454]

Hypolipidaemic
In vivo—A number of clinical trials on patients with diabetes and/or hyperlipidaemia reported reduced cholesterol levels of between 15–33%,[447,455,456] reduced LDL and serum triglycerides and HDL levels that rose[449] or were unchanged.[448,455]

Blood glucose and lipid levels in normal volunteers have been more variably affected by fenugreek with some studies reporting an improvement[447] whilst others found no change.[457]

Galactagogue
In vivo—The traditional use of *Trigonella* in increasing milk production in lactating women has been supported by an observed increase in milk volume of around 20%.[458] Increased lactation was reported as occurring within 24–72 hours of taking the herb.[459]

Other
In vitro—Fenugreek is also:-

- protective of liver cells exposed to alcohol, the effect being comparable to silymarin (*Silybum*)[460]
- anti-oxidant—the seeds, sprouts and aerial parts[439,461,462]
- anti-inflammatory on mucosal cells of patients with inflammatory bowel disease[463]
- bacteriostatic against *Escherichia coli, Staphylococcus aureus* and *Yersinia enterocolitica*[464]

The constituents diosgenin (see *Dioscorea villosa*)[465,466] and protodioscin[427] have anticancer propertites.

In vivo—*Trigonella* was successfully used topically as part of a mixture to treat head lice.[467]

Medicinal uses
Respiratory tract
- bronchitis

Gastro-intestinal tract
- anorexia
- dyspepsia
- gastritis
- constipation

Reproductive tract
- increase lactation/milk flow

Externally
Its local healing and anti-inflammatory effects are used in poultices to treat:

- boils
- myalgia
- lymphadenitis
- gout
- wounds
- crural ulcers

Pharmacy

Three time daily. *The German Commission E* recommendation is:-

Dried herb	– up to 2 g
Tincture 1:5	– maximum 10 ml
Fluid extract 1:1	– maximum 2 ml

Externally as a poultice 50 g seed: 250 ml water, bring to the boil and apply to bruises, swellings, boils, ulcers and suppurating wounds.

The studies conducted on the hypoglycaemic action of the seeds used between 15–100 g a day of powdered seed whilst a dose of 100 g per day of the defatted seed powder was used in treating type 1 diabetes.

Precautions and/or safety

The herb is not genotoxic in standard tests.[468] Clinical trials reported side effects included mild gastro-intestinal discomfort but even long term use of the herb was not associated with significant side-effects.[443]

Although it has been suggested fenugreek could increase bleeding time there are no reports of such adverse reactions and measurements on platelet aggregation and fibrinolytic activity showed no changes.[457]

There have been only 2 reported cases of severe allergy to fenugreek, one due to inhalation of the powdered herb and the other from a topical application.[469]

In cultures where unusually large quantities of seeds may be consumed it is possible they may contribute to the development of anaemia due to the fibre inhibiting iron absorption.[470]

Ingestion of fenugreek can lead to an odour in urine that has been confused with "maple syrup urine disease".[471,472] This disease is due to an inborn error of the metabolism of branched amino acids and causes production of sotolone, also present in maple syrup and fenugreek, which is responsible for the smell. Women using the herb to aid lactation or childbirth may have babies who, because of this odour, are erroneously suspected of having the disease.[473]

Interactions

Trigonella may contribute to excessive hypoglycaemia if used with similar acting pharmaceuticals.

There has been one case reported of an interaction between warfarin and fenugreek-boldo, the coumarin content of both being cited as the likely cause of an increased tendency to anticoagulation (raised INR).[474] Neither herb has significant coumarin levels. Further warnings relate to the potential for interactions with any drug with anticoagulant properties.[475,476] However no drug interactions have actually been reported.[456]

Historical uses

To cleanse breast, chest and lungs; for imposthume, ulcer or stoppage in uterus; to aid childbirth; to prevent fevers; comfort the stomach; diabetes; scrofula; rickets; gout; anaemia; post-infection convalescence; neurasthenia; baldness (All conditions except fever or headache.)

FAGACEAE

The Fagaceae or beech family consists of 6 genera containing about 600 species of deciduous or evergreen trees and shrubs, mostly monoecious, and all but *Nothofagus* native to temperate and sub-tropical regions of the Northern Hemisphere.

- Leaves alternate, simple, entire or variously cleft
- Flowers unisexual, male flowers in catkins or heads, female flowers solitary or in clusters. Perianth 4–7-lobed, stamens 4–20, ovary 3–7-celled
- Fruit a nut enclosed in a cup or burr

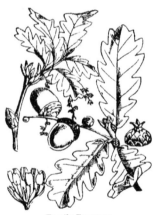

Family Fagaceae

Quercus robur

Oak, English oak

Description
Round-topped deciduous tree to 40 m with a large girth. Bark smooth when young, later rough and furrowed. *Leaves* oblong-ovate with 3–7 lobes each side, fresh green in spring and turning rich brown in autumn. *Flowers* staminate, in small greenish-yellow catkins; pistillate flowers in spikes in the leaf axils. Flowers in spring. *Fruit* acorns, first green, and then brown when falling in autumn, 2–4 cm long growing in clusters of 1–3; oblong-ellipsoid and enclosed by a cup.

Odour—slightly aromatic; taste—slightly bitter and astringent.

Habitat and cultivation
Native to Europe, North Africa and Western Asia. Introduced and naturalised elsewhere. Easily grown from acorns but should be transplanted carefully to ensure the tap-root is intact. Grows in

197

forests or mixed woodlands on clay soil. Drought and frost resistant.

Parts used
The dried inner bark from smaller branches and young stems,[1] most easily collected in spring. Galls, which are excrescences due to the puncture of a hymenopterous insect, *Cynips tinctoria*, and the presence of its deposited ovum have also been used (*Grieve*).

Active constituents
1) Tannins (15–20%) consisting of mainly quercitannic acid, a condensed tannin or phlobotannin, but also the hydrolysable ellagitannins, gallic acid and oligomeric and polymeric proanthocyanidins. More than 20 compounds have been isolated[2,3]

Also contains a small amount of volatiles, mainly as aldehydes,[4] flavonoids (quercetin) and triterpene saponins.[5]

There is a degree of genetic variation within this species.[6]

Actions
1) Astringent
2) Haemostatic
3) Antiseptic

Scientific information
Oak bark was used by early Greeks and Romans, the preparation still appearing in pharmacopoeias around the world until the 20th century.[1] Its modern uses included rectal injections to treat haemorrhoids and as a gargle. *German Commission E* has reported astringent and virustatic activities for *Quercus* and has approved use of the bark, internally, for acute diarrhoea and externally for inflammation of oral, pharyngeal, genital and anal areas.

All the recognised actions of *Quercus* are attributable to the very high level of tannins. Animal based studies are, however, revealing pharmacological activities for the saponins also.

In vitro—Oak bark is to some degree anti-oxidant,[7] antimicrobial—against *Staphylococcus aureus* and other *Staphylococcus* species,[8] *Enterobacter aerogenes* and *Candida albicans*,[9] can stimulate the expression of detoxification enzymes[10] and is antithrombotic.[11]

In vivo the extract has been useful for treating some chronic skin conditions.[12]

Medicinal uses
Cardiovascular system
• haemorrhage
• haemorrhoids

Respiratory tract
• pharyngitis

Gastro-intestinal tract
• diarrhoea (specific indication in *BHP* is acute diarrhoea)

Externally
The tannins help form a protective eschar over abraded tissue and their antimicrobial activity helps ensure that, with the loss of the skin barrier, the site of injury does not become an entry point for infection.

• weeping eczema
• leucorrhoea (douche)
• burns
• bedsores
• tonsillitis (gargle)
• gingivitis
• haemorrhoids

Pharmacy
Three times daily
Decoction of dried herb   – 1–2 g
Fluid Extract (25%)   – 1–2 ml

Potter's indicates a maximum dosage for the fluid extract of 5ml thrice daily whilst *German Commission E* quotes 3 ml or 3 g maximum a day. For the treatment of acute diarrhoea small frequent dosing is indicated and taken in a good amount of water the fluid imbalance will be addressed at the same time.

A decoction of the bark can be effectively used as a compress, the powdered bark can be applied directly to weeping sores.

Precautions and/or safety

The precautions for this herb are usually applied to all herbs containing hydrolysable tannins. They have caused liver damage in animals and there were reported cases of acute hepatotoxicity after tannic acid was added to barium enemas.[13] Recent studies using purified tannic acid on patients with 10% burns however found no abnormalities in liver function tests.[14]

There is insufficient data at present on the absolute safety, or otherwise, of internal use of hydrolysable tannins and some doubt anyway as to the bioavailability of dietary tannins in general as they form insoluble protein-tannin complexes.[15] Hydrolysable tannin-rich foods or herbs should be avoided for long term use. In addition tannins may impair nutrient absorption[16] so their protracted use internally is therefore undesirable.

Historical uses

Vomiting; spitting of blood; agues. As a substitute for quinine in intermittent fevers. Acorns and the bark decocted to antidote poisonous plants (probably because the tannins precipitate out the alkaloids, the constituents most likely responsible for poisoning). Haematuria.

FUMARIACEAE

This family is sometimes included in Papavaraceae. It consists of about 16 genera of mainly perennial herbs of the North Temperate areas of Europe, Asia, North Africa and North America. They are often slender, brittle, weak stemmed, sprawling plants with watery sap. *Corydalis* is included in this family.

- Leaves are much dissected
- Flowers in loose spikes or clusters. Sepals 2, petals 4 in 2 dissimilar whorls

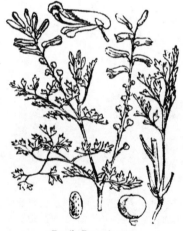

Family Fumariaceae

Fumaria officinalis

Fumitory

Description
A glabrous, scrambling, annual, which flops over other plants. *Leaves* glaucous, crowded to distant; over 8 × 4 cm; lamina dissected with linear or linear-lanceolate segments. *Inflorescense* dense, becoming lax at fruiting, with usually more than 20 flowers. Peduncles 1–3 cm long. Bracts oblong, membranous pale with pink tips. Sepals ovate. Corolla purplish-pink with dark green and purple tips, top petal spurred, lower petal spoon-shaped with widely spreading margins at the tips. *Fruit* broader than long, obovoid, about 2 × 2.5 mm, rugose when dry. Flowers from spring to autumn. There are at least four other species.

Odourless; taste—bitter and salty.

Habitat and cultivation
A weed of cultivated fields and gardens, and waste places, it is found worldwide. It grows from seed, self sows and needs no cultivation.

200

Parts used
The herb, harvested just prior to or during flowering.

Active constituents
1) Alkaloids (around 1%) mainly the isoquinoline alkaloids protopine (fumarine), fumarophycine and cryptopine.[1-3] More than 22 have been identified
2) Flavonoids based on quercetin including iso-quercitrin and rutin[4]
3) Organic acids including chlorogenic, caffeic and fumaric acids

Actions
1) Laxative
2) Diuretic (mild)

Scientific information
Fumaria has been an official medicine and was valued as a depurative from early times. In British herbal medicine fumitory has mainly been used to treat skin conditions however there are more references in the literature to the herb's use as a treatment for biliary disorders, a use for which it is approved in Germany.[5] In Bulgaria it has been used as a cholagogue and is also considered spasmolytic and hypotensive whilst in Italy small doses are used to stimulate circulation and respiration and as a depurative.[6]

Scientific evaluation of this herb is very limited. In treating patients with irritable bowel syndrome it was deemed to have failed to have therapeutic value.[7] However *Weiss* says clinical trials have proven the herb useful for biliary disorders including colic and chronic dyskinesia. The alkaloid protopine, like papaverine, may contribute a spasmolytic effect on biliary vessels.

Much of the remaining studies have been conducted on animals, emerging from these is the potential for the herb to have an amphoteric effect on gall bladder function adjusting bile flow i.e. to either increase it where flow is low or decrease it where it is being over-produced.

Medicinal uses
Gastro-intestinal tract
May function as a gall bladder tonic. The herb has been used to aid elimination and for:-

• cholelithiasis
• cholecystalgia

Skin
As it is an aid to gastro-intestinal and renal elimination i.e. depurative, it would be expected to benefit skin conditions.

• chronic eczema
• cutaneous eruptions

Externally
• conjunctivitis (lotion)

Pharmacy
Three times daily
Infusion of dried herb   – 2–4 g
Tincture 1:5 (45%)   – 1–4 ml
Fluid Extract (25%)   – 2–4 ml

Historical uses
Obstructions of the liver and spleen including jaundice; leprosy, scabs, tetters and itches; melancholy. Also for plague or pestilence. As a gargle for sores of mouth and throat. Externally for skin problems including cradle cap and to remove freckles; affections of the eyes.

GENTIANACEAE

Members of the Gentianaceae are usually hairless herbs with opposite, entire, usually stalkless leaves without stipules.

- Calyx has 4–5 lobes, the corolla tubular with 5–9 lobes, overlapping and twisted in the bud
- There are 5 stamens attached to the tube
- The ovary is superior, usually one-celled
- The many-seeded fruit is usually a capsule with a persistent corolla

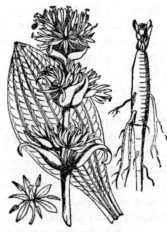

Family Gentianaceae

Gentiana lutea

Gentian, yellow gentian

Description
A perennial herbaceous plant with a very long, thick tap-root and erect, stout, smooth, hollow stems, 50–125 cm high. *Leaves* large, broadly oval, seven-veined, 20–30 cm long, bluish-green. Lower leaves stalked, upper leaves opposite, stalkless and clasping. *Flowers* numerous, short-stalked, golden yellow, about 2.5 cm long, in dense axillary and terminal whorls. *Corolla* with 5–9 lance-shaped lobes, more or less spreading in a star, not tubular; calyx papery.

Habitat and cultivation
Native to southern Europe in mountain pastures. Cultivated elsewhere from seed or root division in deep, rich, moist soil to allow roots to develop. Needs suns and shelter from cold winds and takes up to 3 years to flower. Drought tender, frost resistant.

Parts used
The root and rhizome harvested in the autumn of the second or third year and before the plant is mature

enough to flower. Roots, dug in autumn, should be dried quickly to preserve their white colour. Slow-dried gentian becomes reddish and contains less medicinal properties. However, after 6–8 months the root always seems to darken in colour.

Active constituents[1]
1) Bitter secoiridoids (up to 4%) including predominantly gentiopicroside also amarogentin, sweroside and swertiamarin.[2,3] The level of the bitter secoiridoids is affected by the way the roots are dried, gentiopicroside increases when roots are dried at 40°C,[4] however this is not the official method of preparation
2) Oligosaccharides including gentianose and polysaccharides—inulin and pectin
3) Xanthones (0.1%) mainly gentisin and isogentisin also gentioside, gentisein and mangiferin.[5–9] Xanthones are chemically related to flavonoids and give the root its yellow colour
4) Phenolic acids including gentisic and caffeic acids
5) Triterpenes including β-sitosterol, campesterol, stigmasterol and squalene[3,10]

Also traces of a complex volatile oil and inositol. Alkaloids (e.g. gentianine) are usually reported as being present in *Gentiana* but are now believed to be created by the isolation procedure which uses ammonia.

Nutritional constituents
Vitamins: Vitamin B complex, especially niacin
Minerals: Iron, also calcium, magnesium, manganese, phosphorus, potassium, selenium, sulphur and zinc.

Actions
1) Bitter
2) Gastric stimulant
3) Sialagogue
4) Cholagogue

Scientific information
Gentiana has been an official medicine in a number of countries. It was used as a bitter to stimulate gastric secretions and improve appetite.[11] It was valued from very early times and demand for the roots has meant that in some countries the wild variety has become endangered.[12] *German Commission E* approves its use for digestive disorders including loss of appetite, fullness and flatulence.

Armarogentin, although not the most prevalent glycoside, is 5000 times more bitter than gentiopicroside, the predominant constituent.[2] Amarogentin and swertiamarin are extremely bitter being detectable at concentrations as low as 1 in 50,000. Gentianose, a trisaccharide, also contributes to the bitterness of *Gentiana*. The herb is the standard bitter.

There is little clinical data to support traditional uses but earlier research established its action in stimulating digestive function through increased gastric and gall bladder secretions.[13] The postulated mechanism of the bitter constituents' action is through the stimulation of nerve endings on the tongue, causing a reflex stimulation of saliva and gastric secretions.

In vitro—*Gentiana* has a limited inhibitory effect on *Helicobacter pylori* strains.[14] Gentiopicrin has some fungitoxic activity[15] and isogentisin inhibits monoamine oxidase[16] as well as having antitubercular activity.[17]

Medicinal uses
Gastro-intestinal tract
• anorexia
• atonic dyspepsia
• gastritis
• heartburn
• diarrhoea
• nausea
• gastro-intestinal atony
• flatulence
• bloating

Pharmacy
Three times daily
Decoction (dried root)   – 0.6–2 g
Tincture 1:5 (45%)   – 1–4 ml
The herb should be sipped slowly mixed with water 30–60 minutes prior to meals.
CONTRAINDICATIONS—Peptic ulcers (gastric and duodenal).

Precautions and/or safety

Gentisin and isogentisin are mutagenic in the standard Ames test, they occur in the root at an estimated 0.04% and 0.03% respectively. Their *in vivo* potential to be mutagenic is yet to be established.[18,19] In order to benefit from bitters the taste must not be disguised, however if given in too large a dose they can suppress digestive secretions.

There are a number of recorded poisonings due to the mistaken substitution of *Veratrum album* for *Gentiana lutea*, the two being similar in appearance prior to flowering and often growing side by side.[20-22]

Historical uses

Antidote for many poisons; the bites of mad dogs and venomous beasts. Fevers; lameness arising from cold in the joints; for bruises; as a diuretic and emmenagogue; for cramps and convulsions; for voiding tough phlegm; for a number of skin conditions; jaundice; as a vermifuge. Hysteria; female weakness! To refresh weary travellers; urinary tract stones; cramps and convulsions.

GERANIACEAE

The Geraniaceae or geranium family consists of 11 genera of widely distributed herbs and shrubs. The flowers are bisexual and mostly regular in parts of 5. The botanical name is thought to have been given by *Dioscorides* from the Greek *geranos*, meaning a crane, because the seed pods are like that bird's beak. The European species, *G. robertianum*, *G. molle* and *G. dissectum* were used medicinally from medieval times for their astringent and styptic properties but now only *G. maculatum* is considered important.

Geranium maculatum

American cranesbill

Description
An erect perennial, 30–60 cm tall. A few long stalked 3–5 parted leaves grow from the roots. The flowering *stems* are straight, hairy, with a single pair of opposite short stalked leaves, cut into 5–7 sections, growing near the top. Above the leaves rise the flower stems bearing several conspicuous rose-purple flowers 2.5–4 cm wide, followed by a 3–4 cm tube with a 5–8 mm beak. A white-flowered form is also known.

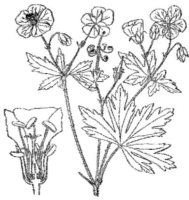

Family Geraniaceae

Habitat and cultivation
Native to North America, *G. maculatum* grows in open woodlands and meadows from New foundland to Georgia and Missouri. It may be grown from seed or root division in any moist, humus-rich soil. Frost and drought resistant.

Parts used
The root and herb are used. The herb is harvested during or just prior to flowering, and the root in the late summer or autumn. The root is stronger than the herb.

205

Active constituents[1]
1) Tannins up to 30%—mainly hydrolysable gallitannins (15–20%)[2]

Actions
1) Astringent
2) Antihaemorrhagic
3) Vulnerary

Scientific information
This herb was at one time an official medicine recommended to treat sore throats, colic, ulcers and diarrhoea. Little is known of its other constituents and therefore the pharmacology is limited to the general features of tannins (see Appendix III).

Medicinal uses
Gastro-intestinal tract
• diarrhoea
• melaena
• dysentery
• haematemesis
• mucous colitis

• peptic ulcers
• haemorrhoids

BHP specific for diarrhoea and peptic ulcers.

Reproductive tract
• metrorrhagia
• menorrhagia

Externally
• haemorrhoids
• leucorrhoea (douche)
• indolent ulcers
• bleeding
• burns

Pharmacy
Three times daily
Infusion of dried herb   – 1–2 g
Decoction of dried root   – 1–2 g
Tincture 1:5 (root 45%)   – 2–4 ml
Fluid extract (root 45%)   – 1–2 ml
    Potter's maximum dosage is much higher being 8 ml fluid extract (root).

GINKGOACEAE

The Ginkgoaceae family belongs to the Gymnosperms and consists of 1 genus and 1 species extinct in the wild but preserved as temple trees in China and Japan.

Ginkgo biloba

Ginkgo, maidenhair tree

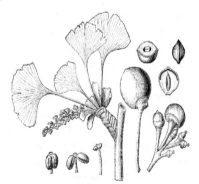

Family Ginkgoaceae

Description

A deciduous, resinous, dioecious tree to 40 × 7 m. Branches stiff with both elongate and spur shoots. *Leaves* alternate or clustered, fan-shaped, cut or divided in the middle, dichotomously veined, long-petioled, 5–7 cm long, soft green in spring, turning rich gold in autumn. Reproductive structures on spur shoots in axils of leaves or bracts; male catkin-like, female consisting of 2 ovules on a long peduncle, usually only 1 maturing but sometimes both. *Fruit* plum-like, yellow, fleshy to 2.5 cm long, seed a kernel, ripening in late autumn.

Odour—weak and characteristic.

Habitat and cultivation

Originally from S-E China the *Ginkgo* is grown as a street or ornamental tree throughout temperate regions of the world. It may be grown from seed, layers and cuttings and several cultivars are grown from buds or grafts. Male trees are most common because the smell of the ripe fallen fruits of female trees is unpleasant. Frost resistant, drought tender.

Parts used

The leaves gathered from mid summer to just prior to their turning yellow in mid autumn, this is when the content of the main active constituents is highest.

Active constituents[1-4]

1) Flavonoids (0.5–1.16%)[5-7]

   a) flavones—mainly derivatives of kaempferol, quercetin and isorhamnetin, also derivatives of myricetin and rutin

   b) biflavones—amentoflavone, bilobetin and ginkgetin[8]

   The flavonoid levels which are influenced by geographical location,[9] are highest in early summer, decrease till the end of summer and then are stable to the end of autumn before rising again just before leaf fall.[10,11]

2) Terpene lactones including diterpene lactones known as ginkgolides (up to 0.23%), mainly A, B and C with much smaller amounts of J, K and L[12]—these are unique chemical entities. Leaves from young trees of either sex are richer in terpenes than those from mature trees.[13]

3) Sesquiterpene lactone—bilobalide (up to 0.26%)

Also contains proanthocyanidins, phenolic acids (mainly protocatechuic acid, also vanillic and caffeic),[14,15] ginkgolic acids (up to 1.5%),[16,17] amino acids (around 9%) including some that are essential,[18] polyprenols and phytosterols.[19] Male leaves have a higher phenolic content than those of the female tree,[10] although the latter have a more beneficial metal ion profile.[20]

Nutritional constituents
Vitamins: A, B_6, C and E[18]

Actions
1) Vasodilator
2) Antispasmodic
3) Anti-inflammatory
4) Anti-oxidant

Scientific information
Ginkgo is one of the most consumed herbs, possibly because of the scientific information available and conversely because of its high usage, there continues to be a significant amount of research into it at all levels. Standardised extracts are registered in a number of countries for the treatment of neurological and vascular problems. Although there is a long history of *Ginkgo* use in Asia it was the seeds (called "nuts") that were used, the first mention of the medicinal use of the leaves occurring in the 15th Century.[21] *Ginkgo* was not part of the European *materia medica* until recent decades. Its modern application is being established by research into its constituents and their unique pharmacological actions. *German Commission E* has approved leaf extracts for use in the treatment of dementia, with symptoms of impaired memory, altered concentration and mood, dizziness, tinnitus and headaches. Also for use in peripheral arterial occlusive disease and vertigo. Research has been conducted on standardised extracts which have a variety of commercial names depending on the particular manufacturer.

Anti-oxidant
The flavonoids, terpenes,[22] proanthocyanidins and organic acids all contribute to this activity[15,23-26] which is comparable to that of vitamin E.[27] The flavonoids are considered the most powerful anti-oxidants[6] being significantly stronger than ascorbic acid.[28]

In vitro—*Ginkgo* has a variety of anti-oxidant mechanisms which include increases in oxygen scavenging, superoxide dismutase activity[29] and cellular glutathione levels.[30]

It protects metabolites[31-34] and cells[35-39] against oxidative stress and using *Ginkgo* in topical preparations helps to stabilise them and may also offer protection to skin from free radical damage.[40]

Ex vivo—*Gingko* improved the anti-oxidant status of erythrocytes from healthy people as well as those with glucose-6 dehydrogenase deficiency,[41] type 2 diabetes[42] and patients with Behçets disease (in which this mechanism is impaired).[43]

In vivo—Oral doses were strongly anti-oxidant as seen in platelets from normal people and those with hypercholesterolaemia,[44] reduced damaging free radicals in serum and erythrocyte membranes of insulin-dependent diabetics[45] and in the serum of ultra-violet exposed sunbathers.[46]

However commercial preparations vary considerably in anti-oxidant potential depending on their method of preparation.[47,48]

Antiplatelet activating factor

Platelet activating factor (PAF) is released from various cells where it mediates reactions which include platelet aggregation, vasodilation, inflammation, vascular permeability, bronchoconstriction and anaphylaxis.

In vitro—The ginkgolides are PAF antagonists, ginkgolide B being the most effective[49,50] and this, combined with their antioxidant capacity, may account for the anti-inflammatory action.[51–54] In addition ginkgolide B enhances white blood cell function via its effect on their PAF receptors.[55] Whole leaf extracts also inhibit platelet aggregation through a variety of mechanisms.[56]

In vivo—Ginkgolide B used in patients prior to kidney transplantation significantly improved their post-operative renal function, due to the anti-PAF activity inhibiting organ ischaemic-reperfusion injury.[57]

Circulatory system

Ginkgo's prime benefit is that it improves blood flow and much research has focussed on how this is achieved.

In vitro—Apart from the anti-PAF effect, the herb and/or some fractions of it:-

- enhance the number and activity of endothelial cells[58,59]
- reduce cytokines associated with endothelial adhesiveness[60] and atherosclerosis development[61,62]
- protect endothelial cells from hypoxic damage via inhibition of the phospholipase A2 cascade[63]
- increase the efficiency and protection of mitochondrial respiration[64,65]
- vasodilate—through the flavonoid fraction (not due to nitric oxide production[66]) and also due to enhanced nitric oxide levels in endothelial cells,[67] mediated by calcium-activated potassium channels[68]

Excessive amounts of nitric oxide in macrophages leads to tissue damage and an exacerbation of atherosclerosis. *Ginkgo* reduces levels of nitric oxide produced by stimulated macrophages[69,70] including that caused by homocysteine.[71]

Ex vivo—It reduces factors in blood indicative of active atherosclerotic plaque formation, in patients with coronary disease.[72]

In vivo—*Ginkgo* improves peripheral and cerebral blood flow,[73] without increasing blood pressure[74] and with a decrease in erythrocyte aggregation.[75] In older adults it not only increased cerebral perfusion and cognitive function but also decreased blood viscosity.[76] Indeed in a variety of vascular-related diseases the extract reduced blood-associated risk factors.[77]

In healthy adults *Ginkgo* protected against hypoxia-induced neurological dysfunction,[78] reduced both systolic and diastolic blood pressure,[79] had a vasoregulatory effect, being capable of either increasing or decreasing blood flow[80] and reduced platelet hyperactivity.[81]

Clinical tests have found *Ginkgo* an aid in the treatment of:-

- chronic venous insufficiency[82,83] and varicose veins[84] including acute haemorrhoids[85,86]
- angina whether stable or unstable improving symptoms and haemorrheology[87,88]
- recovery from heart and cerebrovascular surgery[89,90]
- type 2 diabetes—reducing raised platelet aggregation,[81] improving retinal blood flow and haemorrheology[91]
- intermittent claudication due to peripheral arterial occlusive disease[92–96] with improved haemorrheology.[97] (Not corroborated[98])
- arteritis[99]
- Raynaud's phenomenon[100]
- trophic lesions due to poor circulation[101]
- oedema associated with increased capillary permeability[102–104]
- microcirculation of the skin whether due to arteriosclerosis or other circulatory pathology[105,106]
- cerebrovascular disorders[107,108] and/or insufficiency[109,110] including in children with early forms of the disease[111]
- visual acuity due to impaired retinal flow[112,113]

The majority of trials of *Ginkgo* treatment for cerebrovascular insufficiency have concluded it was an effective treatment for this condition.[114,115] Benefits of *Ginkgo* to help in recovery from acute ischaemic strokes has been questioned, for although trials have reported improvement in neurological deficits in these patients, the methodology has been criticised and one scientifically acceptable study failed to demonstrate any advantage.[116,117]

Given *Ginkgo's* biological actions it was tested as a potential medication to prevent acute mountain sickness. Results have been mixed with several positive trials,[118] two negative trials[119,120] and one trial where it significantly reduced the severity of the symptoms.[121] It may be beneficial in low oxygen environments by reducing nitric oxide-related cerebral vasodilation.[122]

Nervous system

This is the other main system in which *Ginkgo's* use has been extensively examined. Age-related dementia cases are increasing and as yet there is no medical "cure" for them. Oxidative stress is again considered one of the primary factors involved in neurodegenerative diseases causing neuronal loss and dysfunction. Patients with Alzheimer's disease for example have been found to have higher levels of oxidative damage in their frontal cortex.[123]

The aetiology and progression of neurodegenerative diseases like Alzheimer's dementia and Parkinson's disease have been associated with increased levels of particular proteins in brain tissue that accumulate, aggregate and become neurotoxic. In the case of Alzheimer's disease this protein is β-amyloid.[124]

In vitro—*Ginkgo* protects neurons from oxidative damage[123,125-130] decreasing their apoptosis, reducing both the production of β-amyloid protein, via reduced cholesterol levels,[131] and its aggregation.[132] In addition ginkolides protect neurons directly from the toxic effects of β-amyloid protein and also from PAF.[124,133]

Ginkgo has other actions that may affect the nervous system. It inhibits the breakdown of neuropeptides that aid mental function[134] and the ginkgolides and bilobalide are antagonists of inhibitory neurotransmitters, including $GABA_A$, leading to increased neuronal excitability (used therapeutically in some antidepressants).[135-137] It does not

however seem to have any effect on monoamine oxidase activity.[138,139]

In vivo—Many clinical trials have demonstrated *Ginkgo's* efficacy in treating dementia due to multiple infarcts and Alzheimer-type dementia.[140-144] Although the exact mechanisms by which the herb exerts these benefits are still not well understood actions such as protection for nerve cells, including from free radical damage, and increased blood flow no doubt contribute and it is probable that all the constituents of the herb are important in achieving the effect.

Ginkgo has been considered as effective as the current cholinesterase inhibitors used in the treatment of mild to moderate Alzheimer's disease[145-148]—(not corroborated[149]) with the added advantage that loss of improvement did not occur to the same extent on cessation of treatment.[150] *Ginkgo* has in fact been shown to have the same effect on the brain's electrical activity as the cholinesterase inhibitors and drugs called cognitive activators or "nootropics",[151] normalising disturbed electrical activity in the cognitively impaired.[152] It has also been shown to:-

- slow down progression of the more severe forms of the disease[146]
- improve the quality of life of dementia patients[153-155]
- improve cognitive, behavioural and psychological symptoms.[156]

Measurements of amyloid protein in plasma, which increases with age as well as with Alzheimer's disease, were lowered in healthy elderly people on *Ginkgo* supplements[157] so that it may also help prevent the development of the disease.[158] A large prospective trial has begun to evaluate this aspect.[159]

Some clinical trials found *Ginkgo* did not improve Alzheimer's disease,[160] and/or age-related memory impairment[161,162] or showed only slight benefit.[163,164] Overall however the conclusion appears to be it has promise for the treatment of cognitive function in dementia or cognitive decline,[165-167] is apparently as effective as current pharmaceuticals but with a better safety record.[168] *Ginkgo* is regularly prescribed in Germany for the treatment of dementia.[169]

It has also helped in the treatment of other conditions of the nervous system. These include:-

- schizophrenia-improving symptoms, efficacy of antipsychotics[170–173] and immune function which is depressed by the drugs[174]
- generalised anxiety/adjustment disorder with anxious mood[175]
- multiple sclerosis[176]
- Ménière's disease[177]
- mood, sleep and quality of life[178–182] (not corroborated[183]). Also sleep disturbances due to antidepressants[184] or in major depression (used with *Hypericum*)[185]
- memory in mild cognitive impairment,[186] in post-menopausal women[187] and in healthy adults of all ages[188–190] (not corroborated[191])
- visual processing (cognition) in healthy older adults[192]
- colour vision/retinal problems[193] including that associated with diabetic retinopathy[194,195]
- glaucoma, improving visual function and blood flow without increasing intraocular pressure[196,197]
- senile dry macular degeneration[198,199]
- hypoacusis or hearing loss due to poor circulation[200]
- tinnitus[201–204] (not corroborated[205,206])—some reviewers argue that scientifically rigorous studies do not show benefits[207–209]
- vertigo/vestibular dysfunction,[210–216] cochleo-vestibular disorders[217,218] including sudden deafness[219,220] (as effective as pharmaceuticals[221,222])
- mental performance in healthy adults[223–232] (not corroborated[233–236]), in adults with slight to moderate memory impairment,[237–240] cerebral insufficiency[241] or cerebro-organic syndrome,[242] in post-menopausal women[243] and in patients with asthenia[244–246]
- neuropathy—(intravenous administration)[247]
- Attention Deficit Hyperactivity Disorder (ADHD) alone or used with *Panax quinquefolium*[111,248]
- hypoxic-ischaemic encephalopathy in neonates[249]

Cancer protective
In vitro—*Ginkgo* has a biphasic effect on oestrogen and its receptors. It is oestrogenic when low levels of oestrogen are present, which would help in hormone depletion e.g. menopause, but is anti-oestrogenic when oestrogen levels are high and therefore may protect against hormone-dependent cancer.[250,251] It has antiproliferative effects on a number of cancer cell lines[252–256] and is anti-angiogenic.[257] In addition the flavonoids can act as anticancer agents as they are anti-oxidant, alter genetic expression of factors associated with cancer formation and increase detoxification of chemical carcinogens.[258,259]

In vivo—Extracts have inhibited chromosomal damage from radiation and oxidative stress, both being potential cancer-inducers.[257] Chromosomal radiation damage was significantly reduced in workers from the Chernobyl reactor accident after 2 months treatment[260] and benefits persisted for months after cessation of *Ginkgo* therapy.[261]

Intra-venous *Ginkgo* improved the effect of conventional chemotherapy treatment in progressive colorectal cancer, so it may have an adjunctive role too.[262,263]

Endocrine
In vitro—*Ginkgo* inhibits fatty acid synthase which is a new target treatment for obesity.[264]

Fractions of the leaf were good relaxants of penile *corpus cavernosum* tissue and may have significance for treating impotence.[265]

In vivo—studies have indicated *Ginkgo* could also help in the following:-

- sexual dysfunction in women[266–268] although the herb does not appear to affect androgenic hormone levels.[269] It's affect on sexual function in those whose impairment was due to antidepressant medication has been contradictory. No benefit was achieved according to some studies[270,271] and an improvement was found in others, with women benefiting more than men[272,273]
- premenstrual congestion and associated breast tenderness and altered mood, used over 2 cycles[274]

- stress-induced blood pressure increase and cortisol release[275]
- early diabetic nephropathy[276] by improving renal function, lipid levels and haemorrheology[277]

Gingko increased the production of insulin from pancreatic cells in non-diabetics[79] and also in type 2 diabetics (including those with pancreatic exhaustion), although this may not necessarily mean improved glucose tolerance as it may increase insulin catabolism too.[278] The increase in insulin level was not accompanied by increased resistance to the hormone.[279] In addition type 2 diabetics on *Ginkgo* supplements showed a reduced risk of developing vascular problems.[279]

Antimicrobial
Gingko inhibits the growth of *Streptococcus pyogenes*[280] and the cytotoxic enzyme produced by *Porphyromonas gingivalis*.[281] Constituents inhibit *Clostridium perfringens, Escherichia coli,*[282] *Enterococcus faecalis*[283] and *Pneumocystis carinii*[284] and a peptide also has antifungal activity.[285]

Other
In vitro—*Gingko* stimulates production of collagen and fibronectin and enhances growth of skin fibroblasts,[286] reduces platelet aggregation and thromboxane levels suggesting inhibition of COX-1[287] and inhibits T-cell lymphocyte stimulation by inflammatory cytokines.[288]

In vivo—The herb was effective in the treatment of interstitial pulmonary fibrosis[289] and helped in the treatment of moderate chronic asthma,[290] reducing airway inflammation.[291] It also arrested the progress of vitiligo[292] and liver fibrosis due to chronic hepatitis[293] and with co-enzyme Q was reported to benefit fibromyalgia syndrome.[294] Applied topically the flavones inhibited skin inflammation.[295]

Ginkgo has been subject to more research than most other herbs. The inconsistencies in the results of clinical trials above highlight general flaws associated with research into agents as complex as herbal medicines. Reviewers of the trials found large inconsistencies in methodology[296] and often the extracts used were not characterised.[297]

Furthermore by using standardised extracts it may be assumed that the test "drug" is consistent but standardised commercial extracts still vary chemically[1,298–301] and some may have been synthetically fortified.[301,302] Standardisation of one or two constituents also ignores the contribution of other constituents which could still have variable levels and/or variable bioavailability.[303,304]

Medicinal uses
Cardiovascular system
- venous insufficiency
- angina
- recovery from heart surgery
- type 2 diabetes
- arteritis
- recovery from cerebrovascular surgery
- intermittent claudication
- varicose veins
- trophic lesions due to poor circulation
- Raynaud's phenomenon
- haemorrhoids
- oedema, due to increased vascular permeability
- cerebrovascular disorders
- visual acuity
- microcirculation of skin

Respiratory tract
- asthma
- interstitial pulmonary fibrosis

Nervous system
- schizophrenia
- anxiety
- vision
- glaucoma
- improve mental performance
- multiple sclerosis
- memory
- hypoacusis
- neuropathy
- macular degeneration
- Ménierès disease
- tinnitus
- ADHD
- cognitive function

Reproductive tract
- impotence
- pre-menstrual oedema
- sexual dysfunction in women

Endocrine system
- early diabetic neuropathy
- stress-induced hypertension

Pharmacy
Three times daily
Infusion of dried herb   – 2–3 g
Standardised extract   – 40 mg

It may take at least 12 weeks to see improvements.

Standardised extracts used in clinical trials contained a flavone glycoside content in the range of 22–27% and terpene lactone content of 5–7% of which 2.8–3.4% are ginkgolides and 2.6–3.2% is bilobalide.[2] These extracts were not all identical and some may not have contained all the constituents present in the raw leaf e.g. some lacked biflavones.

Pharmacokinetics
In vitro—Studies show that membrane transport may limit cellular levels of the main flavonoids.[305]

In vivo—The flavonoids, quercetin and kaempferol are absorbed at about the same rate and are excreted as glucuronides in urine.[306] The main ginkgolides and bilobalide appear to be well absorbed, ginkgolide A having a half-life of 4.5 hours, ginkgolide B 10.6 hours and bilobalide 3.2 hours.[307] Gingkolide B reaches maximum plasma concentration 2.3 hours after administration of the extract[308] and total ginkgolides peak 2 hours after ingestion.[309] About 70% of ginkgolide A, 50% ginkgolide B and 30% of bilobalide were excreted unchanged in urine following oral doses.[49]

Precautions and/or safety
Ginkgolic acids are potentially toxic and allergenic and *German Commission E* has set maximum allowable level of 5 ppm (5 mg/kg) in standardised extracts.[310,311] Ginkgolic acids have been found in commercial ginkgo products at levels a great deal higher than this.[302,312] Colchicine, as a contaminant,

has also been reported.[313] Possible side-effects are gastric disturbance, vomiting and diarrhoea; restlessness and headache all of which have been reported after using standardised preparations. Their occurrence is rare and the trials above consistently reported good safety and tolerance for *Ginkgo*, adverse events being no different from that reported for placebo.[204,314]

There are more serious anecdotal reports implicating *Ginkgo* in the development of acute generalised exanthematous pustulosis,[315] toxic epidermal necrolysis,[316] ventricular arrhythmia,[317] spontaneous haemorrhage,[318–320] post-operative bleeding,[321–326] sub-dural haematoma[327] and seizures in epileptics.[328,329] The nuts inside the fruit are considered neurotoxic and cytotoxic[330] and have been associated with vomiting and convulsions.[331] Contamination of leaf extracts with ginkgolic acid is cited as a possible contribution to epileptic seizures, particularly in the elderly.[332]

In healthy volunteers, including some who were elderly, *Ginkgo* did not alter bleeding or coagulation times.[333–335] Furthermore the levels of ginkgolides required to produce anti-PAF activity are estimated to be 100 times higher than that found at peak plasma levels when recommended doses of standardised extracts are used suggesting that it is unlikely to cause haemorrhaging.[336] Reviews of data on patients using *Ginkgo* have concluded there is a low but increased risk of bleeding.[337,338]

Extracts have been found to be free of type I allergens.[339]

Interactions
In vitro—*Ginkgo* affected the organic anion-transporting polypeptide B which is involved in intestinal absorption of some drugs,[340] although no related *in vivo* problems have been reported.

In vivo—Studies are not consistent regarding the effects of the extract or its fractions on the various P450 isozymes.[341-345] Where inhibition of P450 has occurred e.g. CYP2C9 indicating a potential interaction between warfarin and *Ginkgo*,[346] which was demonstrated using rats as a model,[347] it did not occur *in vivo* in humans. Specifically, at recommended doses, it did not affect clotting time, pharmacokinetics or pharmacodynamics of warfarin in healthy volunteers.[346-348] Data from either *in vitro* or animal studies are therefore not necessarily predictive of what is likely to occur in humans *in vivo*. Cytochrome-P450 levels are believed to decline with age possibly changing drug metabolism in the elderly in a more marked manner and as this is a subset of the population more likely to use *Ginkgo* this could be a concern. The herb's effect on elderly healthy subjects was tested with a variety of drugs metabolised by different P450 isozymes, no significant interactions occurred.[349]

Another possible area for interaction arises from *Ginkgo's* anti-PAF activity where it has been predicted it would increase bleeding if used with aspirin or other antithrombotic medications.[350] Co-administering *Ginkgo* with antithrombotic pharmaceuticals, including aspirin and warfarin (as above), did not enhance antiplatelet activity.[351-355]

Specific tests failed to produce an interaction with metformin (diabetes),[356] donepezil (Alzheimer's disease),[357] digoxin[358] and antipyrine (anti-inflammatory).[359]

Caution: *Ginkgo* was shown to potentiate the effect on bleeding time of **cilostazol** without enhancing antiplatelet activity.[351] It **may** interact with **omeprazole**[360] and **nifedipine**.[361]

Anecdotal cases have been reported of interactions with the concomitant use of a standardised extract and **ibuprofen** (fatal intracerebral bleed)[362] and low-dose **trazodone** (coma).[363]

Further studies are needed to clarify these potential interactions but to-date no human studies have found a proven interaction between ginkgo and any pharmaceuticals *in vivo*.[364,365]

Historical uses
Chinese use has been long term (4000 years!) to "benefit the brain, coughs, asthma and heart. Also for filariasis, enuresis; leucorrhoea and longevity. Leaves for diarrhoea.

HAMAMELIDACEAE

The witch hazel family consists of 23 genera of deciduous or evergreen trees or shrubs of warm temperate regions of Asia, North America, Africa, Australia and Madagascar. *Liquidambar* spp. and *Hamamelis virginiana* are the best known medicinal plants of this family.

Hamamelis virginiana

Witch hazel

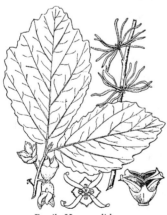

Family Hamamelidaceae

Description
A deciduous shrub or small tree to 5 m often with several crooked, branching trunks from the same root. *Leaves* hazel-like, alternate, elliptic-ovate, short petioled, acuminate, serrate, light green. *Flowers* small, yellow, in clusters in the leaf axils, appearing in late autumn often among the dry autumn leaves. Calyx lobes 4, brownish. Petals 4, strap-like. *Fruit* a woody capsule, ripening in the following autumn.

Odour—leaves slight; bark odourless; taste—leaves astringent, slightly aromatic and bitter; bark astringent and slightly bitter.

Habitat and cultivation
Native to Eastern North America growing in damp, well-drained soils and semi-shade. Propagated by seed or cuttings. Drought and wind tender, frost resistant.

Parts used
The bark, twigs and the leaves, fresh or dried, collected in autumn.

Active constituents[1]
1) Tannins (3–10%) mainly condensed. Leaf tannins are composed of gallic acid (10%),

215

hydrolysable hamamelitannin (1.5%) and condensed polymeric proanthocyanidins (88.5%) and catechins. Bark is richer in tannin, its constituents are similar to the leaf, but the level of hamamelitannin is much higher[2,3]

2) Flavonoids including quercitin, kaempferol and astragalin

Also contains small amounts of saponins, volatile oil, soluble polysaccharides[4] and resin.

Actions
1) Astringent
2) Antihaemorrhagic
3) Anti-inflammatory

Scientific information
Hamamelis is an official preparation in a number of countries[22] and is approved by *German Commission E* for the treatment of local inflammation, haemorrhoids, varicose veins and minor skin injuries. It has mainly been used topically to treat bruises and inflammation and to stimulate wound healing. It is also much used in the cosmetics industry as an astringent.

In vitro—The leaves have a range of good antibacterial activity against periodontal Gram-positive and Gram-negative infective pathogens.[5] A distillate of witch hazel is antimicrobial against *Staphylococcus aureus, Escherichia coli, Bacillus subtilis, Enterococcus faecalis* and *Candida albicans*[6,7] whilst the procynanidin fraction is antiviral against HSV-1.

The whole extract is anti-mutagenic/desmutagenic in the standard Ames assay, an action due to the proanthocynanidin fraction,[8] and the tannins are antigenotoxic partly mediated through increased detoxification by glutathione-S-transferase.[9]

The extract and hamamelitannin have strong anti-oxidant activity[10-13] as does the procynanidin fraction which also inhibits α-glucosidase and leukocyte elastase[14] and increases keratinocyte proliferation.[4]

The anti-haemorrhagic action of the herb seems due partly to the inhibition by hamamelitannin of TNF-α[15] whilst its anti-inflammatory action, and

that of the tannins, may be due to their potent inhibition of 5-LOX.[16]

In vivo—A 10% *Hamamelis* distillate, used as a cream or lotion, showed significant anti-inflammatory properties in the treatment of both UV radiation damage and physically irritated skin.[17-19]

The herb is a vasoconstrictor, an action which would augment its anti-inflammatory effect.[1] Various extracts have been used topically to treat:-

- eczema—it effectively reduced the symptoms associated with endogenous and attrition eczema,[1] giving the same benefits as a pharmaceutical anti-inflammatory cream,[20] although it did not seem to significantly improve atopic eczema[21]
- sodium lauryl sulphate skin irritation—reduced transdermal water loss and erythema[4]
- stage 1 haemorrhoids—symptoms were significantly improved[1]
- episiotomy—the benefit was comparable to that of using an ice pack or hydrocortisone cream containing a local anaesthetic[1]
- HSV-1 infection[1]—inflammation was significantly reduced

Medicinal uses
Cardiovascular system
In all situations where an astringent action would be beneficial e.g. for bleeding and lax vessels:

- haemorrhoids
- haemorrhage
- varicose veins

Respiratory tract
- haemoptysis

Gastro-intestinal tract
The tannins help reduce bowel overactivity.

- diarrhoea
- enteritis
- gastritis
- mucous colitis
- haematemesis

Externally
- bruises
- wounds
- bleeding or infected gums
- nasal catarrh (snuff)
- sprains
- eczema
- sore throat (gargle)
- burns including sunburn
- ulcers
- styes (eyebath)
- leucorrhoea (douche)
- haemorrhoids (suppositories)

Pharmacy
Three times daily

Infusion of dried leaves	– 1–4 g
Decoction of dried bark	– 1–4 g
Tincture 1:5 (25%)	– 2–4 ml (suggested guidelines)
Fluid Extract (45%)	– 2–4 ml

Distilled witch hazel can be used neat or diluted 1:3.[1]

Distilled witch-hazel or *Hamamelis* Water (*B.P.C.*) sold in pharmacies is produced by a fairly complicated process involving steam distillation of a water macerate using the leaves and twigs, collected in spring to early summer, and adding alcohol to a level of 14%.[22] It will have excluded the majority of tannins which are considered central to the herb's action, however an astringent activity is still achieved and must be due to some constituent carried over in this process.

Precautions and/or safety
There are rare cases of contact dermatitis reported.[23]

Historical uses
In America used as a poultice for tumours and painful swellings. Also for phthisis; gleet; ophthalmia; menorrhagia and to aid recovery from abortion; haematuria and kidney pains; epistaxis; as a tonic and for insect bites.

HIPPOCASTANACEAE

The Hippocastanaceae family consists of 2 genera and about 15 species of mostly trees or large shrubs with opposite, compound leaves and large, terminal racemes or panicles of flowers. The fruit is a large capsule, either smooth or spiny, opening by 3 valves and usually containing one seed.

Aesculus hippocastanum

Horse chestnut

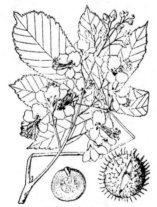

Family Hippocastanaceae

Description

A large deciduous tree 30 × 5 m, with a rounded crown and spreading branches. Trunk erect, stout and columnar; bark smooth, grey-green. Twigs stout, with very large reddish brown sticky buds. *Leaves* opposite, with 5–7 sessile leaflets. Central leaflets about 15–35 × 6–14 cm, obovate, irregularly crenate-serrate. Basal leaflets smaller. *Flowers* in broad-cylindric panicles to 30 cm high. Peduncles and pedicels glabrous or hairy. Calyx 4–6 mm long with fine short dense hairs inside. Petals 1–1.7 cm long with a narrow basal claw and the rest of the petal broad-oblong, very undulate and recurved, white with a yellow to red spot near the base. Filaments slender, hairy and curving downwards. *Capsule* to 6 cm wide, sub-globose, echinate. *Seeds* (conkers) 1–2, 3–5 cm wide, usually asymmetric, dark, shining brown with a prominent, white hilum. Flowers in spring, fruits in autumn.

Odour—slight; taste—bitter, acrid.

Habitat and cultivation

Native to Eastern Europe. Prefers to grow in rich, well-drained sandy loam in sunny, sheltered situations. Grown from seed sown in autumn or stratified, and will self-sow. Widely cultivated in cool climates. Drought and frost resistant.

Parts used

The fresh seed, harvested in autumn, when ripe. The bark and even the leaves have been used.

Active constituents[1,2]

1) Saponins—triterpenoid (up to 13%) containing "aescin" and "protosapogenin" or "prosapo-genin". Aescin itself exists in three forms—α-aescin, β-aescin and cryptoaescin. These are complex mixtures in themselves and β-aescin consists of more than 30 derivatives[3,4] of pro-toaescigenin and barringtogenol-C. Also contains hippocaesculin[5]
2) Flavonoids including quercetin, kaempferol and their derivatives
3) Tannins including proanthocyanidin A_2

The seeds also contain up to 7% fatty oil, triterpenes (including taraxerol, α- and β-amyrin),[6] sterols,[7] coumarins (esculin and fraxin)[2] and a lectin.[8]

Actions

1) Venous tonic
2) Astringent
3) Anti-inflammatory

Scientific information

Aesculus was introduced into Europe in the 16th century from Asia. Its constituent coumarin esculin was officially used in its glycoside form in external preparations for sunscreens and to treat haemor-rhoids and internally for the treatment of capillary fragility.[9] *German Commission E* has approved the herb's use for chronic venous insufficiency includ-ing varicose veins and oedema.

Most of the research on horse chestnut has con-centrated on its effect on veins and the microcir-culation. Extracts of *Aesculus* that have been used clinically have been standardised to around 70% β-aescin (referred to as aescin or escin) content, as this complex is considered to be the most signifi-cant contributor to the herb's activity.[2]

Circulatory system

In vitro—A number of pharmacological activi-ties have been established for aescin which may provide an explanation for the actions of *Aesculus* on vein function *in vivo*.[2] It is:-

- anti-oedematous—through inhibition of hyaluronidase activity (may prevent break-down of, and at the same time strengthen, capillary wall stopping oedematous leak-age[10]), altered membrane permeability, reduced intercellular gaps in veins and reduced hypoxia of endothelial cells which via phopholipase-A2 can lead to inflammation that precedes oedema
- anti-inflammatory—as above and also through inhibition of leukocyte activation, reduced neutrophil adhesiveness and reduced release of inflammatory mediators
- venotonic—through blood vessel contrac-tion, mediated through prostaglandin $F_2\alpha$.[2] This occurs in normal and slightly dilated saphenous veins although not in more severely dilated or overtly varicosed ones, these being unresponsive to vasoactive drugs generally[11]

The above pathogenic processes are closely inter-linked and can exacerbate each other therefore aes-cin could intervene at various levels to ameliorate the development of venous insufficiency.[2]

In vivo—A topical preparation consisting of 1% aescin plus essential phospholipids was beneficial for:-

- acute inflammation due to histamine[12] or dis-turbed venous flow[13]
- severe venous incompetence, reducing capil-lary fragility and fluid leakage[14]
- venous microangiopathy reducing plasma free radical levels[15]
- superficial venous thrombosis[16]
- microcirculation in the skin of people with diabetes[17] including those with neuropathy and small ulcerated lesions[18-21]

This same combination used internally was diuret-ic.[22] Aescin alone improved signs and symptoms of haemorrhoids and varicose veins and helped resolve post-operative oedema.[2]

Aesculus has been tested in the treatment of chronic venous insufficiency (CVI) and varicose veins. Some of its action is achieved by reducing the accumulation of oedematous fluid through decreased trans-capillary filtration.[23] Internal use of the herb decreased the signs (oedema, erythema) and symptoms (pain, fatigue, heaviness of limb, itching) of CVI and improved general quality of life for people with the condition[24-28] (not corroborated[29]). *Aesculus* improved venous insufficiency due to pregnancy too.[1] In early stage CVI it was as effective as compression stockings in reducing oedema, with better patient tolerance.[30] In advanced stages of the condition the stockings were more effective.[31] *Aesculus* gave better improvement in the treatment of varicose ulcers, a consequence of CVI, when used with conventional strategies (compression stockings and dressings) than when conventional therapy was used alone.[32]

Only one study to-date failed to find *Aesculus* of benefit in the treatment of CVI[29] and a number of reviews have concluded in favour of its efficacy for CVI and varicose veins.[33-37]

The herb has also been successfully used:-

- as a prophylactic prior to surgical treatment in those with evidence of deep vein thrombosis[38]
- to reduce oedema induced by flying[1]
- in the treatment and prophylaxis of venous problems caused by the contraceptive pill[39]
- in topical treatment of sprains and bruises.[1]

Other
In vitro—Some of the saponins are cytotoxic[5] and an unidentified glycoside inhibits sweet taste receptors.[40] The whole extract is a very good antioxidant.[2] Aescin is active against the virus responsible for SARS.[41]

In vivo—A gel containing 3% horse chestnut extract, through fibroblast contraction, reduced wrinkles.[42]

Medicinal uses
Cardiovascular system
- varicose veins
- varicose ulcers
- haemorrhoids
- oedema

- arteriosclerosis
- thrombosis
- thrombophlebitis
- prophylactic against thrombosis

Gastro-intestinal tract
- gastritis
- enteritis

Externally
As an ointment it has been used to treat:

- varicose veins
- bruises
- sprains

Pharmacy
Three times daily
Fluid Extract   – 0.5–1.2 ml
Standardised extracts used have been based on 50–150 mg of aescin per day and topical preparations contained 1–2% aescin.[1]

Pharmacokinetics
β-aescin is bioavailable to a variable extent depending on the particular formulation used.[43] It reaches maximum blood levels after 2 hours with a half life of between 6–8 hours,[2] although there appears to be considerable variation even for the same extract[44] and some diurnal variation too.[45]

Precautions and/or safety
The extracts used in clinical trials were found to be safe and well tolerated.[25,28,33,36] Adverse reactions that have been reported for *Aesculus*/aescin preparations include gastro-intestinal disturbances, headaches, itching and dizziness.[2]

The unripe seed has caused poisoning in children. There are anecdotal reports of hepatic injury after intravenous use of an *Aesculus* extract[46] and contact dermatitis from a topical preparation.[47]

A botanical preparation of which horse chestnut was a part was withdrawn from the market after cases of pseudo-lupus were connected to its use, however *Aesculus* was not considered the causative factor.[48,49]

Renal failure has been observed in patients given intravenous[50] or high oral doses of aescin.[1] No cases of renal problems have been attributed to *Aesculus* used at recommended doses.

Interactions

Aescin has been added, with benefit, to the treatment regime of AIDS patients to help prevent the crystallisation of indinavir that can occur in renal tubules.[51]

Historical uses

The bark was used as a febrifuge, tonic and narcotic—used in fevers and externally for ulcers. The seeds for coronary heart disease; dysentery; fevers rheumatism, neuralgia, menorrhagia, bronchitis, wounds, chilblains, prostatitis, constipation. Leaves used for whooping cough.

IRIDACEAE

The Iridaceae or Iris family is a cosmopolitan monocotyledon family of some 60 genera and over 800 species of bulbous, cormous or rhizomatous perennial plants with fibrous roots.

- Leaves are mostly basal, usually 2-ranked and linear to sword-shaped
- Flowers are bisexual, and may be regular or irregular, solitary, in clusters in 2 spathe-like bracts, or in racemes or panicles
- Perianth segments are 6, separate or basally united into a short or long tube
- Stamens 3, ovary usually 3-celled. Fruit a 3-valved capsule
- The family includes many beautiful garden bulbs.

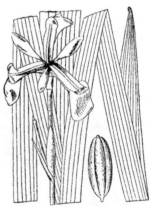

Family Iridaceae

Iris versicolor

Blue flag

Description

Perennial plant with thick rhizomes. *Leaves* sword shaped, matt green, 20–50 cm tall 15 mm-3 cm wide. *Flowers* borne alternately on a stout tall stem, 30–60 cm tall, typical iris shape and blue-violet in colour, blooming late spring to summer. *Seeds* black, layered in a three-compartmented capsule. Dies back in winter.

Odour—slight but peculiar; taste—bitter and acrid.

Habitat and cultivation

Native to North America and cultivated in many other countries in moist swampy situations, pond and river banks. Grown from root division in spring or autumn or from seed. Forms big clumps and will self-sow. Drought and frost tender.

Parts used
The rhizome.

Active constituents[1]
1) Resin—acrid (up to 25%)—("irisin" or "iridin" represents a mixture).[2]

Also contains tannins, small amount of volatile oil including furfural and irone, isophthalic and salicylic acids, gum and triterpenoids.

Actions
1) Cholagogue
2) Emetic (large doses)
3) Anti-inflammatory
4) Diuretic
5) Laxative
6) Anti-emetic (small doses)
7) Dermatological agent

The combined actions suggests *Iris* qualifies also as an alterative.

Scientific information
There is virtually no pharmacology specific to this herb and it has not been well characterised chemically either.

Iris has been an official preparation in the *United States Pharmacopoeia* and *National Formulary*.[2] The Eclectic use of the herb was for chronic skin conditions due to liver and/or gall bladder congestion, oily skin and for yellow clay-coloured stools.[3]

It has been used in the treatment of psoriasis[4] and in Ayurvedic medicine to help with obesity.

Medicinal uses
Gastro-intestinal tract
• nausea with constipation
• liver dysfunction
• vomiting in pregnancy (low dose)

Skin
• skin diseases
• cutaneous eruptions (*BHP* specific)

Externally
As a poultice or ointment for a variety of:

• skin diseases

Pharmacy
Three times daily
Decoction of dried rhizome   –   0.6–2 g
Tincture 1:5 (45%)   –   3.0–10 ml
Fluid Extract (45%)   –   0.6–2 ml
Fresh root preparations are stronger than dried ones and should probably be used at lower doses.

Historical uses
Syphilis; scrofula; dropsy. Also for lung conditions with phlegm (syrup).

JUGLANDACEAE

The walnut family. This family is comprised of 6 genera and about 60 species of deciduous, monoecious trees native to Asia, Europe, North and South America. Their leaves are alternate and pinnate. The male flowers are catkins the female flowers in racemes or in small groups. The fruit is a winged nutlet or a drupe containing a nut or stone. They are grown as ornamental trees and/or for their nuts or wood.

Juglans cinerea

Butternut

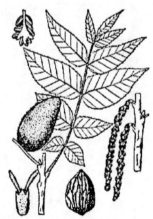

Family Juglandaceae

Description
A deciduous tree growing up to about 35 m. *Bark* grey. *Leaves*, bright green, pinnate with 11–19 opposite leaflets rounded at the base and with minute clusters of downy hairs beneath. *Fruit* egg shaped to 7 cm long, sticky-pubescent. Nuts thick shelled with many broken ridges. Flowers April to June in North America.

Habitat and cultivation
Native to eastern North America, growing in rich woods. Not often grown elsewhere.

Parts used
Dried inner bark.

Active constituents
1) Naphthoquinones including juglone (5-hydroxy-1,4-naphthoquinone), juglandin and juglandic acid.[1] Also contains essential and fixed oil, tannins and a bitter principle[2]

Actions
1) Laxative
2) Mild cathartic
3) Cholagogue

4) Vermifuge
5) Dermatological agent

Scientific information
All three *Juglans* species have much in common, more valued in the past they still have both commercial (nuts, oil) and medicinal value. *J. cinerea* was an official preparation in the *United States Pharmacopoiea* from 1820–1905[2] but has received very little scientific investigation as a medicinal.

In vitro—The bark has very good antimicrobial activity against:

- a range of bacteria including *Staphylococcus aureus, Bacillus subtilis, Mycobacterium phlei, Pseudomonas aeruginosa, Salmonella typhimurium, Klebsiella pneumoniae*
- a range of fungi including *Candida albicans, Cryptococcus neoformans, Trichophyton mentagrophytes, Microsporum gypseum, Aspergillus fumigatus* and *Fusarium oxysporum*, as well as some that have become resistant to standard antifungals[3,4]

The active constituents for the antimicrobial activity are considered to be the naphthoquinones[5] which are common to all the medicinal *Juglans* spp. Juglone is the best known of these. It is a strong oxidant producing hydrogen peroxide in cells, which may account for its abililty to be:-

- cytotoxic to some cell types both normal[5,6] and malignant.[7-9] Possible mechanisms are by causing DNA damage, interferring with transcription and protein synthesis and through altered potassium flow through the cell membrane[10]
- antibacterial—against *Listeria monocytogenes*, MRSA,[11] some cariogenic bacteria,[12,13] *Bacillus subtillis, Mycobacterium smegmatis*[14] and *Helicobacter pylori*[15]
- antifungal—against a number of pathogenic fungi including *Candida albicans, Trichophyton mentagrophytes* and *Microsporum gypseum*[14]
- antiviral—inhibits the growth of HIV through inhibition of reverse transcriptase[16]
- antiparasitic against *Toxoplasma gondii*[11]

Medicinal uses
Cardiovascular system
- haemorrhoids

Gastro-intestinal tract
J. cinerea is considered a gentle laxative and intestinal stimulant in small doses, emetic and cathartic in large doses. It does not cause griping or constipation.

- constipation (chronic)
- liver dysfunction
- dyspepsia

Skin
Through stimulation of liver and bowel function the herb is considered an alterative. Used internally and externally for cutaneous eruptions (exudative) including:-

- eczema
- herpes
- indolent ulcers

Externally
- eye inflammation
- acne

Pharmacy
Three times daily

Decoction of dried bark	– 2–6 g
Fluid Extract bark (25%)	– 2–6 ml
Fluid Extract leaves (25%)	– 0.6–2 ml
Tincture green hulls 1:10 (25%)	– 0.5–2 ml

Historical uses
Dysentery; for rheumatism and arthritis; headaches; syphilis; old ulcers (internally and externally); tonic; fevers and toothache. Used externally as a wash for wounds to stop bleeding and promote healing. The fruit oil as vermifuge for tapeworm though the bark was used for thread and pin worms.

Juglans nigra

Black walnut

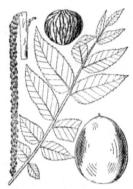

Family Juglandaceae

Description
A taller tree, growing to about 50 m. *Bark*, dark brown, and fissured. *Leaves* pinnate with 15–23 leaflets, ovate oblong, slightly hairy underneath and on leaf stems, but hairs solitary, not in clusters. *Fruits* rounded, strongly ridges and thick shelled.

Odour—leaves aromatic, bark odourless; taste—leaves and bark are bitter and astringent.

Habitat and cultivation
Native to eastern North America, growing in rich woods. Also grown in central Europe but rarely elsewhere. Often planted for timber.

Parts used
Dried inner bark, leaves and fruit husks.

Active constituents
1) Naphthoquinones—mainly juglone,[1] also plumbagin[18]

Also tannins including ellagic acid,[19] volatile oil and flavonoids (based on myricetin and sakuranetin).[20]

Nutritional constituents
Vitamins: B_{12}
Minerals: Manganese, magnesium, silica, calcium, phosphorus, iron and potassium

Actions
1) Alterative
2) Laxative
3) Antimicrobial
4) Vermifuge
5) Sudorific—green hulls

Scientific information
There is very little specific information available in the modern literature relating to *J. nigra*.

The leaf extract scavenges peroxynitrite radicals *in vitro*.[21] The naphthoquinones (as for *J. cinerea*) are cytotoxic and inhibit the growth of malignant cells.[18] Ellagic acid is also cytotoxic and anti-oxidant.[22]

J. nigra has a reputation as an antifungal. For actions of juglone see *J. cinerea*.

Medicinal uses
Skin
Used internally and externally.

- eczema
- herpes
- indolent ulcers

External
- fungal infections
- acne

Pharmacy
Three times daily

Decoction of dried bark	– 2–6 g
Fluid Extract bark (25%)	– 2–6 ml
Fluid Extract leaves (25%)	– 0.6–2 ml
Tincture green hulls 1:10 (25%)	– 0.5–2 ml

Historical uses
Culpeper recommended the fresh leaves for digestive ailments and said the older leaves were heating and drying and harder to digest but may be better for those with a "colder stomach", also for worms. For venomous bites or those of a mad dog; as an astringent for women's courses and falling hair; agues; plague; deafness; earache; old ulcers,

scrofula and carbuncles; as a gargle for inflammations of throat and mouth.

Juglans regia

Walnut, Persian walnut

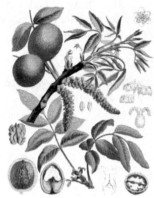

Family Juglandaceae

Description
Deciduous tree, to about 30 m with a broad spreading crown and silvery bark. *Leaves* pinnate with 5–9 leaflets, downy when young but becoming glabrous as they grow older. Aromatic when crushed. Male catkins pendulous, 5–15 cm appear with the young leaves. *Fruit* 4–5 cm, ovoid, green and glandular. Shell thin or thick and wrinkled.

Habitat and cultivation
Native to South-East Europe, and widely cultivated throughout the world for its nuts.

Parts used
Leaves, bark and the green hulls.

Active constituents[23]
1) Napthoquinones-mainly juglone (about 0.5%).[24] Juglone levels are reduced in dried leaves
2) Phenolic acids, based on cinnamic and quininc acids (these were highest in spring-early summer)
3) Flavonoids based on quercetin and kaempferol

4) Tannins based on ellagic acid[25]

Also a number of volatile oil constituents.[26] The fleshly outer part of the fruit is rich in vitamin C.

Actions
1) Alterative
2) Laxative
3) Antimicrobial
4) Dermatological agent

Scientific information
J. regia is the best studied of the three species, this being reflected in the known list of constituents. They all seem to have many uses in common. The leaf has been used medicinally for thousands of years. *German Commission E* has approved the leaves for external use only to treat mild superficial skin inflammation and excessive perspiration of feet and hands.

In vitro—The leaves inhibit the acne-causing bacteria *Propionibacterium acnes* also *Staphylococcus aureus* and *S. epidermis*, the level of activity being similar to that of antibiotics.[27] They are also active against *Helicobacter pylori*.[28] *J. regia* has very good antifungal activity against a number of pathogenic fungi including *Microsporum canis*, *Trichophyton mentagrophytes* and *T. violaceum*.[29]

The bark too is antimicrobial with activity against *Staphylococcus aureus*, *Streptococcus mutans*, *Escherichia coli*, *Pseudomonas aeruginosa* and *Candida albicans*.[30] (There are ethnobotanic reports of the bark being used to "clean teeth").[31] It is also antiproliferative for a number of cell lines, is antimutagenic and anticarcinogenic.[32,33]

Many of the parts of this species have been used in traditional systems of healing. Walnut, the edible nut itself has potential benefits for cardiovascular[34,35] and Alzheimer's disease.[36]

For actions of juglone see *J. cinerea*.

Weiss suggests this herb is suitable for the treatment of skin conditions in children.

Medicinal uses
Gastro-intestinal tract
• constipation
• liver dysfunction

Skin
• eczema
• herpes
• inflammation of the eyelids

Externally
• ulcers
• cutaneous eruptions
• fungal infections
• acne

Pharmacy
Three times daily

Decoction of dried bark	–	2–6 g
Fluid Extract bark (25%)	–	2–6 ml
Fluid Extract leaves (25%)	–	4–8 ml
Tincture green hulls 1:10 (25%)	–	0.5–2 ml

Precautions and/or safety
Juglans spp. have been implicated in toxicity in animals however there are no reports in the literature of poisoning in humans. *In vitro* the leaf extract of *J. regia* was not toxic to hepatocytes[37] nor was the herb found to be genotoxic,[38] although juglone itself is mutagenic.[39]

There is a report of the juice of green walnut hulls (*J. regia*) causing acute irritant contact dermatitis, presumed to be due to juglone.[40,41]

Historical uses
See *J. nigra*. Nuts thought to be good for the brain and therefore good for headaches and epilepsy, (doctrine of signatures); good for sexual vigour, associated with Jupiter and love.

LAMIACEAE

[Formerly known as Labiatae]

This is a family of 3500 species worldwide but especially abundant in the Mediterranean region. Many culinary herbs belong to the Lamiaceae and are cultivated in gardens. Lamiaceae are distinguished by their flower form, square stems and often scented leaves. The flowers are all insect pollinated and secrete large amounts of nectar.

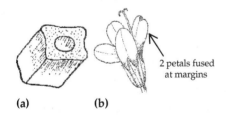

2 petals fused at margins

(a)   **(b)**

General characteristics
- Stems are more or less quadrangular (a)
- Leaves are opposite and usually, but not always, simple
- Flowers are usually small and borne in modified cymes forming verticils or pseudo-whorls which are either spaced along the inflorescence rachis or aggregated into spikes or panicles

- The calyx is tubular with 5 lobes or 2 lips
- The corolla is tubular and usually has an upper lip composed of 2 lobes and a lower lip of 3 lobes (b)
- There are often conspicuous bracts
- There are usually 4 stamens, their filaments attached to the inside of the corolla wall. A few genera have only 2 stamens often with tiny remnants of 2 others (c)
- The pistil has a long style with a forked stigma. Its ovary has 4 compartments each with 1 ovule (d)
- Around the base of the ovary is a fleshy ring—the disk—which secretes the nectar
- The fruit is the same in all Lamiaceae. The ripened ovary splits into four one-seeded nutlets

There are 7 subfamilies:

1. Subfamily Ajugoideae
   - Which is characterised by having the corolla with the upper lip short or absent
   - 2–4 stamens, exserted
   - The style is not gynobasic
   - Seed non-endospermic e.g. *Ajuga* and *Teucrium*

229

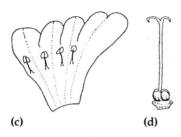

(c)   **(d)**

2. Subfamily Lamioideae
   - Here the corolla is bilabiate to almost regular
   - 2 or 4 stamens, often exserted
   - The style is gynobasic
   - The seed non-endospermic

There are 6 tribes of this sub family:

a) Lamieae—calyx almost regular to bilabiate and tubular bell-shaped. Corolla strongly bilabiate with concave or cucullate upper lip. 4 stamens lying under the upper lip, 1 pair long, 1 pair short (didynamous) e.g:-
   - *Ballota nigra*
   - *Leonurus cardiaca*
   - *Melissa officinalis*
   - *Prunella vulgaris*
   - *Stachys officinalis*
   - *Lamium album*

b) Marrubieae—calyx more or less regular, tubular bell-shaped. Corolla bilabiate with flat upper lip. 4 stamens, didynamous e.g:-
   - *Marrubium vulgare*

c) Monardeae—calyx regular or bilabiate. Corolla with concave or upright upper lip. 2 stamens e.g:-
   - *Monarda didyma*

d) Nepeteae—calyx almost regular to bilabiate. Corolla bilabiate with concave upper lip. 4 stamens sometimes didynamous with posterior pair longer and anterior pair sterile e.g:-
   - *Glechoma hederacea*
   - *Nepeta cataria*

e) Salvieae—calyx bilabiate. Corolla bilabiate with helmet-shaped or cucullate upper lip. 2 stamens e.g:-
   - *Salvia officinalis*

f) Mentheae—calyx regularly 5-toothed or bilabiate. Stamens may be 2 or 4, equal or didynamous e.g:-
   - *Hyssopus officinalis*
   - *Lycopus europeaus*
   - *Mentha x piperita*
   - *Mentha pulegium*
   - *Origanum vulgare*
   - *Thymus vulgaris*

3. Subfamily Lavanduloideae
   - Corolla weakly bilabiate, with the teeth sub-equal
   - 4 stamens, didynamous, included
   - Style gynobasic
   - Seed non-endospermic e.g. *Lavandula*

4. Subfamily Ocimoideae
   - Corolla with 4-lobed upper lip and 1-lobed lower lip
   - 2–4 stamens descending, exserted from corolla tube and lying under the lip or enclosed by it
   - Style gynobasic e.g. *Ocimum*

5. Subfamily Prostantheroideae
   - Upper lip of the corolla very broad, concave or almost flat
   - Stamens 2 or 4, usually included
   - Style not gynobasic
   - Seed endospermic e.g. *Prostanthera, Westringia*

6. Subfamily Rosmarinoideae
   - Corolla bilabiate with upper lip cut into 2 narrow lobes
   - 2 stamens strongly exserted
   - Style incompletely gynobasic e.g. *Rosmarinus*

7. Subfamily Scutellarioideae
   - Corolla limb 2-lipped and upper lip hooded
   - 4 stamens exserted but lying beneath upper lip
   - Style gynobasic e.g. *Scutellaria*

Ballota nigra

Black horehound

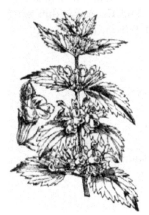

Family Lamiaceae

Description

A dark green, hairy, strong smelling perennial to 40–80 cm. *Leaves*, stalked, lamina 2–5 cm, oval or rounded with coarsely toothed margins. *Flowers* reddish purple in numerous whorls in the axils of the upper leaves. Corolla, 1–2 cm, hairy outside, with tube shorter than the calyx. *Calyx* glandular-hairy with 5 broad pointed tooth-like lobes recurved or spreading in fruit. Flowers in summer.

Odour and taste—foetid.

Habitat and cultivation

Originally from Eastern Europe *Ballota nigra* grows in waste places, along tracks and hedges throughout most of Europe and north-east America. It grows from seed and will self sow. Frost and drought resistant.

Parts used

Aerial parts harvested just prior to, or during, flowering.

Active constituents[1]

1) Diterpenoids including marrubiin, ballonigrin, ballotinone and ballotenol[2,3]
2) Flavonoids including derivatives of luteolin[4]
3) Phenylpropanoids including verbascoside, forsythoside-B, arenarioside, balloteroside and caffeoyl malic acid[5-7]
4) Volatile oil including α- and β-pinene, caryophyllene, linalol and sabinene

Actions

1) Anti-emetic
2) Sedative
3) Antispasmodic
4) Mild astringent

Scientific information

This herb is related to *Marrubium vulgare* and shares some of its chemical constituents, however it is not so well characterised or used. Research undertaken on *Ballota* to-date indicates that it has very good anti-oxidant properties, due at least in part to the phenylpropanoids.[5,8] In addition they have sedative actions (possibly by binding to a number of different receptor sites in neurones)[9] and antibacterial activity against *Proteus mirabilis* and *Staphylococcus aureus*.[7]

Medicinal uses

Gastro-intestinal tract
• nervous dyspepsia
• nausea
• vomiting including that due to pregnancy

Nervous system

As a sedative *Ballota* is also used for:

• nausea of nervous origin
• vomiting of nervous origin

Pharmacy

Three times daily
Infusion of dried herb   – 2–4 g
Tincture 1:10 (45%)   – 1–2 ml
Fluid extract (25%)   – 1–3 ml

Historical uses

Antidote to mad dog bite; vermifuge.

Glechoma hederacea
[Formerly Nepeta hederacea]

Ground ivy, alehoof

Description

Perennial herb with hairy, non-flowering stems creeping and rooting at the nodes, and lax, leafy, ascending, flowering stems. *Leaves* opposite,

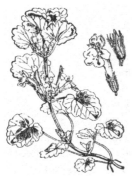

Family Lamiaceae

long-stalked. Lamina 1–3.5 × 1–4.5 cm, sub-orbicular to reniform, sparsely to densely hairy especially underneath, shallowly to deeply crenate; base cordate. A variegated-leaved species is common. *Flowers* in axillary whorls of 6. Calyx about 5 mm long with 15 hairy nerves; teeth triangular-acuminate. Corolla blue or blue violet, 1–1.5 cm long, hairy outside, lower lip with purple spots. *Nutlets* if present are 2 mm long, smooth and more or less obovoid. Flowers in spring and summer.

Habitat and cultivation
Originally from temperate Eurasia, both green and variegated forms grow in many countries in shady/semi-shady places with moist well drained soil. Grown from division by lifting and resetting rooted stolons. Frost resistant and drought tender.

Parts used
Aerial parts harvested just prior to, or during, flowering.

Active constituents[1]
1) Flavonoids mainly luteolin, quercetin, apigenin[10,11]
2) Triterpenoids including β-sitosterol, oleanolic and urolic acids[12]
3) Volatile oil (0.03–0.06%) including germacrene B and D, cis-ocimene and β-elemene[13]
4) Phenolic acids including ferulic and p-coumaric acids[14] and nepetoidins A and B[15]
5) Polyphenols

Also contains choline, marrubiin and a bitter named glechomine, free and esterified unsaturated fatty acids,[16] alkaloids (hederacines)[17] and a non-cytotoxic lectin.[18] *Glechoma* exhibits polyploidy, this may alter the chemical make-up.[19]

Actions
1) Anticatarrhal
2) Expectorant
3) Astringent
4) Vulnerary
5) Diuretic
6) Anti-inflammatory
7) Stomachic

Scientific informaion
The herb has not received much attention, although some pharmacologic information exists on individual constituents. It is used in Spain to treat dysmenorrhoea and hypertension and as an antispasmodic.[20]

In vitro—*Glechoma* is antibacterial and has antioxidant activity.[21]

Oleanolic and ursolic acids have potenitial as hepatoprotective, anti-inflammatory, antitumour, anti-hyperlipidaemic, anti-ulcerogenic, antibacterial and hypoglycaemic agents based largely on studies using animal models.[12,22]

The pseudotannins are low molecular weight derivatives of caffeic acid. There are no other tannins in this herb which nonetheless displays astringent properties.

The flavonoids are anti-inflammatory and expectorant and one of the unsaturated fats is credited with regulation of platelet membranes via prostaglandin receptor sites which may have ramifications for hormone and neurotransmitter modulation of cellular activity.[23]

Medicinal uses
Respiratory tract
• chronic/acute respiratory catarrh
• coughs
• bronchitis

Gastro-intestinal tract
- diarrhoea
- gastritis
- haemorrhoids

Urinary tract
- cystitis

Nervous system
- tinnitus

Pharmacy
Three times daily
Infusion of dried herb   – 2–4 g
Tincture 1:5 (25%)   – 5–10 ml
Fluid Extract (25%)   – 2–4 ml

Precautions and/or safety
In large doses *Glechoma* is toxic to horses but no human toxicity is known.

Historical uses
Lead colic in painters; kidney diseases; nervous headaches; consumption. As a liver stimulant; for poor digestion. Sciatica and bone ache; gout. Externally for the treatment of cancers; ulcers; poor eyesight; poor hearing; fistulas; hollow ulcers. Gargle for sore mouths and throats. Expressed juice used for bruises; black eyes; as an antiscorbutic.

Hyssopus officinalis

Hyssop

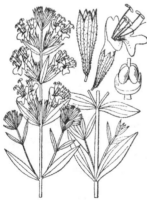

Family Lamiaceae

Description
A perennial, aromatic, nearly hairless, much-branched undershrub 20–60 cm tall. *Leaves* opposite, sessile, narrow, dark green, clustered at the nodes 1.5–2.5 cm, linear or oblong lance-shaped, hairless with sunken glands. *Flowers* in a compact, elongated spike, often interrupted below. Corolla blue, pink or white, 10–12 mm long, the upper lip and middle lobe of lower lip notched; calyx hairless 6–8 mm; stamens 4, diverging and projecting beyond corolla. Flowers in summer.

Habitat and cultivation
Native to Mediterranean, on dry banks or screes, introduced elsewhere. Grown from seed or cuttings in well-drained soil. Likes colder winters and low humidity. Drought and frost resistant.

Parts used
Leafy flowering tops harvested just prior to, or during, flowering.

Active constituents[1]
1) Volatile oil (up to 1%) mainly monoterpenes, including pinocamphone, linalool, α- and β-pinene, camphor, 1,8-cineole, thujone, α-terpineol and limonene[24]
2) Flavonoids including diosmin[25] and hesperidin
3) Tannins up to 8%
4) Terpenoids including marrubiin, ursolic and oleanolic acids[26]

Also contains phenolics including rosmarinic and caffeic acids,[27,28] phenylpropanoids[29] and a polysaccharide with potential medicinal activity.[30] There is a degree of physical and chemical variation amongst cultivated hyssop.[31]

Actions
1) Carminative
2) Sedative
3) Diaphoretic
4) Expectorant

Scientific information
Research specific to *Hyssopus* is limited. It has been used as an anthelmintic in India.[32]

In vitro—The herb inhibits HIV whilst conferring some protection on HIV infected lymphocytes.[30,33] This antiviral activity is not due to the herb's tannins, possible contributors being the phenolic and polysaccharide constituents.[34] The essential oil has some antibacterial[35] and anti-fungal activity.[36]

A phenolic fraction is able to inhibit α-glucosidase activity and this may or may not have relevance for human gastro-intestinal absorption of carbohydrates and therefore hyperglycaemia.[28,37]

Medicinal uses
Respiratory tract
- bronchitis
- chronic nasal catarrh
- coughs
- colds and influenza

Nervous system
- epilepsy (petit mal)
- anxiety states
- hysteria

Pharmacy
Three times daily

Infusion of dried herb	– 2–4 g
Tincture 1:5 (45%)	– 2–4 ml
Fluid Extract (25%)	– 2–4 ml

Precautions and/or safety
Essential oil of hyssop is toxic[38] and pinocamphone is considered to have been responsible for seizures induced by it.[39,40]

Historical uses
Internal and external treatment of "muscular rheumatism"; bruises and cuts; nervous restorative—uplifting to spirit and mind; anthelmintic; "purgeth gross humours by stool"; to restore normal colour after jaundice; dropsy. Externally for wounds; inflammations and bruises. "Excellent" for quinsy or swelling in the throat; toothache. For ear inflammation and "singing noise" (tinnitus?). The oil for lice and itchy scalp.

Lamium album

White dead nettle, white archangel

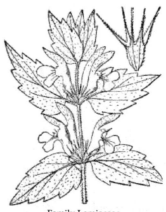

Family Lamiaceae

Description
A hairy perennial with creeping rhizomes and erect stems, 20–60 cm tall. *Leaves* stalked, 3–7 cm, oval heart-shaped, sparsely to densely hairy, pointed and coarsely toothed. *Flowers* white, large in distant whorls, corolla 2–2½ cm, the tube curved with an oblique ring of hairs near the base, longer than the calyx, upper lip with long hairs, bilobed lower lip with small teeth. *Anthers* blackish and hairy. Flowers spring to autumn.

Habitat and cultivation
Native to Britain and Europe, naturalized in other countries. Grows in waste places, along tracks and hedges.

Parts used
The herb used just prior to or at flowering or the flowers used alone.

Active constituents
1) Tannins (around 5%), mainly catechins
2) Flavonoids including derivatives of rutin, p-coumaroyl, quercetin and kaempferol[41,42]
3) Saponins including triterpenoids (ursolic acid)[43]

4) Phenolic acids including chlorogenic acid[44]
5) Secoiridoid glycosides including lamalbid, caryoptoside and albosides A and B.[45-47] Also phytoecdysteroids[48]

Also contains mucilage, amines and phenylpropanoid glycosides (lamalboside and acetoside).[41,49] A 13 carbon glucoside has been isolated from the leaves.[50]

Actions
1) Astringent
2) Haemostatic

The flowers have also been used in some traditions to treat mucous membrane inflammation, as an antispasmodic, antibacterial, diuretic and depurative.

Scientific information
Although this is not one of the best known medicinal herbs it has been found to contain some quite unusual constituents and there has been scientific interest in their structure.

In vitro—Both the flowers and the herb have a good spectrum of anti-oxidant activity.[51,54] The flowers, dried and fresh have a high level of enzyme activity and whilst this may contribute to the therapeutic value of the herb they have not been shown to have specific actions.[52] The flowers have been used traditionally as a vulnerary and anti-inflammatory and extracts of the triterpenoid fraction supported this use by stimulating fibroblast proliferation.[43]

Water extracts have moderate anti-inflammatory activity[53,54] but no antibacterial activity against the organisms tested.[55]

Medicinal uses
Reproductive tract
• leucorrhoea
• menorrhagia
• vaginitis
• dysmenorrhoea
• prostatitis

Externally
• vaginal discharge (douche)

Other possible uses
The herb has been quoted as useful for:[56]

• cystitis
• diarrhoea
• irritable bowel
• catarrh
• bleeding haemorrhoids

Pharmacy
Three times daily
Infusion of dried herb   – 2–4 g
Tincture 1:5 (25%)   – 5–10 ml
Fluid Extract (25%)   – 2–4 ml

Historical uses
As a tonic, for hardness of the spleen; depression. Externally for gout; sciatica; wounds; old ulcers; to draw splinters; bruises; burns and to treat scrofulous lesions.

Lavandula angustifolia subsp. angustifolia

Lavender, English lavender

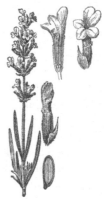

Family Lamiaceae

Description
A very aromatic, greyish-leaved, branched, perennial shrub 36–80 cm high in flower. *Leaves* opposite, sessile, 2–6 cm long, oblong to linear, margins revolute. Young leaves white-hairy, adult leaves grey-green. Foliage is compact. *Flowers* borne in spikes, 3–7 cm long, on long stems. Spikes often

interrupted below. Corolla is hairy outside, 10–12 mm long with large lobes, and is twice as long as calyx which is generally 4–7 mm long. Flowers generally lavender but there are cultivars with flower colour ranging from lavender to violet, pink and white. *Bracts* purple, broadly oval, pointed, papery, seven veined. Small linear bracteoles may be present. No terminal bracts present. Flowers in summer.

Odour—aromatic, intense and pleasant; taste—bitter and pungent.

Habitat and cultivation

Originally from the Western Mediterranean this lavender is now grown throughout the world for its sweet scented flowers. It is often called English lavender because the finest lavender oil is produced in the cooler English climate with its long hours of summer daylight. It is grown commercially in many countries. Can be grown from seed which may hybridise and therefore may not be true to type. So it is generally grown from cuttings. Prefers an open sunny situation and needs free draining soil with lime. Grows better in areas of winter cold. Drought and frost resistant.

Parts used

The flowers.

Active constituents

1) Volatile oil (0.5–1.0%) containing up to 36 constituents, including predominantly the monoterpenes linalool, linalyl acetate, lavadulyl acetate, α-terpineol, geranyl acetate, borneol, thymol and carvacrol.[57,58] Another monoterpene, perillyl alcohol, has also been identified. The constituents vary with the origin of the flowers, growing conditions, time of year harvested and method of extraction. The leaf oil has a different profile and its inclusion would also alter the final make-up.

2) Coumarins including herniarin, umbelliferone and santonine

3) Tannins

Also triterpenes, flavonoids,[59] sesquiterpenes (caryophyllene)[58] and phenolic acids including rosmarinic acid.[60]

Actions

1) Carminative
2) Spasmolytic
3) Rubefacient
4) Antidepressant
5) Antirheumatic
6) Insect repellent

Scientific information

The antiseptic properties of *Lavandula* were known in all ancient traditions. The tincture and essential oil have been official preparations in pharmacopoeias around the world finding uses as carminatives to treat flatulence and colic internally and as an insect repellent externally (oil[141]). *German Commission E* has approved use of the flowers to treat restlessness, insomnia and nervous stomach, Roehmheld's syndrome and meteorism, and as a bath to treat functional circulatory disorders.

Whilst the essential oil has been subjected to some analysis in terms of its pharmacology the whole extract is not well studied. The oil probably contributes largely to the herb's actions.

In vitro—The oil has antimicrobial properties and has displayed some degree of activity against a number of pathogens:-

- bacteria[61]—including *Gardnerella vaginalis, Atopobium vaginae* (from vaginal infections);[62] *Helicobacter pylori* strains,[63] oral pathogens,[64,65] MRSA[66] vancomycin-resistant *Enterococcus faecalis*[66]
- fungi—*Candida albicans* (linalool also active),[67] *C. glabrata* and *C. tropicalis*,[62] *Aspergillus* spp.[68,69] and *Trichophyton* spp.[66]
- protozoa—*Trichomonas vaginalis* and *Giardia duodenalis*[70]

Inconsistency in antimicrobial activity (some research reports limited activity)[71,72] may be associated with the great variability possible in the constituents of *Lavandula* essential oil.[66] However its *in vitro* activity has been considered comparable to that of tea tree oil.[66]

Constituents other than the essential oil are good anti-oxidants[73,74] although the oil itself does have limited activity.[76]

The whole extract as well as the essential oil also has some inhibitory action on acetycholinesterase activity, and they may improve neuronal function.[73,76]

Perillyl alcohol has shown potential in a number of different studies as an anticancer agent *in vitro*[77–79] and *in vivo*.[80]

In vivo—Clinical trials have been conducted on the use of the essential oil mostly in the practice of aromatherapy where massage may add to any benefits achieved.

The aromatic oil alone was found to:-

- improve the sleep quality in insomniacs[81] and depth of sleep (slow wave sleep) in normal volunteers[82]
- reduce the rise in diastolic blood pressure associated with muscle exertion[83]
- reduce signs of depression[84]
- improve psychological well-being[85,87] and increase a sense of "happiness"[86] although it was also found to decrease cognitive function in healthy volunteers[87]

Lavandula tincture taken with a standard antidepressant also gave better outcomes for patients than using the antidepressant alone[88] whilst ingestion of the oil improved the state of relaxation and mental "regeneration" of healthy volunteers suggesting an improvement in their ability to cope with stress.[89,90]

The discovery, *in vitro*, of acetycholinesterase inhibition, has prompted trials using the oil in aromatherapy to treat Alzheimer's disease. It provided some improvement in the aggressive behaviour and emotional state of sufferers of this disease and in those with severe dementia.[91,92]

The oil's aromatic effect appears to occur at a level within the central nervous system higher than the brain stem[83] and through changes to autonomic nervous system function.[86,93]

Used in the bath water of new mothers the oil helped relieve perineal discomfort associated with childbirth.[94,95]

In combination with other herbal extracts lavender, was used topically to treat alopecia areata with some success[96] and as an anti-inflammatory on oral mucosa,[97] an activity for which the oil and leaves have been used in Iranian herbal medicine.[98]

Linalool applied topically decreased systolic blood pressure.[99]

The herb is considered to be a choleretic and cholagogue.

Medicinal uses

Cardiovascular system
- vasospastic conditions

Gastro-intestinal tract
- flatulent dyspepsia
- colic

Nervous system
The volatile oil can directly affect this system by smell as it goes from the olfactory nerve into the brain:

- headaches
- restlessness
- insomnia
- depression
- irritability
- excitability
- Musculoskeletal
- rheumatism

Externally
- myalgia
- neuralgia
- rheumatism
- burns
- insect bites and stings

Pharmacy
Three times daily
Infusion of dried herb   – 1–2 g
Tincture 1:5 (60%)   – 2–4 ml

The oil is widely available and is safe to use neat on the skin (see Precautions) but it has not been traditionally used internally. (Essential oils are very concentrated partial extracts and they should not be used internally.)

Precautions and/or safety
The widespread topical use of lavender oil prompted safety studies into its potential muta-genicity. Standard bacterial tests found it was in fact anti-mutagenic.[100]

In vitro—The essential oil, linalool and linalyl acetate are toxic to endothelial and fibroblast cells however the significance of this is unclear unless this is a contributory factor to the development of allergy (see below).[101]

There has been a reported case of eczema due to contact with a lavender pillow.[102] Over a period of 9 years the recorded cases of contact allergy to the oil at one centre was found to occur on average in 3.7% of those who were known to suffer with contact allergy problems. Contact with dried lavender flowers may precipitate the development of allergy to the oil[103] and a known allergy to one member of the Lami-aceae family may result in sensitivity to others.[104]

The rate of allergic reaction does appear to be low considering lavender oil is the one most commonly used for cosmetic and aromatherapy purposes.

Historical uses
"All griefs and pains of the head and brain that proceed a cold cause"; apoplexy; epilepsy; dropsy; cramps; convulsions; palsies. To strengthen the stomach and liver; spleen congestion. As a diuretic. As a gargle for toothache; to restore a lost voice; "passions of the heart and its tremblings, faintings and swoonings". Internally and externally for bites of mad dogs, serpents and other venomous crea-tures. Oil used externally for varicose ulcers and sores.

Leonurus cardiaca

Motherwort

Description
A perennial herb forming a basal clump from which rise 1 or more stout, square, erect, and

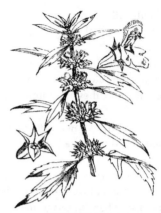
Family Lamiaceae

sometimes branching flowering stems to 1 m. *Basal leaves* on long petioles to 20 cm. Lamina 6–10 × 5.5–10 cm, broad ovate and usually 7-lobed, dark green and hairy with a cordate base. *Upper leaves* and bracts opposite, similar but 3–5 lobed, becom-ing smaller and entire towards the top of the spike. *Inflorescence* a spike of 6–15 flowers in dense verticils in crowded or distant axillary whorls. Calyx tube 3–4 mm long with 5 spinose teeth. Corolla 8–10 mm long, pale pink with tiny purple spots on upper and lower lips, and a ring of white hairs inside the tube. *Nutlets* about 2 mm long, sharply angled with an api-cal tuft of hairs. Flowers from summer to autumn.

The biennial *L. siberica* has compound leaves with narrow oblong lobes.

Habitat and cultivation
Originally from Europe, *Leonurus* is cultivated and sometimes found wild elsewhere. It is generally grown from seed and self-sows freely, preferring well-drained soils and open, sunny situations. It is frost resistant but drought tender.

Parts used
The herb gathered during or just prior to flowering.

Active constituents
1) Alkaloids including stachydrine (also called proline betaine)[105] and leonurine
2) Iridoid glycosides[105]—leonuride, ajugol and galiridoside
3) Bitter glycosides[105]

4) Flavonoids including quercetin, kaempferol and apigenin[105,106]
5) Terpenes
   a) diterpenes of labdane type[107] including leocardin[108]
   b) triterpenes (ursolic acid)[26]
6) Tannins (5–9%) both hydrolysable and condensed—pseudotannins

Also contains phenolic acids (caffeic acid[109]), phenyl-propanoids (verbascoside,[110] lavandulifolioside[111]) and terpenoids (caryophyllene and α-pinene).[112]

Actions
1) Sedative
2) Hypotensive
3) Cardiac tonic
4) Antispasmodic

Scientific information
The common name of the herb indicates its traditional use as a female reproductive remedy. *German Commission E* has approved its use for nervous cardiac disorders and as symptomatic treatment for hyperthyroidism.[113]

There are a number of different *Leonurus* species that are used medicinally, it is unclear to what extent they are interchangeable, but traditionally their uses were very similar. The Chinese herb (*L. heterophyllus*) has been better studied in recent times, there being very little new information available for *L. cardiaca*.

In vitro—*Leonurus* has some anti-oxidant activity.[114,115] Further research is based on isolated constituents and their pharmacological actions in animals. Lavandulifolioside and verbascoside appear to have a hypotensive effect[111] and leonurine is vasorelaxant[116] and uterotonic.[117] Leonurine is also an inhibitor of creatine kinase.[118] Stachydrine is oxytoxic.

Studies on the Chinese species have shown the intravenously administered herb reduces platelet aggregation.[119]

Medicinal uses
Cardiovascular system
• cardiac disorders due to nerves
• palpitations
• simple tachycardia
• cardiac disorders in pregnancy
• cardiac debility
• arrhythmia of nervous origin

BHP specific for cardiac symptoms associated with neurosis.

Gastro-intestinal tract
The tannin content is high enough to make the herb astringent.

• diarrhoea
• colic
• flatulence

Reproductive tract
The action on the uterus aids labour, giving rise to effective contractions, and it also aids menstruation. It is considered safe for use in pregnancy.

• dysmenorrhoea
• amenorrhoea
• fibroids
• menopausal nervous problems

Pharmacy
Three times daily
Infusion of dried herb   – 2–4 g
Tincture 1:5 (25%)   – 4–10 ml
Fluid Extract (25%)   – 2–4 ml

Historical uses
Fevers with delirium; "to strengthen and gladden the heart"; hysteria; for labour and "to settle wombs". For tremors; "faintings"; spinal disease and cramps. For phlegm in the chest; to dry damp cold from the body as a diuretic. Also for green wounds and as an anthelmintic.

Lycopus europaeus

Gypsywort, bugleweed

Description
L. europaeus is a perennial herb with creeping rhizomes. *Stems* square, erect, hairy and branched up

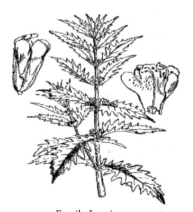

Family Lamiaceae

to 1 m tall. *Leaves* shortly petiolate or sessile, opposite, 2.5–10 cm long, lanceolate-ovate to elliptic and deeply crenate-serrate. Basal leaves with narrow oblong lobes extending to midrib. Upper leaves and bracts smaller without basal lobes, hairy especially on veins beneath. *Flowers* in many-flowered verticils in dense, discrete, globose whorls. Calyx bell-shaped about 3 mm long and hairy. Corolla 3.5–4 mm long, white with purple dots on lower lip and in the throat. *Fruit* 4 small tetrahedral nutlets. Flowers from summer to autumn. Other species such as *L. americana*, *L. lucidus* and *L. virginicus* are used in similar ways in North America.

Habitat and cultivation
Originally from Britain, Europe and cold temperate Asia, *Lycopus* is naturalised in wet areas around the world. It may be grown from seed or root division and dies back completely in winter. It prefers rich, moist soils in sun or semi-shade and is frost resistant but drought tender.

Parts used
The herb gathered during or just prior to flowering.

Active constituents
Not well characterised.

1) Phenolic acids including caffeic, rosmarinic, chlorogenic, ellagic and lithospermic acids[120–122]
2) Flavonoids—luteolin derivatives[123]
3) Diterpenoids—isopimarane derivatives[124,125]

Also contains volatile oil and tannins. *L. virginicus* is very similar to *L. europaeus* but the latter has an additional pimaric acid ester.[126]

Actions
1) Cardioactive diuretic
2) Peripheral vasoconstrictor
3) Antihaemorrhagic
4) Sedative
5) Thyroxine antagonist
6) Antitussive

Scientific information
The active constituents of both species of *Lycopus* are poorly investigated but are believed to derive from oxidation of the phenolic acids by intrinsic plant enzymes.[121,127–129]

In vitro—*Lycopus* spp. and oxidised phenolics from the herb decrease the activity of TSH.[121,130] They also bind to, and inactivate, the auto-antibodies produced in Graves' disease patients and inhibit iodine metabolism and the release of thyroxine from the thyroid, probably via inhibition of cyclic AMP at the thyroid membrane.[130,131] Extracts have antigonadotrophic properties in animal models[123,128] an action to which lithospermic acid is likely to contribute.[122]

Leaf extracts have good inhibition of xanthine oxidase[132] and good anti-oxidant activity, possibly due to rosmarinic acid which is present in significant amounts.[120,133]

The isopimarane diterpenoids potentiate the activity of antibiotics to which *Staphylococcus aureus* has become resistant without having any antibacterial activity themselves.[134]

In vivo—Low dose *Lycopus* improved the cardiac function—palpitations, arrhythmia and extrasystoles—of patients with hyperthyroidism without altering hormone levels.[135]

Medicinal uses
Cardiovascular system
• nervous tachycardia

Respiratory tract
• haemoptysis
• irritable coughs with copious sputum

Endocrine system
- Graves' disease
- hyperthyroidism
- thyrotoxicosis[†]

Pharmacy
Three times daily

Infusion dried herb	–	1–3 g
Tincture 1:5 (45%)	–	2–6 ml
Fluid Extract (25%)	–	1–3 ml

Marrubium vulgare

Horehound, white horehound

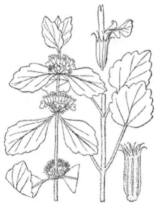

Family Lamiaceae

Description
Much branched, aromatic perennial herb. *Stems* square, more or less lanate, to 50 cm high. *Leaves* opposite, petioles slender, lanate or densely hairy. Lamina 1–3.5 × 1–4.5 cm, broad ovate to sub-orbicular, rugose, white-tomentose except for upper surface when mature, crenate; base truncate to cuneate in upper leaves and bracts, sub-cordate in lower leaves; apex obtuse. *Verticils* dense, globose in axillary whorls. Calyx tube 4–6 mm long, teeth 10, rigid, subulate, hooked. Corolla about 1 cm long, white tomentose outside, lower lip broader than long. *Nutlets* 2.5 mm

---
[†]Dyspnoea, tachycardia and tremor.

long, obovoid and sharply keeled. Flowers from spring to autumn.

Taste bitter and somewhat acrid.

Habitat and cultivation
Native to Eurasia and North Africa it is naturalised elsewhere in open, dry pastures, rocky/sandy soil. Grows from seed, cuttings and layers and self-sows. Likes dry climates because its felt-like leaves rot in wet weather. Frost and drought resistant.

Parts used
Leaves and flowering tops.

Active constituents
1) Sesquiterpene bitters including labdane diterpenes—marrubiin and marrubenol[136]
2) Diterpene alcohols including marrubiol
3) Flavonoids including derivatives of luteolin, apigenin and vitexin[137,140]
4) Tannins

Also contains volatile oil,[138] saponins, mucilage, β-sitosterol, alkaloids, phenylethanoid (marruboside),[139] phenylpropanoids (forsythoside B, verbascoside)[140] and PABA.

Nutritional constituents
Vitamins: A, B complex, C and E
Minerals: Iron, potassium and sulphur

Actions[141]
1) Expectorant
2) Bitter
3) Spasmolytic

High doses of the herb are stated to be laxative.[141]

Scientific informaion
Marrubium has a very long history as a cough remedy and has been an official medicine in the pharmacopoeias of a number of different countries.[141] It is approved by *German Commission E* for the treatment of dyspepsia and anorexia.

In vitro—The herb has very good anti-oxidant activity.[142,143] It prevents oxidation of low density lipoprotein (a process believed to be associated with the development of atherosclerosis) and promotes the high density lipoprotein reduction of cellular cholesterol.[144] The phenylpropanoids appear to play a major role in this activity.[145] They are inhibitors of COX-2 and are likely to contribute to an anti-inflammatory action for which the herb has a traditional reputation.[140]

Horehound also has some antimicrobial activity.[146]

Marrubiin, one of the main active constituents, is believed to result from extraction procedures altering the unstable premarrubiin.[147] It has a number of activities including the ability to normalise extrasystolic arrhythmias, is expectorant and a bitter.

In vivo—An infusion of the herb was tested for hypoglycaemic activity as it used for this purpose in Mexican and Moroccan traditional medicine. It had a minimal effect in reducing blood glucose and triglyceride levels in type 2 diabetics.[148] It has also been used in Morocco as an antihypertensive and to treat heart disease[136,149] but there are no further studies on the herb's pharmacological effects in humans.

Medicinal uses
Respiratory tract
It is expectorant (considered to make mucus more fluid) and a general relaxant of bronchial musculature:

- bronchitis (acute and chronic)
- asthma
- whooping cough
- dry coughs
- catarrh of the respiratory tract

Gastro-intestinal tract
- anorexia
- dyspepsia (acute and chronic)

Pharmacy
Three times daily
Infusion of dried herb   – 1–2 g
Tincture 1:5 (25%)   – 3–6 ml
Fluid Extract (20%)   – 1–2 ml

Historical uses
Powdered leaves used as a vermifuge. As an ointment for wounds; an antidote to poison, snake venom or stings. Emmenagogue. Juice used in eyes to clear eyesight; for earache; as snuff for jaundice.

Melissa officinalis

Balm, lemon balm

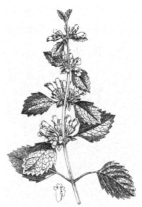

Family Lamiaceae

Description
Perennial, rhizomatous, lemon-scented herb. *Stems* square, erect and branching, reaching 60 cm in flower. *Leaves* opposite, petiolate. Lamina 2–8.5 × 1–7 cm, elliptic to broad ovate, hairy, though sometimes sparsely hairy above. Base more or less truncate in larger lower leaves, cuneate in upper smaller leaves and bracts. *Flowers* in verticils in leaf axils usually 3–10 flowered. Calyx about 8 mm long, nerves prominent, with long white pilose hairs. Upper teeth broad-triangular, aristate, lower teeth narrow-triangular, aristate. Corolla 12–15 mm long, white or cream; lobes hairy outside. *Nutlets* 1.7–2 mm long, almost black. Flowers from summer to autumn.

Odour—aromatic, lemony; taste—pleasant and lemony

Habitat and cultivation
Native to Eurasia and is naturalized elsewhere. Grows from seed, cuttings and division, selfsows

freely in sun or semi-shade. Should be cut back after flowering and is prone to rust in poor draining soils. Frost resistant, drought tender.

Parts used
Fresh or dried leaves or aerial parts collected just before or during flowering.

Active constituents[150]
1) Volatile oil (0.02–0.37%) including predominantly citral (a mixture of geranial and neral)[151] also citronellal, geraniol, linalool[152] and β-caryophyllene. The essential oil may be very variable altering with leaf position on the stem,[153] age of plant,[151] time of harvest and method of processing.[152] Fresh leaves have a higher content of oil than those that are dried.[154] The yield of essential oil from *Melissa* is low and it therefore has a high value[151]
2) Phenolics (around 12%)[155] including rosmarinic (up to 6%), p-hydroxybenzoic, gallic, vanillic, protocatechuic,[156] caffeic and chlorogenic acids[157,158]

Also contains terpenes—ursolic, oleanolic and carnosic acids,[159,160] tannins and flavonoids including luteolin and its derivatives.[161,162]

Actions
1) Carminative
2) Antispasmodic
3) Sedative
4) Diaphoretic

Scientific information
Melissa was used in ancient Greece and Rome and has been an official medicine in a number of countries.[141] *German Commission E* has approved its use for nervous sleep disorders and gastro-intestinal functional problems.

Anti-oxidant
In vitro—*Melissa* has one of the best anti-oxidant activities amongst medicinal herbs, probably due to its high level of phenolic constituents.[163–169] This activity has been demonstrated in the protection of lipids from oxidation after exposure to UV irradiation.[170]

Constituents including oil,[171] rosmarinic acid[172] and terpenes[160] are also anti-oxidant.

Nervous system
In vitro—Aqueous and ethanolic extracts of the herb, as well as the essential oil, have good inhibition of the enzyme acetylcholinesterase and may be of use in treating Alzheimer's Disease.[165] *Melissa* has also shown cholinergic activity via muscarinic and nicotinic receptor sites in cerebral cortical cells, up regulating these sites that become deficient in Alzheimer's disease. The constituent(s) responsible is/are unknown at present and the level of this activity appears to vary from one extract to another.[173,178]

In vivo—There is good clinical evidence for the use of *Melissa* in the treatment of Alzheimer's disease. It improved cognitive function and reduced agitation in patients with mild to moderate forms of the disease.[174,175] The aromatherapy use of the essential oil was also beneficial in cases of severe dementia by reducing levels of agitation and improving quality of life.[176]

In healthy volunteers it improved the mood and level of "calmness" induced by acute stress and also improved memory performance.[177–179] At higher doses however, it may reduce the speed of performance on some mental tasks.[178,179]

Valeriana and *Melissa*, given in combination, were both effective and well tolerated in treating children with restlessness and insomnia and in improving the sleep quality and anxiety levels of healthy adults.[181,182] In combination with other nervines it was shown, via measurements of brain activity, to increase relaxation and mental function.[183]

Antimicrobial
In vitro—Aqueous extracts have antiviral activity,[150] particularly against HIV-1,[184] HSV-1 and 2 and against an HSV-1 strain resistant to acyclovir.[185,186] HSV viral inhibition by whole extracts occurs prior to cellular entry suggesting its effect is likely to be confined to topical use[185] however the volatile oil inhibits the replication of HSV-2.[187] *Melissa* has some antibacterial activity[188,189] including against *Helicobacter pylori* species.[190]

The essential oil is antibacterial, antifungal[171] and antiprotozoal,[191] rosmarinic acid is antiviral and antibacterial[172] and citral is antibacterial.[192]

In vivo—A cream containing lemon balm improved the healing of herpes simplex lesions, shortening healing time, preventing the spread of viral infection, rapidly relieving symptoms and increasing the time between recurrent infections.[193,194]

Endocrine

In vitro—Aqueous extracts are inhibitory to α-glucosidase which may be of use in the treatment of diabetes.[195]

An anti-thyrotropic activity has also been demonstrated. TSH activity was inhibited by *Melissa* through direct binding to the hormone and indirect binding to TSH-receptor sites.[196] This latter effect also occurs in the presence of autoantibodies generated by Graves' disease.[131]

Gastro-intestinal

In vivo—Herbal combinations containing *Melissa* have been used in clinical trials for a variety of gastro-intestinal problems. They have reduced abdominal discomfort experienced by patients with irritable bowel syndrome,[197] symptoms of functional dyspepsia[198,199] and chronic colitis.[200] It effectively reduced infantile colic in breast-fed babies when combined with *Foeniculum* and *Matricaria*.[201]

Other

In vitro—*Melissa's* essential oil has antitumour properties, inhibiting growth in a number of different cancer cell lines[202] and citral has anticancer properties even at low doses.[203] Constituents (caffeic acid and an unknown glycoside) from leaves can inhibit protein synthesis and may contribute to this antitumour effect.[204,205]

Rosmarinic acid is anti-inflammatory.[206]

Medicinal uses

Cardiovascular system
- palpitations
- fever

Gastro-intestinal tract
- heartburn
- indigestion
- flatulent dyspepsia
- nervous dyspepsia
- nausea due to nerves

Nervous system
- restlessness
- excitability
- nervous headaches
- anxiety
- depression
- dizziness
- herpes
- insomnia

The anti-oxidant and acetylcholinesterase inhibiting potential may give it a place in the treatment of Alzheimer's disease, an added advantage being that of reducing associated agitation.

Reproductive tract
- morning sickness
- headaches in pregnancy

Endocrine system
Given the anti-thyroid effects of *Melissa* shown *in vitro* it may have a use in the treatment of:

- Graves' disease
- hyperthyroidism

Externally
- cutaneous lesions of herpes simplex (cream)

Pharmacy
Three times daily

Infusion of dried herb	–	2–4 g
Tincture 1:5 (45%)	–	2–6 ml
Fluid Extract (45%)	–	2–4 ml

The cream used to treat *Herpes labialis* contained 1% of a 70:1 extract of the leaves and was applied 4 times a day for 5 days.[193]

Precautions and/or safety

Safety studies found no genotoxic activity in standard assays.[207]

Historical uses

Longevity; to strengthen brain and memory; for melancholy and sadness; for difficult breathing. To help expel the afterbirth. Externally for scorpion stings and bites of mad dogs; as a bath to bring on menstruation; as a wash in toothache. For wens, kernels and hard swellings in flesh and throat. To clean sores. Gout. To ripen boils.

Mentha x piperita var. piperita

Peppermint

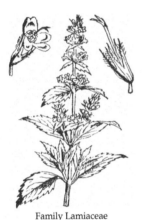

Family Lamiaceae

Description

Mentha x *piperita* is a hybrid of *M. aquatica* and *M. spicata*. It is a rhizomatous perennial with glabrous or sparsely hairy stems, often submerged, to 60 cm tall. Aerial stems are erect and often purple. *Leaves* opposite, very variable but usually distinctly petiolate: lamina 1–6 × 1–3.5 cm, with finely serrate margins. Leaves on flowering shoots elliptic-lanceolate or narrow elliptic, smelling of peppermint when bruised; base cuneate to rounded, apex acute. *Flowers*—terminal inflorescence is an oblong spike, often longer than wide, rarely interrupted. Calyx 3–4 mm long, tubular, purple, dotted with oil glands, teeth equal, ciliate, narrow-acuminate.

Corolla 5–6 mm long, mauve or lilac, glabrous; stamens small, included. *Nutlets* not formed. Flowers from mid-summer to autumn.

Odour—strong, characteristic; taste—aromatic, characteristic and cooling.

Habitat and cultivation

Peppermint is a hybrid first recorded and named by the botanist John Ray in 1696. Its growth is widespread and it is cultivated commercially. The best essential oil comes from areas at latitude 40° north or south. It prefers rich, damp, well-drained soils and dies back in winter. It is prone to rust. Mints hybridise so should be grown from cuttings/root division, not seeds. Frost resistant and drought tender.

Parts used

Leaves or aerial parts just prior to flowering.

Active constituents[208,209]

- Volatile oil (1–3%) including predominantly the monoterpenes menthol (30–55%), menthone (14–32%) and menthyl acetate (3–5%). Also neomenthol, monomenthyl succinate,[210] isomenthone, menthofuran, pulegone, limonene, 1,8-cineole,[211] α- and β-pinene. The level of menthol is inversely related to the level of menthone.[211] The composition of the essential oil varies with the maturity of the plant— menthol is maximal when the plant is in full bloom and increases with the number of leaves and biomass of the plant.[211–214] It also varies with genotype[215] and conditions of light and temperature.[216] In young leaves limonene and menthone are the main monoterpenes.[212]
- Flavonoids (about 12%) including derivatives of eriodictyol, luteolin, hesperidin and apigenin.[217] Also various flavones[217–219]
- Phenolic acids, including those based on hydroxycinnamic acid and rosmarinic acid (1.4%)[217]
- Bitter principle

Additional constituents include triterpenes, carotenoids, inositol, choline and betaine.

Nutritional constituents

Vitamins: A,[220] C and niacin

Minerals: Iron, magnesium, calcium, potassium, copper, iodine, silicon, sulphur, manganese and zinc.[221] Infusions of the herb are not considered a good source of the majority of these minerals.[222]

Actions

1) Carminative
2) Spasmolytic
3) Choleretic
4) Diaphoretic
5) Anti-emetic Locally
6) Antiseptic
7) Antipruritic

Scientific information

Mentha has a history of medicinal use spanning thousands of years. Its well established carminative properties ensured its place in the pharmacopoeias of many countries.[141] *German Commission E* has approved its use for spasms in the gastro-intestinal tract, gallbladder and bile ducts. The chemistry of *Mentha* essential oil has been well characterised as it is widely used as a flavouring agent in the food and dentifrice industries. Whilst this fraction undoubtedly is important to the herb's action, there are other significant chemical constituents and in herbal medicine essential oil alone is not used internally.

Antimicrobial

In vitro—The herb has antibacterial (*Salmonella typhimurium, Staphylococcus aureus, Vibrio parahaemolyticus,* and *Helicobacter pylori*),[223] antimycobacterial[224] and antiviral activity (herpes simplex, Newcastle disease, vaccinia).[209,225] Extracts of *Mentha*, though not infusions, are also antiprotozoal with activity against *Giardia lamblia.*[226]

The essential oil and its main constituent, menthol, are much stronger antibacterial agents. They act via increased membrane permeability and disruption of cellular activity to inhibit bacterial growth and enterotoxin production, Gram-positive bacteria appearing to be more sensitive than Gram-negative ones to the oil.[227] Both may enhance the efficacy of some antibiotics.[228] *Mentha* oil has antibacterial activity against a number of different food related,[227,229,230] respiratory tract[231] and anaerobic oral pathogens.[232] It also has antifungal activity (*Candida albicans* and *Trichophyton tonsurans*)[233–240] and is directly active against HSV-1 and 2.[241]

Mentha oil combined with essential oil of nutmeg was effective against *Pediculus humanus capitis* (head lice).[242]

Anti-oxidant

In vitro—The herb and its constituents have very good anti-oxidant activity, especially the phenolic constituents[233,243–247] and monoterpenes.[236] Anti-oxidant activity contributes to an anti-inflammatory effect by reducing free radical damage.[248,249]

Gastro-intestinal tract

In vitro—Peppermint oil and menthol are considered central to the pharmacology of the herb and they induce relaxation in isolated colon muscle tissue, due apparently to calcium channel antagonism.[250] Both are also able to reduce gastric and intestinal foaming, which is indicative of a carminative effect.[250]

In vivo—There are no clinical trials into the effect of *Mentha herba* on its own. However a combination which included peppermint did significantly improve the symptoms of functional dyspepsia.[251–253]

The majority of recent studies have been conducted using the oil. This used alone or in combination with other agents was effective as a/an:-

- muscle relaxant to aid endoscopic and colonoscopic examination, proving to be safer and more effective than some currently used pharmaceuticals[254–259]
- spasmolytic on gastro-intestinal smooth muscle,[260,261] ameliorating diffuse oesophageal spasms[262]
- treatment for irritable bowel syndrome[263–265]—reviews of data concludes it is beneficial[266,267]
- treatment for functional dyspepsia[265,268–270]
- aid in prolonging the transit time in the small intestine[271]
- treatment to reduce post-operative nausea[272]
- stimulant of salivary flow via olfactory nerve[273]

There is also anecdotal evidence suggesting the essential oil may reduce the overgrowth of bacteria in the small intestine associated with irritable bowel syndrome, fibromyalgia and chronic fatigue syndrome.[274]

Respiratory tract
In vivo—Inhaled peppermint oil reduced the level of inflammation and severity of infiltrative pulmonary tuberculosis.[275]

Nervous system
In vitro—The characteristic cooling effect of menthol occurs via induced release of stored calcium which enters, and triggers, sensory neurons.[276] The oil is protective of astrocytes.[277]

In vivo—Studies of the effect of the essential oil on mental function have found that on inhalation it reduces sleepiness,[278] improves the level of focus and performance for some tasks[279] and improves vigilance in people with brain injury.[280]

A 10% solution of peppermint oil applied to the forehead and temples was as effective as acetaminophen (paracetamol) in relieving tension headaches[281] and there is also anecdotal evidence that topical use relieves post-herpetic neuralgia.[282]

Other
In vitro—The herb has anticancer properties[283] and induces cytokine release from intestinal cells indicative of enhanced immune function.[284]

Using an *in vitro* model low dose peppermint oil protected against the absorption of toxic chemicals but at higher doses this benefit may be out-weighed by a reduction in cell membrane integrity.[285]

Medicinal uses
Respiratory tract
Used as a diaphoretic:

- fever
- influenza
- colds

Gastro-intestinal tract
- flatulent dyspepsia
- ulcerative colitis

- irritable bowel syndrome
- cholelithiasis
- colic
- Crohn's disease
- indigestion
- vomiting (safe in pregnancy)
- cholecystitis

Nervous system
- nervous tension
- insomnia
- vertigo

Reproductive tract
- dysmenorrhoea

Externally
Mentha oil can be used in creams or ointments:

- pruritus
- inflammatory skin conditions

Pharmacy
Three times daily
Infusion of dried herb   – 2–4 g
Tincture 1:5 (45%)   – 2–3 ml
After infusing the resultant tea comprises about 21% essential oil and 75% phenolics[208,217]

A safety assessment declared it safe to use in cosmetics but the oil should be used at the recommended levels of less than 0.2% for products that remain in contact with the skin and at 3% for ones that are used as rinses.[286]

CONTRAINDICATIONS—The oil should not be applied neat to skin or mucosal surfaces.

Pharmacokinetics
Studies have been conducted on the metabolism of menthol. It is absorbed relatively quickly reaching peak levels 1.7 hours after ingestion,[287] is metabolised to its glucuronide and excreted by the kidneys reaching maximum levels in urine after 3 hours.[288]

Precautions and/or safety
In tests for genotoxicity the infused herb was not only non-toxic in the model used but protective of

gene damage from reactive oxygen radicals[289] however the essential oil may have some genotoxicity and cytotoxicity.[290]

Peppermint tea may inhibit dietary iron absorption.[291] The whole herb is safe and well tolerated. Internal use of the essential oil has generally given rise to few minor side-effects, notably heartburn, anal/perianal burning or general gastrointestinal discomfort[266] however there are also reports that it has caused burning mouth syndrome, recurrent oral ulceration, a lichenoid reaction, glossitis, stomatitis and/or cheilitis.[292,293,297]

Some sensitive individuals may have a systemic allergic reaction to the members of the Lamiaceae family including *Mentha*.[104] Again the majority of reported cases of contact sensitivity have been to the oil and/or menthol used in foods and toothpastes.[294-298] Given the widespread use of the herb and its constituents as a flavouring the incidence of reported allergic reactions seems low.[299]

A small percentage of samples of peppermint tea that have been tested in Europe have been found to contain unacceptable levels of pesticide residues.[300]

Interactions
Mentha essential oil can inhibit a number of cytochrome P450 enzymes *in vitro*[301] and interacted with a drug metabolised by CYP3A4, increasing its bioavailability without altering its half-life *in vivo*.[302] No interactions have yet been reported for the herbal extract.

Historical uses
Believed to increase lust; for venereous dreams (possibly by drying seminal fluid). As an anti-haemorrhagic including for menorrhagia; for hiccoughs, childbirth; gravel; strangury. Externally to dissolve imposthumes; repress lactation; mad dog bites; for earache; rough tongue; for headache applied to temples; skin eruptions and sores; as mouthwash for sore gums and mouth.

Nepeta cataria

Catnip, catmint

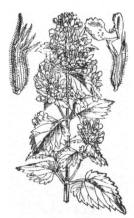

Family Lamiaceae

Description
Densely hairy, aromatic perennial with square, branching, downy, erect stems to 1 m high. *Leaves*, opposite, petioles to 3 cm long. Lamina 4–6 × 3–4 cm, ovate or triangular-ovate, often grey-to-mentose, serrate or crenate-serrate; base cordate or sub-cordate; apex mucronate; upper cauline leaves smaller. *Inflorescence* terminal, dense, spike-like with lower verticils distant. Calyx 6–7 mm long, tomentose outside on nerves; teeth linear-subulate, often purplish tipped. Corolla about 7–10 mm long to apex of upper lip, white with pinkish-purple dots on lower lip; tube somewhat curved, not exceeding calyx, tomentose outside. Upper lip with 2 rounded lobes. Anthers usually purplish, sometimes green. *Style* white or pale mauve. *Nutlets* 1.5 mm long, broad-oblong, dark brown, faintly ridged. Flowers from summer to autumn.

Odour—aromatic; taste—bitter and pungent.

Habitat and cultivation
Originally from Eurasia, *Nepeta cataria* both grows wild and is cultivated elsewhere. It grows easily from seed and self-sows. It prefers free-draining soil but adequate moisture, and grows in sun or semi-shade. Frost resistant but drought tender.

Parts used
Tops and leaves gathered just before, and during, flowering.

Active constituents
1) Volatile oil (up to 0.7%) including predominantly the iridolactones α- and β-nepetalactone (80–90%), also caryophyllene, camphor, humulene,[303] thymol, carvacrol, citronellal and sesquiterpenes.[304] The constituents of the oil vary according to the variety, location and conditions in which the herb is grown.[304] This fraction is at its maximum during flowering[303]
2) Tannins
3) Bitter principle—iridoids[305,306]

Also contains a total phenolic content of around 2%, including caffeic and ferulic acids,[307] flavonoids (predominantly luteolin), terpenes and sterols.[308]

Nutritional constituents
Vitamins: A, B complex and C
Minerals: Magnesium, manganese, phosphorus, sodium and traces of sulphur

Actions
1) Diaphoretic
2) Carminative
3) Spasmolytic
4) Sedative
5) Antidiarrhoeal
6) Antipyretic

Scientific information
Nepeta cataria has been an official medicine[309] and was used as a beverage in England prior to the introduction of tea from China. Recent scientific research is lacking although there is information on some constituents.

In vitro—The herb is antifungal and antibacterial including against resistant strains of *Staphylococcus aureus*.[310]

The phenolic fraction is anti-oxidant[307] and the oil is a strong insecticidal.[311–313] The nepetalactones

are considered to contribute significantly to the known relaxant effect of the herb. Most investigations have involved animals and/or insects, there are no human trials on its pharmacological effects.

Medicinal uses
It is considered an ideal children's remedy.

Cardiovascular system
• fevers (especially of childhood illnesses)

Respiratory tract
• colds

Gastro-intestinal tract
• nervous dyspepsia
• colic
• flatulence

Nervous system
• headaches
• insomnia (especially in children)
• restlessness

Externally
• haemorrhoids (ointment)

Pharmacy
Three times daily
Infusion of dried herb   – 2–4 g
Tincture 1:5 (25%)   – 3–6 ml
Fluid Extract (25%)   – 2–4 ml

Precautions and/or safety
There is a reported case of a child developing gastro-intestinal discomfort, irritability and lethargy after ingesting large amounts of catnip.[314]

Historical uses
Insanity; as an emmenagogue (expressed juice); nightmares; hysteria; scarlet fever; smallpox; bruises; coughs. Locally for painful swellings and scabs.

Rosmarinus officinalis

Rosemary

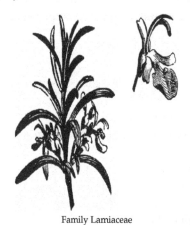

Family Lamiaceae

Description
A dense, much-branched, aromatic, evergreen perennial shrub 1–3 m high. *Leaves* opposite, numerous, narrow, dark-green 2–3.5 cm long, linear, leathery, margin involuted, white-hairy beneath. *Flowers* are stalkless, lilac-blue, and grow in leafy axillary clusters. Corolla two-lipped, upper lip somewhat hooded, tube longer than the calyx; stamens and style curved and much longer than the corolla. It flowers throughout the year. It is a variable species and upright and prostrate varieties are common.

Odour—camphorous, aromatic; taste—strong, bitter, somewhat pungent.

Habitat and cultivation
Native to Mediterranean Europe in well-drained rocky soils. Cultivated elsewhere in gardens and as hedges. Generally grown from cuttings but will also grow from seed. Prefers open, sunny, well-drained situations. Drought and frost resistant.

Parts used
The aerial parts of the herb including twigs.

Active constituents
1) Volatile oil (up to 1.75%) including verbenone (27%), camphor (24%), borneol (12%), 1,8-cineole (10%) and also linalool, α-terpineol and caryophyllene.[315,316] Content varies with geographical location[317]
2) Diterpenes including predominantly carnosic acid, carnosol (picrosalvin) and 12-methoxycarnosic acid,[315,318] others have been identified[319,320] and some, like rosmanol, may be extraction artefacts.[318] Carnosic acid levels are higher in younger leaves, increase with exposure to light[321] and also vary with geographical location[322]
3) Flavonoids including eriocitrin, hesperidin, diosmin, genkwanin, scutellarein, cirsimaritin and luteolin[323–326]

Also contains tannins, a number of phenolic acids including rosmarinic, p-hydoxybenzoic and vanillic acids, resin, salicylates[327] and triterpenes—oleanolic, ursolic and betulinic acids.[328]

Nutritional constituents
Vitamins: A,[329] C and E[330]
Minerals: High in calcium with some iron, magnesium, potassium, phosphorus, sodium and zinc

Actions
1) Carminative
2) Spasmolytic
3) Mild analgesic
4) Thymoleptic
5) Tonic
6) Rubefacient
7) Diuretic
8) Antimicrobial Topically
9) Rubefacient
10) Analgesic (mild)
11) Parasiticide

Many other actions are ascribed to *Rosmarinus*, but the above represents the main basis of the herb's effects.

Scientific information
Rosemary was valued in ancient times for its memory enhancing properties as well as playing a significant part in ceremonial life through the generations. It has been an official medicine in a number of countries and its oil was officially used

into the 20th century. *German Commission E* has approved its internal use for dyspepsia and external use to aid the treatment of rheumatic and circulatory disorders. In Morocco it is used for diabetes mellitus and hypertension.[331]

Current interest in the herb relates to its strong anti-oxidant and antimicrobial potential, both activities being useful for extending the shelf-life of food and cosmetics and especially so as the herb is non-toxic. It no doubt has a much wider application for improving health than the scientific studies to-date would indicate.

Anti-oxidant
In vitro—Many of the individual constituents, especially carnosic and rosmarinic acids,[332,333] and the whole herb have very strong anti-oxidant activity.[315,334] Unusually carnosic acid appears not to lose its anti-oxidative potential as generally occurs once anti-oxidants have reacted chemically.[335] The high level of phenolics in the herb has also been linked to rosemary's ability to inhibit low density lipoprotein oxidation.[336,337] Rosemary itself can inhibit the oxidation of cholesterol in foods, the by-products of which are considered atherogenic, cytotoxic and possibly carcinogenic once consumed.[338] This anti-oxidant activity occurs in both aqueous and lipid mediums.[339]

Antimicrobial
In vitro—The herb and its constituents, particularly carnosic acid and the essential oil, have significant antimicrobial activity against:-

- Gram-negative strains,[340] including *Escherichia coli*,[315,341] *Klebsiella pneumoniae*,[341] *Vibrio parahaemolyticus*[342] and *Helicobacter pylori*[343,344]
- *Gram-positive* strains[340,344,345] including *Staphylococcus aureus*[315,341] *Bacillus subtilis*,[341] *Pseudomonas aeruginosa*[341] and *Proteus vulgaris*.[341,333] The diterpenes may also increase the susceptibility of resistant strains of *S. aureus* to antibiotics[346]
- *fungi*[347] including *Candida albicans*[315,340,344,348]
- viruses including HSV-1 and 2 (before their cellular entry, suggesting an effect in topical

preparations rather than for internal use)[185] and HIV[349] (carnosol), the major diterpenes also inhibit HIV protease[350]
- trypanosomes[328]

Cell protection
In vitro—As an anti-oxidant, rosemary helps protect lipids in the cell membrane from free radical damage.[351] In addition the diterpenes:-

- physically strengthen cell membranes[352]
- protect nigral dopaminergic cells from chemical damage (potential for treatment of Parkinson's disease)[353]
- protect chromosomes from damage including from oxidants, visible light and γ-irradiation[354,355]
- protect DNA through inhibition of cytochrome activated procarcinogens and improved detoxification via glutathione S-transferase[356,357]
- protect cells from damage by chemicals and/or ionizing radiation[358-360]—whole herb and volatile oil

Gastro-intestinal
In vivo—Animal experiments have pointed to a hepatoprotective effect, possibly due to anti-oxidant and cell protecting actions, but there is no confirmation of this action in human studies.[361] However, in combination with other herbs, *Rosmarinus* was used to benefit the treatment of patients with hepatic encephalopathy due to liver cirrhosis.[362]

Nervous system
In vitro—The reputation of *Rosmarinus* in the treatment of poor memory may be partially accounted for by its moderate inhibition of acetylcholinesterase activity, the level of acetylcholine being relevant to memory and cognitive function.[363] The herb and diterpenes are also able to significantly stimulate nerve growth factor (NGF).[364]

In vivo—The inhalation of the aroma of rosemary essential oil improved mental performance and alertness, reduced anxiety and improved mood.[365-367]

Other
In vitro—Rosemary increases the sensitivity of drug-resistant cancer cells to chemotherapeutic agents transported via P-glycoprotein through the cell membrane.[368]

Carnosic acid and carnosol, through activation at the nuclear level,[369] may reduce blood lipid and glucose levels, act as anti-inflammatories and contribute an antiproliferative activity.[370-372]

Rosmarinic acid is anti-inflammatory[373] and the essential oil is insecticidal.[374,375]

Diosmin has a range of activities including acting as a strong antiproliferative,[376] improving venous tone[377] and lymphatic flow,[378] protecting blood vessels,[379] anti-inflammatory,[380] anti-oedema[381] and may be of help in treating the symptoms of diabetes.[382,383]

In vivo—A combination of iso-alpha acids from *Humulus*, oleanolic acid and rosemary was effective in relieving arthritic pain, reducing elevated levels of C-reactive protein (a biochemical marker for inflammation).[384] This same combination however failed to relieve the pain of fibromyalgia.

Rosemary and *Calendula* applied topically helped to prevent irritant contact dermatitis induced after applying sodium lauryl sulphate to healthy volunteers.[385]

The essential oils of lavender, thyme, rosemary and cedarwood, in a carrier oil, were massaged into the scalp of people with alopecia areata resulting in significant improvement.[386]

Medicinal uses
Cardiovascular system
Rosmarinus is a circulatory stimulant and considered beneficial for blood vessels:

• poor peripheral circulation
• hypotension
• arrhythmia
• circulatory weakness
• hypertensive headaches

It may also be of benefit in the treatment and prevention of arteriosclerosis.

Gastro-intestinal tract
• flatulent dyspepsia
• indigestion
• colic

Nervous system
It is described in the old texts as a thymoleptic. Used for:

• migraine headaches
• nerve weakness
• depression
• impaired memory
• poor concentration

The herb may also benefit the circulation to the nerves themselves.

Externally
• baldness (rinse)
• dandruff (rinse)

As a liniment the essential oil is used in:

• myalgia
• sciatica
• neuralgia

Pharmacy
Three times daily
Infusion   – 2–4 g
Fluid Extract (45%)   – 1–4 ml

Precautions and/or safety
The herb appears to be well tolerated. Rosemary extract, carnosol and carnosic acid are all antimutagenic according to standard tests.[387] Phenolic-rich foods, probably through their anti-oxidant action, can chelate metals and the addition of rosemary to meat decreased the absorption of non-haem iron.[388]

Rosemary has been reported to have caused allergic contact dermatitis,[389-391] there may be a cross-reaction with other members of the Lamiaceae family[392,393] but the incidence appears to be low. The herb may not be suitable for those with an allergy to salicylates.[327]

The essential oil should not be applied directly to the skin.

Interactions

In vitro rosemary was tested for its potential to interact with a number of drugs including verapamil, metoprolol, ketoprofen, paracetamol and furosemide. Only the latter was seen to have enhanced permeability although this effect was apparently minimal.[394] No drug/herb interactions have been reported.

Historical uses

All cold diseases of head, stomach, liver and belly; to strengthen memory; paralysis. Gout (externally); as part of herbal smoking mix for asthma and consumption. Appetite stimulant; gum and tooth aches; to improve eyesight (internally); jaundice; pestilence (burnt in sick rooms); to remove spots, marks and scars (the distilled oil).

Salvia officinalis

Sage

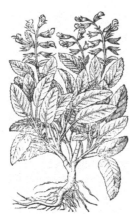

Family Lamiaceae

Description

A very aromatic, short-lived perennial undershrub, 20–70 cm high. *Stems* erect, quadrangular, woody at base, branching, finely hairy. *Leaves* stalked, opposite, simple, thick, greyish and wrinkled, oblong-oval or lance-shaped, and finely round-toothed. *Flowers* grow in terminal spikes in several rather lax whorls of 3–6 large, violet-blue flowers. Corolla 2–3 cm long, 2–3 times as long as the calyx. The upper lip nearly straight. Calyx often violet flushed, not glandular, with adpressed hairs. *Bracts* papery, oval-acute. Flowers late spring to early summer. A red-leaved cultivar "Purpurescens" (red sage) is often grown for medicine too.

Odour—spicy and aromatic; taste—spicy, astringent, bitter.

Habitat and cultivation

Native to Mediterranean Europe on dry banks and sunny places with limey soil. Grown from seed or cuttings and cultivated in gardens for cooking and medicine. Drought and frost resistant.

Parts used

The leaves.

Active constituents

1) Volatile oil including α-thujone (approx. 28%), camphor, α-humulene, 1,8-cineole (eucalyptol), viridiflorol, manool, β-thujone, α- and β-pinene.[395–397] Total thujone levels are lowest when the herb is flowering,[398] camphor content decreases as the herb matures[399]
2) Terpenes including the triterpenes oleanolic and ursolic acids[26] and the diterpenes carnosic acid[400] and carnosol[401]
3) Phenolic acids including rosmarinic,[400,402] epicatechin, gallic, vanillic, catechin, caffeic and salvianolic acids[403–406]
4) Tannins (3–8%) of condensed type
5) Flavonoids including mainly derivates of apigenin and luteolin[406,407]

Also contains phytosterols—β-sitosterol and stigmasterol,[408] polysaccharides[409] and resin.

The chemical content is variable depending on geographical location, extraction procedure,[397] maturity of the plant[410] and time of year when harvested.[411]

Nutritional constituents
Vitamins: A, C and B complex
Minerals: Calcium (significant level),[412] magnesium, iron, potassium and small amounts of manganese, zinc, copper, sulphur, silicon, phosphorus and sodium

Actions
1) Antiseptic
2) Astringent
3) Spasmolytic
4) Carminative
5) Anti-hidrotic

Scientific information
Salvia is another herb with a long history of medicinal use, it has been an official medicine in the pharmacopoeias of many countries. *German Commission E* has approved its internal use for dyspepsia and the symptomatic treatment of excessive perspiration and its external use for mucous membrane inflammation of the nasopharynx. Its genus name derives from the Latin *salvere* reflecting the healing nature of the herb and its ability "to save". It, like rosemary, is being viewed by commercial interests as a safe and effective preservative for food and cosmetics. It is used for diabetes mellitus in Jordan.[413]

Anti-oxidant
In vitro—As with other members of this family the herb has a number of constituents that give it a strong anti-oxidant potential, the flavonoids, diterpenes and phenolic acids all contributing.[414–419] The anti-oxidant activity is measurable in simple infusions of the herb.[420]

The diterpenes are the same as those found in *Rosmarinus*.

Antimicrobial
In vitro—Sage has some inhibitory effect on the bacterial organisms responsible for periodontal disease[421] and strongly inhibits the collagen destroying enzyme of *Porphyromonas gingivalis*.[422]

The essential oil has both bacteriostatic and bacteriocidal properties[423] and significantly inhibits the growth of the urinary tract pathogens *Klebsiella* and *Enterobacter* spp., *Escherichia coli*, *Proteus mirabilis* and *Morganella morganii*.[424] This antibacterial action seems to arise from the altered membrane permeability of the bacteria and/or from disruption of their enzymes, to which Gram-positive organisms are more susceptible.[423,425]

The herb is antiviral against HSV-1 (including against an acyclovir-resistant strain) and 2, before their cellular entry, suggesting the effect would occur in topical preparations rather than after internal use.[185] Diterpenes from the herb also have antiviral activity.[426]

Thujone, 1,8-cineole and camphor all have established antibacterial and antifungal activity.[423] The polysaccharide fraction is associated with immunomodulatory activity *in vitro*.[427]

In vivo—Topical antimicrobial use in clinical trials has been positive. A 15% sage throat spray significantly relieved the pain of acute viral pharyngitis[428] and a cream containing an aqueous extract of sage and tincture of *Rheum* was as effective as acyclovir in the treatment of herpes labialis, the combination was also more effective than sage extract on its own.[429]

Nervous system
Historically *Salvia* was known to be beneficial for the head and brain (memory) and it has been subjected to some testing in this area.

In vitro—*Salvia* and/or its essential oil inhibit both acetylcholinesterase and butyrylcholinesterase activities, which could theoretically improve cognitive and memory function.[430–432] Both flavonoid and diterpene fractions have demonstrated benzodiazepine-receptor/$GABA_A$ binding activity, suggesting it could increase relaxation/reduce anxiety.[433]

In vivo—In healthy volunteers sage improved mood and cognitive function.[430] Treatment of patients with mild-moderate Alzheimer's disease showed significant cognitive improvement after 4 months use without suffering side-effects.[434] The action is likely to be due to a combination of anti-oxidant and anti-cholinergic activities.

Other
In vitro—The essential oil has anti-mutagenic activity protecting cells from damage by UV light.[435,436]

Rosmarinic acid has been well studied in isolation and has a number of pharmacological actions. It is anti-inflammatory, antiviral, antibacterial, anti-oxidant, astringent and also anti-mutagenic.[437]

A methanol extract has strong larvicidal activity.[312]

In vivo—A combination of *Salvia* and *Medicago sativa* (alfalfa) was an effective treatment for menopausal symptoms, including excessive sweating, a symptom for which *Salvia* has a long been used. The only hormone changes detected were increased levels of prolactin and TSH.[438]

Essential oil inhalation of several herbs including *Salvia* helped reduce inflammation in the respiratory tracts of patients with chronic bronchitis.[439]

Medicinal uses
Respiratory tract
- sore throat
- tonsillitis
- quinsy
- pharyngitis
- uvulitis
- gingivitis
- glossitis
- mouth ulcers
- stomatitis

All the above conditions can be treated with washes or gargles as well.

- asthma
- bronchitis
- catarrh
- night sweats of tuberculosis

Gastro-intestinal tract
- gastroenteritis
- indigestion
- flatulent dyspepsia
- anorexia
- sialorrhoea
- colic
- diarrhoea

Nervous system
It has a general relaxant and restorative effect:

- nervousness
- excitability
- dizziness
- trembling

Reproductive tract
Salvia has been used for various gynaecological problems:

- to regulate menstrual cycle length and flow
- dysmenorrhoea
- to aid cessation of breast feeding
- menopausal night sweats

Externally
- throat inflammation (gargle)
- oral inflammation (gargle)
- antisepsis of new cuts/abrasions

As an ointment:

- rheumatism
- arthritis
- neuralgia
- myalgia

Fresh leaves used as a rub:

- to strengthen gums and prevent tooth loss

Pharmacy
Three times daily

Infusion of dried herb	– 1–4 g
Tincture 1:5	– 2–4 ml (suggested guidelines)
Fluid Extract (45%)	– 1–4 ml

CONTRAINDICATIONS—Lactation and pregnancy—*Salvia* will dry up breast milk and thujone is an emmenagogue.

Precautions and/or safety
In high doses the herb may cause irritability. The essential oil did not have mutagenic activity in standard tests.[435] There are reported cases of epileptic seizures from ingesting the essential oil. Internal

use of essential oils should be avoided. There are recorded cases of allergy to the Lamiaceae family, although not to *Salvia* itself, but cross-sensitivity is possible.[104]

Interactions
Salvia had an inhibitory effect on cytochrome P450 isozymes CYP1A2, CYP2D6 and CYP3A4 *in vitro* however there are no reports of drug interactions *in vivo*.[440]

Historical uses
For liver diseases; as a diuretic; to staunch bleeding and clean sores and ulcers. Aching of the testicles (externally); promotes fertility if the womb is "slippery"; haemoptysis; all pains of the head due to cold/rheumatic humours; epilepsy, lethargy; palsy; diseases of chest and breast. For the bloody flux; for the stinging and biting of serpents; to kill worms in the ears and in sores. Improve memory; warm and quicken the senses; plague; stitch or pain in the side due to wind.

Scutellaria lateriflora

Skullcap

N.B. In some books the specific name is given incorrectly as *laterifolia*, *lateriflora* means flowers on the side.

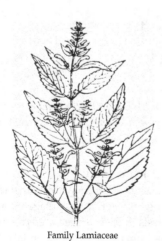

Family Lamiaceae

Description
Fibrous rooted perennial growing 30–60 cm in flower. *Stems* smooth, upright, much-branched or simple. *Leaves* opposite, dark-green, ovate-lanceolate or ovate oblong, pointed, closely serrate and rounded or cordate at the base. Petioles ¼ length of blade. *Inflorescence* in opposite, axillary, unilateral, leafy racemes with first pair of leaves similar to those of stem and the rest gradually reduced to bracts. *Flowers* small, blue, single, in the axils of the floral leaves in pairs facing the same way. Calyx 2-lipped, campanulate, lips entire. Corolla bilabiate, erect, tube elongated, curved upward, dilated at throat and naked within: lips short, equal in length; the upper arched and having 2 lateral divisions connected with the basal sides; the lower spreading, convex, notched at the apex. *Stamens* 4 parallel, ascending under the upper lip, the superior pair shorter. *Fruiting calyx* closed, the upper lip with a concave and enlarged appendage on the back. Nutlets—4. Flowers from spring to autumn.

Habitat and cultivation
Indigenous to North America from Canada to Florida, in moist woods or thickets. Cultivated but not naturalized elsewhere. Grown from seed or division. Dies back in winter. Needs moist soil and shade in dry summer weather. Frost resistant, drought tender.

Parts used
The herb harvested in the late flowering period.

Active constituents
1) Flavonoid glycosides (up to 24.5%) including predominantly baicalin, dihydrobaicalin, lateriflorin, ikonnikoside I, scutellarin and the aglycones oroxylin A, baicalein and wogonin[441]
2) Bitter iridoid—catalpol
3) Volatile oil mainly sesquiterpenes[442] (trace)
4) Tannins

Also contains diterpenes (scutelaterins A–C, ajugaptin and scutecyprol A),[443] amino acids particularly GABA and glutamine[441] and a small amount of melatonin.[444]

Nutritional constituents
Vitamins: C and E
Minerals: High in calcium, potassium and magnesium with some iron and zinc

Actions
1) Sedative
2) Anticonvulsant
3) Antispasmodic
4) Nervine

Scientific information
Scutellaria is not well investigated however it has some flavonoids in common with *S. baicalensis* which is a much better studied medicinal herb.

In vitro—Some of the flavonoid constituents and the amino acids are neuroactive binding to benzodiazepine/GABAA receptor sites.[441] GABA inhibits neurotransmission and can therefore be sedative/relaxant and anticonvulsive (see *Valeriana*) and although it may not cross the blood-brain barrier, glutamine, which can be metabolised to GABA, can do so and may account for some of the herb's activity.[445] The flavonoids also appear to bind to serotonergic receptor sites (5-HT$_7$) which may provide further insight into its mode of action on the nervous system.[446]

The individual flavonoids have been, and are being, investigated. They display a number of pharmacological activities including antioxidant,[447] anticancer,[448] anti-inflammatory[449] and antiviral[450,451] and have potential benefits for cardiovascular function.[452]

In vivo an anxiolytic effect was demonstrated in healthy volunteers given *Scutellaria*.[453]

Medicinal uses
Nervous system
• nervous exhaustion
• tension
• anxiety
• chorea
• epilepsy including grand mal
• restless sleep
• hysteria
• insomnia
• neuralgia
• headaches of nervous origin

Pharmacy
Three times daily
Infusion of dried herb   – 1–2 g
Tincture 1:5 (45%)   – 1–2 ml
Fluid Extract (25%)   – 2–4 ml

Precautions and/or safety
Older references warn of possible hepatotoxicity associated with the herb. This is based on cases where tablets containing *Scutellaria lateriflora* and *Valeriana officinalis* were consumed by people who then developed liver damage.[454] The direct connection between *Scutellaria* and liver toxicity has never been established and it is believed that any causal link was due to the substitution of *S. lateriflora* with *Teucrium* spp. which has known hepatotoxicity.[455,456]

Interactions
In vitro Scutellaria inhibits cytochrome CYP3A4 but to-date there are no reported herb-drug interactions *in vivo*.

Historical uses
Hydrophobia (rabies); alcoholism; headaches from incessant coughing; rickets.

Stachys officinalis
[Formerly *Stachys betonica*]

Betony, wood betony

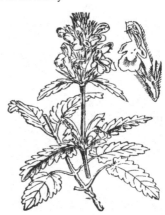

Family Lamiaceae

Description

A hairy perennial with a basal rosette of long-stalked leaves and erect, nearly leafless flower stems in summer. *Leaves* opposite, all stalked and roughly hairy, lower oval-oblong with a heart-shaped base, margins with regular rounded teeth. Upper leaves few, narrower. *Flowers* in dense whorls, sometimes interrupted below. Corolla about 1.5 cm, bright reddish-purple, or rarely white; the tube longer than the calyx, the upper lip more than twice as long as the stamens. Calyx hairless or hairy in the throat, 7–9 mm, lobes with awn-like apex, half as long as the tube; anthers yellow. A variable species. Flowers mid-summer to autumn.

Habitat and cultivation

Native to Europe in meadows, heaths and woods. Cultivated elsewhere. Grown from seed or root division in any moist garden soil. Needs summer shade to prevent wilting. Frost resistant and drought tender.

Parts used

The herb, gathered when the plant is flowering.

Active constituents

1) Alkaloids including stachydrine, betonicine, trigonelline
2) Tannins (up to 15%) including pyrogallol[457]
3) Flavonoids mainly based on quercetin and apigenin[457]
4) Phenolic acids including caffeic acid[457]

Also contains terpenoids[458] including ursolic and oleanolic acids,[26] phenylethanoid glycosides—betonyosides A–F[459] and volatile oil containing germacrene D, caryophyllene and humulene.[460,461]

Nutritional constituents

Minerals: Magnesium,   manganese   and phosphorus

Actions

1) Sedative
2) Bitter
3) Astringent
4) Nervine

Scientific information

The phenolic constituents—tannins, phenolic acids and flavonoids all contribute to the herb's antioxidant[457,462] and antimutagenic activities.[463] Little other scientific information is available.

Stachydrine (like that found in *Leonurus*) is, in isolation, oxytocic.

Medicinal uses

Nervous system

The indications for *Stachys* as a trophorestorative are for the nervous system depleted by chronic illness:

- neuralgia
- vertigo
- anxiety
- headaches including migraine
- tension
- hysteria
- nervous disability

Pharmacy

Three times daily

Infusion of dried herb	–	2–4 g
Tincture 1:5 (45%)	–	2–6 ml
Fluid Extract (25%)	–	2–4 ml

Historical uses

A heal-all. For prophylaxis of epidemic diseases; poor/weak digestion; palpitations; jaundice; epilepsy; palsy; fits; shrinking sinews; gout; dropsy; continual headache. For coughs; colds; wheezes; dyspnoea. Agues; blood cleansing to clear sight; rheumatism; worms; scrofula; stitches and pains in back or sides; griping pains in bowel; flatulence. As a purgative and aid to menstruation. To ease labour and childbirth. Kidney and bladder stones. Internally and externally for the bite of mad dogs. As an anti-haemorrhagic and tissue healing agent. As a gargle for toothache. To draw, e.g. splinters. For earache.

Thymus vulgaris

Thyme, common thyme

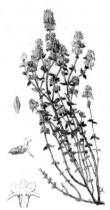

Family Lamiaceae

Description
A small, hairy, perennial, aromatic shrub growing to 30 cm high. Shoots dense, erect or sub-erect, densely clothed in short hairs. *Leaves* opposite, sessile, greenish-grey, 3–8 × 0.5–3 mm, elliptic but appearing linear because of revolute margins, densely hairy with abundant oil globules. *Flowers* in dense terminal heads; lower verticils often interrupted. Bracts green, similar to leaves, often somewhat wider. Calyx 3–4 mm long, bell-shaped, green or purplish, hairy, dotted with oil globules. Corolla 4–6 mm long, white or pinkish-mauve, upper lip with large broad oblong-elliptic to obovate lobes, sparsely/hairy or glabrous; lower lip at right angles to upper. Stamens not or scarcely exserted, anthers purplish. *Nutlets* 6–8 mm diameter, broad ellipsoid to sub-spherical, dark brown. Flowers from spring to midsummer. N.B. *Thymus serpyllum* is also medicinal, but it is not found in many countries.
   Odour and taste aromatic.

Habitat and cultivation
Native to the Mediterranean but found wild on dry slopes in many places and cultivated worldwide. Grown from seed or cuttings and will self-sow. Prefers free-draining, sunny situations with adequate water. Needs a pH of at least 6 so add lime to the soil if necessary. Drought and frost resistant.

Parts used
The herb harvested just prior to, or during, flowering.

Active constituents
1) Volatile oil (1.0–2.5%) contains at least 97 constituents, predominantly monoterpenes and their precursors, including thymol (36–55%), its isomer carvacrol, γ-terpinene, p-cymene also 1,8-cineol, linalool, α-thujene, borneol, β-pinene, camphor.[396,464] These constituents are variable as the herb hybridises easily. They vary with the genetic make-up[465] (there are at least 6 chemotypes),[466] geographical location, environmental conditions, time of harvest, plant part[467] and method of extraction.[468] Thymol levels are highest in young plants and when the herb is in full bloom.[464,469] The volatile oil of *T. serpyllum* has a quite different composition.[470]
2) Flavonoids including apigenin, luteolin, epicatechin and methoxylated flavones[467,471,472]
3) Tannins (up to 10%)
4) Phenolic acids including caffeic, gentisic, syringic and P-coumaric acids[471]

Also contains polysaccharides,[473] small amounts of phytosterols including campesterol and β-sitosterol,[467] salicylates[327] and acetophenones.[474]

Nutritional constituents
Vitamins: B-complex, C, D and E[467]
Minerals: Rich in iodine, smaller amounts of sodium, silicon and sulphur

Actions
1) Antimicrobial
2) Carminative
3) Antitussive
4) Expectorant
5) Spasmolytic
6) Astringent
7) Anthelmintic

Scientific information
Thymus vulgaris has a very long tradition of medicinal use and has been an official medicine in

countries all over the world. *German Commission E* has approved its use to treat the symptoms of bronchitis, whooping cough and upper respiratory catarrh. The food industry has generated a detailed examination of thyme's constituents in the search for safe and effective preservatives.

Anti-oxidant

In vitro—The phenolic constituents all contribute to the anti-oxidant capacity, the extract and culinary herb having shown a strong activity.[168,471,475-478,495] Of the medicinal Lamiaceae *Thymus* is the strongest anti-oxidant.[479,480]

Thymol neutralises and absorbs free radicals and inhibits the release of the enzyme elastase, by blocking calcium channels, suggesting it may also have anti-inflammatory activity.[481,482] Carvacrol is a more potent anti-oxidant than thymol.[495]

Antimicrobial

In vitro—Water and alcohol extracts of thyme have:

- antibacterial activity against pathogenic bacteria including *Vibrio parahaemolyticus*,[483] *Escherichia coli, Staphylococcus aureus* (also MRSA),[485] *Bacillus subtilis, Pseudomonas aeruginosa, Enterococcus faecalis, Helicobacter pylori* and *Mycobacterium tuberculosis* (and an antibiotic resistant strain).[484-488] A crude extract also increased the sensitivity of MRSA to the antibiotic tetracycline, an action attributed to the methoxylated flavones[489]
- antiviral activity against HSV-1 (including an acyclovir-resistant strain) and HSV-2, prior to cellular entry[185] and against influenza A virus and respiratory syncytial virus[490]

The essential oil and/or thymol have wide ranging and strong antimicrobial activity. The oil from the flowering herb shows the strongest activity[491] and the chemotypes rich in phenolic monoterpenes (thymol and carvacrol) are stronger than those rich in the monoterpene alcohol linalool.[492] Antimicrobial action appears to be due, at least in part, to the disruption of the bacterial cell wall/cytoplasmic membrane.[493,494,497] Effective activity has been reported against:-

- many Gram-positive and Gram-negative bacteria including *E. coli, S. aureus, S. epidermidis, Pseudomonas aeruginosa, Salmonella typhus, S. typhyimurium* and *S. enteritidis, Bacillus subtilis, Streptococcus pyogenes, S. pneumoniae, Haemophilus influenzae, Listeria monocytogenes, Aspergillus fumigatus* and others.[495-504] The essential oil also inhibited the ability of *L. monocytogenes* to become infectious.[505] An *in vitro* study using a range of Gram-positive and Gram-negative organisms isolated from severely infected children, all of which displayed some drug resistance, showed that thyme oil had a broad antibacterial activity[506]
- fungi including species of *Trichophyton, Candida* and *Aspergillus*[494,495,507,508] (as well as a clotriamazole-resistant *C. albicans*).[509] The oil also increased the effective inhibition of *C. albicans* by amphotericin B[510]
- protozoa including *Trypanosoma cruzi, T. brucei* and *Leishmania major*[511,512]

The oil is an effective insecticide[513,514] and pediculocide against head lice.[242]

Other

In vitro—Thyme may promote detoxification and antioxidant activity by up-regulating the relevant cell enzymes[515] and at low doses thymol and carvacrol are protective of chemical and oxidative damage to DNA.[516,517] These activities contribute to a cancer protective effect. The polysaccharides isolated from thyme also have potential anticancer properties.[473] Thyme binds to both oestrogen and progesterone receptor sites on breast cancer cells.[518]

The essential oil and its main constituents inhibit acetylcholinesterase.[519] The oil and thymol have some ability to enhance the sensitivity of $GABA_A$ receptors, with possible relevance for anxiolysis and epilepsy prevention.[520,521]

Thyme helps reduce the malodour produced by saliva protein putrefaction[522]—thymol is used in commercial dental preparations.

Thymol inhibits platelet aggregation probably via inhibition of COX.[523]

In vivo—*Thymus* in combination with other herbs was effective and safe at resolving the irritable cough associated with bronchitis, following a cold or due to respiratory tract problems where a viscous mucus was produced.[524–526]

There is an anecdotal report of the successful treatment of vulval lichen sclerosis using a cream containing the herb.[527]

Medicinal uses
Respiratory tract
- bronchitis
- pertussis
- aspergillosis
- coughs
- pleurisy
- laryngitis
- dry coughs
- bronchial catarrh
- asthma
- nervous coughs

Gastro-intestinal tract
In France the bitter properties of *Thymus* are valued and it is used for liver dysfunction.

- enteritis
- acute and chronic gastritis
- dyspepsia
- diarrhoea
- colic
- worms (large doses)

Urinary tract
- cystitis
- enuresis in children

Externally
- vaginal thrush (douche)
- fungal infections
- emphysema (inhalant)
- oral thrush (mouthwash)
- skin infections
- tonsillitis (gargle)

Pharmacy
Three times daily
Infusion of dried herb	–	1–4 g
Tincture 1:5 (45%)	–	2–6 ml
Fluid Extract (45%)	–	0.6–4 ml

The essential oil at a concentration of 3% preserves topical preparations from bacterial and fungal growth.[528]

Pharmacokinetics
Studies using healthy volunteers showed that, after ingesting thyme, thymol is not found in its free form but occurs in plasma as thymol sulphate and in urine in either the sulphate or glucuronide form. Plasma levels rose quickly after ingestion suggesting absorption occurs in the upper part of the digestive tract, peaked after 2 hours, and was eliminated slowly from the kidneys with a half-life of 10.2 hours. Plasma thymol sulphate persisted for up to 41 hours after initial administration.[490]

Precautions and/or safety
Thyme preparations used in the above clinical trials were without side effects and the standard bacterial assays used to test for genotoxicity showed the essential oil is safe.[529] At antimicrobial levels the oil, but not thymol, was cytotoxic to intestinal cells *in vitro*.[496] The essential oil should be used as an inhalant, not as an internal medicine.

There are reports of allergies to thyme resulting in reduced lung function and contact dermatitis after occupational exposure to its dust,[530–533] cross-reactivity to it from a contact allergy to rosemary[534] and a systemic allergic reaction from its ingestion.[104] Those sensitive to salicylates may need to use this herb with caution.[327]

Interactions
Thyme inhibits isozymes CYP2C9, CYP2C19, CYP2D6 and CYP3A4 *in vitro* suggesting a potential for drug/herb interaction although there are no reports of any interactions to-date.[535]

Historical uses
Aid to labour and delivery; to bring on menstruation. Leprosy; epilepsy; to promote perspiration so for colds, fever. As an ointment for hot swellings; warts; sciatica; dull sight; hard, painful spleen. Gout; swollen testicles. As a tobacco for improving digestion, headaches and drowsiness.

LAURACEAE

A dicot family of about 47 genera of which the most familiar is *Laurus nobilis*, the bay tree, the leaves of which are used in cooking. Most members of this family are aromatic trees and shrubs, growing in tropical or sub tropical regions. Leaves, mostly evergreen and leathery; flowers small, inconspicuous, green or yellowish. Fruits a one-celled berry.

Cinnamomum zeylanicum [Synonym *Cinnamomum verum*]

Cinnamon

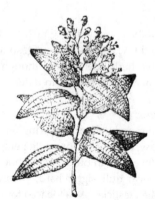

Family Lauraceae

Description

An evergreen tree growing between 10–20 m in the wild but kept much smaller in cultivation. Bark reddish brown and soft. *Leaves* ovate-obovate, about 16 cm long, marked by 3 parallel veins, tips pointed. *Flowers* yellowish, inconspicuous, growing in panicles which are as long as the leaves.

Odour—characteristic and aromatic, taste—slightly sweet, characteristic and fragrant.

Habitat and cultivation

Native to Sri Lanka and south-west India. Growing in tropical forest up to an altitude of 500 m. Cultivated as a spice in other tropical countries e.g. the Philippines and West Indies.

Parts used

Inner bark separated from cork and underlying parenchyma and branches.

Active constituents

1) Volatile oil (min. 1.2%) mainly aldehydes, predominantly cinnamaldehyde (around 65%) also cinnamyl acetate and alcohol, 2-methoxycinnamaldehyde, benzaldehyde, eugenol, methyleugenol, β-caryophyllene, linalool, β-phellandrene, limonene, α-humulene and

262

p-cymene.[1] Although the same chemical make-up exists in leaf, tree and root bark their relative proportions vary. The volatile oil from the inner bark is distinguishable from that of the leaf and the root bark as the predominant constituent in the leaf is eugenol and in the root bark its camphor.[2] The chemical make-up is also altered with age.
2) Tannins

Also contains arabinoxylan[3] and mucilage. *C. cassia*, Chinese cinnamon, has a different chemical make-up to *C. zeylanicum*, for example the volatile oil of the former contains coumarin and very little eugenol whilst the latter contains only traces of coumarin.[1]

Nutritional constituents
Minerals: Manganese, calcium, phosphorus, potassium and sulphur

Actions
1) Spasmolytic
2) Carminative
3) Stimulant
4) Antimicrobial
5) Anthelmintic
6) Astringent (mild)

Scientific information
Cinnamon is one of the oldest spices known to man and *C. zeylanicum* has been an official medicine in many countries of the world.[4] *German Commission E* has approved its use for the treatment of gastrointestinal problems (see under Medicinal Uses).

Other species of cinnamon are also medicinal and have formed part of the traditional medicine of the countries in which they grow. *C. zeylanicum*, called true cinnamon, is considered by some to be the best quality cinnamon. The whole spice, as quills or powder, is used in the baking industry and to make medicine, whilst the oil or oleoresin has been used for the cosmetic, food and pharmaceutical industries. Distillation of the bark produces very small quantities of oil and this with the higher prices demanded for *C. zeylanicum* has led to some adulteration with other species. Furthermore the officially accepted "cinnamon" may vary from one country to the next. For example species other than just *C. zeylanicum* are accepted as cinnamon and given the generic name "cassia" in the United States where they are the commonest types of cinnamon used.[1] This may have lead to discrepancies in recorded constituents of the herb and possibly some of its medicinal actions. Indeed much of the current investigation into the medicinal properties of cinnamon and/or its constituents has focused on *C. cassia* and given the differences between the two cinnamons in terms of their constituents it may be unwise to extrapolate these findings.

Anti-oxidant
In vitro—Aqueous and alcoholic extracts of cinnamon are anti-oxidant[5] and both the volatile oil and eugenol exhibit this activity strongly.[6]

Antimicrobial
In vitro—Cinnamon oil and/or its main constituents are strong inhibitors of a great number of pathogenic organisms. These include both Gram-negative and Gram-positive bacteria, as well as some isolated from children with severe infections in which the causative bacteria had become antibiotic-resistant.[7] Those found susceptible include *Pseudomonas aeruginosa*, *Proteus vulgaris*, *Klebsiella pneumoniae*, *Escherichia coli*, *Salmonella enteriditis*, *Listeria innocua*, *Bacillus subtilis*, *Staphylococcus aureus* and *Helicobacter pylori*.[8-13] The essential oil also inhibits the ability of *Listeria monocytogenes* to become infective[14] and is inhibitory to a broad range of fungal pathogens such as *Aspergillus niger*[15] and *Candida albicans*.[10,16-20] The bark is active against a fluconazole-resistant strain of *C. albicans*.[21]

Cinnamon also has antiparasitic properties. The oil and some of its constituents are toxic to *Pediculus humanus capitis* and their eggs[22] and the herb is anthelmintic with activity against the roundworm *Ascaris lumbricoides*.[23]

In vivo—Although no clinical trials have been conducted using *Cinnamomum* as an antibacterial there is anecdotal evidence of a baby who had become a carrier of *Salmonella enteriditis* being successfully treated with powdered cinnamon bark.[24] Also a small sample of HIV patients were successfully treated for oral thrush with the herb.[21]

Other

In vitro—Cinnamaldehyde has anti-cancer properties[25] and it, and eugenol, have good COX-2 inhibition.[26]

In vivo—*C. zeylanicum* has been traditionally to treat diabetes.[27] Clinical trials have been conducted using *C. cassia* with promising results but animal based comparisons between the two species suggest that *C. zeylanicum* is inferior in its ability to influence insulin and cellular glucose uptake.[28]

Medicinal uses
Respiratory tract
As the oil has a broad spectrum of antimicrobial activity it would be a useful inhalant in the case of infections.

- influenza
- common cold

Gastro-intestinal tract
- nausea
- flatulent dyspepsia
- colic
- diarrhoea
- anorexia
- vomiting

Pharmacy
Three times daily

Infusion of powdered bark	– 0.5–1 g
Tincture 1:5 (70%)	– 2–4 ml
Liquid extract (70%)	– 0.5–1 ml

Cinnamomum is often used to enhance the action of the herbs in a prescription.

Precautions and/or safety
Standard mutagenicity tests have been negative and it is considered safe.[29] Prolonged contact between skin and the essential oil may cause burning.[30] Cinnamon has been cited in a number of allergic reactions in particular to toothpaste and chewing gums containing the oil as a flavouring. They have been reported to have caused contact stomatitis,[31-33] oral erosion[34] and contact eczema possibly with bullous lesions (low incidence).[35-38] Patients with oro-facial granulomatosis who went on a cinnamon and benzoate free diet had a significant improvement in oral inflammation.[39] There is also one report of squamous cell carcinoma of the tongue attributed to prolonged use of cinnamon-flavoured chewing gum.[40]

The species of cinnamon, oil or constituents which gave rise to these reports does not appear to have been determined. It is difficult to know if it is all or a particular cinnamon species, and/or its derivatives, that may be responsible for these reactions or if it is due to processing methods used. However there remains the possibility of allergic reactions to the herb in sensitive individuals.

Historical uses
As for current uses. Also used for menorrhagia and haemorrhages. Used in perfume and incense.

LILIACEAE

The Lily family
There are about 294 genera in the lily family throughout the world mainly in warm and tropical regions. It is the most typical monocot family of mainly perennial herbaceous plants. Many species contain alkaloids and are more or less toxic.

Characteristics
- Stems are often partly underground in the form of bulbs, corms or rhizomes
- Leaves are simple, usually narrow and with parallel veins, alternate and spirally arranged
- Flowers are usually regular, insect pollinated, solitary or in racemes, spikes, panicles or umbels
- Perianth—the calyx and corolla are not distinguishable with 6 tepals, free or united, arranged in two whorls of 3
- Stamens usually 6 in two whorls of 3
- Gynoecium—ovary superior with 3 united carpels divided into 3 loculi with numerous ovules in each loculus
- Fruit usually a capsule

Aletris farinosa

True unicorn root, colic root

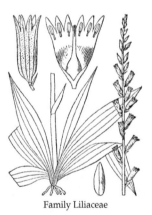

Family Liliaceae

Description
A perennial growing from a stout rhizome, up to a 1 m tall in flower. *Leaves* in a basal rosette, lance shaped over 15 cm long, yellowish green. *Flowers* white, tubular swollen at the base and with a mealy surface grow in a long raceme up a tall, leafless stalk. *Fruit* shorter than the perianth. Flowers in late spring to summer.

265

Odour—faint; taste—sweet then bitter and soapy.

Habitat and cultivation
Aletris grows in grassy woods in dry or moist peat or sandy soils, throughout the eastern states of USA. It is grown commercially in North Carolina, Virginia and Tennessee.

Parts used
The dried roots and rhizomes harvested when flowering is over.

Active constituents
This herb is very poorly characterized.

1) A saponin has been suggested as the major constituent[1]—this could be the steroidal saponin, diosgenin,[2] or it may be an additional constituent to it
2) Volatile oil

Also contains alkaloids.

Actions
1) Tonic
2) Bitter
3) Spasmolytic
4) Mild sedative

Scientific information
Aletris was an official medicine in the *United States Pharmocopoiea* and *National Formulary* until the mid 20th Century. It has been suggested that it was used interchangeably or in combination with False Unicorn Root (*Chamaelirium luteum*) in the treatment of the female reproductive tract, although they should not have been confused from their physical appearance.

The early American herbalists used the herb to treat a broad range of female issues including amenorrhoea, dysmenorrhoea, threatened and habitual miscarriage, uterine prolapse, uterine weakness for example due to "too frequent child bearing", infertility, leucorrhoea and as a menstrual cycle regulator. *Weiss* too states that *Aletris* is a uterine tonic. However due to the confusion surrounding the purity of the herb and its common substitution, or contamination, by *Chamaelirum* it is possible that it is a digestive and not a female tonic (*King's American Dispensatory*).[3] Although its chemistry would suggest it may have an influence on the reproductive tract.

The true value of *Aletris* may have to await future scientific study of its constituents and pharmacological actions. There has been no modern research.

Medicinal uses
Gastro-intestinal tract
The herb's actions would have given rise to one of its common names—colic root.

• flatulent colic
• anorexia
• dyspepsia

Pharmacy
Three times daily
Decoction of dried root/rhizome   – 0.3–0.6 g
Fluid Extract (45%)   – 2–4 ml

Precautions and/or safety
The fresh root in large doses can cause vomiting and diarrhoea and may be narcotic, in small doses it can cause hypogastric discomfort and vertigo.

Historical uses
See above. Also rheumatism; as a diuretic.

Allium sativum

Garlic

Description
A perennial bulb, ovoid or globose, usually divided into several cloves within the multi-layered membranous coat which later dries to form a protective papery layer. The cloves are swollen buds formed in the leaf axils at the base of the bulb. The cloves are pointed at the top, swollen in the middle and narrower and flat at the base. *Scape* to 60 cm with 4–6 flat leaves about 1–1.5 cm

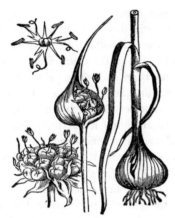

Family Liliaceae

wide, which form a sheath from the base of the plant. *Flowers* are pedicellate, small and white or pinkish, borne in a terminal umbel, interspersed with bulbils. *Seeds* are not usually fertile but bulbils may be used as seed though garlic is usually grown from cloves.

Odour—strong; taste—persistently pungent and acrid.

Habitat and cultivation

Originally native to Asia, garlic is now grown throughout the world for use in food and medicine. Garlic is usually grown from individual cloves and the larger the clove the bigger the mature garlic bulb will be. The cloves should be set, pointed end up, about 5 cm deep and 15 cm apart, in fertile, slightly alkaline soil with good drainage. The plot must be kept weed free. The cloves are usually planted in mid winter because garlic requires a period of chilling below 10°C before hours of long daylight and hot dry conditions in spring and summer. This means that it often does not grow well in wetter areas. It is frost resistant but drought tender.

It is generally harvested when the tops die back in late summer and should be dug with its stems left on and dried, being turned regularly. It must be protected from dew and rain while it is drying. Once properly dried it should keep until the following harvest. If it is not dug, garlic will continue to grow but the bulbs will become smaller.

Parts used

The bulb harvested in mid to late summer when leaves have died back. The bulb is divided into cloves.

Active constituents

1) Volatile oil (about 0.2%) including:
   a) sulphur containing compounds (more than 90%) as S-alk(en)yl-L-cysteine sulphoxides (alliin, isoalliin, methiin and cycloalliin)[4] and γ-glutamyl-S-allyl-L cysteines.[5] Derivatives of vinyldithiin have recently been isolated in fresh garlic.[6] Thiosulfinates arise from the sulphoxides once it is crushed, eg. allicin from alliin, they are not present in intact garlic[5]
   b) other—citral, geraniol, linalool
2) Flavonoids including myricetin, quercetin and apigenin[7]
3) Steroidal saponins (based on erubroside and sativosides)[5,8]

Also scordinins which are sulphur containing glycosides, mucilage, adenosine, organo-selenium compounds, predominantly selenomethionine[5,9,10] (when garlic is grown in soil rich in selenium it tends to replace sulphur),[11] lignans,[12] fructans[13] and proteins including allivin[14] and/or alliumin[15] (the protein may vary with the sub-species of *Allium sativum*, of which three have been identified).[16] Also contains a number of essential amino acids.[16]

The chemistry of garlic is complicated by the reactive and unstable nature of its main constituents and their conversions as the tissue cells are disrupted, a process which is influenced by the particular processing method used to achieve the end product.[17] Even within the fresh, intact herb the chemistry is variable, alliin being present at higher levels in the outer cloves.[18] Further alterations result from duration and temperature of storage.[4]

Alliin (S-allylcysteine sulfoxide) is itself stable but on crushing fresh garlic or adding water to garlic powder the enzyme allinase, which occurs in a separate compartment in the intact bulb, comes together with alliin which it converts to thiosulfinates. This process is rapid and occurs in about 10 seconds at room temperature.[19] Of the thiosulfinates produced 70–80% is allicin, which is unstable, unless dried, and has a half-life of 2.5 days at room temperature.[19] Allicin subsequently decomposes to form a number of other sulphur containing compounds including allyl sulfides—diallyl sulphide (DAS), diallyl disulfide (DADS) and diallyl trisulfide (DAT or allitridin)—vinyldithiins and ajoenes (isomers called E and Z) depending on the temperature and pH. These compounds are themselves very reactive and form complexes with cellular proteins and fatty acids.

The γ-glutamyl-S-allyl-L cysteines are converted to:

a) sulfoxides when bulbs are hydrolysed, oxidised or stored at low temperatures[20] or to
b) S-allyl-cysteines via another enzyme conversion if the herb is extracted into water.

Commercially produced aged garlic is prepared by adding minced garlic to 15–20% alcohol, incubating for 20 months and then concentrating the resulting extract.[21] Odourless garlic has had the allinase inactivated or is deodorised by the addition of chlorophyll.

Nutritional constituents
Vitamins: A, B_1,[22] B_2, B_6, nicotinic acid, biotin, C[23] and E
Minerals: Selenium (good source),[24,25] germanium, sulphur, calcium, magnesium, manganese, copper, potassium, zinc and some iron[26,27]

Actions
1) Antimicrobial
2) Anthelmintic
3) Anti-inflammatory
4) Hypolipidaemic
5) Spasmolytic
6) Diaphoretic
7) Expectorant
8) Hypocholesterolaemic
9) Antithrombotic
10) Hypotensive

Scientific information
The use of garlic dates back to our earliest history and written records of its medicinal use were found in ancient Egypt in the *Codex Ebers* ca. BC 1550. The herb has been, and still is, valued across many cultures not only as a medicine but as a food flavouring and preservative. In more modern times it was used as an antimicrobial during World Wars I and II and it is still an official medicine in a number of countries. In Europe where garlic is sold mainly as a powder 156 different garlic preparations are licensed.[28] *German Commission E* has approved its use to aid the reduction of serum lipid levels and as a preventative for age-related vascular changes.

The investigation into garlic, its constituents and their therapeutic effects began in the mid-20th century and still continues at a rapid rate today. Where at one time many of garlic's actions were thought to relate to its allicin content it is now recognised that many of the constituents are biologically active. Alliinase appears to be irreversibly inactivated below pH 3.6 which has raised some doubt about the enzyme's ability to survive exposure to stomach acid and to enable allicin to be produced and absorbed further down the gastro-intestinal tract. Allicin also binds easily to protein and fatty acids so that it may be trapped in the cell membrane, being unavailable for absorption, a proposal borne out by the fact that allicin is not detectable in either blood or urine after consuming garlic or pure allicin.[5] Moreover, when allicin is added directly to blood it is undetectable after a few minutes suggesting its rapid chemical alteration.[29] However the body does seem to have some limited alliinase-like activity.[30] It is probable that allicin alone is not responsible for the known medicinal benefits of the herb *in vivo* and that other constituents, in particular the organo-sulphur compounds that result from allicin's breakdown, are the pharmacological agents.

There is a lack of consensus on some aspects of garlic's medicinal benefits and effects and a number of significant reasons could explain these contradictory results:-

1) Chemical complexity. Constituents can vary with geographical origin,[31] method of storage, age of the garlic and processing of the

bulb e.g. allicin levels are lower in powdered garlic than in the fresh herb.[32] As allicin has been assumed to be garlic's main active constituent preparations have been standardised on it. However it has been estimated that the amount of allicin released from the type of tablet most used in clinical trials from 1994–2000 varied between 14–18%,[30] leaving the majority of the chemistry uncharacterised. In actual fact more than one hundred constituents have been isolated from garlic so far[33] of which the organo-sulphur compounds have variable stability[20]

2) Biological complexity. A great many of the known constituents and their derivatives are biologically active. In addition the volatile constituents are inherently unstable and may change or react *in vivo* with the metabolites found within the cells or at the cell membrane. There are therefore a great many unknowns in garlic's activity and whilst some of the activities of particular metabolites have been assigned biological functions[34] the whole preparation is too complex to be easily standardised. Clearly it becomes very difficult to unify one preparation on all of the active constituents let alone all the different commercial products that have been used in the multitude of trials. Therefore each clinical trial is really assessing a particular garlic product rather than garlic as a single entity

3) Bio-availability. Even within similarly prepared garlic products that may be expected to have similar chemical profiles e.g. garlic powders the bio-availability can be very different. For example enteric-coated garlic tablets designed to preserve allinase from stomach acid were tested for the bioavailability of their allicin, this was found to vary between 3–94% across 24 different brands.[30,35,36] There are many other constituents for which this comparison has not yet been made

4) Experimental variability. Trials have varied from the baseline health of the subjects used, their gender, duration of treatment, experimental design and dosage, all of which may have influenced the trial outcomes[37,38]

There is a large volume of research and reviews into this herb and some of the older information has been superseded by more recent work. Research from the last decade has therefore provided the main basis of the information below but this in turn is based on earlier work.

The process used to produce aged garlic alters its chemistry and possibly its actions compared to the fresh or dried herb. Aged preparations have also been intensively researched but data cannot necessarily be extrapolated to the non-aged herb and has, therefore, not been included.

Anti-oxidant
Garlic exhibits a spectrum of strong anti-oxidant activity due to the polyphenols, tocopherol, protein and volatile oils within it.[39–43] Cooking for less than 20 minutes does not diminish the activity of the non-volatile constituents significantly[10] but microwave heating and pickling do significantly weaken it.[44,45] Water extracts of the fresh bulb provide the strongest anti-oxidant preparations.[46]

Antimicrobial
In vitro—An extensive range of antimicrobial actions exists for the fresh herb, powder, water extract and/or its constituents with ethanol extracts having the strongest activity.[47] Actions to date include:-

• antibacterial against a broad range of organisms, both Gram-positive and Gram-negative, some of which are antibiotic-resistant.[48–52] These include *Staphylococcus aureus, Escherichia coli, Salmonella typhi, Bacillus cereus,*[53,54] *Neisseria gonorrhoeae,*[54] *Enterococcus faecalis,*[54] *Pseudomonas aeruginosa, Salmonella typhimurium, Klebsiella pneumoniae, Streptococcus pneumoniae, Helicobacter pylori,*[55–58] *Bacillus anthracis,*[59] *Clostridium* spp., *Mycobacterium tuberculosis,*[60] oral/periodontal pathogens[61,62] and many others.[63] Not only does garlic inhibit this great range of bacteria, it does not seem to induce resistance in them and can be effective against some bacterial toxins too.[64] The antibacterial activity is apparently 10 times stronger against pathogenic bacteria than against gut flora[47,64] the growth of the latter being additionally encouraged by the fructans present in the herb

Garlic works synergistically with some antibiotics[65] but was found to increase the minimum inhibitory concentration of others (ampicillin and norfloxacin) when the two were co-administered.[66]

Powders are more effective antibacterials than oil extracts,[67] powder from the fresh bulb being stronger than that derived from stored bulbs.[68]

- antifungal[15,69] against a range of fungi including *Candida* spp. (*C. albicans*),[49,63,70–72] *Cryptococcus neoformans*,[60] *Scedosporium prolificans*[73] (which is resistant to orthodox antifungals), *Aspergillus* spp.[74] and other pathogenic fungal species.[75–77] It also enhanced the activity of pharmaceutical antifungals against *C. albicans*,[78] *Aspergillus fumigatus*[79] and *Trichophyton* spp.[80] Fresh garlic seems to be a better antifungal against *Candida* than garlic powder[81]
- antiviral against human cytomegalovirus,[82–84] the enteroviruses coxsackie and ECHO virus;[85] HIV in the early part of its life cycle,[86] influenza A and B, HSV-1 and 2, parainfluenza virus type 3, vaccinia virus, vesicular stomatitis virus and human rhinovirus type 2[60]
- antiprotozoal against *Giardia lamblia*,[87] *Entamoeba hystolytica*,[60] *Trypanosoma* spp.[88] and *Leishmania* spp.[89] and inhibitory to *Plasmodium* sporozoites (malaria)[90]

In vivo—The clinical trials conducted on garlic are limited given its broad spectrum of activity *in vitro*.

Topical preparations effectively treated:-

- oral candidiasis (paste), comparable results to clotrimazole[91]
- otalgia associated with acute otitis media (combined with other herbs) as ear drops, comparable benefits to orthodox therapy[92,93]
- tinea infections (ajoene)[94,95]
- recurrent mouth ulcers (powder)[96]
- warts (both aqueous and lipid fractions of fresh garlic, the latter being much more effective and faster acting).

Furthermore use of the preparation on larger warts resolved smaller untreated warts in the same vicinity[97]

Garlic's systemic antibacterial activity was epidemiologically assessed by checking the occurrence of *Helicobacter pylori* amongst regular garlic eaters compared with non-garlic eaters. Although its prevalence was not reduced by garlic,[98] the bacterial population size was significantly lower[99] suggesting its consumption may confer some protection. However garlic oil failed to reduce signs of *H. pylori* infection in a small group of dyspeptic patients.[100]

Other studies have shown that garlic:-

- reduced the incidence of the common cold and hastened recovery from infection when used daily[101]
- treated giardiasis successfully[47]
- reduced the incidence of acute viral infections of the respiratory tract[102]

The mode of action as an antimicrobial is not only one of immune stimulation (see below). It seems likely that the sulphur content disorders the cellular activity of pathogens without disturbing human cells which are protected by their glutathione content.[87,103]

Anticancer
In vitro—The herb and its sulphur constituents inhibit a number of cancer cell lines, the lipid soluble fraction being more effective than the water soluble one[104] and the action of alliinase apparently playing a significant role in the development of this activity.[105]

Mechanisms contributing to the anticancer activity of the herb and/or its constituents probably involve:-

- anti-oxidant activity[23,106,107]
- direct anti-proliferative effects—many studies show increased apoptosis and arrest of division of cancer cells.[15,106–112] Cell lines that have been inhibited include nasopharyngeal carcinoma,[113] neuroblastoma,[114] prostate[115,116]—including the unresponsive androgen-independent type,[117–119]

gastric[120–123] lung,[124,125] skin,[126] melanoma,[127] leukaemia,[128–132] liver,[133–135] colon,[136–138] oesophageal,[139] bladder[140,141] and breast cancer cells whether hormone-dependent or not[130,142,143]

- induction and maintenance of detoxification enzymes against potentially damaging chemicals.[23,106,107,144–146] This prevents damage to DNA (genotoxicity) including from asbestos,[147–149] aflatoxin,[150] chemical carcinogens[151] or mutagens[152–154] and radiation[154–156]
- increased immune activity[23,107] (see below)

In addition research has shown that *Allium* and/ or its constituents can induce some cancer cells to differentiate,[157] inhibit their invasiveness,[158] inhibit angiogenesis[159,160] and can act synergistically with conventional chemotherapeutic drugs, increasing cancer cells susceptibility to them.[161]

In vivo—Epidemiological evidence indicates that garlic users may have protection against a range of cancers[23,162,163]—breast,[164] ovarian,[165] colorectal,[166] oropharyngeal,[162] laryngeal,[162] oesophageal,[167] stomach,[166–170] prostate[162,171] and renal cancers.[162] Protection was linked to the consumption of garlic, either raw or cooked, more than three times a week.[163]

Garlic juice reduced levels of an endogenously produced chemical carcinogen derived from a high level of dietary nitrate[172] and ajoene has been used with success in the topical treatment of basal cell carcinoma to reduce tumour size.[173]

Cardio-vascular effects
In vitro—Actions that have been demonstrated for garlic preparations and/or its constituents include:-

- inhibition of platelet aggregation[21,174–177] the thiosulfinates are stronger than aspirin at equivalent doses.[178] (Raw garlic is stronger than cooked[179] and steam-distilled garlic oil and garlic oil macerates have a very much reduced activity. Aged garlic may be devoid of anti-platelet activity.)[180]
- protection of erythrocytes[181] and neutrophils[182]
- reduced cytokine induced endothelial inflammation and monocyte adhesion—early factors in the development of atherosclerosis and

atherothrombosis[183]—and decreased arteriosclerotic plaque formation[184]
- protection of LDL from oxidation[185] and glycation[186,187]
- inhibition of cholesterol and fatty acids synthesis[188–191] and reduced production and secretion of chylomicrons[192]
- activation of nitric oxide production—vasodilation[21,160]
- inhibition of angiotensin converting enzyme (γ-glutamylcysteines)
- reduced lipid accumulation in aortic cells derived from arteriosclerotic plaque[193]

At high enough doses garlic modulates the cytokines involved in pre-eclampsia in placental cells[194] although to-date this effect has not been borne out *in vivo*—see below.

In vivo—Early work on garlic suggested it had hypolipidaemic and hypotensive activity however it is here that a lack of consensus on garlic's benefits is most apparent. Results of clinical trials have been reviewed over a number of years.[21,37,195–199] The averaged results of the positive data showed a reduction in cholesterol of 9.9%, LDL 11.4% and triglycerides 9.9%.[188] However less than half of the studies assessed in a 2006 critical review found garlic preparations lowered cholesterol.[188]

The hypotensive activity of garlic preparations have been tested in clinical trials—the majority of these were positive[21,200] and a pilot epidemiological study also associated regular garlic consumption with lower systolic blood pressures.[201] There are negative studies here too though.[188,202]

Other circulatory benefits that have been reported are[188]:-

- reduced oxidative stress[200]
- prevention and some reduction of arteriosclerotic plaque formation[203,204]
- protection of elasticity in aging blood vessels[205]
- inhibited platelet aggregation (garlic is a possible substitute for aspirin-intolerant patients)[206,207]
- increased peripheral blood flow[21,208,209] with benefits for treating peripheral arterial occlusive disease[21] (reviewed[210])

- reduced incidence of myocardial infarction in men with a high risk for coronary heart disease[21,211]
- increased tolerance for exercise in patients with coronary artery disease[212]
- increased fibrinolytic activity in patients with atherosclerosis, this increases with regular use of the herb[21]
- improved arterial oxygen levels and reduced dyspnoea in cases of hepatopulmonary disease[213-215]
- improved skin temperature as well as reduced erythrocyte and thrombocyte aggregation in patients with systemic sclerosis[216]

A review of garlic's use to prevent pre-eclampsia, and its complications, concluded the herb was safe for pregnant women and may help reduce hypertension, but there was insufficient data to recommend its use to treat this condition.[217,218]

With the current discrepancies in clinical trials, the true and full extent of the benefits of garlic for cardiovascular problems must await further evaluation.

Immunomodulatory
In vitro—Garlic and its constituents have demonstrated potential benefits by:-

- increased activity and protection of macrophage and lymphocyte activity[219] including against chemotherapeutic agents and UV radiation[220]
- increased levels of natural killer cells[220]
- cytokine modulation associated with inflammation and immune function[221-226]
- modulation of membrane-dependent immune cell functions[227]
- modulation of T-cell function associated with chronic inflammation[228]

Other
In vitro:-

- some of the sulphides are COX-2 inhibitors[229]
- the oil is a good solvent for gall stones[230]
- aqueous garlic extracts can immobilise sperm (membrane disruption)[231]

- garlic and/or its constituents have insecticidal activity[232] and are anthelminitic against roundworms and hookworms[21]
- garlic has some phyto-oestrogenic potential (lignans)[12]

In vivo garlic:-

- with vitamins improved chronic atrophic gastritis[233]
- was carminative in patients with gastro-intestinal discomfort[21]
- was beneficial (anti-inflammatory) for patients with rheumatoid arthritis[234]
- decreased blood glucose by over 11%,[206] in men only[38] but not in non-insulin dependent diabetes[21]
- reduced apparent nephrotoxicity of cyclosporine in renal transplant patients[235]
- effectively treated corns (lipid fraction)[97]
- as a 1% topical application of garlic oil was a deterrent to sand flies (97% protection)[236] but ingestion of a single dose did not reduce mosquito bites.[237]

Medicinal uses
Cardiovascular system
Because of the effects on serum lipids, platelet activity and hypotensive activity as well the action on the blood vessel walls themselves, it may be used for:

- hypertension
- hypercholesterolaemia
- hyperlipidaemia
- thrombosis
- varicose ulcers
- atherosclerosis (prophylaxis)
- atheroma
- phlebitis

Respiratory tract
- influenza
- whooping cough
- infections (lungs, throat and tonsils)
- asthma
- recurrent colds
- respiratory catarrh
- bronchitis (chronic and acute)

Gastro-intestinal tract
As an antimicrobial in the gut, it is effective in treating all infections in this area. It is believed to have a normalising effect on beneficial gut flora.

- typhoid
- food poisoning
- worms
- dysentery (amoebic and bacillary)
- cholera
- flatulence
- colic
- increased assimilation of vitamin B_1

Externally
- infected wounds
- otitis (drops)

Pharmacy

Dosage   – for long term maintenance 3–8 perles or 1 clove
          – for acute infections 2–6 good sized cloves a day
Daily (*BHP*) – 4–12 mg of alliin (approximately 2–5 mg allicin)
          – 400–1200 mg fully dried powder
          – 2–5 g fresh bulb
          – 0.03–0.12 mg garlic oil

Tinctures may have very variable compositions due to the instability of the constituents.[238]

The macerated oil can be dropped into the ears to treat ear infections. The fresh clove can be swallowed whole, after cutting if necessary, crushed or chopped and added without cooking to food. Cooking will cause loss of at least some of the active, volatile constituents. Garlic should be taken with food to avoid gastro-intestinal problems.

CONTRAINDICATIONS—Warfarin and **saquinavir** users or those with an allergy to the herb or *Allium* family.

Pharmacokinetics
After consuming garlic a complex series of chemical transformations occur and many elements of the pharmacokinetics are still to be elucidated.

Although allicin has been shown to diffuse easily through cell membranes *in vitro*,[239] no allicin is detectable in serum, urine or stools *in vivo* even after the consumption of large amounts of raw garlic. It seems likely that allicin is converted by stomach acid to DAS and DADS[240] and that these substances are further metabolised to produce the sulphur constituents found in the breath namely allyl mercaptan, methyl mercaptan and the predominant allyl methyl sulphide (AMS)—cooking garlic reduces these breath-detectable metabolites.[241] (DADS has also been reported to occur in breath after eating garlic[5] and *in vitro* it is converted by liver microsomes to allicin[242]). Apart from the sulphur containing compounds, non-toxic levels of acetone are also detectable on the breath which may result from increased triglyceride metabolism.[32] Although the immediate breath odour is from sulphur constituents produced in the mouth these are subsequently replaced by AMS produced in the gut.[243] Cysteine metabolites (S-allyl-cysteines) are excreted in urine after being further modified to S-allyl-mercapturic acid.[244]

Precautions and/or safety
Its use by breastfeeding mothers has not been associated with any adverse effects in their infants.[245]

In standard test constituents of garlic were strongly anti-mutagenic due to the induction of detoxifying enzymes.[246] The most frequent side-effects is that of a perceptible odour on the breath and body that is not always acceptable. Raw garlic in particular can also cause flatulence, heartburn, diarrhoea[247] and possibly stomach irritation if taken on an empty stomach.[32] Skin contact with raw herb can cause burns.[248,249]

It has been established that there is a food allergy to members of the onion family and an enzyme has been isolated from them that evokes an immunoglobulin-E-mediated (type-1 hypersensitivity) response in sensitive individuals.[250] Skin prick tests on patients with suspected food allergies found a 4.6% reaction in children and 7.7% reaction in adults to the herb.[251]

Other reported allergic reaction include urticaria,[252] contact dermatitis,[253-257] occupational rhino-conjunctivitis and asthma from exposure to garlic dust[258] and one case of anaphylaxis in a patient with multiple allergies.[259] However immediate allergic reactions, either by contact or ingestion, are considered to be rare.[252]

There is a suggested link between garlic consumption and the exacerbation of pemphigus,[260] one case of surgical haemorrhage[261] and one of spinal epidural haematoma.[21]

Interactions

In vitro—Garlic and its constituents can affect cytochrome P450 isozymes. These include CYP2C9*1, CYP2C19, CYP3A4,[262] CYP3A5, CYP3A7[263] and CYP2A6.[264] Both the herb and allicin had low to moderate interaction with P-glycoprotein, a cell membrane transporter.[262,265] Organo-sulphur constituents in garlic altered the transport of cisplatin (chemotherapeutic), suggesting a potential to either increase or decrease levels of this drug.[266] It does not interfere with the activity of the antibiotic gentamicin.[267]

In vivo—Co-administration of garlic with the chemotherapeutic drug docetaxel found no interaction occurred however there is a possibility that it could decrease clearance of the drug.[268]

Garlic reduced levels/bioavailability of saquinavir a protease inhibitor when the two were taken together[269] but did not significantly affect the level of another protease inhibitor, ritonavir.[270] However two cases of gastro-intestinal toxicity have been reported where ritonavir and garlic were used together by HIV patients.

There are only two reports to-date of garlic and warfarin causing increased clotting time when used together[271] and one of an interaction between garlic and the antithrombotic, fluindione.[272]

CYP3A4 activity was not affected by concomitant garlic use.[273]

CYP2E1 activity represented by chlorzoxazone (muscle relaxant) metabolism was reduced by garlic oil in elderly volunteers[274] and by DAS in healthy volunteers (protective?) although no therapeutic interactions have been reported.[275]

No other interactions have been reported.[276]

Historical uses

As a treatment for worms; tumours; arthritis and heart disorders. An ancient heal-all; diuretic; emmenagogue; a cure for all poisons; removes spots and blemishes; jaundice; epilepsy. Bites of mad dogs and venomous creatures; cure for lethargy! Prophylactic for the plague; piles; smallpox; hoarseness; tuberculosis; rheumatism.

Aloe barbadensis
[Formerly *Aloe vera*]

Aloe

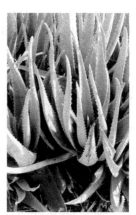

Family Liliaceae

Description

A stemless, stoloniferous, drought-resistant succulent which forms a clump over time. First leaves upright growing in a fan shape. Older leaves spiral round the plant. *Leaves* narrowly lanceolate, 30–60 cm long, smooth, rubbery, succulent, glaucous green. They are flat on the upper surface, curved beneath and dotted with small white stripes. Margins armed with whitish-reddish teeth. A mature aloe has about 15 leaves forming a basal rosette and the leaves are held upright by the water pressure of the gel. *Flowers* yellow-red, tubular, about 2 cm long in a long raceme up to about 1 m tall, blooming intermittently throughout the year. Plants growing in full sun may be stunted and/or have pinkish-red leaves which curve at the tips or lack gel.

Latex odour—characteristic and unpleasant; taste—nauseating and very bitter. Gel—odourless; taste—slightly bitter.

Habitat and cultivation

Originally from southern and eastern Africa and introduced to the Mediterranean,[291] it is cultivated throughout the world. It is usually propagated from "pups" or young suckers which grow from the main root stock. They may be easily separated and reset when they have some roots of their own. Aloes need a frost-free situation and well-drained soil. They do best in semi-shade with adequate water in hot weather when they are growing strongly. They need drier conditions in winter. When transplanting, it is important not to water them for 7–10 days or they will rot and die. They are best potted and brought inside for winter in frosty areas.

Parts used

There are two different fractions of the herb that are used medicinally. The latex or juice, known as aloes, is an exudate derived from the outer part of the leaves after they have been cut transversely near the base. It is collected for a period of 6 hours and evaporated to a yellow residue. Latex levels vary within the plant for instance younger leaves have more than older ones.[277] The other fraction is the gel derived from the inner central part of the cut leaf, which is usually used or processed when fresh—the leaf automatically seals itself so may need to be cut again several times.

Active constituents[278]
Latex

1) Hydroxyanthracene derivatives (min. 28%) of anthrone type including barbaloin (15–40% consists of the isomers aloin A and B),[279,280] emodin, aloe-emodin[281] and chrysophanol[282,283]
2) Chromone derivatives[284-286] including aloeresins of which up to 30% is aloeresin B or aloesin[287]

Also contains coumarins/dihydrocoumarins[288] and a number of aromatic substances mainly aldehydes.[289]

Gel

1) Carbohydrates (0.3%)
   a) polysaccharides (10%) consisting of units of mannose, glucose and galactose.[290]

Mannose, as mannose 6-phosphate,[291] is the predominant one and gives rise to the name mannans.[292-294] It includes the acetylated mannan, acemannan, which may have one or more polymers of various chain lengths.[277] Other polysaccharides include aloeride which contains predominantly glucose units.[295] The make-up is dependent on a number of variables such as subspecies, geographical location,[290] growing conditions[382] and extraction process[296]
   b) glucans (malic acid acylated carbohydrates)[297]
2) Glycoproteins[298] including lectins—aloctin I and II[299]

Also contains some hydroxyanthracene glycosides, triterpenoids including lupeol, phytosterols[300] including β-sitosterol[301] and campesterol, salicylic acid, prostanoids including arachidonic acid,[302] cholesterol,[302] choline,[302] a phthalate[303] and tannins. A number of amino acids[291] and enzymes have been identified in the gel including a peroxidase,[304] carboxypeptidase[305] and superoxide dismutase isozymes.[306]

There are four main medicinal species of Aloe although *A. barbadensis* is considered the most potent.[277]

Nutritional constituents
Vitamins: A, C, E and B vitamins including thiamine, riboflavin, niacin and folic acid
Minerals: Zinc, sodium, copper, potassium, manganese, iron, calcium and traces of chromium[307] and germanium[308]

Actions
Latex

1) Laxative

Gel

2) Vulnerary
3) Anti-inflammatory
4) Emollient

Scientific information

Aloe has been used for many centuries and in many different cultures, the latex as a purgative and food flavouring (bitters) and the gel for external healing. In recent times the gel has been of interest to the medical and cosmetic industries and this in conjunction with its widespread public use has generated a body of research. The gel has yielded contradictory results in the scientific literature and this may be explained by a number of factors as is the case with garlic. Firstly it is chemically complex, there are more than 75 biologically active constituents in the gel[277] and over 200 in the leaf, some of which are volatile and oxidise/degrade very rapidly on exposure to air.[309] In addition preparations may have varying levels of "contaminants" like hydroxyanthracene glycosides depending on the starting material and processing used,[382] indeed some preparations are actually derived from the whole leaf and contain both fractions.[277] Even though the gel is treated to stabilise it chemically (heated/treated with antioxidants), and keep it free of bacterial contamination, this does not necessarily ensure a stable product and new compounds may form during storage.[310]

Secondly the constituent(s) responsible for the pharmacological activity of the gel are uncertain and although acemannan has been assumed to be the main active there are a number of different constituents that have activity.[309] *In vitro* the polysaccharides are immune modulatory and anti-inflammatory, the glycoproteins are vulnerary with possible anti-tumour and anti-ulcer effects, the hydroxyanthracenes are purgative, anti-inflammatory, anti-oxidant and anti-proliferative. This makes standardisation a very complex task and as yet there are no accepted protocols for the extraction, processing and stabilisation of the raw material so that the end-products are inconsistent.[309,311] Not only has variable quality of commercial gel[312,313] (and latex[282]) products been reported but adulteration of the gel also occurs.[314]

Finally the fresh gel is pharmacologically different from that produced by processing. Gel preparations lose their UV protection activity as early as one month after processing[277] and whilst the fresh gel promoted cell growth and attachment, the processed gel was cytotoxic to normal as well as cancer cells.[291]

In vivo the mechanism behind the herb's actions is yet to be fully determined but it seems certain that the results of each trial product cannot easily be extrapolated to another due to their great variation. Currently there is greater interest in, and investigation into, the gel rather than the latex, particularly for topical use.

Immunomodulatory
In vitro—Different cells respond to the polysaccharide fraction, particularly acemannan,[315] by releasing cytokines[316] that stimulate immune function, However humans lack the necessary enzyme to break down acemannan[277] and its seems to pass through the digestive tract unchanged. Whilst it may have a local effect in the digestive tract it is considered unlikely that acemannan is responsible for any immunomodulatory effects attributed to aloe.[295] Aloeride, a potent immune stimulator/macrophage activator, although present at low concentration, possibly as a contaminant may in fact be responsible.[295]

Components of the gel activate complement and stimulate polymorphonuclear neutrophil activity whilst reducing the damage associated with free oxygen radicals.[317] However low molecular weight constituents in the gel may be cytotoxic.[318]

Antimicrobial
In vitro—As well as stimulating macrophage activity the latex has direct activity against *Leishmania* spp.[319] and the anthraquinones, aloin in particular, have antibacterial[320] and antiviral properties.[321] Aloin inhibits bacterial collagenase and may help moderate host cell damage during infection.[322]

The gel is active against *Shigella flexneri, Streptococcus pyogenes*[323] and *Trichomonas vaginalis*[324] and acemannan enhances macrophage destruction of *Candida albicans*.[277]

In vivo—Aloe was part of a preparation used to successfully treat HPV infections topically.[325]

Anticancer
In vitro—Constituents of *Aloe* (mostly hydroxyanthracene derivatives but also the phthalate) are anti-proliferative in a number of cancer cell lines,[326-332] inhibit angiogenesis,[333] are anti-mutagenic[303,334] and may have anti-carcinogenic[335]

activity. However emodin and aloe-emodin are both potentially genotoxic.[334]

In vivo—*Aloe* tincture added to melatonin seemed to be a promising treatment for intractable solid tumours.[336]

Vulnerary

Aloe gel has been subject to a number of tests related to wound healing and skin protection.

In vitro—Vulnerary actions that have been established for the gel or its constituents include:-

- increased growth of various connective tissue cells, including those derived from healthy and diabetic sources[337–341]
- protection of cells from radiation damage[342,343]
- promote angiogenesis (new blood vessel growth)[301]
- anti-oxidant activity[304]

Whole leaf extracts and aloe emodin[344] may however increase the potential for UVA light to cause oxidative damage to skin even though some of the anthraquinones are themselves anti-oxidants during irradiation.[345]

In vivo—Plant derived complex carbohydrates, including those of *Aloe*, protect the skin's immune system from UV damage.[346] However *Aloe's* vulnerary and cell-protection activities have produced contrary results possibly for reasons highlighted above. Benefits from topical application include:-

- aid to prevention of skin ulcers due to impaired circulation[347]
- increased skin hydration i.e. it is an effective moisturiser[348]
- improvement in occupational irritant contact dermatitis using gel-coated latex gloves[349]
- anecdotal resolution of a case of lichen planus[350]
- improvement in healing time, with reduced infection, in burns treatment[351,352]
- improvement of psoriasis,[353] (not corroborated)[354]

A preparation containing acemannan used topically after tooth extraction reduced the incidence of alveolar osteitis.[355]

Negative trials claim no clear benefit in treating aphthous ulcers,[356] pressure ulcers[357] or protecting or treating sunburn due to UVB light.[358] One study found the gel apparently delayed healing of surgical wounds.[359]

Aloe gel's use for radiation burns dates back to the 1930s when its benefits were reported in a number of cases. Some recent attempt has been made to validate these protective effects against radiotherapy damage. Again results have been mixed ranging from success[291,360] to no benefit either in topical form[361–363] or orally for mucus membranes.[364] These results have been reviewed.[365,366]

Anti-inflammatory

In vitro—Individual constituents of *Aloe* are anti-inflammatory—glucans,[297] chromone,[284] glycoprotein,[367] carboxypeptidase (inactivation of bradykinin)[305] and trace elements.[368] The whole leaf extract also inhibits 5-LOX activity[369] and the gel is anti-inflammatory in inflamed colorectal mucosal biopsy cells, through cytokine inhibition and anti-oxidant activity.[370] In fact leaf extracts of plants older than 2 years have exhibited stronger anti-oxidant activity than vitamin E[371]—an activity linked to the chromones[285] and dihydrocoumarins.[288]

In vivo—Aloe gel had no significant benefits for irritable bowel syndrome although it helped improve diarrhoea or alternating bowel habit whilst it was being taken.[372] It did however give some improvement, with apparent anti-inflammatory effects, in ulcerative colitis.[373]

Other

In vitro—The whole leaf extract inhibits cholinesterase activity[369] whilst the trace elements seem responsible for anti-spermicidal[374] and anti-diabetic[307] properties (this is a traditional use).[375]

In vivo—aloe gel preparations were found to:-

- slow down the rate but increase the level of absorption of vitamins C and E[376]
- increase excretion of precursors to kidney stone formation, so may be a prophylactic for lithiasis[377,378]

- reduce hyperlipidaemia particularly triglyceride levels[379]
- reduce blood sugar in diabetic patients[379] (not corroborated.[380] Reviewed[381,382])

The laxative actions are associated with the hydroxyanthracene derivatives—see *Cassia* spp. (senna).

Medicinal uses
Gastro-intestinal
- constipation (latex)

Externally
- burns
- wounds

Pharmacy
Once daily (latex)
Powder   – 50–200 mg
Tincture 1:40 (45%)   – 2–8 ml[383]

The laxative effect of aloe is due to aloin which passes through the digestive tract unchanged until it reaches the bowel where it is transformed to aloe-emodin-9-anthrone by intestinal bacteria,[277] an action that occurs 6–12 hours after ingestion. The laxative action involves increased water and electrolyte secretion in the colon which stimulates peristalsis[384]—(see *Cassia*).

Gel applied topically is best used fresh. The gel used orally to treat ulcerative colitis was a commercial product used at a dose of 100 ml twice a day but introduced at doses of 25–50 ml twice daily for 3 days to establish tolerability.[373]

CONTRAINDICATIONS—Intestinal obstruction and **abdominal pain** of unknown origin. Patients with haemorrhoids should rather be given bulk laxatives.

Precautions and/or safety
Latex—Should be combined with a carminative to reduce griping. This stimulating type of laxative should not be used for longer than 10 days. Possible minor side-effects are diarrhoea, *pseudomelanosis coli* (see *Cassia*), red coloured urine. More serious effects can result from overdose or chronic use such as hypokalaemia, electrolyte imbalance and renal damage. Steatorrhoea, hypoalbuminaemia and osteomalacia have also been reported.[291]

Gel—The incidence of contact allergy to aloe gel appears to be quite low[385] but there are reports of hypersensitivity,[386] disseminated dermatitis in a patient with stasis dermatitis,[291] photodermatitis[387] and severe dermatitis when used on skin that had been subjected to dermabrasion.[388] Internal gel use has been reportedly associated with *Henoch-Schonlein purpura*,[389,390] acute toxic hepatitis[391,392] and thyroid dysfunction (topical and internal use).[393]

Aloe gel may have genotoxic properties but it is not cytotoxic and does not appear to cross cell membranes.[394]

Pregnancy and lactation—anthraquinone metabolites of *Aloe* are secreted in breast milk and should be used cautiously[291] although more recent reviews have cleared *Cassia* and *Rhamnus* for use in this situation (see *Cassia*).

Interactions
There is a reported interaction between *Aloe* tablets taken prior to surgery and sevoflurane, an anaesthetic drug, which lead to increased bleeding during surgery.[395]

Other cautions are hypothetical rather than actually reported. One is the possibility that aloe may lower blood sugar and therefore care should be taken by those using hypoglycaemics. The other is that the latex may reduce the absorption of other drugs by decreasing intestinal transit time. Chronic use or abuse of *Aloe* latex which leads to hypokalaemia could potentiate the effect of cardiac glycosides, (like digitalis), or anti-arrhythmics and exacerbate potassium deficiency induced by thiazide diuretics or adrenocorticosteroids.

Historical uses
As for modern uses. Applied to fingernails to stop children biting them.

Chamaelirium luteum

Helonias root, false unicorn root

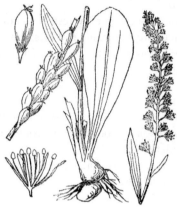

Family Liliaceae

Description
An erect, dioecious, perennial herb with tuberous roots, growing from 60–100 cm tall. Female plants taller and more leafy than male plants. *Basal leaves* spatulate to obovate, 7–15 cm long, in basal rosette. Stem leaves progressively reduced and narrowed upward along the stem. *Flowers* yellowish, in crowded spikes, usually drooping at the top, flowering from May to July in their native woods in North America.

Habitat and cultivation
Native to rich woods in West Massachusetts, New York to Florida, Arkansas to Illinois and Michigan. Also sometimes planted in shady places in American gardens.

Parts used
Rhizome and root, collected in autumn.

Active constituents
Little information is available as it is not a well studied plant.

1) Steroidal saponins, including diosgenin and its derivatives chamaelirin[1] (9.5%), helonin.

Also contains starch, calcium oxalate and an oleoresin.

Actions
1) Uterine tonic

Scientific information
There are no modern investigations into this herb. Its western history is closely allied to that of *Aletris farinosa* for which it seems to have been used interchangeably.[3] With the degree of confusion between the two and no scientific study into either herb it is difficult to know to what extent their actions have been confused and interchanged too. It is possible that *Chamaelirium* substituted for *Aletris* gave the latter herb its reputation for treating gynaecological problems. Likewise *Chamaelirium's* usefulness in treating gastro-intestinal problems may have been due to the presence of *Aletris*. This herb comes from the American Indian tradition.

Medicinal uses
Reproductive tract
The action is presumed to derive from the steroidal saponins:

- dysmenorrhoea[†]
- amenorrhoea
- infertility
- irregular menstruation
- leucorrhoea
- uterine prolapse
- pelvic congestion
- pelvic inflammatory disease

The herb is also reported to be useful for morning sickness in pregnancy and in threatened miscarriage, due to atony of the uterus.

Pharmacy
Three times daily

Decoction of dried root	– 1–2 g
Tincture 1:5 (45%)	– 2–5 ml
Fluid Extract (45%)	– 1–2 ml

[†]Associated with a dragging sensation.

Precautions and/or safety
In large doses it can cause nausea and vomiting. Chamaelirin is suspected of being cardiotoxic, large doses of the herb should be avoided.[1]

Historical uses
Anthelmintic; tonic for urinary and reproductive tracts; emetic and diuretic. A liver remedy to improve anabolism. Also for dyspepsia, colic, indigestion. Purported to alkalinise urine.

Convallaria majalis [Restricted Herb]

Lily-of-the-Valley

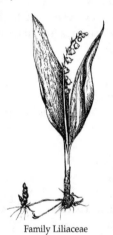

Family Liliaceae

Description
A perennial with a creeping rhizome. *Leaves* usually 2, elliptic, glabrous, glossy green 8–20 cm topping stems with papery sheathing bracts. *Flowers*, 5–10, pure white, sweetly scented and pendulous growing on one side of the curved stem, above a pair of leaves. Perianth broadly bell-shaped 6–8 mm with short, recurved, triangular lobes. *Fruit* bright red, globular, poisonous berries. Flowers mid spring to early summer.

Habitat and cultivation
Native to most of Europe and Britain, growing in dry woods and thickets on calcareous soils. Naturalized in north eastern North America. Cultivated in gardens for its beauty and fragrance. Grown from separated crowns and forms large patches if undisturbed.

Parts used
Leaves or whole plant harvested in flower. The fresh leaves are, according to *Weiss*, the strongest medicine followed by the flowers. The berries are highly toxic.

Active constituents[2]
1) Cardioactive glycosides (0.1–0.5%) including the cardenolides convallatoxin, convalloside, convallatoxol[396-399]
2) Steroidal saponins—progesterone has been reported in the leaves[400,401]
3) Flavonoids[402]

Other constituents include an analogue of the amino acid, proline[403] and chelidonic acid.[404]

Actions
1) Cardioactive
2) Cardiac tonic

Scientific information
Convallaria has been an official medicine in a number of countries.[383] Its acts like *Digitalis* to increase the excitability of heart muscle and its force of contraction and slows ventricular contraction, these actions being effected through electrolyte changes. It is considered a much safer remedy than *Digitalis*. The main active constituent is convallatoxin but its bioavailability is aided by some of the apparently non-active constituents of the herb. Used in Denmark to treat epilepsy, an extract was shown to have some affinity for GABA receptors in animal tissue *in vitro*.[405] **It is now a restricted herb**.

Medicinal uses
Traditional uses of the herb includes:-

• arrhythmia
• congestive heart failure[†]
• atrial fibrillation

[†]Especially that associated with bradycardia.

- oedema of cardiac origin and cardiac asthma
- angina
- coronary insufficiency
- hypotension

Precautions and/or safety
Convallaria is apparently a common cause of plant poisoning in children.[406] It can cause respiratory allergies due to the strong scent of the flowers.[407] Its main side-effects in overdose include arrhythmias, nausea, vomiting, diarrhoea, intestinal colic, headache, lethargy and visual disturbances (it is reported to affect colour perception[408]). However the herb is not known to have caused any human fatalities.[409]

Interactions
It is likely to interact with other cardiac glycoside containing medicines.

Smilax ornata and spp.

Sarsaparilla

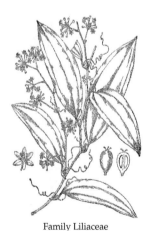

Family Liliaceae

Description
Evergreen vines to 4 m. *Stems* twining and trailing with paired tendrils growing from leaf axils. *Leaves* alternate, orbicular-ovate. *Flowers* small, greenish, in axillary umbels.

Taste—sweet and acrid, mucilaginous and almost odourless.

Habitat and cultivation
Native to tropical America in rich, moist soils in semi-shady, sheltered situations. Propagated from cuttings. The medicinal species are both drought and frost tender.

Parts used
Root and rhizome of spp. Those used are:
  S. aristolochiaefolia (*S. medica*)—Grey or Mexico Sarsaparilla
  S. febrifuga (*S. officinalis*)—Ecuador or Guayaquil Sarsaparilla
  S. ornata—Jamaica, Costa Rica or Red Sarsaparilla
  S. regelii—Honduras or Brown Sarsaparilla

Active constituents
1) Steroidal saponins (up to 3%) based on either smilagenin or sarsapogenin. Parillin and smilacin are glycosides of the latter, possibly formed as a by-product of processing[1,410,411]
2) Phytosterols including β-sitosterol and stigmasterol
3) Flavonoids including astilbin and its derivatives, smitilbin, resveratrol, dihydroxyquercetin and taxifolin[412–416]

Also contains proteins (smilaxin[417] and a lectin[418]), essential oil, phenylpropanoids, resin, starch, calcium oxalate and sarsapic acid.

Nutritional constituents
Vitamins: A, B complex, C and D
Minerals: Potassium (approx. 1.25%), iron, manganese, sodium, silica, sulphur, copper, zinc and iodine

Actions
1) Alterative
2) Anti-inflammatory
3) Antipruritic
4) Diuretic
5) Antiseptic
6) Antirheumatic

Scientific information
S. ornata was part of the medical tradition in a number of countries including China and

has been an official medicine throughout the world.[383,410]

Much of the chemical analysis of the steroidal saponins was undertaken many decades ago. However there is still ongoing research into the herb's constituents and their actions although this has comprised either *in vitro* or animal based studies. There are no modern clinical trials reported.

In vitro—*Smilax* was used traditionally to treat infectious conditions. It inhibits pathogenic dermatophytes[419] and the steroidal saponins have some antifungal activity against *Candida* spp.[410,411]

A decoction of *Smilax* is cytotoxic to liver cancer cells[420] (it has been used in combination with other herbs, to treat cancer in Sri Lanka).

Some of the constituents have been tested *in vitro*. Astilbin inhibits delayed type hypersensitivity and may reduce the inflammatory damage of auto-immune diseases[414] whilst smilaxin attenuates HIV-reverse transcriptase[417] and the lectin has antiviral activity against HSV-1 and respiratory syncytial virus.[418]

In vivo—Animal studies suggest *Smilax* may have hepatoprotective properties[415,421] and that it is anti-inflammatory, modulating cytokine release.[422]

Other research is now somewhat dated but includes its use in a herbal combination to benefit patients with chronic hepatitis B[423] and on its own to help in the treatment of leprosy[424,425] and psoriasis.[426]

Chinese uses of *Smilax* include detoxification, relief of dampness and joint problems and it has also been used to treat and prevent syphilis, leptospirosis, acute bacterial dysentery, acute and chronic nephritis.[414]

Medicinal uses
Musculoskeletal
- gout
- arthritis
- rheumatoid arthritis
- chronic rheumatism

Skin
- psoriasis
- eczema
- skin conditions

Pharmacy
Three times daily
Decoction of dried root   – 2–4 g
Fluid Extract (50%)   – 2–4 ml

Precautions and/or safety
May cause gastric irritation. It has been suggested the herb could lead to a temporary impairment of the kidneys although there is no apparent evidence to support this, it may relate to its calcium oxalate content. Contrary to this is the traditional understanding that it aids excretion of chlorides and uric acid (*BHC*), is a noted diuretic and is used in traditional Chinese medicine to treat nephritis.

Historical uses
As above. Also used in passive dropsy and venereal diseases. Asthma (smoke inhalation).

Trillium erectum

Bethroot, birthroot

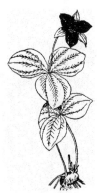

Family Liliaceae

Description
A perennial with a short thick rootstock, growing to 60 cm tall in flower. *Leaves* sessile, triangular oval, to 12 cm long, 3 in a single terminal whorl, subtending a flower on a peduncle 10 cm long. Sepals 3, green; petals spreading from the base, brownish-purple or purple, sometimes white, yellow or green, to 5 cm long, nearly erect, ill-scented. Ovary purple, fruit a dark red 6-angled berry with 3 seeds. Flowers from April to June in North America.

Habitat and cultivation
Originally native to North America in rich wood-lands from Nova Scotia to Georgia in mountain-ous regions, Florida, Tennessee to Michigan, and Ontario. It prefers rich, damp soils in protected shaded situations and may be grown from seed although germination is poor. It is generally trans-planted from the wild after flowering and may also be grown from division. Grown in similar situations to *Paeonia* (peony). Frost resistant but drought tender.

Parts used
The roots and rhizomes.

Active constituents
1) Steroidal saponins including trillarin, trillin, kryptogenin and diosgenin[427]
2) Steroidal glycosides
3) Tannins
4) Fixed oil

Actions
1) Antihaemorrhagic
2) Mild expectorant
3) Astringent

Other actions ascribed to the herb include partus praeparator, antiseptic and tonic.

Scientific information
The herb, used by American Indians to facilitate childbirth, was an official medicine in the USA. The chemical analysis was carried out many decades ago and the pharmacology is largely unexplored but the steroidal constituents must account for its action on the female reproduc-tive tract.
    While its haemostatic properties are largely employed in the reproductive tract it was also used to staunch bleeding elsewhere e.g. in the urinary and respiratory tracts.

Medicinal uses
Respiratory tract
In the symptomatic treatment of:

• haemoptysis

Urinary tract
In the symptomatic treatment of:

• haematuria

Reproductive tract
Used in the treatment of uterine bleeding but also as a tonic and astringent:

• menorrhagia
• metrorrhagia
• leucorrhoea

BHP specific for menopausal menorrhagia with depression.

Externally
• leucorrhoea (douche)
• vaginal infections (douche)
• indolent ulcers (poultice/ointment)

Pharmacy
Three times daily
Decoction of dried herb   – 0.5–2 g
Tincture 1:5 (40%)   – 1–4 ml
Fluid Extract (25%)   – 0.5–2 ml
    Used in combination with *Ulmus rubra* and *Lobelia inflata*, as powders, for ulcers.

Historical uses
Internally used for diarrhoea and dysentery; bron-chial problems—coughs—was called "cough root", diabetes. Externally for halting gangrene; tumours, insect stings.

Urginea maritima

White squill

Description
A large perennial bulb 10–15 cm across, from which arise, in autumn, long, leafless, unbranched flower stems 1–1½ m tall, bearing spikes of numer-ous spirally arranged flowers in a cylindrical clus-ter about 30 cm or more long. *Perianth* 8 mm long, white, with green or purplish midveins; anthers short and greenish. Flower stalks spreading and

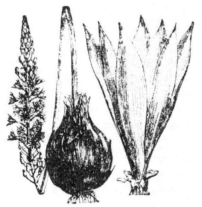

Family Liliaceae

2–3 times as long as bracts. *Leaves* appear only after flowering and persist into the following summer. They are large, lance-shaped 15–30 cm × 2½–10 cm slightly fleshy, smooth, flat and glossy. Bulbs are often partly exposed. Flowers in autumn.

Habitat and cultivation
Native to Mediterranean Europe, the Canary Islands and South Africa growing in sandy rocky places along the coast. Cultivated for medicine in Italy and Malta.

Parts used
The bulb collected soon after flowering, sliced and dried.

Active constituents
1) Cardiac glycosides of the bufadienolide type based on scillaren and scilliphaeosidin. There are also bufadienolides that are not glycosides[428–430]
2) Flavonoids based on quercetin and kaempferol and also glycosylflavones.[431,432]

Also contains mucilage, sinistrin (a fructan) and calcium oxalate.

Actions
1) Expectorant
2) Cardioactive
3) Diuretic
4) Cathartic
5) Emetic

Scientific information
This herb was known and used by ancient civilisations. The use of squill for treating coughs was supposed to have been discovered by Pythagoras in the 6th Century BC.[433] It was also used in medieval times to treat dropsy/oedema.

The cardiac glycosides like those of *Digitalis* and *Convallaria*, increase the force of contraction of the heart (inotropic)[434] thereby improving circulation and kidney function. However these glycosides are not well absorbed and the action of *Urginea* is much weaker than that of *Digitalis*.[383]

Its acts on the respiratory tract by reflex irritation of the gastric mucosa causing an increase in mucous secretions.[383]

Medicinal uses
It was used traditionally for treating:-

- chronic bronchitis
- pertussis
- mild cardiac insufficiency
- pulmonary catarrh
- asthma
- emetic (in large doses)

There is a variety of *Urginea maritima*, called red squill, which contains the toxin scilliroside, that was used at one time as a rat poison.[383]

CONTRAINDICATIONS—Hypokalaemia and **impaired renal function.**

Precautions and/or safety
The herb can cause nausea, vomiting, diarrhoea and reduced heart rate. In large enough doses it may be fatal[435] although the emetic action should offer some protection against the cardio-toxicity that would occur from overdosing.

Interactions
Should not be used with *Digitalis* or other cardiac glycoside medications.

LINACEAE

The Linaceae or flax family consists of about 14 genera of annual or perennial herbs or sometimes shrubs, of mainly temperate regions worldwide. Leaves simple, entire and usually alternate. Flowers mostly in cymes though sometimes corymbose, racemose or panicled; regular, in 4 or 5 parts. Fruit usually a capsule but sometimes a drupe.

Linum usitatissimum

Flaxseed, linseed

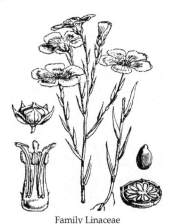

Family Linaceae

Description
A thin annual growing from 30–130 cm tall in flower. *Stems* erect, usually glabrous and simple but sometimes branching at the base. *Leaves* alternate, sessile, simple, linear to lanceolate, entire, glaucous green, 3–5 cm long and marked with 3 veins. *Flowers* pale to dark blue, sometimes white, 5-petaled, to 3 cm across in terminal leafy panicles, sepals ovate, half as long as the petals. *Capsule* longer than the calyx, containing 5 or 10 cells packed with shiny brown oblong, oval seeds narrowed at one end, 4–5 mm long. The capsule does not shatter to release seed. Flowers from late spring to early autumn.

Habitat and cultivation
Flax has been cultivated for its fibre and linseed oil for so long that no one knows its origin. It is an introduced crop in the southern hemisphere. It is also widely naturalised. It is always grown from seed sown where the plants are to stand and prefers a rich, moist soil and sunny situation. It is drought and frost tender. An improved type of *L. usitatissimum* containing omega 3 fatty acids is also available and is grown in the same way.

Parts used
The seed harvested when ripe.

Active constituents

1) Fixed oil (30–40%) mainly based on α-linolenic (55%) and linoleic acids—the proportions change according to growing conditions.[1] As the seed develops the former increases and the latter decreases[2].

2) Cyanogenic glycosides including mainly linus-tatin and neolinustatin[3,4]

3) Mucilage (up to 10%) mainly arabino-xylans[5,6] and galactoglucan[7] as part of dietary fibre

4) Lignans (0.7–1.5%)[8–11] mainly secoisolaricires-inol diglucoside[12,13] in the form of a polymer, also glycosides of matairesinol,[14] isolaricires-inol and pinoresinol[15]

Also contains dietary fibre (both soluble and insoluble up to 28%),[16] cinnamic glycosides[8] (p-coumaric and ferulic acids),[17] proteins (25%) and cyclic peptides,[18] a phenylpropanoid (linusitamarin),[19] β-sitosterol,[19] wax and sugar.

Nutritional constituents

Vitamins: B$_3$ (nicotinamide)[19]
Minerals: Calcium and potassium

Actions

1) Laxative
2) Demulcent
3) Antitussive
4) Emollient

Scientific information

Linum was an ancient Roman medicine although its origins are likely to pre-date this period. It has been an official medicine throughout the world, being used internally as a demulcent to treat coughs and as a bulk laxative and externally as a poultice to reduce inflammation.[20] *German Commission E* has approved its internal use for the treatment of chronic constipation, irritable bowel, diverticulitis, gastritis and enteritis and externally for local inflammation.

In traditional medicine linseed is used for conditions that benefit from the action of mucilage. The seeds which contain high levels of unsaturated fatty acid, particularly α-linolenic acid (ALA), have good nutritional value also. However the lignans

and their metabolites have been studied in recent times as they have been linked to benefits for the cardiovascular system, reduction of aromatase activity (an enzyme involved in hormone production) and possible inhibition of prostate and breast cancer.[21] As linseed has become a commercially successful health supplement it has been preferentially referred to as flaxseed possibly to disassociate it from its other uses—protecting wood and as a component of paint.

Cardiovascular effects

The oil has a very high level of ALA, one of the omega-3 fatty acids, which can be converted *in vivo* to the longer chain poly-unsaturated fatty acids associated with protection against cardiovascular disease.

In vivo—Long chain fatty acid levels in erythrocytes and plasma rose after 4 weeks supplementation of 50 g a day of ground linseed.[74] ALA supplementation from linseed has resulted in:-

• decreased levels of inflammatory markers[22]
• a reduction in markers of atherosclerotic development in dyslipidaemic patients[23]
• raised levels of eicosapentaenoic and docosahexaenoic acids[24] although levels may be lower than that achieved by using fish oil[25]
• small benefits equivalent to fish oil on haemostatic factors in dyslipidaemic patients[26]

There appears to be little benefit from using plant derived unsaturated omega-3 oils to treat raised serum lipids[22,27–29] although one study in which flaxseed oil was used with an appropriate diet, lipid profiles in overweight men did improve.[30]

The use of whole ground flaxseed to alter cardiovascular disease risk factors has yielded mixed results. Positive benefits in serum lipid levels were shown in:-

• young healthy women[74]
• post-menopausal women[31] including a group with mild hypercholesterolaemia[32]
• hyperlipidaemic patients[33,34]
• type 2 diabetes where it also reduced their blood clotting tendency[35]

Other trials showed there was no benefit to lipid profiles or cardiovascular health in already healthy people, from supplementing with lignans or ground flaxseed.[36-40]

Phyto-oestrogen

Linseed contains the highest levels of plant lignans in the edible plants so far studied.[41] These are metabolised by gut flora to the "mammalian lignans", predominantly enterodiol and enterolactone, via intermediate metabolites that are also likely to be bioactive.[42] These compounds are structurally similar to oestrogens and tamoxifen and appear to be both weakly oestrogenic and anti-oestrogenic.[43]

In vitro—Enterolactone and/or lignans induce apoptosis and inhibit the growth of colon cancer cells[44] and hormone dependent tumour cells.[45]

In vivo—The potential for the phyto-oestrogenic lignans to act as a natural HRT in post-menopausal women has been assessed. Studies failed to find any advantage in healthy post-menopausal women in reducing menopausal symptoms[36,46] or improving bone density[31,36,47] from supplementation with *Linum*. However flaxseed may be as effective as HRT in women with mild symptoms[48] and did reduce blood pressure in post-menopausal women with cardiovascular disease who were subjected to stress.[49]

Flaxseed alters hormone metabolism. Postmenopausal women who supplemented with it daily had decreased levels of 17 β-oestradiol and oestrone sulphate, increased prolactin levels[50] and increased excretion of oestrogen metabolites[51] all of which could be protective against breast cancer. (Diets rich in ALA and dietary fibre have been associated with a decreased incidence of some cancers.)[52,53] Flaxseed supplements given to women with primary breast cancer had reduced levels of proliferation and invasiveness of their tumours.[52]

Phyto-oestrogens are also potentially useful for prostate disease. A pilot study using a low fat diet and flaxseed supplement reduced proliferation of prostate cancers[53] and benign prostatic hyperplasia, growth rates were reduced without changing testosterone levels.[54] More information on these potential benefits is required as another study failed to corroborate benefits for prostate cancer treatment.[55]

Glucose control

In vivo—*Flax* meal increased bowel function (bulk laxative), improved postprandial blood glucose[48,56,74] and reduced insulin levels[48] whether taken in baked products or as ground meal.

Other

In vitro—Other actions for *Linum's* constituents include:-

- a cyclic nonapeptide with immunosuppressive,[57,58] antimalarial and anti-lipaemic activity[59]
- lignans,[60,61] their metabolites[62] and flaxseed oil[63] are anti-oxidant
- ALA may have anti-allergic, anti-atherogenic and anti-arrhythmic effects[64]
- secoisolariciresinol diglucoside has anticancer activity[61]

Ex-vivo—ALA from flaxseed oil does not seem to have the same beneficial anti-inflammatory potential as γ-linolenic acid of animal or plant origin.[65]

In vivo—Additional clinical data:-

- flax oil with vitamin C improved the symptoms of children with Attention Deficit Hyperactivity Disorder[66]
- the mucopolysaccharide fraction was successfully used in a mouth rinse to improve oral dryness due to Sjögren's syndrome[67]
- phyto-oestrogens including the lignans were beneficial in the treatment of chronic renal disease[68-70]

Medicinal uses
Respiratory tract
- respiratory catarrh
- bronchitis
- coughs

Gastro-intestinal tract
As a tonic laxative it may be used safely and long term for an over-relaxed bowel. Also for:

- pharyngitis
- gastritis

- mucosal inflammation
- chronic constipation from laxative over-use

Externally

As a poultice *Linum* is used to soothe:

- pleuritic pain
- bronchitis
- boils
- burns
- scalds

Pharmacy

Three times daily

Crushed or entire seeds	– 3–6 g
Infusion of the seeds	– 3–6 g

Ground flaxseed doses used in the above clinical studies have varied between 5–50 g per day with most using 20–40 g daily. *German Commission E* recommends 20–30 g daily.

The seeds of *Linum* can be used either whole or crushed however the bio-availability of lignans is greatly increased by crushing or better still by grinding them.[71] The lignans are heat stable, appear to store well, survive being baked[72] and if eaten with dietary fibre, their absorbance from the digestive tract is not impeded.[73] The fatty acids are also very well absorbed from the ground seeds.[74]

To achieve the bulk laxative effect the seeds should be taken whole or crushed, followed by drinking at least 1–2 glasses of fluid as this releases their mucilage. The seeds may need to be taken for a long time before bowel tone is restored and the immediate laxative effects too may require several days continuous intake to become effective.

The other way of using *Linum* is to first soak the seeds to extract the mucilage and then to use this internally as a demulcent or externally as an emollient. They may be applied after soaking in hot water (as a poultice), to draw boils.

CONTRAINDICATIONS—Stenoses of gastrointestinal tract or **ileus**.

Pharmacokinetics

After ingestion of flaxseed the gut flora convert lignans to enterolignans, the main one being enterolactone. They are absorbed by the intestinal cells and conjugated there or in the liver, mainly with glucuronide, becoming detectable in plasma some 8–10 hours later[75] and reaching peak plasma levels after 24 hours.[76] They occur with a variety of their metabolites in this conjugated form in plasma, serum and urine[77,78] but are present in faeces in their free form.[79] The plasma level of enterolignans attained varies from person to person[75] but is dose-related.[80]

Precautions and/or safety

There have been cautions issued regarding flaxseed use and studies have examined their veracity:-

1) The cyanogenic glycosides can degrade to release cyanide—these levels were non-toxic to humans[81]
2) Long chain fatty acids could delay spontaneous births—flaxseed oil did not effect delivery dates[82]
3) The lignans may alter female hormone levels— serum hormone levels of pre-menopausal women were unchanged after consuming flaxseed[73]

Flaxseed oil fed to fruit flies was genotoxic although the significance of this for humans is uncertain.[83] There are reported cases of anaphylaxis to the herb.[84,85]

Interactions

There is an anecdotal report of haematuria after flaxseed oil was used with aspirin, omega-3 fatty acids could have altered prostaglandin levels.[86]

Historical uses

In coughs and colds; for urinary tract irritations.

LOBELIACEAE

The Lobeliaceae is a family of about 25 genera of mainly herbs, mostly native to tropical regions. Leaves are alternate, sometimes in rosettes and without stipules. Flowers may be solitary or in racemes, spikes or panicles. Calyx and corolla both 5-lobed and the corolla petals are variously united, 1 or 2 lipped. There are 5 stamens and the fruit is fleshy and berrylike or a capsule containing many small seeds.

Lobelia inflata [Restricted Herb]

Lobelia, Indian tobacco

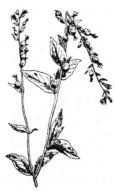

Family Lobeliaceae

Description
A hairy annual or biennial, often branched herb, 15–45 cm tall in flower. *Basal leaves* obovate to lanceolate, serrate, usually less than 7 cm long, hairy beneath. *Stem leaves* alternate, sessile, becoming smaller up the stem. *Flowers* small, inconspicuous, solitary, in racemes in the axils of the upper leaves. Corolla white to pale blue. The calyx tube inflates to 1.5 cm after the flower dies, enclosing the capsule containing many tiny, rough seeds. Flowers from mid summer onwards.

Habitat and cultivation
Lobelia is native to North America in fields, waste places and open woods from Nova Scotia to Georgia, Arkansas, east Kansas and north to Saskatchewan. It was introduced to other countries and is always grown from seed sown in autumn or spring and will self-sow in open sunny situations. Drought and frost resistant.

Parts used
The herb gathered when the lower fruits are nearly ripe.

Active constituents
1) Alkaloids over 20 of the piperidine type (0.2–0.6%) mainly lobeline also lobelanine, lobelanidine and allosedamine[1]
2) Carboxylic acids—chelidonic acid
3) Bitter glycoside—lobelacrin

Also contains a derivative of β-amyrin,[2] volatile oil, resin and gum.

Nutritional constituents
Vitamins: C
Minerals: Magnesium, phosphorus, potassium and calcium

Actions
1) Respiratory stimulant
2) Expectorant
3) Emetic
4) Spasmolytic
5) Diaphoretic
6) Anti-asthmatic

Scientific information
Lobelia has been an official medicine,[4] was used widely in North America and had enjoyed a prized place in herbal medicine as a respiratory stimulant but its effects were apparently unpredictable and it fell out of favour.[3] It was called Indian tobacco because it was smoked by Native Americans to get the same effect as that derived from nicotine in tobacco. **It is now a restricted herb.**

Lobeline, the main active alkaloid, has similar actions to nicotine, binding to the same receptor sites in nerve cells (nicotinic agonist) although it can also act as a nicotinic antagonist.[3] It is a neural depressant for autonomic, central and neuromuscular synapses although its initial effect is stimulating.[4] Lobeline stimulates the cough reflex,[5] is a respiratory stimulant (has been used to counter respiratory depression from narcotic overdose), broncho-relaxant, aid to expectoration, has cholinergic properties, increases dopamine levels, is emetic, may increase mucosal and lacrimal secretions, has mild appetite suppressant properties[6] and may be of use in the treatment of psycho-stimulant abuse.[7] However it has low bioavailability unless it is absorbed through the sublingual mucosa.

Medicinal uses
Lobelia is used for treating:-

• asthma
• chronic bronchitis
• pneumonia
• croup
• irritable bowel disease

Externally used as a lotion for:-

• muscle spasms
• myositis
• rheumatic nodules
• sprains

Externally as a plaster for:-

• acute bronchitis
• pleurisy
• intercostal myalgia

Precautions and/or safety
Lobelia in large doses can have side effects including diarrhoea, increased diuresis, nausea, vomiting, increased sweating, paresis, tachycardia, hypotension and coma. Over dosing is however rare as it induces vomiting and no fatalities due to it alone have been recorded.[8]

LOGANIACEAE

A dicot family of about 800 species of herbs, shrubs or trees, native to warm temperate or tropical regions. Some such as Buddleia, are grown as ornamentals and food for butterflies and others yield drugs and poisonous substances.

Gelsemium sempervirens [Restricted Herb]

Carolina jasmine, yellow jasmine

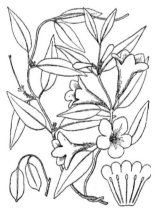

Family Loganiaceae

Description

An evergreen twining shrub growing to 6–7 m. *Leaves*, opposite, entire, lanceolate, narrow at the base, glossy green above and about 10 cm long. *Flowers* trumpet shaped, bright yellow, fragrant 4 cm long. Flowers most of the year.

Habitat and cultivation

Native to North America, from Virginia to Florida, west to Texas, and Central America. Grown as an ornamental vine over porches and trellises in many parts of the world. Propagated by seed or cuttings. Prefers a damp situation.

Parts used

Root and rhizome best collected in autumn and dried.

Active constituents

1) Alkaloids predominantly of indole type (min. 0.32%)[1] mainly gelsemine,[2] a number of others have also been characterised.[3]

Also contains coumarins, anthraquinones, volatile oil, resins and fatty acids.[4]

291

Actions
1) Analgesic
2) Sedative
3) Hypotensive

Scientific information
Gelsemium was an official medicine in the *United States Pharmacopoeia* from 1860 to 1926 although its historical use does not appear to date back much further than this time. There is no relevant modern research into this herb.

It was used to treat fever, inflammation of the gastro-intestinal tract, hypertension, asthma, whooping cough, croup, dysmenorrhoea, chorea, epilepsy and urinary retention. Its main use was due to its action as a nervous system depressant. **It is now a restricted herb.**

Medicinal uses
Gelsemium is used to treat:-

* migraine
* neuralgia particularly trigeminal neuralgia

CONTRAINDICATIONS—In hypotension, heart disease and myasthenia gravis.

Precautions and/or safety
It can cause dizziness, diplopia, ptosis, mydriasis and respiratory depression. These symptoms may take some hours to develop and can occur even with small doses. The herb has been associated with fatalities caused by respiratory arrest.

LORANTHACEAE

The Loranthaceae or mistletoe family consists of about 20 genera of erect or pendant
shrubs mainly semi-parasitic on both deciduous and evergreen trees. Mistletoes have green
leaves so they can produce some of their own food
by photosynthesis, but they gain water and inorganic nutrients by penetrating the host plant with
modified roots called haustoria. Their flowers are
pollinated by insects or birds and their fruits are
usually specialised for bird dispersal. The medicinal mistletoes are the European *Viscum album* and
the American *Phoradendron serotinum*.

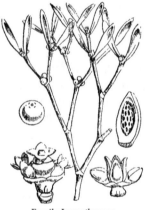

Family Loranthaceae

Viscum album

Mistletoe

Description
An evergreen semiparasitic plant found mainly
on the branches of deciduous trees. The green
branches are 40–60 cm long and regularly branching where flowers form in the branch axils. The
leaves are opposite, narrowly obovate, yellow-
green and leathery, to 8 cm long. *Flowers* sessile,
unisexual, pale yellow or green, in axillary inflorescences appearing from March to May in the

Northern Hemisphere. The female flowers develop
into sticky, translucent white berries which ripen
from September to November.

Habitat and cultivation
Viscum is native to Britain and parts of Europe and
Asia. It commonly grows on deciduous trees such
as apple and pear trees, as well as hawthorn, poplar and rarely oaks. It is also sometimes found on
evergreens such as larch. It is generally collected
from the wild and is spread by birds which eat the
berries and either excrete the seeds onto branches

293

or rub the seeds off their beaks onto branches when cleaning off the sticky fruit pulp. It may be semic-ultivated by squashing the berries onto branches to stick the seeds to the bark of host trees.

Parts used
The young leafy twigs harvested in early spring. **N.B.** *The French Pharmacopoeia specifies leaves only.*[1]

Active constituents
1) Cardioactive polypeptides—viscotoxins or thionins[2]—the composition of these varies with the host plant on which the mistletoe has grown[3,4]
2) Glycoproteins—lectins[4,5]
3) Triterpenes inlcuding oleanolic, betulinic and ursolic acids[6,7] and saponins based on oleanolic acid
4) Flavonoids including derivatives of naringenin[8]
5) Lignans including syringin and eleutheroside E[9]

Also contains mucilage, alkaloid,[10] choline,[11] tyramine, phenolic acids (21 different ones have been identified varying somewhat with the host plant),[12] a monoterpene glucoside,[13] polysaccha-rides[14] and a muco-inositol called viscumitol (mini-mum content 2.3%).

Nutritional constituents
Vitamins: B_{12}
Minerals: Calcium, sodium, magnesium, potas-sium, iron, iodine and copper

Actions
1) Hypotensive
2) Cardiac depressant
3) Sedative
4) Immunostimulant
5) Anticancer
6) Antispasmodic

Scientific information
Mistletoe has been used as a medicine for hundreds of years and was official in some European phar-macopoeias.[1] Although research into the traditional

uses of this herb does exist it was conducted some time ago and there is very little current information relating to oral extracts. The predominant modern interest is based on its anticancer potential. Aque-ous extracts of the herb e.g. *Helixor* and the better known fermented extract *Iscador* (developed by Rudolf Steiner, registered since the late 1960s) have been produced commercially and tested exten-sively both *in vitro* and in clinical trials.

Anticancer
In vitro—Various of *Viscum*'s constituents have displayed antitumourigenic properties includ-ing oleanolic, betulinic and ursolic acids,[6,7] the viscotoxins,[15,16] lectins,[15–17] alkaloids[10] and oligo-saccharides/polysaccharides.[18,19] Non-toxic levels of viscotoxins stimulate natural killer cell lysis of tumour cells.[20]

Whole herb extracts also have anticancer properties although this activity may alter with the host tree on which the herb was grown[21] and its time of harvest.[22] The whole aqueous extract enhances DNA repair following exposure to either γ-irradiation or genotoxic chemicals.[23,24]

It had been reported that low dose lectins seemed to stimulate the growth of six different human cancer cell lines but the action of the whole aqueous extract was subsequently found to be anti-proliferative in a dose and time dependent manner for these same cells.[25] A more recent *ex-vivo* study using leukaemia cells from children again showed that *Viscum* extracts *(Iscador)* at concentrations likely to be achieved *in vivo* seemed to increase the survival of these cells prompting safety concerns for its use in cancer.[26]

In vivo—The anticancer properties of *Viscum* have been strongly linked with the level of lec-tins which are considered to increase apoptosis,[27] inhibit angiogenesis and act as immunomodu-lators.[28] Clinical trials conducted to-date relate to aqueous preparations, whether fermented or not, being given by injection which is a dosage form that is not used by medical herbalists. Lec-tins are not stable in the gastro-intestinal tract and are not absorbed orally, hence the need to inject them although oral preparations in which they can survive digestion may become available.[28] These preparations are showing some promise in treating cancers (it is usually used with or after chemo- or radio-therapy) although more clinical data appears to be needed to make a definitive judgement. Clinical data has been reviewed periodically.[29-34]

Immunostimulant
In vitro—Aqueous fermented extracts and *Viscum* succus do not enhance phagocyte activity[35] however viscotoxins[36] do and whole extracts also increase chemotaxis[37] and modulate lymphocyte activity.[38] Immunostimulant activity is demonstrated by the polysaccharides.
In vivo—Injectable extracts of *Viscum* alter immune function however this action cannot be extended to oral use without further investigation.[39,40]

Other
In vitro—Extracts of *Viscum* are:-

* anti-oxidant—the level of which varies with the host tree on which the herb was grown and the time of year it was harvested[41]
* vasodilatory by inducing nitric oxide production[42]—human models demonstrating this are lacking
* inhibitory to platelet aggregation[43]
* inhibitory to α-glucosidase[44] (traditionally used in Turkey and the West Indies to treat non-insulin dependent or type 2 diabetes)
* inhibitory to human parainfluenza virus type 2, a water extract being the most effective[45]

In vivo—Although no current investigations have been conducted with respect to the effect of *Viscum* on blood pressure *Martindale* specifies it has a vasodilatory action that peaks after 3–4 days.[1]

Medicinal uses
Cardiovascular system
Used in the treatment of high blood pressure. *Weiss* says of this herb that it will not lower blood pressure markedly if it is very high but it gives very good symptomatic relief of symptoms of hypertension. He says also that it is effective with moderate to slight hypertension and advocates it be used as a tea:

* hypertension
* arteriosclerosis
* hypertensive headaches
* nervous tachycardia

Nervous system
* hysteria
* chorea

Pharmacy
Three times daily
Infusion of dried herb	–	2–6 g
Tincture 1:5 (45%)	–	0.5 ml
Fluid Extract (25%)	–	1–3 ml

Precautions and/or safety
The berries have been known to cause gastroenteritis. Normal medicinal preparations used at the recommended doses are not toxic or genotoxic.[46,47]

Historical uses
A heal-all; for spleen; tumours; epilepsy for which it was specific; apoplexy; palsy; delirium; neuralgia; nervous debility; urinary disorders; sterility; heart tonic in typhoid fever; internal haemorrhage. Externally to cure ulcers and sores; to draw out "bad nails".

MALVACEAE

There are about 200 species of Malvaceae in the world. They consist of shrubs and trees or herbaceous annuals and perennials with mucilage canals, fibrous stems and usually star-shaped hairs.

The most important member of the Malvaceae is *Gossypium herbaceum*, cotton, and the most commonly grown ornamentals are *Hibiscus* and *Abutilon*.

A number of wild mallows grow in pastures and waste lands but only *Althaea officinalis* and *Malva sylvestris* are used in herbal medicine.

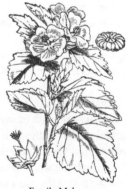

Family Malvaceae

Althaea officinalis

Marshmallow

Description

A perennial herb which dies back in winter. The whole plant is covered with soft, dense, velvety down. *Root* white, thick, long, tapering, pliant and sweet-tasting. *Leaves* alternate, stalked, broadly ovate, undivided or 3-lobed, lower leaves 8 cm long, often cordate at the base, upper leaves narrow. *Flowering stems* erect, branched to 1–1.5 m in flower. Individual flowers small, pale rose coloured, growing on short pedicels in axils of the upper leaves and in almost leafless terminal spikes. Calyx 5-lobed. *Fruit*, called a cheese because of its rounded wheel shape, consists of kidney shaped brown seeds packed tightly together. Flowers mid to late summer.

Odour—root faint, characteristic and somewhat mealy; taste—mucilaginous and sweet, leaves taste mucilaginous.

Habitat and cultivation

Native to Southern Europe, Britain and Northern Asia in marshes, mostly by the coast. Widely cultivated elsewhere and naturalised in North

296

American salt marshes. Grown from seed and self-sows, it also grows from root division in winter when dormant. Grows in gardens in open, sunny situations with moist soils. Frost resistant but drought tender.

Parts used
The leaves gathered when the plant is in flower. The root collected from the second year onwards, in autumn.

Active constituents
Roots
1) Mucilage (up to 20%) consisting of polysaccharides including galacturonan[1]
2) Tannins (2%)
3) Volatile oil
4) Pectin (up to 35%)

Also flavonoids,[2,3] phenolic acids[2] and asparagine (1–2%)

Leaves
1) Mucilage (up to 10%) consisting of polysaccharides[4] including glucan and glucuronoxylans[5]
2) Flavonoids[3]—kaempferol and quercitin
3) Coumarin—scopoletin
4) Polyphenolic acids including caffeic, salicylic and vanillic acids

N.B. The *BHC* states that the content of mucilage in the root is about 11% in late autumn declining to 6% in mid summer and that the levels reported in other sources are invariably overstated, possibly from inclusion of the polysaccharide fraction.

Nutritional constituents
Vitamins: Very high in vitamin A. It also contains vitamin B complex
Minerals: Calcium, zinc, iron, sodium and iodine

Actions
Leaf and root
1) Demulcent
2) Emollient
3) Diuretic

In addition:

4) Vulnerary (root)
5) Expectorant (leaf)
6) Antilithic (leaf)

Scientific information
Althaea has been used medicinally for thousands of years, first recorded use occurring in the 9th Century BC. *German Commission E* has approved use of leaf and root for irritation of oral and pharyngeal mucosa and associated dry cough and the root for mild gastric inflammation.

There are few current studies available although both leaves and root have been official preparations all over the world.[6]

In vitro—The herb is active against periodontopathic bacteria[7] and reduces the development of melanin pigmentation and melanocyte proliferation after UVB irradiation.[8] The polysaccharides are anti-oxidant[5] and immunostimulating.[9]

In vivo—Marshmallow has been used traditionally for the symptomatic relief of coughs, the mucilage being considered the main active constituent. A herbal mix which included marshmallow root mucilage helped alleviate coughs[10,11] including that associated with the use of angiotensin-converting enzyme (ACE) inhibitors.[12]

Medicinal uses
Respiratory tract
• coughs
• bronchitis
• respiratory catarrh

Gastro-intestinal tract
The mucilage content in the root is in sufficiently high quantities to directly soothe the intestinal mucosa. Mucilage also reduces peristalsis and the sensitivity of the mucosa to irritants:

• gastritis
• peptic ulcers
• enteritis
• ulcerative colitis
• colitis

Urinary tract
• cystitis
• urethritis
• urinary calculus

Externally
Both parts of *Althaea* can be used locally to soothe, and in the case of the root, to aid healing too:

• abscesses
• boils
• ulcers
• lacerations
• inflammation of pharynx/mouth (root, as a gargle)

Pharmacy
Leaf and root
Three times daily
Infusion/decoction   –   2–5 g
Tincture 1:5 (25%)   –   5–15 ml (suggested guidelines)
Fluid Extract (25%)   –   2–5 ml

As an ointment/cream the root or leaf can be added, powdered, to the base to give a 5–10% concentration of herb.

Interactions
It is possible the mucilage may delay absorption of other medicines consumed at the same time.

Historical uses
A cure-all; speed and ease delivery of babies; as a compress with honey for all swellings of the eyes; as a poultice to soften tumours, a hard liver and spleen; for swellings of the testicles; for skin problems and to stop hair falling out; gentle laxative; to ease the passage of stones; to soothe a sore chest and help hoarseness and coughs; to stimulate the kidneys. Also for bruises and sprains; aches in muscles or sinews.

MENYANTHACEAE

This is a family of 5 genera of aquatic or subaquatic perennial herbs with free-floating or rooted stems. They are native to tropical, subtropical or temperate regions especially of Asia and were, until recently, included in the Gentianaceae. Leaves are usually alternate, but may be opposite on flowering shoots, and the petioles are sheathed at the base. Flowers may be in bunches, or in racemes or cymes, and are in parts of 5.

Menyanthes trifoliata

Bogbean, buckbean

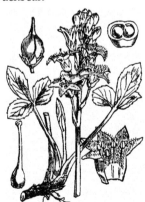

Family Menyanthaceae

Description
A glabrous perennial herb with a stout rhizome. Petiole may be up to 40 cm long in water but only 5–10 cm long in drier conditions: basal sheaths purplish. *Leaves* alternate and entire with 3 leaflets, 5–13 × 2.5–9 cm, obovate to elliptic, lateral leaflets somewhat asymmetric; apex rounded or obtuse, base cuneate. *Flowers* in racemes produced on a leafless scape with pedicels greater than the calyx. *Calyx* lobed nearly to the base, about 4 mm long, lobes narrow-triangular, obtuse. *Corolla* 12–14 mm long, white, flushed with pink on the back of the petals which are longer than the tube and reflexed with a fimbriate crest 1–3 mm long. *Capsule* is ovoid, 2-valved. Flowers from spring to autumn.

Habitat and cultivation
Native to northern temperate Europe, Asia and North America in still, shallow water in marshes and bogs. Grows from seed in spring or root division in spring or autumn, in acid, peaty soil in permanently wet places. Frost resistant but drought tender.

Parts used
The leaves, collected after flowering.

299

Active constituents[1]

1) Iridoid glycosides including dihydrofoliamen-thin, loganin and menthiafolin[2,3]
2) Flavonoids including rutin, hyperoside and trifolioside[4]
3) Coumarins including scopoletin and scoparone
4) Phenolic acids[5] including caffeic acid also van-illic and ferulic acids
5) Alkaloids including gentianine and gentialutin
6) Saponins including the triterpenoid menyanthoside
7) Essential oil

Also contains sterols, polysaccharides[6] and pectin.

Nutritional constituents
Vitamins: C and carotene
Minerals: Manganese and iodine

Actions
1) Bitter
2) Diuretic
3) Laxative in high doses

Scientific information
Buckbean has been an official medicine in a number of different European pharmacopoeias as a recognised bitter.[7]

In vitro—It inhibits prostaglandin production[8] and its polysaccharides are immunostimulating.[6]

Medicinal uses
Gastro-intestinal tract
Through its bitter taste:

- anorexia
- dyspepsia
- loss of appetite

Musculoskeletal
- rheumatism
- rheumatoid arthritis
- muscular rheumatism

Pharmacy
Three times daily
Infusion of dried leaves   –   0.5–2 g
Tincture 1:5 (25%)   –   2–6 ml
Fluid Extract (25%)   –   0.5–2 ml
  CONTRAINDICATIONS—Diarrhoea, colitis, dysentery.

Precautions and/or safety
Large doses may cause vomiting.[7]

Historical uses
Internally to treat scurvy; skin diseases; ague. Externally to dissolve glandular swellings. Fresh leaf succus for dropsy and gout.

MONIMIACEAE

This family consists of about 30 genera of tropical and subtropical trees and shrubs with usually opposite, simple, aromatic leaves and inconspicuous flowers. The fruit is an achene or drupe.

Peumus boldo

Boldo

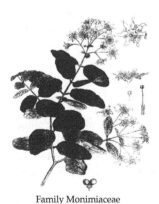

Family Monimiaceae

Description

An aromatic evergreen shrub to 8 m. *Leaves* opposite, entire, broadly ovate to ovate-elliptic, to 5 cm long, somewhat revolute, grey green. Young leaves pilose on both surfaces; mature leaves glabrous and dotted with oil glands on the upper surface. *Flowers* in terminal cymose panicles, perianth tube campanulate with 10–12 spreading segments. Stamens many, 3–5 carpels and fruit 2–5, each 1-seeded.

Odour—strongly spicy and characteristic; taste—pungent spicy and somewhat bitter.

Habitat and cultivation

Native to the Chilean Andes, Boldo has been introduced elsewhere and grows on sunny slopes in the Mediterranean region.

Parts used

The leaves.

Active constituents

1) Volatile oil (2%) including mainly p-cymene and ascaridole the proportions of each varying with genetic make-up.[1] Also cineole, limonene and β-phellandrene[2]
2) Alkaloids[3,4] (up to 0.7%) including the predominant aporphine alkaloid, boldine (0.009%[1]–0.14%[5])
3) Flavonoids including the phenolic catechin[6–8]
4) Glycoside (0.3%)—boldoglucin

Also contains tannins and resins.

Actions
1) Cholagogue
2) Diuretic
3) Liver stimulant
4) Sedative
5) Mild urinary antiseptic/demulcent

Scientific information
It seems *Peumus* was known for its medicinal properties thousands of years ago. *German Commission E* has approved it for the treatment of mild dyspepsia and spasms in the gastro-intestinal tract.

Although it has been an official medicine both as a diuretic (herb) and to treat liver congestion (boldine)[9] recent interest has been rekindled in this herb based largely on the exploration of the properties of boldine.

In vitro—*Peumus* is a strong anti-oxidant.[10,11] This action appears to be due to both catechin[6] and boldine[5,12] and whilst the latter is the stronger it occurs at much lower levels than catechin. The herb is protective against oxidative damage due to visible light[13] and boldine is protective against UVB irradiation.[14]

Catechin is an inhibitor of both COX-1 and COX-2 and therefore has anti-inflammatory potential.[6]

Boldine, in addition, appears to have cyto-protective[12] and hepato-protective properties,[15] is active against the organism responsible for Chagas' disease—*Trypanosoma cruzi*[16]—and has immuno-modulating activity.[17]

Ascaridole is anthelmintic[18] and potentially toxic. The essential oil is antimicrobial.[2]

In vivo—The herb slows intestinal transit time probably by acting as a local muscle relaxant in this system.[19]

Medicinal uses
Gastro-intestinal tract
• cholelithiasis (*BHP* specific)
• gall bladder and liver pain

Urinary tract
• cystitis

Musculoskeletal
• rheumatism

Pharmacy
Three times daily
Infusion dried leaves – 60–200 mg
Tincture 1:10 (60%) – 0.5–2.0 ml
Fluid Extract (45%) – 0.1–0.3 ml

Precautions and/or safety
Peumus and boldine are considered to have low toxicity.[15] Tests conducted to-date found boldine is not teratogenic.[20,21] Due to its tannins, boldo tea may inhibit iron, zinc or copper absorption if consumed around meal times.[22]

There is a reported case of anaphylaxis occurring after drinking boldo tea.[23] There are also two anecdotal reactions reported, one of cardiac disturbance[24] and one of raised liver enzymes levels in a fatty liver patient.[25] Both had used over-the-counter products containing boldo, which was cited as the suspected cause.

Interactions
The INR was increased in a patient who was taking warfarin concurrently with a variety of natural products, one of which contained fenugreek and boldo. Although nothing untoward occurred, this combination was held to be the most likely culprit.[26]

Historical uses
Headache, earache; nervous weakness, dropsy, dyspepsia, menstrual cramps; as an antiseptic. In its native South America also used to treat gonorrhoea. Boldine was used by veterinary doctors for jaundice. *Potter's* suggest this herb is an aid to slimming.

MYRICACEAE

The Myricaceae, bayberry or wax myrtle family consists of 2 genera of widely distributed monoecious and dioecious trees and shrubs.

- Leaves alternate, simple or pinnatifid
- Flowers small, unisexual, in axillary spikes or catkins; perianth lacking; stamens 2–16; ovary 1-celled
- Fruit a small drupe or nutlet

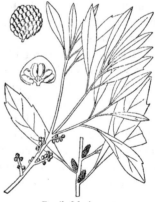

Family Myricaceae

Myrica cerifera

Bayberry

Description
Fragrant perennial, more or less evergreen, branching shrub or tree from 1–10 × 3 m, with smooth, greyish bark. Male or female. *Leaves* alternate, oblong-lanceolate, acute, entire to sharply serrulate above the middle, glabrous, shining above and resinous with oil glands, 3–7.5 cm long. *Flowers* short globular (female), or conical (male), scaly, yellowish catkins. *Fruit* green at first then greyish-white, waxy, spherical, one-seeded berries appearing in clusters in late spring to mid-summer and persisting for 2–3 years on female shrubs.

Habitat and cultivation
Native to eastern North America from New Jersey to Florida, on poor, moist, sandy soils, in fields, woodlands and thickets near the sea. It is grown from seed or cuttings. It is a wild plant not generally cultivated. Frost resistant, drought tender.

Parts used
Root bark collected in late autumn. The berries and occasionally leaves may also have been used but are not commonly part of the *materia medica*.

Active constituents
1) Tannins, mostly of hydrolysable type; also the phenolic tannic and gallic acids[1]
2) Resin—myricinic acid
3) Triterpenes including taraxerol, taraxerone and myricadiol[2]
4) Flavonoids including myricitrin[2]

Also contains trace amounts of volatile oil and gum.

Nutritional constituents
Vitamins: C

Actions
1) Astringent
2) Circulatory stimulant
3) Diaphoretic

Scientific information
Myrica was an officially recognised astringent.[1] The tannins and their physiological properties must contribute largely to its actions.

In vitro—It is a good inhibitor of thrombin.[3] Myricitrin is a strong anti-oxidant.[4]

There is no modern research into the herb although related species have been studied.

The use of the herb has been wide ranging especially in the physiomedical tradition. It was, and is, used in combination with other herbs to enhance their actions. It can be used in any situation requiring astringency and a stimulant effect.

Medicinal uses
Cardiovascular system
• fevers
• haemorrhages

Respiratory tract
• colds

Gastro-intestinal tract
• diarrhoea
• mucous colitis (specific *BHP*)

Externally
• leucorrhoea (douche)
• sore throat (gargle)
• wounds (poultice)
• indolent ulcers (poultice)
• nasal congestion (snuff)

Pharmacy
Three times daily
Decoction of dried herb   –   0.6–2 g
Fluid Extract (45%)   –   0.6–2 ml
Potter's quotes larger doses for dried bark and fluid extract to a maximum dose of 4 g and 4 ml respectively, three times daily.

Precautions and/or safety
Large doses of *Myrica* are emetic.[1]

Historical uses
Many uses including jaundice; scrofula; eruptive fevers; dysentery; cholera; goitre; boils; cankers; carbuncles and catarrh. The powder in snuff is sternutatory. Also used as a tonic, vermifuge, anti-inflammatory and analgesic.

Used in Thomson's Composition Powder (no. 6).

NYMPHACEAE

A dicot family of 8 genera of aquatic plants. The long-stemmed leaves are usually large and arise from submerged roots to float on the surface of ponds and lakes. Flowers solitary, regular and beautiful.

Nymphaea odorata

White water lily, white pond lily

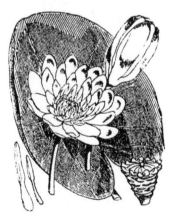

Family Nymphaceae

Description

A hardy robust perennial aquatic plant which dies back in winter. *Leaves* simple, orbicular apart from a cleft where the stalk is attached, growing singly on long petioles from a horizontal rhizome to float on the surface of the water. Green above, reddish below and when young. *Flowers* large, 8–20 cm in diameter, with 3–5 green-backed sepals. Petals white, numerous, united to the ovary. Stamens many, carpels many with yellow stigmas. Single buds develop under water and rise to float on the surface when they open. Flowers close at night and open for 2–3 days before withdrawing under water again. Blooms in summer.

Odour—slight; taste—mucilaginous and slightly pungent.

N. odorata is native to North America and is considered synonymous with *N. alba*.

Habitat and cultivation

Native to Great Britain and Europe except in the extreme north. Grows in sheltered parts of lakes, slow moving streams, ponds, canals and dykes. Also grows in North America and elsewhere as an ornamental pond plant. Propagated by seed or division of rhizomes in winter. Prefers slightly acid water rich in nutrients up to 3 m deep. It may be increased from seed or by dividing the rhizomes. Duck and other water birds eat the foliage and kill the lilies and fish will loosen the roots if containers of rich soil are not weighted down with stones.

Parts used
The dried rhizome and/or root collected in autumn or spring.

Active constituents
The roots and rhizomes have not been well studied or characterized.

1) Polyphenols mainly tannins (hydrolysable) and derivatives of gallic and tannic acids[1]
2) Flavonoids

Also mucilage and probably some alkaloids (*Nymphaea* species have been used historically as hallucinogens all over the world).[2] The roots and rhizomes readily accumulate ions of elements like iron, manganese, copper, phosphorus, calcium, chromium but may also take up undesirable heavy metals like cadmium.[1,3,4]

Nutritional constituents
Vitamins: C

Actions
1) Astringent
2) Demulcent
3) Antimicrobial

Scientific information
There are no human-related studies into the medicinal benefits of this herb and only a very few animal studies that indicate potential benefits due to its anti-oxidant activity.[5,6] This would accord well with the suggested high levels of polyphenols, known to be strong anti-oxidants, which are found in *Nymphaea*.[1] The tannin and mucilage content probably account for the modern uses listed.

Anecdotally, it has been recorded as an effective treatment for uterine cancer.

Medicinal uses
Gastro-intestinal tract
• chronic diarrhoea

Externally
• pharyngitis (gargle)
• boils (poultice)
• leucorrhoea (douche)
• vaginitis (douche)

Pharmacy
Three times daily
Decoction of dried herb   – 1–2 g
Fluid Extract (25%)   – 1–4 ml

Historical uses
Dysentery, gonorrhoea, scrofula; bronchial and urinary problems; fluxes in men and women. Externally: inflamed mucous membranes and skin.

OLEACEAE

A dicot family of about 29 genera of trees or shrubs, growing in temperate or tropical regions in both hemispheres. The olive is the best known and many other members of the family are grown in parks and gardens as ornamentals.

Chionanthus virginicus

Fringe tree

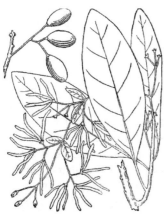

Family Oleaceae

Description
A deciduous shrub or small tree growing from 2–7 m tall. *Leaves*, opposite, entire, oval, over 20 cm long, glabrous or downy, glossy green, turning yellow in autumn. *Buds* on previous year's growth develop into long stems with numerous delicate, fringe-like white flowers in 10–20 cm long panicles. (*Chionanthus* means "snow flower".) *Fruits* blue-black oval elongated fleshy drupes with 1–3 seeds. Flowers from late spring to mid-summer.

Odour—none; taste—very bitter.

Habitat and cultivation
Native to North America from Pennsylvania to Florida and west to Texas. Available from garden centres and cultivated in all temperate regions. Propagated by seed or cuttings and grown in moist, sandy, loam soils in sunny situations.

Parts used
The root bark collected in autumn.

Active constituents
1) Lignans including phillyrin, pinoresinol and their glucosides[1]

307

2) Secoiridoids including oleuropein, ligustroside and angustifolioside B[1]
3) Saponins including chionanthin

The bark constituents are very poorly characterised.

Actions
1) Cholagogue
2) Laxative
3) Anti-emetic
4) Hepatic stimulant

Scientific informaion
The herb was an official medicine in the USA however there is very little scientific research available on any aspect of it. Its use is therefore reliant on tradition where it was considered of great value in treating liver-related diseases predominantly but also feverish conditions.

In vitro—The lignans have good anti-oxidant properties.[2]

Medicinal uses
Gastro-intestinal tract
Used for:-

• cholelithiasis
• hepatitis/jaundice
• portal hypertension
• glycosuria of hepatic origin
• duodenitis
• cholecystitis
• splenomegaly

Pharmacy
Three times daily

Decoction of dried herb	– 2–4 g
Fluid Extract (25%)	– 1–3 ml
Tincture 1:5 (45%)	– 2–3 ml

Historical uses
Fevers (typhoid, intermittent and bilious); dyspepsia including that of infants, gastritis due to alcohol, pancreatic disease; scrofula; syphilis; as a diuretic, nephritis; as a tonic, cachexia; to aid recovery from exhaustive illness. Externally for wounds, ulcers and inflammations.

Olea europaea

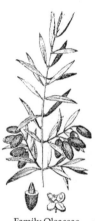

Family Oleaceae

Olive

Description
A long-lived evergreen tree growing to 10 m with a greyish deeply grooved trunk. *Leaves* elliptic-lanceolate over 7 cm long, leathery, green above, silvery beneath growing in opposite pairs. *Flowers* small, greenish-white in panicles, corolla tube short with 4 lobes. *Fruit* an oblong drupe, to 4 cm long, fleshy, green at first becoming glossy black when ripe. Many cultivars are available for oil.

Habitat and cultivation
Olives are native to the Mediterranean area where they have been cultivated for centuries as a source of oil. They are also cultivated worldwide in areas with a similar Mediterranean-type climate. Trees may be propagated by softwood cuttings or from suckers taken with a heel from around the tree trunk. They may also be grown from seed but seedling-grown trees are usually grafted later. They need a deep fertile well-drained soil to thrive. Drought resistant, frost tender.

Parts used

Leaves gathered throughout the year. Historically it has been the fruit and its oil that was valued in medicine. Both are still recognised in modern medicine for their contribution to a healthy diet although the oil is no longer used directly as a medicine. The fruit gathered green or ripe for pickling and ripe to be pressed for oil.

Active constituents

1) Phenolics[3] including mainly:-
   a) secoiridoids[4,5] predominantly oleuropein (6–9%),[6] also derivatives of elenolic acid and hydroxytyrosol—actual levels of these vary particularly with the age of leaf (green leaves are richer in oleuropein)[7] but also to some extent with variety of olive,[8] method of processing and time of harvesting[8]
   b) flavonoids mainly derived from luteolin, also rutin and apigenin derivatives[6,9–11]
   c) phenylpropanoids including verbascoside,[9] caffeic,[6] p-coumaric and ferulic acids[12]
2) Triterpenes of oleanane type including oleanolic and betulinic acids[13]
3) Volatiles including aldehydes, sesquiterpenes and monoterpenes[14,15]

Also contains a xylitol (0.5–1%)[16] and β-sitosterol.[17] Apart from the unsaturated fatty acids, the oil also contains phenolics similar to those found in the leaf[18] and melatonin, the levels of the latter being higher in virgin than refined oil.[19]

Nutritional constituents

Vitamin: A and E

Actions

1) Hypotensive
2) Diuretic
3) Antiseptic
4) Spasmolytic

Scientific information

The oil has been an official preparation and is much better documented for medicinal use. The leaves have enjoyed a limited reputation in traditional medicine without having been registered officially. Recent studies on the leaf extract and/or its constituents have driven some of its current applications in proprietary natural medicines. However these uses are not supported by traditional medicine and are yet to be fully validated.

Anti-oxidant

In vitro—All the phenolic constituents are very good anti-oxidants,[20,21,35] they appear to work synergistically,[22] giving the whole leaf a very strong activity.[23] This action protects cells from oxidative damage.[24] Oleuropein, the main active constituent (also considered the bitter principle of the herb),[12] slows down the aging of fibroblasts.[25]

As the processes of oxidation are believed to be behind the initiation of a number of diseases it is the anti-oxidant action that forms the basis of a good deal of the recent research into Olea.[12] It is likely that this action, found in the oil and fruit also, is at least in part responsible for its epidemiological link of reduced risk of heart disease in the Mediterranean countries where they are routinely consumed.

Antimicrobial

The leaf has antiviral activity against HIV-1[26] as well as providing cells with protection from infection by the virus. The secoiridoids contribute to this activity by blocking viral attachment to host cells.[27,28]

Aqueous leaf extracts have broad spectrum antibacterial activity[29,30] including against Staphylococcus aureus[31] and dermatophytes including Candida albicans.[29] Hydroxytyrosol, oleuropein, elenoate and the aldehydes all have a wide range of antimicrobial activity.[14,32–35]

Other

In vitro—The leaf inhibits the growth of leukaemia cells and encourages them to differentiate.[36] It inhibits platelet aggregation and may be anti-inflammatory.[37] The phenolic fraction is also anti-inflammatory.[20]

Some of the phenylpropanoid acids are well absorbed through the skin where they can prevent oxidative damage due to ultra-violet irradiation.[38]

In vivo—One clinical trial undertaken in 1996 showed the leaves were hypotensive[39] an action for which they have been used traditionally.[40] This may be due in part to the spasmolytic effect on blood vessels which has been demonstrated in animals only so far. Leaves have also been used in some traditions to treat diabetes.[40]

There are no *in vivo* studies reported into the effectiveness of the leaf in preventing or treating microbial infections, the claims for this action appears to be by extrapolation from *in vitro* research and/or anecdotal reports. The *in vivo* absorption of some phenols, particularly oleuropein, is still to be established, and it has been suggested that the large size and particular configuration of this molecule may mean that this is poor[37] (see Pharmacokinetics).

Medicinal uses
Cardiovascular system
The vasodilatory effect of the leaves would explain its traditional use in fevers and for aiding:

• hypertension

Weiss has described the herb as being suitable for "labile and medium-severe hypertension".

Gastro-intestinal tract
The combination of the bitterness of oleuropein, which should encourage digestive secretions, and the established *in vitro* research of its antimicrobial activity may indicate a use for the leaf extract in treating infections in this tract.

• gastro-intestinal infections
• constipation

Endocrine
Based on tradition the leaves may be useful for:

• diabetes

Externally
The antimicrobial activity indicates a wash of leaf extracts may be used for:

• skin infections
• mucosal infections
• protecting skin from sun damage (topically)

Pharmacy
There are no official guidelines for dosage of *Olea folia*.
Three times daily suggested dosage[41]
Infusion of dried leaves   – 5–15 g
    However there is this precaution from *Weiss*—the leaves may cause gastric irritation and should be taken after food.
    Oil as a laxative single dose 15–60 ml.

Pharmacokinetics
Some preliminary studies failed to detect either oleuropein or its metabolites in plasma after the consumption of leaf extracts,[42] however hydrotyrosol and tyrosol have been detected as glucuronides in urine.[43]

Historical uses
Leaf—fevers including malaria. **Oil** used as a nutrient, demulcent and purgative. The oil was used "to retard the flow of gastric juice" in the treatment of peptic ulcers[44] and to treat constipation and/or impacted stools. Externally—as an emollient to soften crusty lesions, to soothe burns.

PAPAVERACEAE

A nnual or perennial herbs with watery sap or milky or coloured latex.

- Leaves spiralled, exstipulate, variously lobed to dissected
- Flowers solitary or sometimes in lax leafy cymes, rarely in axillary umbels. Sepals 2. Petals 4–6, all similar, sessile, not spurred. Stamens many, free
- Fruit a capsule opening by valves or pores. Seeds many, small

There are 26 genera world-wide and about 200 species, mostly from the temperate Northern Hemisphere. Some plants of the family contain narcotic and medicinal alkaloids.

Chelidonium majus

Greater celandine

Description

A perennial herb with a branched, woody orange-coloured rootstock, releasing orange latex when broken. *Stems* erect, slender, sparsely hairy at

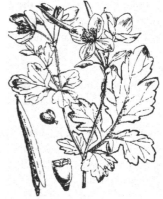

Family Papaveraceae

nodes, brittle, 30–90 cm tall in flower. *Leaves* pinnate, lamina 5–15 × 5–12 cm. Lateral leaflets in 3–5 pairs, ovate to elliptic, bicrenately lobed. Midrib and petioles narrowly winged, and wing expanded at the base of the petiole. Terminal leaflet ternate. Stems and leaves also contain orange latex. Foliage often blue-green. Peduncles 2–10 cm long with 2–6-flowered umbels. Sepals obovate, 8 × 5 mm. Petals yellow, obovate and up to 1 cm long. *Capsule* linear, somewhat constricted between seeds, 20–50 mm long. Plant flowers and fruits in spring and summer.

Odour—peculiar and unpleasant; taste—bitter and pungent.

Habitat and cultivation
Native to temperate Europe and Britain and naturalised elsewhere. Grows easily from seed in light soils in sun or semi-shade. Drought and frost resistant.

Parts used
Fresh or dried herb gathered at, or just prior to, flowering. The fresh latex.

Active constituents
1) Alkaloids (0.6–1.75%)—at least 20 have been identified.[1,2] They are of the isoquinoline type mainly coptisine[3] also chelidonine, homochelidonine, berberine, protopine, stylopine and smaller amounts of chelerythrine and sanguinarine.[1,4,5] (These latter alkaloids are found in higher concentration in the root of the herb.[6]) The content of alkaloids is dependent on temperature and light conditions[7] and stage of development of the plant[8]
2) Flavonoids
3) Phenolic acids including those derived from caffeic, p-coumaric and ferulic acids[9]

Also contains proteins[10] (content varies with time of year[11]) but includes enzymes—oxidases,[11,12] proteolytic enzymes and nucleases[11,13]—lectins[13] and a proteinase inhibitor (chelidocystatin),[14] a bitter principle—chelidoxanthin, volatile oil and the plant acids chelidonic, succinic, citric and malic acids.

Nutritional constituents
Vitamins: Nicotinic acid
Minerals: Calcium, potassium, magnesium, phosphorus, sulphur and some iron[1]

Actions
1) Spasmolytic
2) Cholagogue
3) Diuretic

Scientific information
Chelidonium has been used medicinally at least since the middle ages. It has been an official medicine in both western and eastern traditions. There are a number of biologically active components, including the alkaloids. The proteins in the latex are also considered likely to be pharmacologically active.[11] Constituent levels vary according to plant maturation, possibly altering the herb's observed actions.[8]

Antimicrobial
In vitro—The herb and/or its constituents have the following activities:-

- antibacterial against Gram-positive organisms[6] including resistant strains of Staphylococcus and Enterococcus,[15] Streptococcus mutans responsible for dental caries[16,17] and strongly active against Mycobacterium tuberculosis[18]
- antiviral against some types of human tumour viruses and adenoviruses,[6] herpes,[6] retroviruses (preventing cell infection and viral spread)[19] and polio viruses.[6] Chelidocystatin may inhibit viral protein production[14]
- antifungal against a range of dermatophytes including Trichophyton spp., Aspergillus fumigatus and Candida spp. including C. albicans[6] and some Fusarium spp.[20]

The peroxidase and nucleases, which protect the plant from pathogens, have general antimicrobial activity.[11]

In vivo—Clinical trials with toothpaste containing sanguinarine reduced plaque and gum disease.[21,22] Both sanguinarine and chelerythrine may reduce halitosis by reducing the oral production of volatile sulphur compounds.[23]

Celandine was used to treat chronic tonsillitis in children improving their immune function, including their non-specific resistance, and decreasing disease recurrence.[24]

Anticancer
In vitro—The anticancer properties of some of the alkaloids particularly sanguinarine, chelerythrine

and chelidonine have been noted.[25-28] Sanguinarine and berberine can interact with DNA which may contribute to their cytotoxicity.[6] The alkaloids are toxic to cancer cells[29] whilst the whole extract is cytostatic.[30]

A chemotherapeutic agent has been produced based on the modified alkaloids of *Chelidonium*. Called *Ukrain* it has been subject to fairly extensive testing *in vitro* and *in vivo*, the results of which have been reviewed and are considered promising.[31] The actions of *Ukrain* cannot be extrapolated to *Chelidonium* itself.[26]

In vivo—As part of a Chinese preparation it had an antitumour effect in patients with oesophageal cancer.[32]

Other

In vitro—*Chelidonium* and some of its alkaloids inhibit acetylycholinesterase,[33,34] the herb also modulates binding to $GABA_A$ receptor sites.[35]

Anti-inflammatory activity has been demonstrated in whole extracts[36,37] as well as by alkaloids, in particular sanguinarine[38] (also inhibits platelet aggregation,[39] COX-1[39] and 5-LOX[37]).

The extract is anti-oxidant[36] (although this action may not be very strong[40]) and it is capable, *ex vivo*, of stimulating an immune response in blood samples from patients with infections who had low immune function.[41]

In vivo—A preparation containing *Curcuma longa* (turmeric) and *Chelidonium* gave symptomatic relief of right upper abdominal colic attributed to biliary dyskinesia.[42]

Apart from those using *Ukrain* there are no other modern clinical trials.

Medicinal uses
Respiratory tract
- pertussis (China)
- bronchitis

Gastro-intestinal tract
Weiss claims that *Chelidonium*, if not used within 6 months, loses efficacy giving inconsistent results. However the spasmolytic action and the cholagogue effect (which he says has been shown to increase pancreatic enzyme secretion) aid:

- cholecystitis (*BHP* specific)
- cholelithiasis (*BHP* specific)
- jaundice

Externally
The fresh latex from the broken stem is applied directly to the skin where it may inactivate wart viruses:

- warts
- verrucae
- eczema
- tinea
- malignant skin conditions

Pharmacy
Three times daily

Infusion of dried herb	– 2–4 g
Tincture 1:10 (45%)	– 2–4 ml
Fluid Extract (25%)	– 1–2 ml

Precautions and/or safety
In vitro—Studies using tinctures with up to 6.2 mg/g of total alkaloids were not toxic to hepatocytes,[43] and in standard bioassays.[2]

In vivo—Recorded minor side-effects include a dry mouth and dizziness.

There are a number of cases in the literature linking the use of *Chelidonium* to reversible hepatitis albeit in a relatively small number of cases (10 people over 3 years).[44] The hepatitis may be due to an idiosyncratic reaction[44-46] or possibly a herb-induced auto-immunity.[47] These cases were mainly in Germany and occurred after either using extracts standardised on chelidonine or preparations of which *Chelidonium* was a part.[48] As preparations containing *Chelidonium* have been very widely used in Germany under the assumption the herb is safe, it is suggested the number of untoward events may be under recorded.[45] One unusual case of *Chelidonium* causing haemolytic anaemia[49] and one of contact dermatitis to the latex have also been reported.[50]

Historical uses

Blood cleanser; diaphoretic (hot infusion). Torpid liver conditions. Cure for sore eyes and films in the eyes. Also used for dropsy; itch; scurvy; ringworm; corns; tetters; old sores and ulcers. The juice taken, with fasting, for the pestilence; rubbed on the abdomen for griping and post-partum pains. Applied to the breasts to reduce heavy menstruation. Toothache (gargle); haemorrhoids (ointment). In Traditional Chinese Medicine it is used as a pain-killer, antitussive, alterative and anti-inflammatory.

Eschscholzia californica

Californian poppy

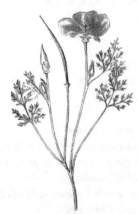

Family Papavaraceae

Description

A fast-growing, slender, erect annual or perennial with much dissected blue green leaves growing to 60 cm. Stems branched, and glabrous. *Flowers* solitary, showy yellow or orange-red. Sepals 2, forming a hood-like cap, pushed off upwards by the 4 petals as they open. *Capsules* slender to 10 cm long. Sap colourless. Flowers throughout summer.

Habitat and cultivation

Native to western North America. Always grown from seed and self-sows freely in suitable situations. Prefers full sun and well-drained soil.

Parts used

The herb gathered during flowering.

Active constituents

1) Alkaloids—isoquinoline type including californidine, californine (escholtzine), protopine, allocryptopine, lauroscholtzine (*N*-methyllaurotetanine) also sanguinarine, chelerythrine, laurotetaine and caryachine derivatives[51-53]
2) Flavonoids including those based on rutin, quercetin and isorhamnetin[54]

Actions

1) Sedative
2) Anxiolytic
3) Analgesic

Scientific information

Research into this herb is occurring at present, being driven by the interest in the alkaloids which are related to those in *Papaver somniferum*—opium poppy—and also because of their particularly antimicrobial and anticancer potential (sanguinarine, chelerythrine and protopine).[51,55-57] Protopine also has anti-inflammatory[58] and nematocidal[59] properties *in vitro*.

The western use of the herb, adopted from the Native Americans' understanding, is for its actions on the nervous system, an action due predominantly to the alkaloids.

In vitro—The alkaloids may act via benzodiazepine receptors and/or via inhibition of the degradation of catecholamines. They also interact *in vitro* with serotonin receptors.[52]

In vivo—The herb either by ingestion or smoking can supposedly create a state of mild euphoria lasting 20–30 minutes.[53] A clinical trial using a medicine, registered in France, which combines *Cratageus* and magnesium with *Eschscholzia* was beneficial in the treatment of mild to moderate anxiety.[60]

Weiss says of the herb its action is gentle and an aid to "establishing equilibrium and it is not narcotic".

Medicinal uses
Urinary tract
Weiss recommends its use as an aid to treating:

• enuresis

Nervous system
The main use of *Eschscholzia* is to treat:-

• anxiety
• insomnia
• neuropathy

Pharmacy
There are no current guidelines on dosage for this herb. *Weiss* recommends one teaspoonful per cup of dried herb as an infusion. He considered the herb to be safe and suitable for use in children.

The formulated medicine in the above clinical trial used two tablets twice daily and contained 20 mg of an aqueous extract of *Eschscholzia*.[60]

King's Dispensatory recommends a dose of between 12–185 grains which converts to 0.8–12 g of herb, as a single dose.

In animal studies doses between 25–200 mg per kg were used, the lower doses being considered anxiolytic and the larger ones sedative.[61] This equates to 1.5–6 gm for a 60 kg adult if the action were to be the same in humans.

Three times daily (suggestion based on *Chelidonium* with similar alkaloids)
Infusion of dried herb   – 2–4 g
Tincture 1:10 (45%)   – 2–4 ml
Fluid extract (25%)   – 1–2 ml

Interactions
In vitro—Some of the alkaloids inhibit CYP3A4[52] although no interactions of the herb with drugs metabolized by this enzyme have yet been reported.

Historical uses
An analgesic used in toothache. To stop lactation by topical application of the crushed seeds. Children's sedative. As a compress for healing wounds.

Sanguinaria canadensis

Blood root

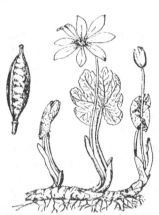

Family Papavaraceae

Description
Perennial, 15–30 cm tall. Rhizome horizontal, extending 5–10 cm, cylindrical, slightly branched with numerous tender rootlets underneath, brownish red externally and exuding a blood-red juice when cut. Previous year's shoots leave scars on the rhizome. *Stems* simple, smooth naked scapes each topped by a single flower which appears before or with the leaves in early spring. *Leaves* palmately seven-nine lobed, upper surface light green, underside whitish, glaucous. Ribs prominent. *Flowers*—sepals two, forming an ephemeral calyx. Petals 8–12, white, to 5 cm in diameter, spatulate, not crumpled. Stamens usually 24, unequal, arranged more or less distinctly in 2 rows. Pollen golden yellow. Style, short, thick, rounded. *Pod* oblong, sharp-pointed, turgid, opening by 2 uplifting valves to allow the escape of numerous seeds. Seeds poisonous. Flowers in spring.

Odour—slight; taste—acrid, bitter and nauseating.

Habitat and cultivation
Native to rich, open woods of North America from Manitoba and Nova Scotia to Florida and east Texas. Grows in a moist, shady places under deciduous trees. Cultivated in similar places elsewhere.

Propagated by root division in autumn. Frost resistant, drought tender.

Parts used
Rhizome, gathered in autumn. The rhizome is ready for harvesting about 6 years after growing from seeds or 4–5 years from cuttings. Wildcrafting may lead to this herb becoming endangered.

Active constituents
1) Isoquinoline alkaloids including mainly sanguinarine (up to 4%) and chelerythrine (up to 2%), also chelirubine, sanguirubine, sanguilutine, protopine and allocryptopine.[62–65] Oxysanguinarine is produced when sanguinarine is exposed to light. Levels of sanguinarine are highest in plants harvested at higher altitudes, in early spring just after flowering[63]
2) Red resin

Also chelidonic, malic and citric acids, gum, starch and sugars.[66]

Actions
1) Expectorant
2) Spasmolytic
3) Emetic
4) Cardioactive
5) Cathartic
6) Antiseptic Topically
7) Irritant
8) Escharotic

Scientific information
The name of this plant, *Sanguinaria*, derives from the red blood-like latex that oozes when rhizomes are cut. It was an official medicine in the *American Pharmacopoeia* until 1926.

In the 1980's the root extract was used in toothpastes because of its anti-plaque properties but it fell out of favour when possible links to an increased cancer risk were reported. It is again receiving interest for use in animal feeds, as a natural antibiotic, and because it increases the weight of livestock. There are moves to encourage the cultivation of *Sanguinaria* in the United States.[63] Whilst the alkaloid content of wildcrafted rhizomes is higher than that of cultivated plants they are also more variable.[63]

Antimicrobial
In vitro—An extract and/or the main alkaloids have good antimicrobial activity against a range of strains of *Helicobacter pylori*,[67] some species of *Mycobacterium* including *M. tuberculosis* (traditional use of herb)[68] and a range of Gram-positive and Gram-negative plaque bacteria[69] in which sanguinarine seems to specifically accumulate and be retained.[70]

In vivo—A number of clinical studies have been conducted using an extract in mouth rinses and toothpastes. Many have shown these preparations reduced plaque and gingivitis safely,[71–78] although not all trials were in agreement as to its efficacy.[79–82] It was used in commercial products for this purpose until it was apparently linked to an increased incidence of leukoplakia, a precancerous condition.[83–85] Reviews of data by an expert panel concluded that *Sanguinaria*, at normal concentrations was, and is, in fact safe and effective and not causally related to leukoplakia development.[86–88] Design flaws in research methodology may have contributed to the conflicting results obtained.[89]

Anticancer
In vitro—Sanguinarine inhibits the proliferation of various types of cancer cells—epidermal,[90] prostate (whether androgen-dependent or not),[91] keratinocytes,[92] cervix[93] and lymphoma.[94] It was also effective against some cancer cells resistant to current chemotherapeutic agents.[93,94] The alkaloid inhibits DNA transcription,[95] selectively causes apoptosis and necrosis of cancer but not normal cells,[96] and may inhibit angiogenesis an important stage in the progression of cancer.[97]

In vivo—A paste containing *Sanguinaria* with zinc chloride and antimony sulphide has been marketed for the treatment of skin cancers including melanoma. The safety and efficacy of such preparations has been called into question because of poor outcomes in anecdotal cases.[98,99] A similar preparation (called Mohs paste) had been in use, as an injection in the 1930's, in the orthodox treatment of tumours but has since been superceded.[100]

Other
Sanguinarine is anti-oxidant,[101] anti-inflammatory[102] and has antiplatelet activities.[102] The alkaloids would seem to be responsible for most of the observed actions of the herb.

Medicinal uses
Cardiovascular system
Used for improving:

• circulation of capillaries

Respiratory tract
It is expectorant in small doses and also seems to relax bronchial muscles:

• asthma
• pharyngitis
• croup
• laryngitis
• bronchitis (sub-acute or chronic)

BHP specific indication—asthma and bronchitis with feeble peripheral circulation.

Gastro-intestinal tract
• to promote emesis (in large doses)

Externally
More recently external preparations have included *Sanguinaria* to treat:

• epithelial tumours
• skin infections
• buccal infections
• sensitive teeth

As a snuff for:

• nasal polyps
• nasal infections

Pharmacy
Three times daily

Dried rhizome	– 0.06–0.5 g
Tincture 1:5 (60%)	– 0.3–2 ml
Fluid extract (60%)	– 0.06–0.3 ml

As snuff a pin-head size quantity of powdered rhizome is all that should be used for a single dose.

Single dose for emesis

Dried rhizome	– 1–2 g
Tincture	– 2–8 ml
Fluid extract	– 1–2 ml

Sanguinaria was used in anti-plaque toothpastes at concentrations of 0.075% and in mouthwashes at 0.03%. It is no longer used in dentifrices.

Precautions and/or safety
In vitro hepatocyte cytochrome P450 isozymes reduce the potential toxicity of sanguinarine[103] which at high enough doses is toxic (the same is true for chelerythrine). The alkaloids are not believed to be toxic *in vivo*[104] however recommended doses of the herb should not be exceeded.

In excess it may cause intense thirst, vomiting, faintness, vertigo, burning in the stomach, prostration and dimness of vision.

Historical uses
For fevers; atonic dyspepsia; dysentery; torpid liver; tuberculosis; scrofula; heart disease and palpitations. Used externally for fungal infections including ringworm; eczema especially when associated with varicose ulcers; cancers; skin growths.

PASSIFLORACEAE

The passionflower family consists of about 12 genera of herbaceous or woody vines or erect shrubs with tendrils, native to tropical and warm temperate regions of both hemispheres.

- Leaves are alternate, simple or lobed
- Flowers regular, usually with a conspicuous fringed crown in the centre
- Fruit a berry or capsule with many seeds

Passiflora incarnata

Passionflower

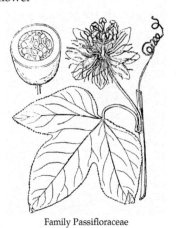

Family Passifloraceae

Description
A perennial climbing vine to 10 m with spring-like tendrils and extensive rootstock, which dies back completely in winter. *Stems* cylindrical, or angular when young. *Leaves* alternate, deeply 3-lobed, serrate, about 10–15 cm long, dull green above on petioles with 2 glands. *Flowers* solitary, with 5 green sepals and 5 petals, white or pale lavender with outer 2 rings of the corona consisting of pink or purple filaments. *Fruit* to 5 cm long, ovoid, yellow and edible. Flowers in summer and autumn.

Odour—slightly aromatic; taste—bland.

Habitat and cultivation
Native to North America from Virginia to Florida and cultivated in other countries. *Passiflora* prefers a sheltered sunny situation and needs support for its climbing vines. It may be grown from seed or from root cuttings and likes a light soil. It is frost and drought tender but survives because it dies back completely in winter.

Parts used
The aerial part of herb harvested during the flowering and fruiting period but excluding flowers and fruit. Leaves and stems are the most pharmacologically active.[1]

318

Active constituents

1) Flavonoids (0.8–2.5%) based on luteolin and apigenin including vitexin, iso-orientin and schaftoside and their isomers, rutin and chrysin.[2-5] A tri-substituted benzoflavone compound has also been reported[6]

2) Alkaloids (around 0.1%),[7] small amounts, levels dependent on time of harvesting, including norharman, harman also harmalol and harmol

Also contains chlorogenic acid, maltol (benzopyrone derivative),[8] gynocardin (a cyanogenic glycoside),[9] sterols and traces of volatile oil.[10]

Actions

1) Sedative
2) Anodyne
3) Antispasmodic
4) Hypnotic

Scientific information

Various species of *Passiflora* are used medicinally throughout the world but *P. incarnata* is the main one used in Europe. It may have been confused in the past with *P. edulis* as the two are morphologically very similar and at one time they were considered synonymous.[11] However *P. edulis*, an edible variety, lacks significant anxiolytic activity.[12] Passionflower has a very long traditional use in conditions of the nervous system and has been an official medicine in pharmacopoeias worldwide[13] having been introduced to Europe by Spanish explorers of Mexico. It is used for asthma and worms in Brazil. It has been approved by *German Commission E* for the treatment of nervous restlessness.

Nervous system

Scientific studies have generally failed to identify the constituents responsible for the neurological activity of *Passiflora*. Maltol at high enough concentration has some activity in animals but is not present in the plant at required levels. The alkaloids have MAO inhibitory activity but they too are present at very low concentrations. The flavonoids are the most likely pharmacological agents, (chrysin is anxiolytic in animal models) and the more recently characterised benzoflavone constituent may be significant.[6]

In vitro—In animal cells the herb acts via GABA[14] and serotonin[15] receptors but there is little confirmation of this in human models.

In vivo—There are a few small clinical trials using branded combinations of herbs which include passionflower that have shown benefits for patients with anxiety related problems.[16,17]

The herb has been used in India in the treatment of morphine addiction. A clinical trial found *Passiflora* significantly helped control the mental symptoms associated with opiate withdrawal.[18] It was also as effective as benzodiazepines when used to treat patients with generalised anxiety disorder[19,20]—reviewed.[21]

Other

In vitro—*Passiflora* has a good level of antibacterial activity against a number of strains of *Helicobacter pylori*.[22]

The herb may have some potential in preventing cancer.[23]

Medicinal uses

Cardiovascular system
• nervous tachycardia

Respiratory tract
• spasmodic asthma

Nervous system
• insomnia (*BHP* specific)
• nervous stress
• restlessness
• epilepsy
• neuralgia
• anxiety

Pharmacy

Three times daily

Infusion dried herb	– 0.25–1 g
Tincture 1:8 (45%)	– 0.5–2 ml
Fluid Extract (25%)	– 0.5–1 ml

May be more effective as a hydro-alcohol extract than as an infusion.[12]

Precautions and/or safety

Safety data on passionflower has shown that it is not genotoxic using standard assays.[24] Harman and norharman can enhance mutagenicity of other compounds and may intercalate with DNA[25] but are only present in trace amounts.[26]

The only reports of side effects associated with *Passiflora* relate to over-the-counter preparations and include:-

- gastro-intestinal disturbance (nausea and vomiting), drowsiness, bradycardia and arrhythmia in one individual—classed as likely to be idiosyncratic[27]
- altered consciousness in 5 cases (product described as containing mainly *Passiflora* fruit[28])
- ventricular tachycardia in an infant (product containing 5 different herbs, *Passiflora* assumed the likely cause)[29]
- vasculitis (combination herbal extracts containing passionflower)[30]

Around 15 cases of toxicity have been reported to the FDA in total but they have all involved preparations of herbal combinations, which include *Passiflora*.[31] The herb has "safe for general use" status throughout the world although in Australia long-term use of the harmala-type alkaloids has been prohibited.[31]

Interactions

There is a potential for interaction between *Passiflora* and warfarin, due to its content of vitamin K which may reduce the drug's effectiveness.[32] It has also been pointed out that because the alkaloids can act as MAOIs, the herb should not be used with these types of drugs as it may have an agonist action.

To date no interactions between *Passiflora* and any drug have been reported.

Historical uses

Diarrhoea; dysentery and dysmenorrhoea through actions on the nervous system.

PEDALIACEAE

The Pedaliaceae or pedalium family contains about 16 genera of annual or perennial plants native to the tropics and subtropics.

- Leaves are opposite, the upper leaves sometimes alternate; simple or deeply lobed and covered with slime-secreting hairs or glands
- Flowers are bisexual, irregular, axillary and usually solitary
- Calyx 5-parted, corolla 5-lobed and broadly tubular, stamens usually 4 in 2 pairs borne on the corolla tube
- Fruit a nut or capsule, often hooked or horned

Sesamum is the best known member of the family.

Harpagophytum procumbens

Devil's claw

Description
A perennial growing up from large globular tubers. *Flowers* trumpet shaped, red or violet coloured. *Fruit* large, hooked claw-like.

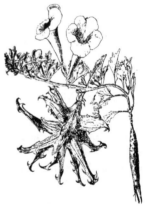

Family Pedaliaceae

Habitat and cultivation
Native to eastern and southern Africa, in the desert mainly around Namibia, South Africa and Botswana. It does not grow in other places.

Parts used
The secondary tuberous roots.

Active constituents
1) Iridoid glycosides including harpagoside (about 2%), harpagide and 8-O-p-coumaroyl-harpagide[1-3]

321

2) Phenylpropanoids including acteoside
3) Sugars—mainly tetrasaccharides[4,5]

In smaller amounts:

4) Terpenes mainly diterpenes[1] but also triterpenes—ursolic and oleanolic acids[6]
5) Aromatic acids including cinnamic,[1] caffeic[7] and chlorogenic acids[6]
6) Phytosterols including β-sitosterol and stigmasterol[6]
7) Flavonoids derived from luteolin and kaempferol[6]
8) Harpagoquinone[6]

Nutritional constituents
Minerals: Phosphorus, potassium, calcium, manganese, iron, copper and zinc

Actions
1) Anti-inflammatory
2) Analgesic
3) Diuretic
4) Sedative
5) Antirheumatic

Scientific information
Harpagophytum reached Europe in the early 20th century and since then its use has grown, particularly in Germany, for the treatment of joint pain. Such was the demand that the roots were becoming endangered and efforts are now being made to cultivate the herb commercially.[8] There are two species of Harpagophytum, H. procumbens and H. zeyheri, that have been used in southern Africa for medicinal purposes. They have similar chemical constituents and pharmacological properties but are distinguishable by their iridoid profiles but commercial preparations probably consist of both species.[9] It is approved by German Commission E for loss of appetite, dyspepsia and musculoskeletal degenerative problems.

Harpagophytum was traditionally used to treat joint inflammation and has been investigated in this context. The active constituents responsible and mechanism of action have not been fully established although harpagoside level is used as a marker for the strength of the herb.

Musculoskeletal
In vitro—Devil's claw modulates a number of different cytokines and this may be one of the mechanisms by which it is able to reduce inflammation.[10–13] Harpagoside itself can inhibit both 5-LOX and COX-2[14,15] however ex vivo studies indicate it is not the only constituent contributing to an anti-inflammatory activity, the whole extract being stronger than harpagoside alone.[12]

In vivo—The herb has been effective in the treatment of pain associated with various joints including:-

• low back pain of a chronic and non-specific nature[16,17] and not due to spinal nerve irritation.[18] It gave much the same relief as the anti-inflammatory rofexcoxib[19]
• arthroses of hip and knee—signs and symptoms measurably reduced[20]
• arthritis of hip and knee[16]—comparable in efficacy and with fewer side effects than diacerhein[21,22] and required less concurrent analgesia[22]
• slight to moderate pain of back, neck and shoulders of non-specific nature, reduced muscle stiffness[23]

It also improved mobility and reduced pain in degenerative rheumatism.[24] However a small trial using arthritic patients unresponsive to pharmaceutical therapy found no improvement on introducing an aqueous based tablet of the herb.[25]

Healthy people who took the herb for 3 weeks had no change in arachidonic acid metabolism, an effect that occurs with non-steroidal anti-inflammatory drugs.[26]

There are a number of reviews of clinical trials where Harpagophytum was used to treat osteoarthritis and chronic low back pain and the evidence strongly supports its effectiveness at doses of 50 mg harpagoside or more a day.[6,27,28] Reviewers have been critical of the quality of many of these trials and they conclude better research is necessary before drawing firm conclusions.[29,30]

Other
In vitro—The herb is inhibitory to a number of microorganisms particularly aerobic bacteria including

Staphylococcus aureus and also to *Candida* spp.[31] Diterpenes show strong anti-plasmodial activity (effective against a chloroquine-resistant strain of *Plasmodium falciparum*) whilst having no cytotoxicity to human cells.[32]

Water soluble components of *Harpagophytum*[33] and the whole herb[34] are strongly anti-oxidant due at least in part to the phenols, harpagoside being only weakly so. The herb has potential to treat inflammatory bowel disease.[34]

Devil's claw is used in some parts of South Africa to treat type 2 diabetes.

Medicinal uses
Gastro-intestinal tract
The iridoid fraction is bitter and therefore stimulates digestive secretions.

- dyspepsia
- anorexia

Musculoskeletal
The actions make it particularly effective in the treatment of problems in this system:

- arthritis
- rheumatism
- fibrositis
- myalgia
- painful arthrosis
- lumbago
- tendonitis
- pleurodynia
- gout

BHP specific for rheumatic disease.

Pharmacy
Three times daily
For dyspepsia and anorexia

Decoction	–	0.5 g or as dried tuber
Tincture 1:5 (25%)	–	1 ml

Other applications

Decoction	–	1.5–2.5 g or as dried tuber
Tincture 1:5 (25%)	–	2.0–4 ml
Fluid Extract (25%)	–	1.0–2 ml

Dosage recommendations differ slightly from one study group to another as do commercial preparations. Most commercial processing increases the proportion of harpagoside.

ESCOP's recommended dosage is 2–5 g daily rising to 4.5–9 g for low back pain. *Chrubasik*, who has contributed many papers on the subject, suggests that a minimum daily dose of 50 mg of harpagoside is required for effective pain relief[35,36] and that even though the iridoids are equally soluble in water and alcohol, water extracts may be more effective based on the results of clinical trials.[37] Interestingly doubling the dose of harpagoside from 50 mg to 100 mg did not give greater relief of back pain.[17] ESCOP recommends treatment with the herb be continued for 2–3 months to achieve results.[19]

Pharmacokinetics
Studies show harpagoside reaches peak plasma levels 1.3 to 2.5 hours after ingesting whole extracts.[12] *In vitro*, bacterial flora metabolised the iridoids, converting them into the alkaloid aucubinine B.[38]

Precautions and/or safety
Many of the clinical trials report good tolerability with few side effects using the equivalent of 3 ml per day of a 1:2 extract or 60 mg of harpagoside,[16,23,24] even after one year's continuous use.[19]

Care should be taken with patients who have peptic ulceration—due to the stimulation of digestive secretions. Minor gastro-intestinal side effects have been noted including diarrheoa.[17,21]

Interactions
In vitro a commercial extract inhibited some cytochrome P450 isozymes.[39] *In vivo* there are no reports of any interactions although there is one anecdotal report of purpura in a patient taking warfarin and *Harpagophytum* concomitantly.[40]

Historical uses
Fevers, blood diseases including malaria, digestive disorders, allergies, skin problems including cancer; complications of pregnancy.

PHAEOPHYCEAE

All seaweeds are classified as belonging to the plant sub-kingdom Thallophyta and are usually identified primarily by colour. All have chlorophyll as their photosynthetic base so all are green, but the green is then covered by another pigment such as brown or red. Some colours seem to overlap, and shade can change with the season or age of the weed. Green light penetrates further into the water than red so brown seaweeds can live in deeper water. They also prefer cooler water temperatures. The Phaeophyceae are a family of large brown algae, (macro algae), the largest and longest of the seaweeds. They absorb medium wavelength green light and contain the pigment fucoxanthin.

Fucus vesiculosus

Bladderwrack, kelp

Description
A tough, leathery, brown and olive green seaweed with branching, flat, wavy-edged but not toothed offshoots, and a conspicuous midrib. Each branch has 2 or sometimes 3 gas bladders grouped together in the body of the frond, and in season,

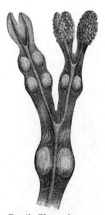

Family Phaeophyceae

reproductive bodies at branch tips—yellowish in male plants and more green in female plants. The holdfast is a blob or lumpy disc with cells on the underside which secrete a kind of glue which sticks the plant to the rock.

Odour—fishy; taste—mucilaginous and salty.

Habitat and distribution
A middle shore species growing in more sheltered sites where the waves have lost much of their power, in cooler waters of the Atlantic and Baltic seas.

Parts used
The whole thallus or plant, harvested at any time of the year.

Active constituents
1) Trace metals (up to 0.4%) especially rich in iodine (up to 0.2%),[1] some of which is bound organically to proteins or amino acids and the rest occurs as iodides
2) Phenols predominantly phlorotannins (around 10%—these are water soluble phenolic compounds composed of polymers of phloroglycinol[2,3]). Also fucols, fucophlorethols, catechin and gallic acid[3]
3) Polysaccharides of various types including alginic acid and fucoidans.[4,5] (Fucoidans contain sulphated units of the sugar L-fucose, they are found in other seaweeds and vary in their chemical structure.) Mucilage is composed of these polysaccharides
4) Sterols (around 0.3%) mainly as free fucosterol[6]

Also contains pigments and polar lipids.[7] Polypeptides referred to as phytochelatins have been identified—the plant uses a process of chelation by these sulphur-rich polypeptides to protect itself from toxic metals and the level of polypeptides therefore changes in response to the concentration of metals present.[8]

Nutritional constituents
Vitamins: β-carotene
Minerals: Calcium, manganese, potassium, zinc, iron, copper and molybdenum.[3,9] Metal content depends on levels present in environment.

Actions
1) Anti-obesic
2) Thyroid modulator
3) Antirheumatic

Scientific information
Fucus has been an official medicine in some countries, used in the treatment of obesity. It has been fairly well characterised chemically in recent times, as it is a monitor of sea pollution because of its ability to accumulate metal ions.

There are not many studies on the medicinal properties of the whole herb but constituent polysaccharides and phlorotannins have shown a range of pharmacological activities.

Endocrine
In vitro—*Fucus* has anti-oestrogenic activity both by reducing oestrogen levels in cell cultures and by competing with oestrodiol binding at both α- and β-oestrogen receptor sites.[10]

In vivo—A pilot study has indicated that *Fucus* lengthened the cycle of pre-menopausal women experiencing abnormal menstrual cycles, reduced their oestrogen and increased their progesterone levels.[11] This has led to the suggestion that dietary intake of kelp by Japanese women may be a factor in their reduced risk of hormone-dependent cancers.[11]

In diets deficient in iodine it seems that *Fucus* may aid weight reduction due to increased thyroid function and therefore an increased metabolic rate.[12] The use of the herb to help with weight loss is historical and was shown in studies conducted some time ago but there is no modern research into this effect.[13,14]

Antimicrobial
In vitro—Various isolated fractions of bladderwrack are bactericidal,[15,16] have a limited antifungal activity[17] and are antiviral to HIV,[18,19] herpes, vesicular stomatitis virus and cytomegalovirus.[20]

Fucoidan reduces the adhesion of *Helicobacter pylori* to gastric cells[21] and inactivates pepsin.[22]

Other
In vitro—There is current interest in fucoidan from several sources and various properties have been found for the type found in *Fucus*. It complexes with toxins from snake venom, inactivating them;[23] may help wound healing;[24,25] may inhibit angiogenesis,[26] is anticoagulant[26,27] and fibrinolytic, can inhibit fertilisation and alters macrophage cytokine production.[29]

Both fucoidan[30] and phlorotannins[31] have antioxidant activity.

In vivo—The herb decreased skin thickness and increased its elasticity when applied topically as a 1% gel and may help reduce the effect of aging.[32]

Medicinal uses
Gastro-intestinal tract
Fucus contains a high content of soluble fibre. In powdered form, it acts as a very beneficial and gentle bulk laxative:

• constipation

Endocrine system
• hypothyroidism
• myxoedema
• obesity
• lymphadenoid goitre

Musculoskeletal
The herb has been used for joint problems:

• rheumatism
• rheumatoid arthritis

Externally
• rheumatism

Pharmacy
Three times daily

Infusion of dried thallus	– 0.8–10 g
Tincture 1:5 (25%)	– 4–10 ml
Fluid Extract (25%)	– 1–2 ml
Powder	– 15 ml or three teaspoons daily as a laxative

CONTRAINDICATIONS—Cardiac problems, pregnancy, lactation and hyperthyroidism.

Precautions and/or safety
As *Fucus* is able to accumulate metals it can also accumulate toxic waste that may be in the surrounding seawater.[33–35] In particular the existence of high levels of arsenic[36] are a potential source of concern and a case of nephrotoxicity linked to arsenic levels in *Fucus* tablets has been reported.[37] The herb should only be gathered from unpolluted waters and should be screened for toxic metals.

There is a report of an obese patient developing ventricular tachycardia/fibrillation after using a herbal preparation containing a mixture of dandelion, boldo and bladderwrack.[38]

In excess it can, according to the *BHC*, cause hyperthyroidism, tremor, increased pulse rate and elevated blood pressure. The current safe level for iodine intake in the USA is 1000 micrograms a day.

Historical uses
Used externally for scrofula; scrofulous tumours; rickets; to strengthen limbs; enlarged or hardened glands.

PHYTOLACCACEAE

The Pokeweed family consists of about 20 genera of herbs, shrubs, trees and sometimes climbers, mostly native to tropical or sub-tropical America and Africa.

- Leaves are alternate and entire and sometimes ill-scented
- Flowers are mostly in racemes and bisexual, sometimes unisexual, with a 4–5-parted calyx and usually no petals
- Stamens may be 3 to many, pistils united or separated
- Fruit dry, fleshy or drupe-like

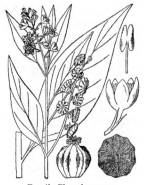

Family Phytolaccaceae

Phytolacca americana
[Formerly known as *Phytolacca decandra*]

Poke root

Description

Erect, branched, glabrous, semi-succulent herb growing up to 3 m high in flower, with thick, softly woody stems. *Leaf* stalks stout, 1–3 cm long; leaf blades 6–30 × 2–12 cm, ovate, ovate-oblong to more or less elliptic. *Flowers* grow in erect racemes which elongate to about 20 cm at fruiting. Peduncles and pedicels are whitish at first and become rose pink later. *Perianth* 5–7 mm in diameter; tepals 2–3 mm long, more or less broad ovate, persistent, white or greenish white at first becoming rose pink later. Stamens 10, filaments and anthers white. Ovary usually 10-carpellate, green with white raphides. *Fruit* about 10 mm in diameter when fresh, depressed globose, with prominent grooves when dried, glossy black, succulent with dark red juice. *Seeds* 2.5–3 mm, sub-spherical and glossy black. Flowers from spring to autumn.

Habitat and cultivation
Native to Eastern USA and introduced elselwhere for culinary use though it is known to be poisonous unless properly prepared. Found wild and cultivated in parts of Southern Europe and elsewhere. Grows from seed in free-draining garden soil and in sun or semi-shade. There are three species of *Phytolacca* which grow wild and look similar. They may be distinguished by the number of carpels and/or colour of their filaments and anthers. *P. americana* has 10 carpels and white filaments and anthers. *P. clavigera* has 6–8 carpels and pink filaments and anthers. *P. octandra* has 8 carpels and white filaments and anthers.

Parts used
The root collected in autumn (see Precautions).

Active constituents
1) Triterpenes:
    a) triterpenoid saponins derived from phytolaccagenin and phytolaccic acid (the phytolaccosides), jaligonic and esculentic acid[1-3]
    b) steroidal saponins including α-spinasterol[1,4]
2) Proteins including phytolacain G, a protease[5] and glycoproteins or lectins A, B, C, D1 and D2[6-8]

Also contains histamine,[9] resins, alkaloids (phytolaccine) and tannins.

Nutritional constituents
Vitamins: A and C
Minerals: Calcium, iron and phosphorus

Actions
1) Alterative
2) Anti-inflammatory
3) Anticatarrhalal
4) Parasiticide
5) Antifungal
6) Anodyne (mild)
7) Antirheumatic

In large doses:

8) Emetic
9) Cathartic

Scientific information
Pokeroot was once an official medicine listed as an emetic, purgative and mild narcotic and used in the treatment of chronic rheumatism.[10] There is an absence of modern scientific research into the whole root.

In vitro—The herb prevents glomerular cell changes induced by high glucose levels.[11]

The lectins are actually chemically complex but are referred to as "pokeweed mitogen". They are immunostimulatory, causing both B and T lymphocyte proliferation and also inducing immunoglobulin production.[12-14] Previous studies that showed these lectins to be immunomodulatory via cytokine and nitric oxide release have questioned whether the action was due to contaminants rather than a property of the mitogen itself.[12] The protease, phytolacain G, contributes to lymphocyte proliferation.[5]

Saponin phytolaccosides appear to improve absorption across intestinal epithelial cells and may be good carriers of pharmacological agents across the gut wall.[15]

Proteins isolated from the leaf have been well-studied due to their antiviral activity, including to HIV, but they do not seem to occur in the root.

In vivo—A combination of *Phytolacca, Guaiacum* and *Capsicum* was effective in alleviating the symptoms of acute tonsillitis.[16]

The herb is much valued and often used by medical herbalists.

Medicinal uses
Respiratory tract
In the treatment of mumps, lymphadenopathy and inflammation within the upper respiratory tract, conditions that often occur together, *Phytolacca* is considered specific (*BHP*):

- adenitis
- chronic respiratory catarrh
- laryngitis
- tonsillitis

Reproductive tract
• mastitis

Musculoskeletal
• chronic rheumatism

Externally
• scabies
• tinea (ringworm)
• sycosis
• acne
• mammary abscesses
• mastitis

Pharmacy
Three times daily
Decoction of dried root   –   0.06–0.3 g
Tincture 1:10 (45%)   –   0.2–0.6 ml
Fluid Extract (45%)   –   0.1–0.5 ml

As an ointment in the ratio of 4 g to 30 g of base, or as a poultice.

Precautions and/or safety
It is toxic in large doses and care must be taken to stay within the recommended dosage. Apart from vomiting and purging associated with large doses, the herb can cause prostration, convulsions and possibly even death. Gloves should be worn and direct contact with the skin should be avoided when handling fresh root for processing. Drying of fresh root reduces its potential toxicity.[17]

Historical uses
Used as a wash to treat cattle, (for parasites and fungal infections). "Headaches of many sources"; cancers of uterus and breast. Granular conjunctivitis; cathartic in bowel paralysis; leucorrhoea; haemorrhoids.

PIPERACEAE

The Piperaceae or pepper family are shrubs, small trees, climbers or herbaceous plants of mainly tropical and subtropical regions. Leaves simple, mostly entire. Flowers very small, simple, and crowded together in narrow, erect inflorescences. They may be unisexual or bisexual, each flower subtended by a bract and minus a perianth, but having both stamens and pistils. Each flower ripens into a single seed usually covered with a fleshy coat. *Piper*, *Macropiper* and *Peperomia* are the main genera.

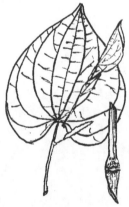

Family Piperaceae

Piper methysticum

Kava

Description
An evergreen shrub to 2 × 2 m. *Stems* fleshy, rising from a stout rhizome, erect and branching. *Leaves* alternate, heart-shaped, 25 × 20 cm, green, unevenly deeply cordate at the base, pointed at the tips and with 9–13 radiating veins. *Flowers* whitish in short, axillary spikes. *Fruit* small drupes.

Habitat and cultivation
Native to the Polynesian Islands and Northern Australia, *P. methysticum* grows in rich, moist soils and semi-shade. It is propagated from seed and is drought and frost tender.

Parts used
The roots and rhizomes, usually harvested after 4 years of growth.

Active constituents
1) Kavalactones—also called pyrones (3.5%–8.3%), at least 18 have been identified,[1,2] 96% of this fraction is made up of kavain, dihydrokavain, dihydromethysticin, methysticin,

330

desmethoxyyangonin and yangonin[3-5] occurring in a resinous form. The kavalactone

2) Chalcones (precursors of flavonoids)—flavokavins (also called flavokawains) A-C (around 1%) with flavokavin A being the predominant one[2,8,9]

3) Alkaloids—the piperidine, pipermethysticine (this is a minor constituent of roots and rhizomes occurring in higher amounts in stem peelings and leaves[10,11])

Also contains amino acids (around 35%), fats, essential oil[12] and stigmasterol[9,12] although the chemical details differ according to chemotypes.

Commercial kava extracts may contain between 30–70% kavalactones these having been identified as the active constituents, their extraction is favoured.[6]

Nutritional constituents
Minerals: Potassium, calcium, magnesium, sodium and iron

Actions
1) Antimicrobial
2) Diuretic
3) Spasmolytic
4) Sedative
5) Carminative
6) Anxiolytic

Topically:

7) Rubefacient

Scientific information
Piper has been used both as an integral part of social and ceremonial life in the South Pacific and as a traditional medicine for thousands of years. It has been known to the western world for two centuries, has been well studied pharmacologically and became an official medicine in a number of countries.

Kava was held to be a very effective treatment for anxiety (in the 1990's it was one of the most prescribed herbal medicines) avoiding many of the side effects like dependency, cognitive impairment, sedation and withdrawal associated with its pharmaceutical equivalents. Commercial *Piper* extracts

were being widely used until around 2002 when reports linking it with hepatic toxicity emerged (see Precautions). In recent years much research has concentrated on trying to validate and understand the link between the herb and/or its constituents and hepatic injury as it is still seen by many as a potentially valuable therapy. *German Commission E* has approved the use of kava for nervous anxiety, stress and restlessness.

Nervous system
In vitro—Animal studies on the herb's action on the nervous system have so far indicated that *Piper* and/or its constituents interact with $GABA_A$,[13,14] opioid,[13] dopamine,[13] histamine,[13] MAO[15] and serotonin[16] receptor sites and that it may have anticonvulsant activity by altering electrolyte channels[16] and glutamate release.[17] The relevance of the above actions to human biochemistry is uncertain.

In vivo—A number of clinical trials have been conducted using *Piper* to treat anxiety of various origins. It was found beneficial in:-

• peri- and post-menopausal women[18-22]
• non-psychotic patients[23-27] which included agoraphobia, simple phobias, adjustment mood disorder and generalised anxiety disorder (meta-analyses[28,29]). *Piper* also reduced the withdrawal symptoms of benzodiazepine therapy,[30] reduced restlessness and tension,[31] improved heart rate[32] and was considered as effective a treatment as the pharmaceuticals buspirone (anxiolytic) and opipramol (antidepressant)[33] and possibly better than benzodiazepines[30]
• helping patients awaiting cytology reports for suspected cancer[34]

Reviews of clinical data have concluded that *Piper* is effective for treating anxiety[35-39,46] with the exception possibly of generalised anxiety disorder.[40-42]
    Piper also:-

• enhanced cognitive function improving accuracy and speed[43]
• improved sleep quality in those with anxiety, tension and restlessness[44-46] (not corroborated[47])
• reduced measured levels of stress.[45] In contrast to drugs like benzodiazepines which

can impair cognitive function, *Piper* left this unchanged or improved[48-50]

It may also reduce the cravings associated with addiction to alcohol, tobacco, cocaine and heroin.[51]

Other

In vitro—Kava and/or its constituents have anti-inflammatory potential via inhibition of both COX-1 and COX-2[52-54] antioxidant,[52] antithrombotic[55] and immunomodulatory activity.[54]

The whole extract and flavokavains also have anticancer properties,[56] inhibiting the growth of bladder cancer cells.[57]

Aqueous extracts have limited antifungal activity[58] but the hydroalcoholic extract is broader and stronger in this action inhibiting *Candida albicans*, *Trichophyton mentagrophytes* and *Aspergillus fumigatus*.[59]

In vivo—Epidemiological studies in South Pacific countries indicate the incidence of cancer is lower the greater the amount of kava drunk, in spite of the higher levels of cigarette smoking in these populations.[60]

Medicinal uses

Genitourinary tract
- cystitis
- prostatitis
- urethritis
- benign prostatic hyperplasia
- neurogenic bladder
- dysuria

BHP specific for infections of the genitourinary tract.

Nervous system

The above research validates the traditional use of this herb for treating states of stress.

- anxiety
- mild depression
- nervous tension
- insomnia

Musculoskeletal
- rheumatism

Externally

As a rubefacient can be used for:

- arthritis
- gout
- joint pain

Pharmacy

Three times daily
Decoction dried root   – 2–4 g
Fluid Extract BPC (1934)   – 2–4 ml

Alcohol extracts are stronger than traditional cold aqueous extracts, in that they contain higher levels of kavalactones.[61]

Commercial preparations in clinical trials contained, for daily use, between 60–400 mg of a standardised extract. However analysis of these products revealed a great variation in kavalactone content from levels stated on the packaging.[62]

All trials reported that *Piper* was well tolerated with minimal side-effects[24,27,28,31,33,34] furthermore benefits were achieved fairly quickly—with improvement possible after just one week of treatment.[30]

Pharmacokinetics

Studies in humans are not very detailed. *In vitro* it has been shown that lactones should be well absorbed, from both water and alcohol extracts and although alcohol seems to enhance absorption it does not affect the relative levels of lactones or their potential bioavailability.[63]

In vivo—Kavain reaches a peak plasma level 1.5–2 hours after ingestion[64] and all major kava-lactones undergo renal excretion after metabolic modifications.[65]

Precautions and/or safety

Clinical studies reported side effects of kava comparable with that of placebo (even using 280 mg kavalactones daily for 4 weeks[66]). Noted side-effects are mostly minor and include dizziness, gastric discomfort,[45] headache, restlessness and/or drowsiness.

Chronic kava use, usually found amongst indigenous populations where kava drinking may be associated with other factors that could impact on health, has been noted to:-

- cause yellow pigmentation, dryness and scales in skin—called kava dermopathy[67,68,73] (attributed by one researcher to possible niacin deficiency[69])
- reduce lymphocyte count[67,73]
- cause hair loss
- cause anorexia[46] and weight loss[73]
- raise lipid levels (total cholesterol as well as LDL and HDL)[70]

In these populations there was no apparent increase in the risk of ischaemic heart disease,[71] infections[72] or brain dysfunction[73] and the above side-effects were reversible on abstaining from further kava use.

Overdoses however may result in depression of nerve function leading to visual[74] and/or hearing impairment, breathing and swallowing difficulties, ataxia,[75] tremors, sedation[76] and paralysis. There are in addition isolated reports of other adverse reactions including acute urinary retention,[77] meningismus (neck rigidity, photophobia and headache),[78] parkinsonism,[79] allergic systemic dermatitis,[80,81] athetosis,[82] sebotropic drug reaction[83] and myoglobinuria (a combination that included kava[84]).

Hepatotoxicity
The question of kava's hepatotoxic reactions still remains unanswered.

In vitro—Extracts of kava in alcohol and to a lesser extent water extracts, kavalactones, pipermethystine and flavokavain B have shown varying levels of cytotoxicity including to hepatocytes.[85-88] Pipermethystine was much more toxic than the tested kavalactones.[87] Flavokavain B also has some cytoprotective activity.[54]

Kavalactones co-administered with alcohol did not inhibit alcohol dehydrogenase activity, an action that, had it existed, may have explained an hepatotoxic effect if they were used together.[89]

In vivo—There have been a number of reported cases of hepatotoxicity assumed to be linked to kava use,[90-98] mostly occurring 3 months after initiating treatment with extracts but in some occurring

after just 14 days use of between 60–120 mg kavalactones a day.[99]

Statistics from 2003 indicated around 100 cases of hepatoxicity had been reported worldwide but closer analysis of available data led to the conclusion that only around 14 could be accepted as "probably" causally related to *Piper*.[100-102] The majority of these were linked either to large doses, longer than 3 months use, co-medication (natural or pharmaceutical) with known hepatotoxins or individuals with pre-existing liver problems.[103,104] A small number of patients required liver transplants and some subsequently died.[105] There followed a withdrawal of medicinal kava products in many countries. Since then substantial research has directly sought answers as to how kava, with its long history of apparently safe use, had resulted in these serious health problems.

A number of explanations have been suggested[100,102,104,105,112,119]:-

- commercial kava products contained kavalactone levels much higher than that found in traditional preparations
- the high demand for *Piper* in the late 1990's may have led to immature or incorrect plant material like the leaves or root peelings being used as well (higher levels of pipermethysticine)
- extraction with high concentrations of alcohol or acetone, the commercial processing chosen to maximise kavalactone recovery, may have introduced toxic changes. This type of processing changes the ratio of the individual kavalactones present, but not the qualitative chemical make-up[106]
- some commercial products were augmented with synthetic kavain including racemic kavain which does not occur naturally in the root
- as kavalactones may interfere with cytochrome P450 isozymes (see Interactions), the high kavalactone commercial extracts may have altered this route of drug metabolism of kava itself or drugs taken concomitantly[107,108]
- there are genetically determined variations in ability to handle drugs through variability of Cytochrome P450 isozymes[109] especially

CYP2D6 and this isozyme is deficient in some Caucasians but not in Polynesians[110]

- non-aqueous kava extracts do not extract root glutathione which is present in water extracts. Kavalactones deplete glutathione and may therefore alter cell protection[105,111]
- inherent toxins in the root hitherto not identified

Whilst liver function tests on groups using water-based kava extracts for over 12 years have shown reversible elevation of some enzymes there have been no signs of liver damage[112] and the profile of elevated enzymes are quite different to that found in drug-induced damage.[113] Rare cases of hepato-toxicity have been reported with use of traditional aqueous preparations too[114] but even very heavy consumers, drinking over 600 g of kava weekly, have not resulted in an increased incidence.[115] Many of the above clinical studies included liver function checks but no evidence of changes were found,[31] neither has a review of safety on kava trials found evidence of serious adverse events.[116]

Reviews of the cases of hepatotoxicity and their potential causes[117-119] conclude no one explanation can account for all the events. At present these cases have been put down to an idiosyncratic drug reaction as the reported incidence of hepatotoxic-ity for kava is very similar to that found for other psychoactive drugs.[91,92,103,111,120,121]

The ban on kava's use has not been lifted across all countries. In Germany where kava medicinal use was highest, it can be prescribed again, but with limitations on dosing (120–210 mg of kavalac-tones per day) and the duration of use limited to a maximum of 2 months.[120]

Interactions

In vitro—*Piper* and its constituents have inhibited some of the P450 cytochrome isozymes[85,122-127] and can also affect P-glycoprotein activity.[128] This gives the herb the potential to cause interactions with other drugs.

In vivo—Studies on drug interactions with kava are currently lacking and are for the most part theoretical.[129]

In contrast to the *in vitro* studies *Piper* was shown **not** to interfere with drugs metabolised by CYP3A4,[130,131] CYP1A2[131] or CYP2D6[131] nor did it affect P-glycoprotein drug handling.[132] In tra-ditional long-term high-consumption kava users (7–27 g kavalactones per week) CYP1A2 does seem to be inhibited and this could confer protec-tion against environmental carcinogens on kava drinkers.[133]

Kava and alcohol used together increased the alcohol-induced impairment of cognitive function in one study[134] but not in another.[135] Concomitant use of kava during withdrawal of benzodiazepines did not result in interactions.[30]

Anecdotal interactions have been reported for kava and **alprazolam** (patient was also using two other pharmaceuticals) that resulted in lethargy and disorientation[136] and with **levodopa** causing reduced drug control of Parkinson's disease.[137]

Historical uses

Gonorrhoea; vaginitis; leucorrhoea; nocturnal incontinence; gout and bronchial problems associ-ated with heart dysfunction; asthma.

PLANTAGINACEAE

The Plantaginaceae or plantain family consists of three genera of widely distributed herbs and sub-shrubs of the temperate region.

- Leaves all basal, but may be alternate or opposite if cauline
- Flowers small, bisexual, inconspicuous in heads or spikes
- Sepals 4-parted, petals 4-lobed and stamens 4 in number
- Fruit a capsule or nutlet enclosed by the calyx

There are many native and naturalised species of plantain. Three species of *Plantago, P. lanceolata, P. major,* and *P. psyllium* are commonly used in traditional western medicine as well as the less well-known *P. indica* and in India *P. ovata.*

Plantago lanceolata

Ribwort, narrow-leaved plantain

Description

A perennial herb with a persistent taproot. *Leaves* all radical, rosulate, hairy with a 1–7 cm long

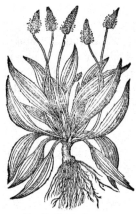

Family Plantaginaceae

petiole, channelled, and with a silky white tuft of hairs and often purplish at the base. *Lamina* 2–20 × 0.5–4.8 cm, linear lanceolate to elliptic-lanceolate, 3–7 veined, glabrate or hairy especially on the veins beneath, entire or slightly toothed. *Scape* (flower stalk), 12–70 cm long, sparsely or densely hairy, strongly ribbed. *Flower* spike very congested, more or less oblong and about 6 cm long. Bracts 3–6 mm long, acuminate with a green keel and the upper part of the bract otherwise brown. Sepals 4, 2.7–3.5 mm long, unequal with the anterior pair fused, midrib green otherwise brown. Corolla tube equal to calyx with lobes about 2 mm long, ovate. Stamens glabrous, exserted, with either white or yellow anthers. Styles exserted up to 15 mm long, densely hairy. *Capsule* usually 2.5–3.5 mm long, ellipsoid and two-seeded. Seeds 2–3 mm long, ellipsoid, medium to dark brown. Flowers present except in winter. In warmer regions of many countries it flowers more or less all year round.

Taste—mucilaginous and somewhat salty and bitter.

Habitat and cultivation
Native to Europe and naturalised elsewhere in open areas, river beds and coastal areas. Grown from seed or transplanted from the wild when small into any garden soil. Frost and drought resistant.

Parts used
The leaves harvested just prior to, or at the start of, flowering.

Active constituents
1) Iridoids (max 9%) including mainly aucubin and its metabolite catalpol[1] as well as asperuloside and verbenalin.[2] These vary with genetic profile and growth conditions.[3,4] Also damage to the plant induces increased levels of iridoid glycosides.[5] Aucubin levels are highest in mid-autumn.[6]
2) Phenylethanoids including acteoside (verbascoside) and plantamajoside[7,8]
3) Flavonoids including luteolin and its derivatives[9]
4) Mucilage (2–6.5%) composed of polysaccharides[10]
5) Tannins (6.5%)

Also contains phenolic and silicic acids. Enzymes occur in the fresh juice and in water extracts.[11]

Nutritional constituents
Minerals: Silicon, zinc and high levels of potassium

Actions
1) Diuretic
2) Anti-inflammatory
3) Antihaemorrhagic

Scientific information
Both *P. lanceolata* and *P. major* are valued as medicinal herbs with some practitioners favouring one over the other. *P. lanceolata* has been especially associated with treatment of the respiratory tract whereas *P. major* is more favoured for treatment of urinary problems. However, they are probably very similar in their pharmacological actions and are considered identical as far as *German Commission E* monographs are concerned.

Both species have a long history of medicinal use throughout the world having been used to treat a multitude of health problems. There has been very little modern scientific validation of these uses. *German Commission E* has approved the internal use of *P. major/P. lanceolata* for catarrh of the respiratory tract and inflammation of oro-pharyngeal mucosa, and external use to treat skin inflammation.

Interest has been shown in the use of *P. lanceolata* as a pasture feed for animals as it has proved beneficial to their health and may reduce the need for antibiotic growth promoters.[12]

In vitro—The polysaccharides have good anti-oxidant activity,[13] in the whole extract this activity has been somewhat variable.[12,14] The herb also inhibits COX-2 activity[15] and this together with any anti-oxidant capacity could help explain its historical use as an anti-inflammatory.

The *Plantago* spp. have been used traditionally for treating cancer and both *P. lanceolata* and *P. major* have activity against cancer cells, an action also displayed by a major flavonoid constituent, luteolin-7-O-β-glucoside, present in both.[16]

Aucubin is known to have bactericidal, bacteriostatic, hepatoprotective, anti-inflammatory, antitumoral and collagen synthesis stimulating activities.[17] Acteoside also has a range of physiological activities, it is anti-inflammatory,[7] antioxidant,[7] anticancer[18] and cytoprotective.[19]

In vivo—The fresh juice of the herb has been used to treat parasitic worms but both water and ethanol extracts may also be effective based on animal studies.[20]

Medicinal uses
Respiratory tract
• all coughs
• asthma

- hoarseness
- haemoptysis
- hayfever
- sinusitis
- nasal catarrh
- bronchitis (acute or chronic)

Gastro-intestinal tract
- peptic ulcers
- colitis
- diarrhoea
- haemorrhoids

Urinary tract
- cystitis
- prostatitis
- haematuria
- calculus

The seed may be used in the treatment of cystitis too.

Externally
The leaf can be applied locally to:

- wounds including slow healing ones
- conjunctivitis (eyewash)
- haemorrhoids
- oral inflammation (mouthwash)
- mouth ulcers (mouthwash)
- blepharitis (eyewash)

Pharmacy
Three times daily
Infusion of dried herb   – 2–4 g
Tincture 1:5 (45%)   – 2–4 ml
Fluid Extract (25%)   – 2–4 ml

Precautions and/or safety
In a standard test *P. lanceolata* was not genotoxic.[21]

Historical uses
Blisters, ulcers, stings, bites, conjunctival congestion, inflammation; anthelmintic.

Plantago major

Rat-tail plantain, broad-leaved plantain

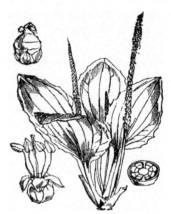

Family Plantaginaceae

Description
A short-lived perennial herb with a stout caudex and many large adventitious roots, or occasionally, with persistent, well-developed primary roots. *Leaves* all radical, rosulate with 1–20 cm long petioles, channelled at the base. *Lamina* 21 × 16 cm, ovate to sub-orbicular, generally puberulent, at least on the main 5–7 veins beneath, generally glabrous, entire or remotely dentate. Base truncate to cordate, apex rounded to obtuse. *Scapes* 5–80 cm long, not ribbed, and generally hairy especially near the base. Spikes dense 1.5–30 cm long, narrow-cylindric. Bracts ovate, larger than calyx. Sepals 1.5–2 mm long, broad ovate. Corolla tube about the same size as the calyx. *Capsule* usually 2.4–4 mm long, broad-ellipsoid, 6–16 seeded. *Seeds* 1–1.8 mm long, rugose; dark red, brown, dark brown or black. Flowers early spring to autumn.

Habitat and cultivation
Native to Eurasia and naturalised elsewhere in moist situations. Grows and seeds freely and may be transplanted into gardens. It is a very variable species in some countries.

Parts used
The leaves harvested just prior to, or at the start of, flowering.

Active constituents

1) Iridoids including aucubin[22]
2) Phenylethanoids including plantamajoside[23]
3) Flavonoids including apigenin, luteolin, baicalein and their derivatives[24]

Also contains tannins and organic acids including caffeic, ferulic and chlorogenic, the triterpenoids ursolic[25] and oleanolic acids,[24] an enzyme that has collagenase activity (named plantagolisin) in fresh juice[26] and some fatty acids.[27]

Nutritional constituents

Vitamins: B-carotene and carotenoids, C and K[24]
Minerals: Calcium, potassium, sulphur and also a high content of trace minerals

Actions

1) Anti-inflammatory
2) Diuretic
3) Antihaemorrhagic

Scientific information

In vitro—Although the aqueous extract of the herb has weak antibacterial, antifungal and antiviral activity against some test organisms,[28-30] a few of the individual constituents are strongly antimicrobial.[30] The herb has antibacterial activity, including against *Salmonella typhimurium*, *Staphylococcus aureus*, *Escherichia coli* and *Bacillus subtilis*, the extracting medium may determine the level of this activity.[31] It also has antiprotozoal activity against *Giardia duodenalis*, comparable to that of a pharmaceutical preparation.[32]

Water extracts inhibit cancer cell proliferation (a number of its constituents are also cytotoxic)[33,34] and are immunomodulatory.[28,33]

A number of constituents are anti-inflammatory, through inhibition of COX activity, including ursolic and oleanolic[25] and the fatty acids.[27]

In vivo—The herb was beneficial in the treatment of chronic bronchitis.[35]

Although there are no modern studies *in vivo* into the effects of *P. major* a review suggests it has antimicrobial (antiviral and antibacterial) action when used topically even though *in vitro* studies indicated low activity.[24]

Medicinal uses

Gastro-intestinal tract
• haemorrhoids

Urinary tract
• cystitis
• prostatitis
• calculus
• haematuria

The seed may be used in the treatment of cystitis too.

Externally
The leaf can be applied locally to:

• wounds (slow healing included)
• conjunctivitis (eyewash)
• haemorrhoids
• oral inflammation (mouthwash)
• mouth ulcers (mouthwash)
• blepharitis (eyewash)

Pharmacy

Dosage three times daily

Infusion of dried herb	– 2–4 g
Tincture 1:5 (45%)	– 2–4 ml
Fluid Extract (25%)	– 2–4 ml

Precautions and/or safety

Most standard tests show *P. major* is not genotoxic[21,36] with the exception of one non-human based assay.[37]

Interactions

There has been a report of *P. major* elevating serum digoxin levels which has since been ascribed to contamination of a commercial preparation of the herb with *Digitalis lanata*.[38] Measurements of levels of digoxin and 13 other drugs including tricyclic antidepressants, anti-epileptics, antibiotics and analgesics showed that *P. major* does not affect their therapeutic monitoring.[39]

Historical uses

P. major was used to stop bleeding from many areas—reproductive tract, lungs, urinary tract and digestive tract including from ulcers; as an antidote to the poison of snakes and mad dogs and the stings of insects and nettles; to cool hot conditions ranging from burns to gout to fevers; dislocated joints. Coughs due to heat; ague; to treat worms. The powdered seeds were given to treat "epilepsy, vomiting, lethargy, dropsy, jaundice, strangury and liver obstructions". The juice of the herb was mixed with Rose oil for headaches and lunacy; eye and ear pain; to restore hearing; toothache. Externally also for scabs; itch; tetters; ringworm; shingles; malignant and leishmanial ulcers; oral thrush.

Plantago psyllium

Psyllium, flea seed[†]

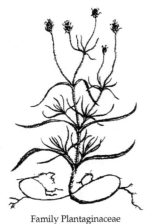

Family Plantaginaceae

Description

A branched annual 35–60 cm tall in flower. *Leaves* linear, entire, sticky-hairy, grey-green, to 7.5 cm long, opposite or in whorls of 3–6 leaves. *Flowers* small, numerous, white, in globose spikes to 1–1.5 cm long, on long peduncles. Flower bracts scarious-margined, rounded at apex. *Seeds* 2–3 mm long, flea-shaped and dark glossy brown.

[†]From the Greek *psylla*—flea because the seeds are the shape and colour of fleas. Apothecaries called the seed *Pulicariae* from the Latin for flea.

Habitat and cultivation

Native to the Mediterranean it grows freely in North Africa, France and Spain, in poor, dry, sandy soils and full sun. May be grown elsewhere from seeds sown in spring in light soil and full sun. Self-sows freely.

Taste—bland and mucilaginous.

Parts used

The seeds (rubbed out of their coats when ripe) and the husks.

Active constituents

1) Mucilage (up to 30%) consisting predominantly of polysaccharides.[40,41] The husk or outer seed coat contains around 85% mucilage[42]
2) Monoterpene alkaloids (seeds)
3) Triterpenes including stigmasterol and β-sitosterol (husks)[43]
4) Phenylethanoids including acteoside and iso-acteoside (seeds)[44]

Also contains a small amount of acubin (seed), sugars and fixed oils rich in polyunsaturated fatty acids—linoleic, oleic and palmitic (husks).[43]

Actions

1) Bulk laxative
2) Demulcent

Scientific information

Seeds of the three species *P. ovata*, *P. indica* and *P. psyllium* have been official medicines.[45] These plus *P. ovata* husks are approved by *German Commission E* for the treatment of chronic constipation, irritable bowel syndrome and diarrhoea.

These species of the western *Plantago* family have been best studied in recent times as they have become important medicines particularly with regard to bowel function. The husks are preferred because they contain more fibre, 67% of which is soluble. (The soluble fraction in the seeds is only 47%.) The mucilage in the husk is composed of 3 main fractions—one representing about 55% is a highly branched arabinoxylan polysaccharide, believed to be a key factor to the herb's activity as a laxative and in helping with lipid reduction.

The second of about 15% is viscous in nature and the rest is composed of insoluble fibre.[41]

Many studies have been conducted into the medicinal benefits of psyllium, some of them driven by commercial interests so that the dosage form used can be variable and may account for some of the discrepancies found.

Gastro-intestinal function

The seeds of all the medical *Plantago* species may be used to help bowel function, however it is usually *P. psyllium*, *P. indica* and *P. ovata* seeds or husks that are used for this purpose. The husks of the first two species are known as psyllium whilst the latter is referred to as ispaghula. In practice this distinction is not necessarily made and the species are often used interchangeably.

The particular structure of the branched arabinoxylan confers activity on the herb as it is resistant to human enzyme digestion and fermentation by gut flora.[41,46] This part of the mucilage, which is capable of holding a good proportion of water, reaches the colon intact where it bulks up the stools and makes their passage easier[47] as well as encouraging better peristalsis and bowel motility.[48-51] Stools become more hydrated, more frequent, have increased weight[48] and are more viscous,[51] providing a lubricant effect so that the consequent laxative action of the husks is both gentle and non-irritating.

The viscous fraction of the mucilage does not alter moisture content of stools or affect lipid metabolism but is fermentable by flora, as is a small proportion of the arabinoxylan and insoluble fractions. This process results in the production of short chain fatty acids as well as gas.[52] Psyllium is considered a prebiotic as it favours the growth of beneficial intestinal flora.[53]

One of its main uses has been to treat constipation. It does not seem to alter gastro-intestinal transit time in healthy individuals[54] but increases it in those with constipation[55] and decreases it in those with diarrhoea.[56,57]

Chronic constipation has been defined as difficulty in passing motions, infrequent motions or both, persisting for a minimum of 3 months in the preceding 12 months.[58] Studies have shown that psyllium fibre gives good improvement in this condition.[59-61] It was more effective than many other laxatives resulting in better formed motions[62] with less side-effects.[63] It can be safely used to treat constipation in elderly people (where it has often been combined with senna)[64,65] and promoted more frequent bowel function in patients with Parkinson's disease.[66]

The mucilage can also improve loose motions in diarrhoea by binding the fluid contents of the colon and psyllium has been successfully used in clinical trials to treat diarrhoea whether chronic (better effect than loperamide),[67] in children,[68] due to radiation therapy or drugs such as anti-obesity lipase inhibitors or[70] protease inhibitors.[71] It has also been effective in reducing faecal incontinence.[72]

It has been used with benefit in the treatment of:-

- bleeding haemorrhoids[73,74]
- tenesmus and pain after haemorrhoidectomy[75] (more effective than glycerine oil[76])
- inflammatory bowel disease—in ulcerative colitis it improved gastro-intestinal symptoms during remission[77] as effectively as mesalamine[78] and improved the condition of patients suffering from Crohn's disease when used with high dose probiotics[79]
- irritable bowel syndrome (IBS)[80,81] where it also reduced constipation and abdominal distension.[82] Soluble fibre can give significant improvement in IBS but insoluble fibre like bran may worsen the condition[83]

Endocrine

Sufficient dietary fibre eaten several hours before or as a part of a meal can reduce postprandial blood glucose and insulin levels.[84,85] The process may in part be due to an increased transit time through the small intestine which reduces carbohydrate digestion and the opportunity for glucose absorption[86] or perhaps by reducing enzyme contact with carbohydrates thereby slowing glucose uptake (see *Avena*). In addition a "second meal" effect has been described where eating a second meal after the initial ingestion of the fibre can still reduce plasma glucose levels from this later meal[87,88] (not corroborated in another study[94]). Furthermore a high soluble fibre diet also seems to improve peripheral insulin sensitivity in normal people.[88]

These actions would be expected to have particular benefits for treating diabetes and a large number of studies have established that using the herb produces a dose-dependent improvement in glucose control. When used in conjunction with standard pharmaceuticals and/or diet psyllium improved blood glucose and associated factors like serum lipid levels and glycated haemoglobin in type 2 diabetics.[89–94] Bowel function in those diabetics with hepatic encephalopathy[95] was improved and uric acid levels also decreased.[91] An additional advantage for type 2 diabetics may be weight loss[96] as it appears to reduce feelings of hunger and give a subjective feeling of fullness[97,98] without slowing gastric emptying.[99]

Psyllium also improved blood glucose (and serum) lipid levels in obese young people.[100]

Serum lipid levels
Dietary fibre has been shown to benefit serum lipid levels although the extent of this is controversial. The mechanism by which serum cholesterol is lowered is not fully understood but seems to be due to the fibre binding bile acids in the intestinal lumen which both prevents their re-absorption and increases their consequent excretion.[101] The loss of bile acids increases their synthesis from cholesterol, effectively reducing serum levels. Increased excretion of bile acids has also been somewhat controversial, some researchers finding no evidence of it, and this proposed mechanism may therefore be too simplistic.[103] However there are other ways by which psyllium may affect lipid levels. It increases the excretion of fatty acids and decreases fat absorption when the two are eaten in the same meal;[102] the short chain fatty acids produced as byproducts of mucilage fermentation may further reduce serum cholesterol by inhibiting its dietary absorption.[103]

Psyllium has been considered one of the more effective fibres for lipid reduction in people with normal or raised cholesterol.[104,105] There are many trials showing lowered levels of total cholesterol and LDL cholesterol in patients with hyperlipidaemia and hypercholesterolaemia[106–112]

(not corroborated[113,128]). Reviews of available data suggest psyllium can alter LDL cholesterol but the range varies between –24% to +3%.[88,114] In children with hypercholesterolaemia it reduced LDL-cholesterol by between 7–22.8%.[100,115] Some trials found cholesterol reduction by psyllium was as good as that achieved through lowering dietary fat intake,[116,117] and may be as effective as statins in reducing LDL cholesterol.[118] It has been suggested that used in conjunction with lipid lowering drugs psyllium may enable the effective drug levels to be reduced[119] also helping to reduce their drug-induced gastro-intestinal side-effects.[120] Whilst a meta-analysis concluded that soluble fibre, including psyllium, does reduce cholesterol levels the large discrepancy across trials was put down to variables like dosage and study design.[104] It has been reported for example that psyllium may be more effective when consumed as part of the meal,[121] that the effects differ by gender and hormonal status—being more beneficial to men[122–124]—and age too may be a factor, being less beneficial in older people (over 60).[125]

There are also conflicting reports of the benefits of husks compared to the seeds in cholesterol reduction. Some research has shown husks improved the lipid profile in patients with cardiovascular disease more effectively than the seeds[126,127] whilst another reported that only the seeds were effective.[128]

Psyllium may help reduce the risk of gallstone formation in people on a low calorie, weight loss diet[129] and may be beneficial when used in conjunction with pharmaceuticals in the treatment of chronic cholestatic liver disease.[130]

Colon cancer
High fibre diets are inversely linked epidemiologically to the incidence of colon cancer.[131] This may be due to the fibre binding potential carcinogens, bile acids and toxins[50] as well as an increased production of metabolites, through fermentation of short chain fatty acids, that have anti-neoplastic potential.[88,132] Because psyllium is not easily digested higher up in the digestive tract it is subject to this fermentation in the colon therefore exerting its protective effect locally.

In vitro—Psyllium fibre protects colon epithelial cells, derived from people at high risk of developing this cancer, from tumour promoting metabolites like the bile acid deoxycholic acid.[133] The short chain fatty acids help the proliferation and differentiation of colonocytes.[133]

In vivo—Using the seed fibre over a period of 3 months the level of the anticancer metabolite, butyrate, increased by 42% in people who had previously had colon cancer.[134] Butyrate production does not persist when fibre use ceases.[134]

The effect of psyllium in patients with a history of adenomas showed that it may actually increase their recurrence especially if combined with a high calcium diet.[135] Adenomas are associated with an increased risk of colon cancer.

Other

In vitro—The polysaccharides enhance proliferation of epithelial cells,[136] reduce bacterial adherence and stimulate macrophage activity, they should therefore aid wound healing and may help limit scar formation.[137]

An extract and some fractions of the husk were inhibitory to *Entamoeba* spp.[138]

In vivo—The addition of psyllium and protein to the diet of hypertensive patients lowered their systolic blood pressure by around 6 mm Hg.[139]

Medicinal uses
Gastro-intestinal tract
• constipation
• chronic diarrhoea
• dysentery
• constipation in pregnancy (*BHC* recommended)[†]
• colitis
• anal fissures[†]
• haemorrhoids[†]
• diverticulosis
• irritable bowel syndrome

Urinary tract
• cystitis

[†]By making the stool softer and easier to pass.

Externally
The seeds can be applied as a poultice to treat:

• boils

Pharmacy

Constipation	5–10 ml (1–2 teaspoons) followed by 250 ml (1 cup) of fluid per teaspoon. Treatment of IBS was effective at a daily dose of 20 g[140]
Hypercholesterolaemia	a minimum of 7.2 g of husks per day has been recommended for reducing cardiovascular disease risk.[108] Many of the studies used 10.5 g daily, as three divided doses of 3.5 g or two divided doses of 5.1 g, taken 15 minutes before meals. Relatively few side effects were recorded across the studies on cholesterol lowering (see under Precautions)[88]
Hyperglycaemia	most studies used 5.1 g two or three times a day taken with or just prior to the meal.[141] One study has reported that lowering of glycaemic index only occurs if psyllium is mixed with food.[141]

CONTRAINDICATIONS:—Stenoses of the gastro-intestinal tract, ileus, difficulty swallowing or **diabetes mellitus** where insulin adjustment is a problem.

Pharmacokinetics
In healthy people most of the mucilage has reached the caecum 4 hours after ingesting the husks.[48]

Precautions and/or safety

Use of husks and seeds does not alter blood biochemistry or most vitamin and mineral levels[91,126] including co-ingested calcium.[142] 10.5 g of psyllium husks were administered daily for a year to a group of healthy people and their nutritional, haematological and biochemical status was checked at the end of this period with no significant changes found other than a small reduction in vitamin B_{12} levels.[143]

Whilst most dietary fibres can alter/inhibit digestive enzyme activity psyllium was shown to either have no effect or to increase enzyme activity *in vitro*.[144]

Possible adverse effects include flatulence (may cause gas retention[145] or a perception of flatulence due to bloating[146]), indigestion, nausea, bloating, retrosternal discomfort and vomiting.[147] These minor side effects may be reduced by introducing fibre gradually, beginning with one dose a day.

There have been reported allergic reactions due to inhalation of psyllium powder[148,149] and ingestion—possibly from proteins from the seed which are often present as contaminants of the husks.[150,151] There have also been more serious cases of anaphylactic shock.[152–154]

Cases of oesophageal obstruction have been reported when treating constipation often due to insufficient water intake[155–157] and in neurologically compromised patients.[158,159] The Food and Drug Administration (America) has recently ruled that granular forms of psyllium are not safe and effective as a laxative for this reason. The ruling does not apply to *Plantago psyllium* in powder, tablet or wafer dosage forms.[160] Other types of gastro-intestinal obstruction have also been reported.[161–165]

There is one case recorded of drug-induced reversible hepatitis to a commercial product containing the herb.[166]

Interactions

It is possible that the fibre can change the absorption and plasma half-life of drugs with which it is co-administered (based on animal data[167]) and it is therefore recommended that psyllium be used an hour after other drugs.

Because of its potential to alter blood sugar, psyllium could interfere with the drug treatment of diabetes.

Actual *in vivo* trials found no change in the absorption of either levothyroxine[168] or digoxin[169] when the drugs were used concurrently with the herb but there is an anecdotal report of it reducing the absorption of **lithium salts**.[170]

Concurrent use of psyllium and **riboflavin** was shown to reduce the apparent vitamin absorption.[171]

Historical uses

Genitourinary catarrh; as an expectorant, antitussive and diuretic. For rheumatic and gouty swellings.

POACEAE

[Formerly known as Graminae]

The Poaceae or Grass family consist of about 9,000–10,000 species world wide. They are:

- Annual or perennial plants; some genera, like bamboo, are woody
- The most significant plant family in the world directly contributing an estimated 60% of the world's food supplies as well as providing food for the meat and milk-producing domestic animals

General characteristics
- Stems are usually cylindrical with swollen nodes and hollow internodes. Many genera have rhizomes

- Leaves are alternate in 2 opposite rows and consist of sheath, ligule and blade which is usually long and narrow. Leaves generally have parallel veins
- Flowers are usually bisexual, small and inconspicuous and called florets. They are usually wind-pollinated
- Inflorescence is compound, with florets arranged in "spikelets" which are in turn arranged in racemes, spikes or panicles (a)
- Each spikelet is enclosed by 2 bracts called **glumes** (b)
- Inside each spikelet each floret is enclosed by 2 bracts—a **palea** and a **lemma** (c)

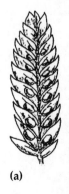 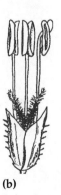 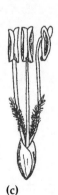 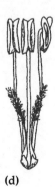

(a)   (b)   (c)   (d)

344

- Petals and sepals have almost disappeared and are reduced and represented by scales called **lodicules**. These lodicules swell and push open the palea and lemma to expose the anthers and stigma (d). Some flowers without lodicules do not open
- There are usually 3 or 6 stamens, with long, slender filaments (d)
- The pistil has one carpel with one ovule and usually 2 large and feathery stigmas (d)
- The fruit is a one-seeded caryopsis or grain, rich in starch and protein (endosperm)

Avena sativa

Oats

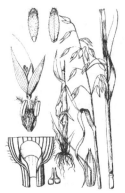

Family Poaceae

Description

A stout annual with an erect, lax inflorescence. *Glumes* 2–2.5 cm long; lemmas hairless or sometimes sparsely hairy and with a twisted jointed awn borne on the lemma of the lower floret only, and about twice as long as it. The florets are not jointed on the axis below and in consequence the spikelets do not shatter on maturity.

Habitat and cultivation

Native to Northern Europe where it is widely cultivated to 60 degrees north, and sometimes grows wild in waste places. It has been cultivated since classical times as a staple food for northern Europeans and the Scots. It is also an important food for livestock. It is grown commercially, from seed, in cooler areas elsewhere.

Parts used

The grain (oats), the green herb and the stalks or oatstraw.

Active constituents

1) Phenolics including
    a. polyphenols derived from hydroxycinnamic acid. They are alkaloids called avenanthramides A-C
    b. small amounts of phenolic acids including ferulic, p-coumaric and caffeic acid[1-4]
2) Saponins (avenacosides)[5]
3) Protein including good levels of the amino acid tryptophan,[6,7] also enzymes including lipase, lipoxygenase and superoxide dismutase[8]
4) Flavonoids including apigenin, luteolin, kaempferol, quercetin and tricin[1]
5) Polysaccharides including β-glucan[9,10]
6) Lipids (min. 0.6%) including predominantly unsaturated fatty acids also choline[11] and γ-linoleic acid (3–11%)[12-15]

Amongst cereal grains oats have one of the highest contents of protein[16] and lipids.[17]

Also contains insoluble fibre (lignin), sterols (mostly β-Sitosterol also avenasterol[18]), silicic acid[19] and some phytic acid.[18] The green herb contains flavolignans.[20]

Nutritional constituents

Both oats and oatstraw are high in:

Vitamins: A, B-complex including thiamine, riboflavin, niacin, folic acid, B_6, C, E (α-tocopherol) and K

Minerals: Silicon, calcium, iron (high in oatstraw), potassium, phosphorus, manganese and zinc

Actions

1) Thymoleptic
2) Cardiac tonic
3) Antidepressant

Scientific information

Earliest signs of oats being used by humans occur around 2000 BC and ancient texts describe the herb's medicinal uses. Apart from a long tradition it was at one time an official medicine in USA. Oatstraw has been approved by *German Commission E* for topical use in inflammatory and sebhorreic skin diseases especially when associated with itching.

Avena is still of scientific interest in the food and cosmetic industries,[8] some of its constituents show interesting physiological activity.

Skin

The use of oats for skin care dates back to earliest times. Finely ground oatmeal (from dehulled oats) produces a colloidal substance after boiling that, since 1945, has been available as a topical preparation to treat itchy and irritated skin. Many of the constituents of oats contribute to its activity as an effective topical preparation. The polysaccharide, starch and β-glucan form the basis of the colloid which can protect skin (its viscous nature forming a protective barrier), helps with hydration and acts as a buffer to maintain normal pH.[8]

Added to this the phenols have anti-oxidant and anti-inflammatory properties, the flavonoids are able to absorb UV light and saponins are soap-like agents that can cleanse the skin.[1,8]

In vitro—The herb is a potential aid to wound healing. It stimulates epithelial growth,[21] reduces inflammation (through inhibition of arachidonic acid metabolism[22]) and reduces oedema.[23]

In vivo—Oat extracts used externally in young children with atopic dermatitis reduced the need for high dose corticosteroid therapy,[24] countered the irritant effects of sodium lauryl sulphate applied to normal skin[25] and reduced the itch associated with burn injuries.[26]

There are a number of older studies showing the soothing effect of the colloid on a variety of dermatoses.[8]

Metabolic

In vitro—The avenanthramides have potential in preventing and/or reducing atherosclerosis by inhibiting vascular cell proliferation, adhesion and inflammation and increasing nitric oxide production.[27,28]

In vivo—B-glucans, as soluble fibre, can reduce postprandial blood glucose levels. One theory is that this occurs by making carbohydrate less accessible to enzyme degradation thereby extending digestion and delaying the absorption of glucose from the digestive tract. Another is that dietary fibre increases small intestine transit time slowing carbohydrate digestion and consequent glucose uptake.[30] This activity was demonstrated in trials where blood glucose and insulin levels were reduced after eating oat products[9,29,30] (not corroborated[32]).

Oat bran, again due to the soluble fibre, increased HDL-cholesterol[9] and lowered both LDL-cholesterol[9,31,32] and total cholesterol.[31,32] Trials have shown the effects of oats on LDL and/or total cholesterol levels ranges from a lowering effect between 3–16% (not corroborated[33]). The mechanism of cholesterol lowering seems to be similar to psyllium. The lignin and β-glucan components of oat fibre bind bile acids,[34] increasing their excretion[35] thereby causing increased bile acid synthesis from cholesterol with consequent reductions in serum levels.[36]

Oats reduced blood pressure[30,37] (not corroborated[38]), reduced body weight[9] and may, by increasing beneficial metabolites like butyrate improve bowel health.[31] Furthermore a diet rich in whole grains increases serum enterolactone, higher levels of which have been found to correlate positively with a decreased risk of heart disease and some cancers.[39]

Other

In vitro—*Avena* is a good anti-oxidant, this activity may be increased after its digestion.[40] Several of the constituents, especially those found in the bran, are likely to contribute.[41–44] Commercial preparation used by the food industry may alter the anti-oxidant potential up or down depending on the method of processing.[45]

Avena may help protect lung cells from nicotine toxicity;[46] and the avenanthramides have antiproliferative activity.[1]

In vivo—Studies done some time ago suggested that *Avena* preparations may help reduce nicotine craving in cigarettes smokers[47,48] (not corroborated[49]); and the avenanthramides are bioavailable and enhance anti-oxidant status.[1]

Traditional uses of the herb to treat the nervous system have not been subject to any recent research.

Medicinal uses
Cardiovascular system
In chronic states of debility it can be used for:

- cardiovascular support

Nervous system
- depression
- melancholia
- general debility
- neuralgia
- neuritis
- convalescence
- shingles
- menopausal neurasthenia
- insomnia

BHP specific for depressive states.

Externally
As an emollient it may be used to good effect for:

- dry skin
- eczema
- wounds
- burns
- neuralgia

Pharmacy
Three times daily
Oatmeal or straw   – 1–4 g
Tincture 1:5 (45%)   – 1–5 ml
Fluid Extract (25%)   – 0.6–2 ml

The herb may be prepared as a decoction of the straw, juice extract of the green herb or tincture of either the seed or green plant. Eating rolled oats as porridge or muesli is also beneficial.

Precautions and/or safety
Avena has been contraindicated in *Coeliac* disease, the necessity of this is uncertain as many gluten-intolerant people have been able to eat oats without problems whilst on a gluten-free diet.[50] The alcohol extract should not cause any reactions in gluten sensitive people.

There is one reported case of contact dermatitis to oats in an atopic individual.[51] Colloidal preparations tested on a group of susceptible children did not induce allergic reactions.[52]

Historical uses
Used externally to treat conditions like leprosy, "the itch" and fistulas; prepared with vinegar as a means of getting rid of freckles and spots; believed to aid withdrawal from addictive substances e.g. opium.

Elytrigia repens
[Formerly known as *Agropyrum repens*;
Agropyron repens; *Triticum repens*]

Couch-grass

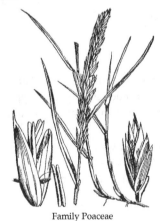

Family Poaceae

Description
A perennial grass spreading extensively by underground stolons and often forming large patches. Rootstock long, jointed and yellowish. Growing rhizomes have strong points which penetrate other plants easily. *Leaves* dull-green, usually sparsely hairy, soft, flat and somewhat drooping, crowded

with fine ribs. *Flower stems* stiff, erect, 30–120 cm bearing a straight, erect, spike-like inflorescence 5–30 cm. Spike not square; 2–9 flowered spikelets, overlapping, 1–2 cm long; bract below spikelets not stiff with slender keel and ribs. (Some *Agropyron* species have square spikes with stiff bracts.) Glumes 3–7-veined, blunt or pointed; lemmas tough, 8–13 mm long, five-veined, blunt or pointed. Hybridises with *A. junceiforme*.

Habitat and cultivation
Native to Europe and Britain in waste ground and rough pasture. Naturalised and a troublesome weed in many countries. It spreads by seed and rooting stolons.

Parts used
The rhizomes harvested in autumn or early spring.

Active constituents
1) Volatile oil (max. 0.05%) including agropyrene
2) Carbohydrates including mannitol,[53] triticin (7–8% this is a complex fructosan[54]), inositol, mucilage and gum[55]
3) Silicic acid
4) Saponins

Also the phenolics vanillin, ferulic[56] and coumaric[57] acids, indole acetic acid, hydroxytryptophan, carboline[58] and a small amount of anthraquinones.[59]

Nutritional constituents
Vitamins: A and some B
Minerals: Potassium and iron

Actions
1) Diuretic
2) Demulcent

Scientific information
Elytrigia has been an official medicine in a number of countries throughout the world.[55] There are no human studies on the rhizomes.

Individual constituents are better characterised than the whole herb. Triticin is a polysaccharide similar to inulin (see *Cichorium intybus*). Mannitol is a well established osmotic diuretic. Its action is based on the fact that it is not re-absorbed from kidney tubules so that it acts via osmosis to draw water into them and in this way increases urine volume.[60] It is possible it has a direct soothing effect on the mucosa too.

Agropyrene appears not to have been studied in recent times but it had been reported to have antibacterial properties.

Medicinal uses
Urinary tract
Its diuretic properties are described as mild[55]:

- cystitis
- nephritis
- urethritis
- prostatitis
- benign prostatic hyperplasia
- calculus

Musculoskeletal
Due to increased kidney output and as a nutritive agent it may be used to help treat:

- gout
- rheumatism

Pharmacy
Three times daily
Decoction — 1–4 g
Tincture 1:5 (40%) — 5–15 ml
Fluid Extract (25%) — 4–8 ml

Historical uses
Food source for livestock; "openeth the stoppings of liver and reins (kidneys) without heat"; jaundice; scirrhous livers; griping pains of the belly; inflammations; worms in children; suppression of urine; stone and ulcers of the bladder; spring tonic and blood purifier; diabetes, heals wounds (external).

Zea mays

Corn silk, maize

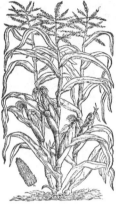

Family Poaceae

Description

A very robust annual growing 2 m or more high. It has a stout stem with many broad leaves and a terminal plume-like inflorescence of male spikelets and several large, lateral, bud-like inflorescences of female spikelets closely invested by overlapping leafy bracts. *Leaves* dull green, 5–12 cm wide, margins rough and finely ciliate. *Flowers* unisexual—male spikelets 6–8 mm arranged closely along many slender branches. Female spikelets densely arranged on swollen lateral branches and completely enclosed in leafy bracts with only the very long stigmas, 12–20 cm, projecting. *Fruit* hard, shining yellow, white or purple, arranged round a much swollen axis and fully enclosed in leafy bracts—the cob.

Odour—faint and characteristic; taste—sweet.

Habitat and cultivation

Native to South America *Zea* is widely cultivated throughout the world. It is grown from seed sown in spring and planted in rich soil in an open sunny situation. Because it is wind pollinated *Zea* produces better corn if planted in squares rather than rows. Drought and frost tender.

Parts used

The fresh or dried styles and stigmas from the female flowers of unripe maize, known as corn silk.

Active constituents

1) Flavonoids including luteolin and its derivatives of which maysin is predominant.[61–63] Also fomononetin[64]
2) Chlorogenic acid[61]
3) Volatile oil including terpineol and geraniol[65]
4) Alkaloids
5) Phytosterols—stigmasterol and sitosterol

Also contains saponins, mucilage, allantoin (around 0.2%),[66] PABA, tannins and proanthocyanidins.[62]

Many hybrids of *Zea mays* exist and the medicinal corn silk is likely to be derived from a number of them.[62]

Nutritional constituents

Vitamins: Rich in vitamin K, also B and C
Minerals: Silicon, potassium, calcium and magnesium

Actions

1) Diuretic
2) Demulcent
3) Antilithic

Scientific information

The herb is listed in a number of pharmacopoeias as a diuretic.[55]

In vitro—*Zea* extracts and its phenolics like the flavonoid, luteolin, are good agents for preventing glycation associated with diabetes and aging.[67] The herb may aid glucose and lipid homeostasis via activation of peroxisome proliferator-activated receptor.[68]

The relatively high content of polyphenols gives it a good anti-oxidant capacity[62] this is particularly so for mature corn silk.[69]

Zea has some antibacterial activity against *Staphylococcus aureus*.[70] It is also a significant inhibitor of cytokine production.[71]

In vivo—A study measuring the diuretic effect of *Zea* found it ineffective over a 12–24 hour period.[72] There is very little other scientific information available on the medicinal action although earlier work suggested the diuretic action may be due to the herb's high potassium levels.

In China it is used to help prevent the complications of diabetes and the Peruvian Indians used it as a narcotic probably due to its alkaloids.

Medicinal uses
Urinary tract
• dysuria
• cystitis
• urethritis
• prostatitis
• enuresis

BHP specific for acute or chronic inflammation of urinary tract.

Pharmacy
Three times daily
Infusion   – 2–8 g
Tincture 1:5 (25%)   – 5–15 ml
Fluid Extract (25%)   – 4–8 ml

Historical uses
For gravel, stones and strangury; gonorrhoea. Poultice for ulcers; swellings; rheumatic pain. Nausea and vomiting.

POLYGONACEAE

The Polygonaceae are mostly wiry-stemmed herbaceous plants, shrubs and lianes of the temperate Northern Hemisphere but there are also a few trees native to the tropics and some grow naturally in the Southern Hemisphere. There are about 1150 species world wide.

The common feature in all members of this family is an ochrea—a peculiar membrane-like sheath which surrounds the stem above each swollen node where leaf stalks are attached. It is formed from modified stipules which in many other families are a pair of flaps at the leaf base.

Many species contain oxalic acid in their tissues which gives a sharp taste to some e.g. sorrel leaves, but is poisonous in others, e.g. rhubarb leaves.

Plants of economic importance include *Fagopyron esculentum* (buckwheat), *Rumex acetosa* (sorrel) and *Rheum* spp. (rhubarbs).

- Leaves are simple and usually entire and alternate; stipules usually united to form an ochrea
- Flowers bisexual and regular; inflorescence racemose but with partial inflorescences usually cymose
- Perianth sepals and petals the same; usually 5–6 segments, often green and in 2 whorls of 3; often persistent, forming a wing in the fruiting stage for wind dispersal
- Stamens usually 6–9 often of 2 lengths; filaments sometimes basally connate
- Ovary superior, unilocular; styles 2–3 more or less united; 1 ovule
- Fruit nearly always a triangular nut or achene; sometimes enclosed in the persistent perianth forming a wing

Rheum officinale

Chinese rhubarb

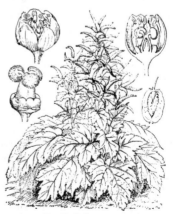

Family Polygonaceae

351

In addition to *R. officinale* and *R. palmatum*, a third species of Chinese rhubarb, *R. tanguticum*, is also officially part of pharmacopoeial *Rhizoma Rhei*, called Dahuang in Chinese.

Description
R. officinale is a taller, larger perennial, more than 3 m in flower. *Leaves* grow on long reddish stems and are up to a 1 m across; ovate, with 5–7 shallow irregular lobes and prominent veins. *Flowers* white in large panicles, blooming in summer.

Odour—characteristic, aromatic; taste—slightly astringent and bitter.

Habitat and cultivation
R. officinale prefers a sunny situation and well drained but moist soils. It can be cultivated in countries with a similar cold climate and soils but does not do well in hot humid areas. It may be grown from seed or division of the roots.

Parts used
Roots and rhizomes harvested, preferably when they are at least 6 years old, in autumn or early spring.

Active constituents[1–3]
1) Hydroxyanthracenes
   a) anthraquinones (about 3%),[4] complex in nature, some free but present mostly as glycosides of emodin (about 2.6%), rhein, aloe-emodin, chrysophanol and physcion[5–7]
   b) dianthrones including sennosides A and B[7,8]
2) Tannins (5–10%) including galloylglucosides, procyanidins and gallic acid[9]
3) Stilbenes including resveratrol[10]
4) Flavonoids including catechin
5) Phenylbutanones including lindleyin[11,12]

Also contains volatile oil including cinnamic acid.[13]

There is geographical variation amongst these *Rheum* species which also alters their chemical make-up[2,14] and there are qualitative and quantitative differences between the species. *R. officinale* appears to have lower levels of the above active constituents[3,15] whereas *R. palmatum* and

R. tanguticum are quite similar. The different species are hard to identify based on their appearance and this is therefore done chemically. In practice the herb is likely to be a mixture of all three official species.[2,15]

Nutritional constituents
Vitamins: A, C and B complex
Minerals: Sodium, potassium, iron, sulphur and phosphorus

Actions
1) Laxative
2) Astringent
3) Tonic
4) Stomachic
5) Aperient

Scientific information
Rheum is a valued and long-established medicine in the East and has been an official preparation in many pharmacopoeias across the world.[16] In the west it has been used mainly as a purgative[16] but the range of uses is much broader in their countries of origin. There are a number of pharmacologically active constituents that have received scientific study although the hydroxyanthracenes are the main ones involved in purgation. A central action that may help give its broad ranging uses as seen in eastern medicine is the fact that it is a strong anti-oxidant[17,18] and this is due to a number of its constituents.[19–21]

Cancer support
In vitro—The anthraquinones have potent anti-tumour properties for a variety of cancer cell lines including liver,[22,23] multiple myeloma,[24] leukaemia,[25–27] oral,[10,28] gastric,[29] ovarian,[30] prostate,[31] epidermal,[31] lung,[32–37] pancreatic[32] and breast.[32,38] Their mechanisms as anticancer agents are multi-factorial and includes the induction of apoptosis and cell-cycle arrest,[39] disruption of mitochondrial function,[26] damage to DNA,[10] protection against chemical mutagens[40–42] and the inhibition of metastatic spread[43–45] and angiogenesis.[46] Tumor cells are more sensitive to these actions than normal cells.[10,47] In addition the anthraquinones may

enhance the activity of cancer chemotherapeutic agents.[47] Stilbene constituents may have anticancer potential too.[10] *Rheum* is one of the four main herbs contained in Essiac tea which has been widely used as part of complementary cancer treatment. Essiac is strongly anti-oxidant and protects DNA from free radical damage.[48]

In vivo—Much of the reported clinical information on rhubarb relates to its use as a supportive treatment in cancer rather than as a treatment on its own. With few side-effects it reduced radiation-induced damage in the treatment of lung cancer through modulation of inflammatory cytokines[49] and it improved the inflammation and return of gastro-intestinal function in patients treated surgically for gastric cancer.[50] To-date there have been almost no reported data from clinical trials on Essiac use in cancer therapy—one recent study failed to find any benefit[51]—although there are anecdotal reports of efficacy.[52,53]

Cardiovascular

In vivo—*Rheum* significantly improved lipid levels[54,55] including in patients with atherosclerosis in whom circulatory flow was increased.[56]

It reduced endothelial damage in women with pregnancy-induced hypertension improving their lipid and immune status.[57] In those women at risk for this condition, low doses of the herb had a protective effect against its development.[58]

Antimicrobial

In vitro—*Rheum* spp. and individual anthraquinones have a range of antimicrobial activity:-

- antiviral and virucidal activity particularly against a variety of enveloped viruses[59] including SARS virus,[60] hepatitis B virus[61–63] (volatile oil also has activity),[64] human cytomegalovirus[65] and HSV[66,67]
- antifungal activity including against *Aspergillus fumigatus* and *Candida albicans* (equally as effective as nystatin[68])
- antibacterial against cariogenic bacteria,[69] *Helicobacter pylori*[70] *Bacteroides fragilis*[71] and *Escherichia coli*.[72] In addition the herb may also increase the efficacy of antibiotics against resistant strains of *Staphylococcus aureus*[73]

Emodin's mode of action is associated with disruption of the micro-organisms' cell membranes.[74]

In vivo—In treating patients with sepsis the addition of *Rheum* helped reduce the incidence of opportunistic fungal infection,[75] decreased intestinal permeability[76] and improved gastro-intestinal perfusion.[77] The herb also improved the outcome of systemic inflammatory response syndrome patients with nosocomial (hospital-derived) Gram-negative bacterial pneumonia.[78]

Rheum and *Salvia officinalis* together in a topical preparation was as effective as *Zovirax* for treating of herpes labialis.[79]

Kidney disease

Rheum has been used in traditional Chinese medicine to help treat renal disease.[80]

In vitro—It inhibits protein glycation[81] (glycation causes nephropathy in diabetes).

In vivo—It was used as part of an effective treatment for nephrotic syndrome complicated by intestinal bleeding.[82] There is evidence from clinical trials that low doses of the herb, in conjunction with orthodox medicine, benefited the treatment of chronic renal failure[83–87] and improved associated hyperlipidaemia.[84,88] This data has been reviewed.[89,90]

Anti-inflammatory

In vitro—A topical gel containing *Rheum* and a pharmaceutical antimicrobial inhibited cytokine release, oedema and vasodilation in simulated inflammation of gingival cells.[91]

In vivo—*Rheum* used with orthodox treatment in patients with systemic inflammation reaction syndrome reduced inflammatory chemical levels in sera, improving patient outcomes significantly compared to orthodox treatment alone.[92]

Other

In vitro—*Rheum* spp.:-

- are phyto-oestrogenic[30] (lindleyin,[93] hydroxyanthraquinones[94]) interacting at both α- and β-oestrogen receptor sites
- help reduce the formation of dental calculus[95]
- inhibit the synthesis of melanin[96]

Individual constituents modulate the excessive production of pro-inflammatory cytokines (emodin),[97] protect neurons from damage by amyloid protein (a stilbene),[98] and may increase insulin sensitivity and energy metabolism in adipocytes (emodin).[99]

In vivo—Clinical studies have reported that *Rheum* was of benefit in:-

- infantile cholestatic jaundice,[100] it has been used traditionally in China to treat neonatal jaundice[101]
- treatment of severe brain injury[102]
- memory in the elderly[103]
- bleeding gastric and duodenal ulcers[104]
- reducing signs and symptoms of endometriosis (it was the main ingredient of a herbal combination[105])

Medicinal uses
Gastro-intestinal tract
This is the recognized western use of *Rheum* and whilst the hydroxyanthracene components are purgative their action is much milder than that of *Cassia* and *Aloe* spp. The tannins help to give the herb an astringent action, and it is additionally bitter with potential antimicrobial and anti-inflammatory activities. It can be used to treat:-

- constipation
- diarrhoea
- gastroenteritis
- haemorrhoids
- anal fissures[†]

Traditional Chinese medicinal uses are listed under Historical uses.

Pharmacy
Daily
Decoction of dried herb   – 0.2–4 g
Tincture *BPC* (60%)   – up to 15 ml
As astringent or stomachic – 0.1–0.3 g
Three times daily

Fluid extract   –   0.5–8 ml (suggested guidelines)

For laxative purposes *Rheum* should be used short term for a maximum of 2 weeks and can be taken as a single or divided dose. It takes from 6–24 hours after ingestion to act and is usually taken at bedtime.

Doses in above trials ranged from 1.5 ml (this is low dose) to 24 ml of 1:2 extract per day (converted from grams).

Constipation is treated with doses in the higher range as at low dose the effect of the tannins predominates.[16]

For pharmacokinetic information on anthraquinones see *Cassia*.

CONTRAINDICATIONS—Intestinal obstruction or **abdominal pain** of unknown origin.

Precautions and/or safety
In overdose it can cause diarrhoea and griping. *Pseudomelanosis coli* is associated with overuse of herbs containing anthraquinones including *Rheum*,[106] it is not considered pathologic and is reversible when usage ceases—see *Cassia*.

Interactions
Because of a decreased transit time through the colon it is possible that *Rheum* may interact with drugs with which it is co-administered and which are absorbed from this area. There are no reported interactions.

Historical uses
Used for conditions of blood stasis and as peripheral vasodilator, anticoagulant, anti-inflammatory and antimicrobial. Internally to treat gastro-intestinal haemorrhage, jaundice; abdominal pain, indigestion, ulcers; amenorrhoea, dysmenorrhoea, hypertension. Externally for scalds and burns.

[†]By making stool easier to pass

Rheum palmatum

Chinese rhubarb, Turkey rhubarb

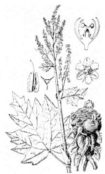

Family Polygonaceae

Description
A stout perennial growing from a thick rhizome up to 2 m high in flower. *Leaves* large, outline rounded, base heart-shaped, with deeply palmate lobes which may be further divided. *Flowers*, small, greenish white, in panicles in summer.

Habitat and cultivation
R. palmatum is native to China, growing on forest margins in wet soils in high mountainous areas. It is wild harvested and also cultivated.

See above (*R. officinale*) for Parts used up to Historical uses.

Rumex crispus

Yellow dock, curled dock

Description
A perennial with a stout taproot growing up to about 1 m high in flower. *Petiole* is shorter than the leaf blade, anterior side flattened with raised margins so that it appears concave. Lamina of lower *leaves* 6–30 × 1.5–6.5 cm, narrow-lanceolate, oblong or ligulate, undulate with curly margins, leaf base attenuate.[†] Upper leaves similar but smaller. *Stem* erect, smooth and slender. *Inflorescence* terminal, nearly simple or with a few erect lateral branches,

------

[†]This distinguishes it from other common docks.

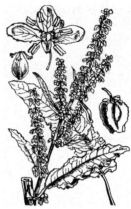

Family Polygonaceae

each subtended by a narrow crisped leaf with whorls of flowers closely bunched. *Flowers* pale green, small and numerous, male or female or both. Perianth 1–2.5 mm long, segments of outer whorl more or less elliptic, obtuse and not reflexing at fruiting. Segments of inner whorl much longer and enlarging at fruiting. *Fruiting valves* 3–4.5 × 3–5 mm broad-ovate with raised veins, entire, sinuate or crenulate; tubercles 1–3, deep red, often 1 being much larger. *Nuts* 2–2.5 mm long, dark brown and sharply angled. Flowers in spring and summer.

Habitat and cultivation
Native to Europe, North Africa and West Asia. Naturalised world-wide in both damp and dry places. It self-sows freely. Deep rich damp soil in full sun produces better roots. Drought and frost resistant.

Parts used
The root harvested after the fruit is ripe, towards the end of summer.

Active constituents
1) Hydroxyanthracenes[107,108]
   a) anthraquinones (3–4%) including nepodin, physcion, chrysaphanol, emodin and 1,5-hydroxy isomers of methylanthraquinone.[109,110] The chemical make-up and levels depend on genetic and environmental factors
   b) anthrone—rumexone[110]
2) Tannins
3) Volatile oil

Also contains resin and oxalic acid.

Nutritional constituents
Vitamins: A and C
Minerals: Iron, manganese, calcium and phosphorous

Actions
1) Mild cholagogue
2) Laxative
3) Alterative
4) Tonic

Scientific information
There has been no recent investigation into this herb however there are many similarities in chemistry between *Rheum* and *Rumex*.

The laxative effects of the anthraquinones are like those found in *Cassia* and *Rheum* and as in the latter they are moderated by the relatively high level of tannins. The bitter quality extends its use beyond just a laxative effect. The purgative effect is gentle.

Medicinal uses
Cardiovascular system
• anaemia

Gastro-intestinal tract
• atonic constipation
• jaundice

Musculoskeletal
• arthritis

Skin
• chronic skin conditions
• psoriasis

BHP specific for skin diseases, especially psoriasis, with constipation.

Externally
• gingivitis (mouthwash)
• laryngitis (gargle)
• slow healing ulcers
• wounds

Pharmacy
Three times daily
Decoction of dried root   – 2–4 g
Tincture 1:5 (45%)   – 1–5 ml
Fluid Extract (25%)   – 2–4 ml

Historical uses
Used "when either the blood or liver is affected by choler", piles; bleeding from the lungs; diphtheria; scurvy; itchy skin conditions; to treat cancer, tonic for weakened constitutions. Seeds have also been employed to treat dysentery. An ointment used for skin problems like itch; scab; eruptions; freckles; morphews; spots and discolouring.

RANUNCULACEAE

The buttercup or crowfoot family is considered to be one of the more primitive of the dicotyledons and contains both common weeds and some important garden plants. There are 1900 species most common in the northern temperate regions. Most of them are perennial herbaceous plants, and may be aquatic or semi-aquatic growing in ponds or damp places, but there are also some shrubs and lianes e.g. Clematis.

N.B. Many species are toxic e.g. the fresh leaves of the genera *Adonis, Anemone,* and *Ranunculus* contain a highly irritant oil called protoanemonin which is poisonous to cattle, sheep and horses, but which breaks down to anemonin when the leaves are dried. Some genera like *Aconitum* contain poisonous alkaloids.

- Leaves usually alternate and may be simple or compound with sheathing bases
- Flowers usually bisexual and insect or wind pollinated. They may be solitary or arranged in cymes
- Calyx consists of a variable number of sepals which may be petal-like or may fall off early
- Androecium: anthers spirally arranged and usually numerous
- Gynoecium: carpels free and usually numerous
- Fruit usually a group of achenes or follicles and occasionally a berry or capsule

Anemone pulsatilla

Pulsatilla, pasque flower

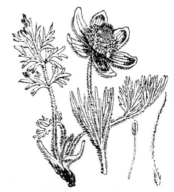

Family Ranunculaceae

Description
A softly hairy perennial to 25 cm growing from a thick woody rhizome. *Basal leaves* finely divided and pinnately cleft at the base with long, linear,

357

pointed segments. *Flowers* solitary, to 5 cm across, erect, with 6 deep purple sepals and many golden stamens, above a ruff of involucral leaves to 2 cm long. *Fruit* small brown achenes with long feathery tails. Flowers in spring and summer.

Habitat and cultivation
Native to central and northern Europe, growing in open, sunny situations and well-drained limey soils. Grown in gardens elsewhere from seed sown as soon as it is ripe, or by root division in spring or autumn. Drought and frost resistant.

Parts used
The herb collected at the time of flowering and **dried before use**.

Active constituents
1) Lactones including ranunculin (around 3%) which, on crushing the plant, is converted to protoanemonin[1] and this, being unstable, is degraded into the stable constituent, anemonin
2) Triterpenoid saponins

Also contains tannins, volatile oil, chelidonic and succinic acids and flavonoids. The flowers have in addition, delphinidin and pelargonidin glycosides.

Actions
1) Anodyne
2) Sedative
3) Antispasmodic
4) Antimicrobial

Scientific information
Very little pharmacological information is available.
In *vitro*—Protoanemonin is antifungal[2,3] including against *Candida albicans*[1] and *Trichophyton mentagrophytes*[4] and antibacterial against both Gram-positive and Gram-negative bacteria including pathogenic cocci, bacilli and also *Mycobacterium tuberculosis*.[1] Anemonin does not have this same activity.[5]
Protoanemonin is also anti-mutagenic[6] and a skin irritant that can cause blistering.[7]

The *BHP* maintains that the herb is a bactericidal and lists the treatment of infections amongst its uses.

Medicinal uses
Respiratory tract
• asthma

Nervous system
• tension headaches
• hyperactivity
• insomnia

Reproductive tract
Used for pain and tension in this tract including:

• epididymitis
• ovarian pain
• orchitis
• dysmenorrhoea, especially with scanty menses (*BHP* specific)

Externally
• earache

Pharmacy
Three times daily
Infusion of dried herb   – 0.1–0.3 g
Tincture 1:10 (40%)   – 0.5–3 ml
Fluid Extract (25%)   – 0.1–0.3 ml
For earache a few drops of the tincture are inserted into the outer ear.
CONTRAINDICATIONS—Pregnancy and lactation.

Precautions and/or safety
The herb must not be used fresh because it causes irritation and blistering on surfaces with which it comes in contact. Excessive doses can cause severe gastritis.

Historical uses
Spasmodic coughs including asthma, whooping cough, bronchitis. Catarrhal conditions—"watery and phlegmatic humours"; as an emmenagogue and for nervous exhaustion in women. Leprosy

and cutaneous conditions including "malignant and corroding ulcers". All afflictions of the eyes and *Weiss* includes here "iritis, scleritis, diseases of the retina, glaucoma and possibly senile cataract".

Cimicifuga racemosa

Black cohosh

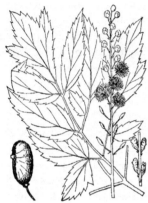

Family Ranunculaceae

Description
A perennial which dies back completely in winter, and grows up to 3 × 2 m in flower. Rootstock thick and blackish. *Leaves* alternate and triternately divided, with the terminal leaflet the largest; dark green and sharply toothed. *Flowers* creamy-white, with long stamens; growing in long, simple or compound spikes, blooming in summer.

Odour—slight; taste—slightly bitter.

Habitat and cultivation
Native to rich woods in Canada and USA from South Ontario to Georgia. Plants are available elsewhere and may be grown in semi-shady situations in good, rich, leaf-mouldy soil. It takes 20 months or more for seeds to germinate.[8] Drought and frost resistant.

Parts used
The root and rhizomes harvested in autumn[8] and **used after drying.**

Active constituents
1) Triterpene glycosides[9-14] (about 2%)[15] many are of the cycloartane type. Over 40 have been reported. The main ones are actein, 23-epi-26-deoxyactein (27-deoxyactein), acetylshengmanol-3-O-xyloside, cimigenol-3-O-arabinoside and cimigenol-3-O-xyloside[16]
2) Isoflavones including formononetin[17] (the presence of this constituent is controversial—it may be present in very low concentrations[15] but has recently been reported as undetectable[18,19])
3) Phenolic constituents (about 0.6%).[20-26] More than 20 have been isolated, either free or as derivatives they include isoferulic, ferulic, caffeic, fukinolic and cimicifugic acids A, B, E and F and a lignan—actaealactone.

Also contains tannin, resin, an alkaloid (cimipronidine[22]), fatty acids, salicylic acid, starch and sugars. *C. racemosa* does not contain cimicifugin or its glucoside.[16]

Interestingly a sample of *Cimicifuga* collected in 1919 had a similar constituent profile, though levels were lower, than a modern specimen suggesting that these constituents are relatively stable.[27]

Nutritional constituents
Minerals: Calcium, iron, magnesium, potassium and zinc[28]

Actions
1) Sedative
2) Antitussive
3) Antirheumatic
4) Emmenagogue

Scientific information
Cimicifuga also known as *Actaea racemosa* is one of a number of this genus that grows in similar habitats in North America. There are also similar species used medicinally in Eastern herbal medicine. Black cohosh, a traditional medicine of the Native Americans, was introduced to early settlers and became an official medicine in the *United States Pharmacopoeia* remaining as such till 1926. It is also recorded as a medicine in the *British Pharmacopoeia*

having been used as a bitter and mild expectorant.[29] *German Commission E* has approved its use for pre-menstrual discomfort, dysmenorrhoea and meno-pausal symptoms.

Cimicifuga has been officially used in Europe for over 40 years for treating menstrual and meno-pausal symptoms. It has become one of the most frequently used herbs which has increased demand and put pressure on its survival as it has mostly been wild-crafted. The chemical profiles of various species in this genus are very similar and there are many triterpenoid constituents. These facts have combined to make species identification difficult[16] so that a large amount of effort has been expended on developing chemical tests to unequivocally identify the different species. It is likely that other species of *Actaea* have been, or are being, substi-tuted for *C. racemosa*,[11] partly to meet world demand and partly through incorrect identification.[20] Fur-thermore in spite of all the trials that have so far been conducted into the pharmacological activities of the herb the active constituents and mechanism of action have not been fully elucidated. Scientific studies may have been confounded by the above factors, further complicated by the usual chemical variations due to geographical conditions, time of harvest and extraction processes. The conflicting results reported on the actions of the herb may be due, at least in part, to these considerations.[11]

Some of the research particularly pertaining to *Cimicifuga*'s use for menstrual problems is rela-tively old and as a result hard to access. The cur-rent focus of its use in hormonal problems has been confined to menopause.

Gynaecological
The unacceptable side-effects of HRT prompted a great deal of interest in natural medicines to achieve relief from what can be quite disabling symptoms for women entering menopause.

In vitro—Early studies reported that *Cimicifuga* was oestrogenic,[30-33] the exact constituents respon-sible were not known although, until doubt arose as to its presence, formononetin was considered the most likely candidate. Many tests have concluded that neither the herb nor its metabolites have activ-ity at α- or β-oestrogenic receptor sites.[34-37]

However a lypophilic extract had some oestro-gen-like activity in endometrial tissue possibly via a postulated third type of receptor, the γ-oestrogen receptor site.[38] The herb reduces oestrogen for-mation in normal breast tissue, tissue from pre-menopausal women being more sensitive to this action. Conversion of circulating pro-hormone by an enzymatic process to produce active hormone in tissues is believed to occur giving rise to local levels different from that in serum. Inhibition of this enzyme could be a possible mechanism by which black cohosh exerts a hormone lowering effect.[39] It is also possible that it could influence menopausal symptoms by acting directly through dopaminergic,[40] serotonergic[41] and/or opiate ago-nist receptors in the central nervous system.[42]

Cimicifuga and its triterpenoids also inhibit osteoclastogenesis.[43,44]

In vivo—A number of trials have been conducted, over a large time frame, into the effectiveness of *Cimicifuga* in treating the physiological effects of menopause. Not all are in accord as to the herb's effectiveness. The positive studies found benefit for:-

- a range of menopausal problems, of vary-ing severity, including vasomotor symptoms, insomnia, nervousness and depression.[45-52] They were equal to oral (tibolone,[46] conjugated oestrogen[53]) and transdermal HRT[54] in effect
- bone metabolism and superficial vaginal tissue (does not increase endometrial thickness)—the herb appears to act as a selective oestro-gen receptor modulator (SERM)[†] beneficially affecting hormone receptors in hypothalamic/pituitary and bone tissue without negatively affecting uterine tissue[53,55]
- hot flushes in pre-menopausal women being treated with tamoxifen for breast cancer[56]
- symptoms in women under 40 years old who had had a hysterectomy but still had at least one intact ovary[57]

The benefits of *Cimicifuga* may be greater in women whose menopausal symptoms are more marked[58]

[†]SERM have a mixed and selective pattern of estrogen agonist–antagonist activity, which largely depends on the tissue targeted.

and in those who have just entered the climacteric period.[59] No changes are observed in endometrial tissue, hormone levels or oestrogenic activity.[51,60]

Combining *Cimicifuga* and *Hypericum* relieved menopausal symptoms, both physical and psychological,[45,61] the improvement in depression was not due to *Hypericum* alone.[45]

The negative studies suggest that *Cimicifuga* was no better than placebo in moderating vasomotor symptoms (hot flushes and night sweats)[62-64] even after 12 months use,[65] although both groups recorded some improvement in symptoms.

Reviews of the various clinical trials of black cohosh to treat menopausal symptoms have found the herb was:

- safe for use in women with breast cancer although its efficacy was inconclusive[98]
- of benefit to otherwise healthy women[66-71] (not corroborated[72])
- beneficial for mood and anxiety levels[73]

The quality of most of these trials has been criticised, however, as not being rigorous enough to draw definitive conclusions.[65,74,75]

Other hormonal effects reported were a herbal combination, which included *Cimicifuga*, reducing the frequency of menstrual migraines[76] and the herb alone reducing LH levels.[77] This latter effect has not been corroborated by more recent trials which found hormone levels were not altered even after 12 months use of black cohosh supplements.[54,64,112,116]

Anticancer

In vitro—Increasing use of black cohosh for treating menopausal symptoms prompted safety checks on its potential to stimulate proliferation of breast cancer cells. *Cimicifuga* and its constituents are devoid of proliferative activity in these cells[78] and have no oestrogenic activity on breast tissue—see above. In fact the triterpenoid fraction,[79,80] the cinnamic acid esters[79] and the whole extract inhibit growth of breast cancer cells, whether oestrogen receptive or not,[81-83] an action occurring at gene-level, through anti-proliferation and apoptotic mechanisms.[84-86] *Cimicifuga* additionally inhibits oestrogen-stimulated proliferation of breast

cancer cells[87,88] and the invasive potential of malignant cells[89] and enhances their effective growth inhibition by chemotherapy treatments like tamoxifen.[87,90,91] It reduces the conversion of oestrone to the more active oestrodiol in breast cancer cells.[92]

The herb and/or its constituents also inhibit the growth of prostate cancer cells,[93,94] whether hormone dependent or not,[95] and oral squamous carcinoma cells.[96] It seems, therefore, that black cohosh may have potential as a cancer preventative.[97]

In vivo—Reviews of trials[52,56,63,64] into *Cimicifuga*'s efficacy for alleviating menopausal symptoms in women who either had breast cancer, a history of the disease or risk factors for developing the disease found it safe for use by them.[98] (It has again been suggested that the studies to-date are not scientifically rigorous enough to be certain).[99] However women who had had breast cancer were not at increased risk from a re-occurrence of the disease after using black cohosh and it may actually have increased their disease-free survival time.[100] Further, a retrospective study of women who had used the herb for menopausal symptom relief suggests it may have had a protective effect against their developing breast cancer.[101]

Other

In vitro—Various other actions have been demonstrated for *Cimicifuga* or its constituents including:-

- good anti-oxidant activity[20,102] and protection of DNA from free radical damage[103] (polyphenolic/triterpenoids)
- a weak antibacterial action (triterpenoids)[104], activity against the malarial parasite *Plasmodium falciparum* (triterpenoids)[105] and very strong anti-HIV activity (acetein)[106]
- anti-inflammatory potential associated with allergy by modifying cytokine release from stimulated mast cells (whole herb)[107] and inhibition of the enzyme neutrophil elastase (cinnamic acid derivatives).[108,109]

In vivo—In some of the above studies checks were also made on any changes to women's risk factors for cardiovascular disease. Again there are conflicting results, some showing no apparent benefit whether *Cimicifuga* was used alone or in combination with other botanicals,[110,111] whilst others found on its own, or combined with *Hypericum*, it improved HDL-cholesterol levels[54,112] and reduced LDL-cholesterol.[54]

Cimicifuga was one of 3 constituents in a cream that reduced wrinkles[113] and it may enhance wound healing, as the triterpenoid fraction can inhibit several collagenolytic enzymes[114] whose excessive activity inhibits normal tissue repair.

Medicinal uses
Respiratory tract
• whooping cough
• bronchitis

Nervous system
As a sensory depressant:

• tinnitus aurium
• chorea
• neuralgia

Reproductive tract
It is a safe alternative to HRT:

• menopausal symptoms
• dysmenorrhoea
• amenorrhoea
• pelvic inflammatory disease
• premenstrual syndrome
• uterine spasm
• fibroids
• aid to labour

Musculoskeletal
• sciatica
• muscular rheumatism
• rheumatoid arthritis
• intercostal myalgia

Pharmacy
Three times daily

Decoction or powdered	– 0.3–2 g of dried root or rhizome
Tincture 1:10 (60%)	– 2.0–4 ml
Fluid Extract (90%)	– 0.3–2 ml

N.B. The *BHC* daily dosage for tincture 1:10 is 0.4–2 ml or 40–200 mg dried herb.

Trials with extracts in tablet-form were based on 40–80 mg/day.

Precautions and/or safety
Standard mutagenicity tests on the herb were negative.[115] No safety concerns arose during the clinical studies and there were no adverse changes in breast, endometrial tissue or reproductive hormone levels in women who used the extract[116,117] even after one year of continuous use.[118] Specific reviews on *Cimicifuga*'s safety conclude it is safe for short term use (up to 12 months).[56,119–121] More studies are needed to assess safety for longer periods of time.

Minor side effects include gastro-intestinal disturbances (nausea and vomiting), rashes, headache, dizziness, mastalgia and weight gain.[74] (These are similar to the side effects reported for placebos[45]). It should be used with caution and only with professional guidance in pregnancy.[122] It use is usually confined to the third trimester or to labour induction.[122]

To-date a total of 42 cases of suspected liver toxicity due to the herb have been reported[66,123–126] but no direct causal link has yet been established.[74,127,128] Only two of these cases have been adjudged to be "probably" related to the use of *Cimicifuga*.[127] There is very high usage of black cohosh world wide, based on commercial sales, so that the likely incidence must be deemed to be very small.[127] Clinical trials that monitored liver function found no abnormalities[54,55,60]—reviewed.[98] However there may be a potential for idiosyncratic reactions of this nature.

There are other reported cases of serious side-effects including reversible cutaneous pseudolymphoma (erythematous plaques on the limbs),[129] autoimmune hepatitis,[130] acute renal transplant rejection,[131] muscle damage leading to reversible myopathy,[132] reversible nocturnal seizure[133] and two cases of cutaneous vasculitis.[134]

Interactions
In vitro—Black cohosh is a moderate inhibitor of organic anion-transporting polypeptide-B, an

intestinal transporter, and could theoretically alter the uptake of medications that use it, if the two are co-administered.[135] It was also a strong inhibitor of CYP3A4 which could potentially increase the serum levels of drugs metabolised by this isozyme.[136] (This was not corroborated *in vivo*).

In vivo—A brand of *Cimicifuga* that was tested was **not** found to have any effect on CYP1A2, CYP2D6 (weak inhibition only), CY2E1 or CYP3A4 drug metabolism[137,138] or on P-glycoprotein transport mechanism (it did not for example interfere with the uptake of digoxin).[139]

Historical uses
Insecticidal; snake bites; sore throats; scarlet fever; scirrhous tumours; backache; colds; constipation; consumption; fatigue; hives; insomnia; kidney problems.

Hydrastis canadensis

Golden seal

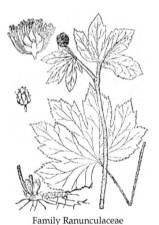

Family Ranunculaceae

Description
A small, herbaceous, perennial herb up to 30 cm tall in flower. *Rhizome* yellowish-brown outside, thick, oblong, irregular and knotted with a bright yellow interior pulp, and numerous roots. *Stem* simple, erect, thick and hairy, growing from the root in spring, surrounded at the base by several sheathing, greenish-yellow bracts. *Leaves* two, alternate, dark green and wrinkled, the lower larger than the upper, growing near the top of the stem, orbicular-cordate at the base, and palmately 5–7-lobed. *Flower* solitary, terminal, with 3 pale rose sepals which fall when the bloom opens. There are no petals but numerous greenish-white stamens and twelve or more short pistils. *Fruit* a succulent, globose berry looking like an enlarged raspberry. *Seeds* obovate, nearly black and glossy. Flowers from April to May in USA and fruits in July.

Habitat and cultivation
Native to North America in moist, rich deciduous woodlands from Vermont to Michigan, Minnesota, Virginia, Tennessee and Arkansas. Now an endangered species due to over-gathering. Grown from stratified seeds or root cuttings planted in autumn 5 cm deep and 20 cm apart in rows. It requires 75% shade and moist, well-drained soil rich in humus and a leafy mulch. It is drought tender.

Parts used
The fresh or dried roots and rhizomes which are generally harvested in the second or third year. In the fourth year the roots may be divided to provide more plants.

Active constituents
1) Alkaloids including berberine (min. 2.5%), (-)-β-hydrastine (min. 2%), canadine (tetrahydroberberine) and hydrastinine,[140–144] highest levels found in rhizomes[143]
2) Chlorogenic acid and other quinic acid derivatives[143,145]

Also contains volatile oil, resin, lipids, sterols (a derivative of β-sitosterol),[143] flavonoids[146] and carbohydrates. Commercial samples of *Hydrastis* have shown great variability.[141,142,147–149] The presence of the alkaloid palmatine is considered indicative of adulteration by other berberine-containing herbs.[147] Hydrastine and canadine are alkaloids specific to *Hydrastis*.[143]

Nutritional constituents
Vitamins: A, B-complex, C and E

Minerals: Calcium, copper, potassium and high content of phosphorus, manganese, iron, zinc and sodium

Actions
1) Antihaemorrhagic
2) Choleretic
3) Antimicrobial
4) Stomachic
5) Oxytocic
6) Laxative

Scientific information

Hydrastis has been an official medicine in many countries, its first reported medicinal use occurring in 1798. It's indicated uses were as an antihaemorrhagic for excessive uterine bleeding, to alleviate dysmenorrhoea and as a bitter.[29]

As one of the top selling herbs in the USA there has been high demand for it resulting in a short supply of roots and rhizomes. As has occurred with *Cimicifuga*, much of the recent scientific study has been directed at correctly identifying the herb and/or part used due to the apparent adulteration of commercial supplies.

The alkaloids berberine, for which there is a relatively large amount of information, and hydrastine are believed to be the major active constituents. The pharmacological actions of berberine include anti-proliferative,[150] antimicrobial, anti-inflammatory, antihaemorrhagic, anticholinergic, anti-arrhythmic and potentially beneficial for hypercholesterolaemia and congestive cardiac failure[151] (see *Berberis vulgaris*). Hydrastine is a peripheral vasoconstrictor with astringent properties and is considered a stimulant to uterine contractractions.[29]

For such a commonly used herb there is very little modern information available on the whole herb.

In vitro—*Hydrastis* has a strong potential for lowering cholesterol and lipids, an effect that is greater for the whole herb than for berberine alone.[152] The herb itself and/or a number of its constituents are antimicrobial to oral pathogens,[146] 15 strains of *Helicobacter pylori*[153]

and a range of bacteria including *Staphylococcus aureus, Pseudomonas aeruginosa, Streptococcus sanguis* and *Escherichia coli*.[154] The extract and berberine are also active against *Mycobacterium tuberculosis*.[145]

It is a good antioxidant.[155]

In vivo—There are no clinical trials using *Hydrastis*. Berberine has been tested in trials and had beneficial cardiovascular effects—preventing ischaemic induced-arrhythmia, increasing heart contractility, lowering peripheral vascular resistance and consequently reducing blood pressure.[156] The whole herb however is contraindicated in hypertension.

Hydrastis is considered a tonic for mucous membranes.

Medicinal uses

Respiratory tract
• upper respiratory catarrh

Gastro-intestinal tract
• atonic dyspepsia
• anorexia
• gastritis
• diarrhoea due to infection
• colitis
• cirrhosis of liver
• peptic ulcers
• constipation
• chronic cholecystitis

Reproductive tract
• infections of this tract
• menorrhagia
• dysmenorrhoea
• post-partum haemorrhage

Externally
• eczema
• inflammation
• catarrhal deafness
• tinnitus
• pruritus
• infections
• conjunctivitis (as eye-bath)

Pharmacy

Three times daily

Decoction of dried herb	–	0.5–1 g
Tincture 1:10 (60%)	–	2.0–4 ml
Fluid Extract (60%)	–	0.3–1 ml

CONTRAINDICATIONS—Hypertension, pregnancy.

Pharmacokinetics

Only a small amount of berberine is measurable in plasma after oral administration.[151]

Precautions and/or safety

The herb is toxic in large doses but it is so bitter that over-dosing is unlikely. Golden seal's alkaloids are phototoxic to keratinocytes,[157] causing damage to DNA,[158] and berberine is phototoxic to lens epithelial cells.[159] This should not present problems for internal use.

There is one case reported of a newly diagnosed type 1 diabetic child suffering reversible hypernatraemia suspected to have been exacerbated by *Hydrastis*[160] and another of a reversible photosensitivity reaction occurring in a woman taking a supplement containing multiple ingredients, of which golden seal was one. It is not known which constituent caused the reaction.[161]

Interactions

In vitro—Golden seal and its alkaloids have strong inhibitory activity on the cytochrome P450 isozymes including CYP2E1,[162] CYP2C8,[163] CYP2D6,[163–165] CYP3A4,[163–166] CYP2C9[164,165] and CYP2C19.[164] Based on calculations and assuming 100% absorption of the main alkaloids, the likelihood of a drug/herb interaction using recommended doses was deemed to be unlikely.[142]

In vivo—*Hydrastis* did inhibit the metabolism of probe drugs using CYP3A4/5[167,168] and CYP2D6[168] suggesting it may significantly affect the handling of other drugs using these enzymes if they are consumed concomitantly. When used with digoxin[169] and indinavir, an antiretroviral,[170] the herb did not affect their pharmacokinetics. No drug/herb interactions have yet been reported.

Historical uses

Varicose veins; haemorrhoids; acne; ringworm; in spring tonics; cancer; cracked and bleeding lips; cankers. Colds; flu; whooping cough; pneumonia; heart trouble. Leaves were used for snake bite and fits.

Ranunculus ficaria

Lesser celandine, pilewort

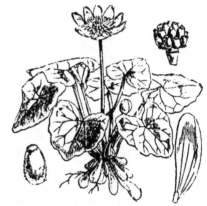

Family Ranunculaceae

Description

A low growing perennial plant, arising from small fig-shaped tubers with fibrous roots. The plant becomes dormant in late summer, and reappears early in the following spring. *Basal leaves* grow in a rosette and are dark green, glabrous, heart shaped and fleshy with long stems, sheathed at the base. *Stem leaves* similar but smaller. *Flowers* have 3 green sepals and 8–12 shining buttercup-yellow petals sometimes white at the tip. *Fruit* achenes finely beaked and keeled, about 2–2.5 mm long. Some sub-species bear bubils at the base of the leaf stalks. Blooms early in spring.

Habitat and cultivation

Native to Britain and Europe, growing along streams and in meadows and woods. Dies back in summer and comes up in autumn. May be propagated from tubers and grown in gardens. Root tubers and mature leaves poisonous to stock. *Ranunculus ficaria* var. *grandiflora* is a larger species whose medicinal use is unknown.

Parts used
Herb harvested when the plant is in flower and dried. The root has also been used for medicinal purposes.

Active constituents
1) Saponins of the triterpenoid type based on hederagenin and oleanolic acid[171-174]
2) Flavonoids[175]
3) Lactones—including anemonin and protoanemonin
4) Tannins

Actions
1) Astringent
2) Demulcent (local)

Scientific information
Ranunculus was valued by early herbalists, its common name, pilewort, indicating the specific use of the herb. This same use is found in the traditional practices from a number of different countries.[176,177] However it did not find favour with *Weiss* who claimed no success using it either internally or as an ointment in the treatment of haemorrhoids.

For actions of anemonin and protoanemonin see *Anemone*. Hederagenin derivatives generally have been examined and found to be biologically active but there are no recent studies on those specifically found in pilewort.

Medicinal uses
Gastro-intestinal tract
For the internal and external treatment of:-

• haemorrhoids

The specific use given in the *BHP* is for prolapsed or internal haemorrhoids with or without bleeding.

Pharmacy
Dosage three times daily
Infusion of dried herb   – 2–5 g
Fluid Extract (25%)   – 2–5 ml
   Ointment 3% in base material.
   Ointment BPC (1934) 30% fresh plant in lard or made into suppositories.

Historical uses
Kernels by ears or throat or scrofula (tuberculous lesions), tumours, wens.

RHAMNACEAE

The Rhamnaceae is a group of 55–58 genera of temperate and tropical regions growing throughout the world. Rhamnaceae are usually trees or shrubs, sometimes spiny, sometimes lianoid.

- Leaves are simple, mostly alternate, mostly stipulate
- The small flowers are usually in cymes with a 4–5 lobed tubular calyx
- Petals may be 3–5 or sometimes absent
- Fruit is usually a drupe

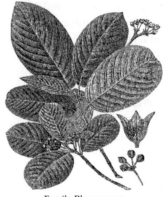

Family Rhamnaceae

Rhamnus purshiana

Cascara, Californian buckthorn

Description

A deciduous tree growing to 8 × 3 m with a trunk diameter to 50 cm. *Trunk* erect and branching. Bark usually under 1 mm thick, close, mottled, dark or light brown, often tinged with red and broken into small thin scales on the surface. *Leaves* alternate, dark green, elliptic-oblong or ovate, to 5 cm wide with a prominent midrib and branching veins. Margins finely serrate. Winter buds naked, hoary or fuzzy.

Flowers relatively inconspicuous growing on slender stems from the axils of the leaves. Corolla 5-petalled, minute. *Fruit* small, black, 2-seeded, less than 1 cm in diameter, with thin juicy flesh. *Nutlets* have a thin grey shell, flattened on inner surface, and the inner surface of the thin seed coat is bright orange.

Odour—faint but characteristic; taste—bitter, nauseous and long lasting.

Habitat and cultivation

Native to the N.W. ranges of North America from British Columbia to central California and the southern slopes of the Grand Canyon in Arizona.

Grown from seed or cuttings in light-medium moist, well-drained soils. It is not usually cultivated. Frost resistant, drought tender.

Parts used
The bark from woody branches more than 12 cm thick, collected in summer and stored for a year before being used.[1] This allows the breakdown of constituents that would otherwise cause griping. Once dried the bark's constituents are stable for a number of years.[1]

Active constituents
1) Hydroxyanthracene glycosides (up to 10%) mainly consisting of anthrone glycosides. 60–70% is made up of cascarosides (which develop on storage), cascarosides A and B are glucosides of aloin (barbaloin) and C and D are glucosides of 11-deoxyaloin (chrysaloin). Another 20–30% are aloins A and B (barbaloin) and 11-deoxyaloins (chrysaloin) A and B. Also glucosides of emodin, chrysophanic acid and aloe-emodin and traces of free anthraquinones[2-4]
2) Tannins (up to 2%)
3) Volatile oil—rhamnol

Nutritional constituents
Vitamins: B-complex
Minerals: Calcium, potassium and manganese

Actions
1) Laxative

Scientific information
Cascara is a recognised purgative and has been an official preparation in pharmacopoeias worldwide.[1] However there is very little recent investigation into the plant itself although the pharmacological actions of constituent anthraquinones have been studied—see *Aloe* and *Cassia*.

In vitro—*Rhamnus* inhibits HSV-1 and it is likely to have activity against other enveloped viruses probably due to its anthraquinones.[5] It also had inhibitory activity against different liver cancer cell lines.[6]

In vivo—Trials with the herb for laxative purposes have shown it to be effective although it was used in conjunction with other agents.[7,8] It was used with safety for colon cleansing in children[9] but was less effective than senna and bowel washes for this purpose.[10] These studies are fairly old and bulk laxatives have largely superseded the use of stimulant laxatives as the preferred method of bowel emptying.

The mode of action of *Rhamnus* is due to the hydroxyanthraquinone glycosides that are hydrolysed by bacterial flora into pharmacologically active metabolites which after partial absorption stimulate colon motility and increase the water content of faeces[11] (see *Cassia*). During the preparation of *Rhamnus* tinctures around 20% of the hydroxyanthracene glycosides may form dimers that have no laxative activity.[12]

Rhamnus purshiana is the gentlest of the stimulating laxatives and its action is considered to be a mild one.[1]

Medicinal uses
Gastro-intestinal tract
The herb, like *Rumex*, has a laxative effect but may also enhance bowel function through its cholagogue action.

- constipation
- dyspepsia
- anal fissures[†]
- haemorrhoids[†]

Pharmacy
Once daily taken at bedtime for laxative purposes
Decoction   – 0.25–1 g
Fluid Extract (BP 1973)   – 2–5 ml

It may take 8–12 hours to be effective. The laxative effect should be tempered by adding a carminative as griping may occur and it should not be used in constipation due to bowel tension. Small doses have been taken before meals as a bitter tonic to stimulate digestion.[1]

CONTRAINDICATIONS—Bowel or intestinal obstruction. Pregnancy and lactation—stimulating laxatives like *R. purshiana* have been contraindicated during in the past but

---

[†] By softening stools.

have been declared safe in recent times (see *Cassia*)—metabolites of anthraquinones are found in breast milk although the levels are too small to be a problem for babies.[1]

Precautions and/or safety
Fresh bark can cause severe vomiting and spasms.[1] Long term use of *R. purshiana* can lead to electrolyte and fluid imbalance (there are recorded cases of hypokalaemia although this occurred after years of herb abuse),[1] metabolic acidosis, weight loss, and malabsorption of nutrients. Used on its own, dependency may occur, causing the bowel to become lax.

A case of cholestatic hepatitis with portal hypertension in which *Rhamnus* was implicated has been reported.[13] There is also one reported case of respiratory allergy due to handling the herb.[14]

Pseudomelanosis coli can occur when using anthraquinone-containing herbs but this is no longer believed to be linked to an increase in colon cancer (See *Cassia*). Anthraquinone metabolites may be excreted in urine causing a non-significant orange discoloration.

Interactions
As with all laxative preparations there is a possibility of reduced drug absorption through decreased gastro-intestinal transit time.[15] Over dosing with the herb may potentiate the action of drugs containing cardiac glycosides like digoxin and anti-arrhythmic drugs like quinidine.

Historical uses
Same as modern usage.

ROSACEAE

The rose family consists of some 3500 species worldwide mainly distributed in temperate and warm regions of the Northern Hemisphere. Most species contain tannins, and only a few contain alkaloids. Because most of the world's temperate fruits belong to this family, it is of great economic importance.

General characteristics
- Leaves may be simple or compound, alternate, usually spirally arranged though they are opposite in one genus
- Stipules are usually present
- Flowers have 5 free petals in a regular circle and are usually bisexual. The floral tube is normally present, the receptacle forming a shallow cup
- The calyx has five free but often overlapping sepals, usually green and often leaf-like
- Stamens usually numerous, and arranged in rings of 5
- Carpels one to many
- Fruits very varied and may be a pome, achene, drupe or, rarely, a capsule

Medicinal plants of the Rosaceae are:

Agrimonia eupatoria   *Fragaria vesca*
Alchemilla vulgaris   *Potentilla erecta*
Aphanes arvensis   *Prunus serotina*
Crataegus spp.   *Rosa eglanteria*
Filipendula ulmaria   *Rubus idaeus*

Agrimonia eupatoria

Agrimony

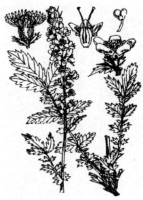

Family Rosaceae

Description
A leafy perennial to 60 cm, which dies back to a rosette in winter. *Leaves* pinnate with 2–4 pairs of larger, oval, saw-toothed leaflets 2–6 cm,

370

alternating with smaller leaflets. Leaves and stem have dense, spreading non-glandular hairs. Stipules leaf-like. *Flowers* borne on long, slender, terminal and often branched, leafless spikes. They are numerous, yellow, stalkless and small, each 5–8 mm across. *Fruit* are about 6 mm across, obconical, deeply grooved, hairy, with spreading hooked bristles above. Flowers from mid-summer to autumn.

Habitat and cultivation
Native to Europe, growing along edges of woods and hedges and in meadows. Grown from seed and will self-sow. It prefers a sunny situation and moist, well drained soil. *A. parviflora* is used in North America. Drought and frost resistant.

Parts used
The herb harvested at or just prior to flowering.

Active constituents
1) Flavonoids including derivatives of luteolin, apigenin, quercetin and kaempferol.[1,2] Also isoflavonoids daidzen and biochanin[3]
2) Oligomeric procyanidins based mainly on catechin and consisting of 2–4 units[4]
3) Tannins (up to 8%)[5]
4) Phenolic acids including p-coumaric and protocatechuic acids[4]
5) Terpenoids

Also contains volatile oil, silicic acid and coumarins.

Nutritional constituents
Vitamins: C,[6] K and niacin
Minerals: Iron and large amounts of silicon

Actions
1) Astringent
2) Diuretic
3) Tonic

Scientific information
There has been very little scientific study of this herb and its use is largely dictated by history. However the recent isolation of oligomeric procyanidins,

which are pharmacologically active (see *Crataegus*), may lead to renewed interest.

In vitro—*Agrimonia* has very good anti-oxidant activity, although the strength of this application may depend on the extracting medium,[7] it is likely due to the phenolic fraction.[4,8,9] This activity is probably linked to the traditional anti-inflammatory action attributed to the herb.[4]

The isoflavonoids have phyto-oestrogenic potential.[3]

Some antimicrobial activity has been established for *Agrimonia*. It is antiviral against hepatitis B virus (this activity was highest in plants harvested when in flower).[10] The seed extract (also anti-oxidant) is antibacterial against *Bacillus subtilis*, *B. cereus*, *Escherichia coli* and *Staphylococcus aureus*.[11] The herb inhibits *Mycobacterium tuberculosis* (based on old research).

Agrimonia has been used traditionally in the treatment of diabetes[12] and whilst this action has been demonstrated in animals *in vivo*, no human studies have been recorded.

In vivo—There is an historical reference to the herb being used with success in the local treatment of cutaneous porphyria (*Potter's*).

Medicinal uses
Gastro-intestinal tract
Its main use is in the digestive tract where it can improve assimilation of nutrients and heal and soothe this tract.

• diarrhoea in children
• mucous colitis
• chronic cholecystopathies with gastric sub-acidity (*Weiss*)
• chronic appendicitis
• chronic gastritis

Urinary tract
• urinary incontinence
• cystitis

Externally
• sore throat (gargle)
• chronic nasopharyngeal catarrh

Pharmacy
Three times daily

Infusion of dried herb   – 2–4 g
Tincture 1:5 (45%)   – 1–4 ml
Fluid Extract (45%)   – 1–3 ml

Historical uses
Internally and externally for a range of conditions including haemorrhages; fevers, coughs; bad breath; relaxed bowels; colic; jaundice; "bad or naughty" livers; skin eruptions; scrofulous sores (with roots); gout; to strengthen joints; "foul, troubled or bloody water"; snake bites; warts; gun shot wounds; sprains; bruises; old sores (ointment), for drawing splinters, ulcers; cancers; ears for "foul and imposthumed" condition of ears (juice as eardrops); all states of heat or cold.

Alchemilla vulgaris

Lady's mantle

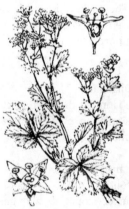

Family Rosaceae

Description
A variable perennial with a woody rootstock and most leaves growing on long stalks in a basal rosette. *Basal leaves* green and often hairy, rounded and with 5–7 pleats which unfold like a fan, and have toothed margins. *Stem* leaves smaller and shorter stalked. *Flowers* tiny, greenish-yellow in terminal clusters, 3–4 mm across with no petals. Flowers from spring to late summer.

Habitat and cultivation
Native to damp meadows, open woods and sometimes rocky places, in Britain and parts of Europe. Grown from seed or division of the rootstock. *Alchemilla mollis* is grown as a garden plant in other countries and has been used in the same way.

Parts used
The herb harvested during or just prior to flowering.

Active constituents
1) Tannins mainly glycosides of ellagic acid (quoted in *Potters'* as 6–8%, it has been reported variously from 3%[13] to 46%[14]) and proanthocyanidins[15]
2) Flavonoids mostly quercetin (0.7%),[15] also luteolin[16] (no flavonoids were found in the herb growing in Iceland)[17]

The total phenolic content has been reported as 6.25%.[13] Also contains triterpenoids—ursolic and oleanolic acids[17] and a small amount of salicylic acid.

Actions
1) Astringent
2) Antihaemorrhagic
3) Styptic

Scientific information
Although the herb has a long tradition of use in a number of cultures not a great deal of modern research into its chemistry or pharmacology exists. The name derives from the Arabic word "Alkemelych" meaning alchemy and is testament to the high regard in which it was held. Indeed *Culpeper* considered it one of the best "wound herbs".

In vitro—The herb has very good anti-oxidant activity, protecting natural biochemicals from free radical damage.[18] Anti-oxidant potential has been shown to be related to the total content of polyphenols (tannins and flavonoids) in a variety of herbs.[19] Quercetin, the main flavonoid, is an established anti-oxidant and anti-inflammatory agent.[15]

The herb also appears to be a good inhibitor of LOX[13] and PAF[20] suggesting a potential mechanism for its observed anti-inflammatory effect. It is a strong stimulant to epithelial cell growth, an action consistent with its traditional use as a wound healing agent.[15] In preliminary tests it inhibited proteases which may give it an angio-protective effect (protecting connective tissues) and possibly also an anti-angiogenesis activity. This has not been tested in human models.[21] However the polyphenol, ellagic acid, has demonstrated inhibition of proteolytic enzymes and protection of elastin fibres in human tissue.[22]

Alchemilla has antibacterial activity against some strains of the gastro-intestinal *Shigella* and *Yersinia* pathogens.[14]

In vivo—The wound healing properties were demonstrated in the treatment of minor types of aphthous ulcers for which the glycetract used was very effective (at 3% concentration).[23]

The herb is a diuretic in Italian folklore, antispasmodic in Swedish folklore and it was used in Arabic medicine for weight loss, abdominal pain and inflammation.[24]

The polyphenols are considered to be responsible for much of the pharmacological activity.[15]

Medicinal uses
Gastro-intestinal tract
The astringency, and probable antimicrobial actions, due to the high tannin content make it useful in treating:-

* diarrhoea
* dysentery

Reproductive tract
Traditionally used to treat female complaints:-

* menorrhagia
* dysmenorrhoea
* leucorrhoea

Externally
* leucorrhoea
* pruritus vulvae

Pharmacy
Three times daily
Infusion of dried herb   – 2–4 g
Fluid extract (25%)   – 2–4 ml

Historical uses
Internally for vomiting; bleeding; ruptures; fertility and threatened abortion, to reduce and firm large breasts (internally and externally). Externally for all wounds including those that are "green" or old or inflamed; bruises, ulcers, eczema, skin rashes.

Crataegus laevigata and *Crataegus monogyna* [C. laevigata formerly known as C. oxyocantha]

Hawthorn

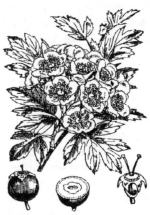

Family Rosaceae

Description
A deciduous shrub or small tree up to 10 m high, armed with axillary spines up to 12–20 mm long, the longest spines being on the short flowering shoots. *Stems* glabrous, smooth and reddish brown when young and grey when older. *Leaves* solitary on new growing shoots but grouped in clusters on short shoots. Petioles short, leaf blades deltoid to rhombic, deeply lobed, glabrous, dark to mid-green above, paler below. *Flowers* many, in flat corymbs, growing on short leafy shoots scattered along the branches. Corymbs subtended by short leafy bracts. Sepals greenish, lobes triangular to oblong, becoming flexed. Petals broadly ovate to orbicular, 4–8 mm in diameter, rounded, spreading, usually white, sometimes pink or red. Stamens greater than petals, filaments white sometimes pale pink, anthers pink. Style usually one. *Fruit* broadly oblong to sub-globose, 7–11 mm diameter, dark red,

shining and crowned by deflexed sepals. Nutlets usually one (monogyna). Flowers in spring, fruits in autumn.

Odour of flowers—faint, strange and often unpleasant; taste—slightly bitter-sweet and astringent. Berries taste of almonds.

Habitat and cultivation
Native to Europe and Britain. Introduced as stock-proof hedging and naturalised elsewhere along roads and grassy places. Grown from seed, but needs frost to germinate, and from rooted suckers separated from the clump and replanted. A variable species. *C. laevigata*, a cultivated double-flowered species has 2 styles in the flower and 2 seeds in the berry. Both species have the same medicinal uses.

Parts used
The leaves and flowers harvested in late spring. The leaves can be harvested without flowers, though the combination of the two is the preferred starting material.[25] Whilst the leaves may be best when the flowers are open (the flavonoid content is highest then),[26] the buds still contain good levels of flavonoids.[27] Leaves may still be harvested through to the summer when the berries are present but still green. The berries harvested when ripe (red) in autumn.

Although the British tradition has tended to use the berries, the leaves and flowers are preferred in Germany and France, and they have a better characterised chemistry and pharmacological activity.

Active constituents
1) Flavonoids.[25,28-30,32] Leaves and flowers—more than 33 have been identified (min. of 1.5%), berries (average around 0.98%). They occur mainly as flavonol-O-glycosides and flavone-C-glycosides and include vitexin-2-rhamnoside, acetylvitexin-2-rhamnoside, hyperoside, isoquercitrin, rutin, quercetin, apigenin, kaempferol and luteolin derivatives. There is little difference in flavonoid content between the two species of *Crataegus*[25]
2) Oligomeric procyanidins (OPCs)—(2–3%).[26,31] These are flavan-3-ols and are related to the condensed tannins and flavonoids. They consist of mainly dimers (two units) up to hexamers (6 units) of (-)-epicatechin and also polymeric procyanidins of more than 6 units.[32] They include (-)-epicatechin and procyanidins B2, B5 and C1. This is a very diverse group that is unstable making analysis difficult.[33,34] Leaves (1.58%) and flowers (1.15%) have a much higher concentration than the berries (0.15%)[35]
3) Anthocyanins including leucocyanidin in the leaves. Anthocyanins give the berries their red colouring[37]
4) Triterpenoids (mainly acidic) up to 3.58%. Includes crataegus lactone, produced on metabolism from crataegus acid (high in fruits); cycloartenol,[36] cinnamic, ursolic and oleanolic acids.[37,38] Highest in leaves and flowers, unripe berries have a higher content than ripe ones[37]
5) Cardiotonic amines including trimethylamine—flowers[39]
6) Phenylpropanoids including chlorogenic, caffeic, ferulic, isoferulic and p-coumaric acids[29,32,40,41]

This chemical breakdown reflects more studies into leaf and flower not necessarily a lack of active constituents in berries. The chemical profile of berries differ in the quality of some of the flavonoid constituents and/or quantity from those found in leaf and flower.[32] The type of OPCs are similar in all parts of the plant but levels differ.[35]

Stressing the plants by restricted water or temperature changes can increase the level of hyperoside and (-)-epicatechin.[42]

Nutritional constituents
Vitamins: C (40–60 mg/100 mg in berries), carotene (5 mg/100 mg), vitamin B_1, B_2, E and P
Minerals: Calcium, magnesium, potassium, iron, zinc, sodium, sulphur, copper, manganese and some chromium[43]

Actions
1) Cardiac tonic and trophorestorative
2) Coronary vasodilator
3) Hypotensive

Scientific information

Crataegus was an official medicine in a number of European pharmacopoeias noted for treating heart disease and for its hypotensive action.[44] Today it is a commonly used herbal medicine in Europe, particularly in Germany. *German Commission E* has approved the use of leaves and flowers for mild forms of heart failure. The flavonoids and proanthocyanidins are considered the important pharmacologically active constituents and commercial products tend to be standardised on OPC or total flavonoid content. Standardisation has however been difficult because there are a number of different *Crataegus* species used medicinally, the same species can be highly variable, one species can hybridise readily with another with little change in morphology, the actual active constituents are still not fully known and likely to be complex and different parts of the plant are harvested viz. stalks may or may not be included, leaves may have flowers and/or buds or have neither.[25] All these variations alter the chemical profile. This is in addition to the usual factors that alter chemical make-up such as geographical location and associated microclimate, time of harvest, method of extraction, storage conditions and year of harvest.[25,26,34,45,46]

Anti-oxidant

In vitro—Both berries[47] and flowers[48,49] have very good anti-oxidant activity, including inhibiting the oxidation of LDL and VLDL (a suspected promoter of atherosclerosis),[50,51] this activity is related to the high level of polyphenolics present.[52] The fresh young leaves are the strongest anti-oxidants followed by fresh flower buds and dried flowers.[53] Leaf activity is related to the content of flavonoids whilst that in flowers and berries depends on levels of proanthocyanidins and catechins.[54]

Circulation

Using hawthorn to treat cardiovascular diseases in the west was first recorded in 1800's although *Culpeper* mentions use of the powdered seeds from the fruit as a treatment for dropsy. Currently only leaf and flower extracts are registered in Germany for the treatment of some types of coronary heart disease and congestive heart failure.[55,56] The action of the herb has been tested in a variety of models which have shown they have a unique combination of actions amongst known cardioactive agents.[57]

In vitro—The extracts and/or constituents:-

- have a protective effect in vascular cells subjected to hypoxia and re-oxygenation[58]
- cause vaso-dilation reducing tension in the wall of both normal and atherosclerotic coronary vessels[59,60]
- help reverse endothelial dysfunction—dysfunction may contribute to heart disease[61]
- dissolve inorganic calcium salts—may be relevant to, amongst other pathologies, that of plaque development[62]
- have some Angiotensin Converting Enzyme (ACE) inhibitory activity[63]
- inhibit neutrophil elastase activity—enzyme suggested to be responsible for ischaemic damage to myocardium[52]
- are positively inotropic by inhibition of the sarcolemmal sodium pump—similar to cardiac glycosides[64,65]
- inhibit thromboxane A2—known vasoconstrictor, inflammatory agent and platelet activator[66]
- may inhibit phosphodiesterase activity,[67] the enzyme responsible for the breakdown of cyclic AMP in heart tissue

All these actions in addition to the anti-oxidant capacity of the herb could contribute to its use *in vivo* for circulatory problems.

In vivo—Extracts of hawthorn containing mostly leaf and flower have been tested in clinical trials. Interest in using hawthorn for the earlier stages of heart failure was generated because at this point treatment may be most effective yet current pharmaceutical options have undesirable side-effects.[68] Although preparations have been used in trials with patients with varying degrees of heart failure from New York Heart Association (NYHA) I to III [levels range from I (least severe) to IV], most have used patients in group NYHA II.[†]

[†]Cardiac disease resulting in slight limitation of physical activity. Symptoms of fatigue, palpitations, dyspnoea or angina pain with ordinary physical activity.

1) In a small 6-week study *Crataegus* was no better than placebo when used in conjunction with conventional medicine for treating heart failure,[69] but in many other trials it was of clear benefit, used alone or with pharmaceuticals, over the longer term—from 8 weeks and up[68] (berries)[70] (leaves and flowers).[71-73] Symptom improvements included increased tolerance to exercise and reductions in ankle oedema, nocturia, dyspnoea, palpitations, fatigue and a modest reduction in blood pressure[74,75]

2) A long-term clinical trial of patients who were already on conventional therapy for heart failure showed *Crataegus* did not reduce levels of morbidity[76] but did offer significant benefits in symptom reduction[77,78]

3) A flower/leaf extract resulted in a small but significant decrease in diastolic blood pressure in hypertensive patients, some of whom had diabetes[79,80]

4) Fresh hawthorn berries in combination with D-camphor effectively treated patients with orthostatic hypotension[‡,81] the effect being significant over a range of age groups.[82] *Crataegus'* contribution is long term by improving the tone of arterioles and cardiac performance[83,84]

Hawthorn's action is positively inotropic and chronotropic, anti-arrhythmic and vasodilatory, and it improves perfusion of coronary vessels and heart muscle, oxygen utilisation and cardiac output.[72,85-88]

Some early work in the 1980s appraised its effect in patients with angina pectoris and though results were positive no further studies have been undertaken.[67]

Direct studies on the anti-arrhythmic and hypolipidaemic activity of *Crataegus* in humans are lacking, however *Passiflora* and *Crataegus* used as a treatment in heart failure reduced serum cholesterol and LDL lipids.[89]

---

‡Defined as a difference in measured blood pressure, within 3 minutes of changing from a prone position to being upright, of 20 mm Hg systolic or 10 mm Hg diastolic pressure. The prevalence of this condition increases with age.

Other

In vitro—Hawthorn inhibits platelet aggregation and consequent 5-hydroxytryptamine release and may therefore have potential application in the treatment of migraine headaches.[90]

A triterpene-rich fraction of the herb is strongly cytotoxic to laryngeal cancer cells.[91]

The berries protect lymphocytes from radiation damage.[92]

In vivo—*Crataegus* was effective when used in conjunction with *Eschscholzia* and magnesium in relieving mild-to-moderate anxiety disorders[93] and in combination with a number of other herbs for adjustment mood disorder with anxiety.[94]

Medicinal uses
Cardiovascular system
Crataegus' actions enable it to normalise heart function so it can be used for two seemingly opposite problems. Used for:

- angina
- congestive heart failure
- hypertension
- hypotension
- tachycardia
- cardiac hypertrophy
- arrhythmia
- ectopic beat
- irregular pulse
- valvular insufficiency
- atheroma
- Buerger's disease
- atherosclerosis
- oedema and dyspnoea of cardiac origin
- chilblains
- intermittent claudication

Pharmacy
Three times daily

Dried herb in any form	– 0.2–1 g
Tincture 1:5 (45%)	– 1.0–2 ml
Fluid Extract (25%)	– 0.5–1 ml

Modern trials used doses ranging from 160–1800 mg of herb a day and the standardised preparation of flowers and leaves used in Germany are based on either 18.75% OPCs (WS 1442/*Crataegutt*) or 2.25% flavonoids (LI 132). In the above clinical trials the herbal preparations were considered safe and without significant adverse effects.[73,81,82,84]

Trials indicate that it may take a minimum of 6 weeks of continuous use to achieve therapeutic benefits.[38]

Pharmacokinetics

In vitro studies on some of the main flavonoids—hyperoside, isoquercitrin and epicatechin—from the fruit indicate they have limited permeability.[95] *In vivo* studies on metabolism of hawthorn and/or its constituents have not been conducted but animal models suggest OPCs are absorbed to some extent.

Precautions and/or safety

The herb has not demonstrated any mutagenic potential in standard tests.[96]

Crataegus has been associated with only minor adverse reactions that are equivalent to those reported for placebos.[69,97] In fact one study found that the extract reduced the number of reported side-effects compared to placebo.[74]

The most frequently reported events have been gastro-intestinal complaints, dizziness/vertigo, palpitation, headache and migraine and less frequently nausea, erythematous rash and somnolence.[77,85] More severe side effects listed but limited to 2 cases each include gastro-intestinal haemorrhage and circulatory failure.[97] No contraindications have been reported.

Interactions

No interactions have yet been reported from clinical trials between *Crataegus* and prescribed hypotensives (ACE inhibitors, diuretics, β-blockers, calcium channel blockers)[69,70,74,79] or various hypoglycaemic[79] medications *in vivo*. There are cautions in the literature about the potential of *Crataegus* to potentiate the effects of cardiac medicines particularly digoxin but this seems to be based either on a "potential" action or on *in vitro* data.[98] In healthy volunteers the pharmacokinetics of digoxin were not altered by hawthorn.[99]

Historical uses

As a gargle in sore throats; kidney stones, colic, digestive problems including vomiting and diarrhoea, externally to draw splinters. In *Chinese Pharmacopoeia Crataegus* spp. are listed and as well as improving heart-related problems, they have been used to treat diarrhoea, dyspepsia, dysentery and hepatitis.

Filipendula ulmaria

Meadowsweet

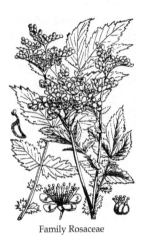

Family Rosaceae

Description

An erect herb up to 50 cm high in flower. *Basal* and *cauline leaves* dark green and glabrous on the upper surface, whitish green and tomentose beneath; pinnate, with 3–5 pairs of large, irregularly 2-serrate leaflets up to 60 mm long, often interspersed with reduced leaflets. *Inflorescence* a many flowered cymose panicle with individual small pale cream flowers, having pinkish or purplish backs to the petals. Flowers in summer.

Odour of flowers—faint and salicylate-like; taste—astringent and quite bitter.

Habitat and cultivation

Native to Europe and Northern Asia, growing in damp meadows, swamps, and ditches. Grown in gardens elsewhere from seed or root division in winter or early spring. Needs a damp, sunny situation to flower. Frost resistant.

Parts used
The herb harvested during flowering.

Active constituents
1) Flavonoids including quercetin, rutin, avicularin, hyperoside, spireoside, kaempferol and their derviatives[100-102]
2) Phenolic glycosides—spiraein, gaultherin (monotropitin), isosalicin and various salicylate derived constituents[100]
3) Volatile oil (about 0.2%) containing salicylaldehyde and methyl salicylate
4) Polyphenols/tannins (10–15%) mainly the hydrolysable group. The major one is rugosin-D
5) Phenolic acids including mainly gallic, p-coumaric and vanillic acids.[100]

Also contains chalcones, mucilage, a small amount of coumarins and a constituent similar to heparin.[103]

Nutritional constituents
Vitamins: C[104]

Actions
1) Anti-inflammatory
2) Diuretic
3) Stomachic
4) Astringent

Scientific information
Meadowsweet was sacred to Druid priests and was well known as a medicine by the 16th century. It has been approved by *German Commission E* to aid the treatment of colds. In Russia the herb has been used for diabetes and cancer.[100] Much of the scientific information relating to *Filipendula* is historical or has been written mainly in Russian and is therefore difficult to access.

"Salicine" was isolated from meadowsweet, formerly called *Spiraea ulmaria*, in 1833 having been reported earlier as the active constituent in willow bark. Apart from the well known content of salicylates, meadowsweet contains a high level of total phenolic constituents and it is probable they contribute largely to its actions.[105]

Anti-oxidant
In vitro—Meadowsweet is a strong anti-oxidant[106,107] (of a similar order to vitamin E) and a strong free radical scavenger.[108,109] It may have promise as a hepatoprotective agent based on this activity and on trials using animals.[110]

Anti-inflammatory
In vitro—This is one of the main actions associated with the herb. However not many studies have been done to suggest its mechanism of action. To-date meadowsweet:

- strongly inhibits 5-LOX[108]
- inhibits complement activation, T-cell proliferation and modulates production of free radicals from polymorphonuclear leucocytes[111]—immune related pro-inflammatory processes[111]
- inhibits prostaglandin synthesis[112]
- strongly inhibits PAF[112]

It has been suggested that although salicylates are established inhibitors of COX, the anti-inflammatory action of *Filipendula* is not likely due to them as their content is minimal.[111] Neither is the action simply due to protein inactivation by tannins. Further research is required to fully elucidate these mechanisms.

Other
In vitro—A limited range of other activities have been found for *Filipendula*. It displays a strong cytotoxic activity to lymphoma cells,[113] has good antibacterial activity against *Staphylococcus aureus* and *Escherichia coli* and some antifungal activity against *Candida albicans* (not due to salicylates),[114] has a strong anticoagulant activity (flowers and seeds)[115] and inhibits the enzyme elastase (due to high tannin content) which breaks down connective tissue.[116]

In vivo—A preparation of the flowers was used as a local treatment for cervical dysplasia with beneficial effects for most women, over half of them showing complete regression of the dysplasia.[117]

For the pharmacological effects of salicylates see Appendix III.

Medicinal uses

Gastro-intestinal tract

The herb is most useful in this system where it addresses a variety of problems:

- atonic dyspepsia
- hyperacidity
- gastritis
- peptic ulcers (*BHP* specific)
- diarrhoea in children
- heartburn

Urinary tract

As a diuretic accompanied by antisepsis (due to salicylate excretion) and astringency:

- acute catarrhal cystitis

Musculoskeletal

Used for the pain of joint problems:

- rheumatic pain
- arthritic pain

Also used topically for the above conditions.

Pharmacy

Three times daily

Infusion of dried herb	–	2–6 g
Tincture 1:5 (45%)	–	2–4 ml
Fluid Extract (25%)	–	2–6 ml

Precautions and/or safety

Some individuals are sensitive to salicylates and may have difficulty tolerating normal doses of *Filipendula*.

Interactions

In spite of the salicylate content and a potential for interaction with anti-coagulant and/or NSAID drugs, there are no reported interactions to-date.[118,119]

Historical uses

For fevers. The distilled water from the flowers as eye drops for burning, itching and to clear the sight. For all bleeding; fluxes and vomiting; colic; with honey as a laxative. Considered a tonic for the digestive tract. Strangury and all pains of the bladder. For dropsy; as a hot infusion to induce perspiration. Externally for cancerous ulcers and for sores.

Prunus serotina

Wild cherry

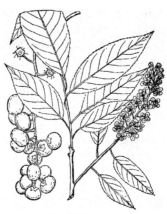

Family Rosaceae

Description

A deciduous, unspined tree to 30 m with smooth, glossy red-brown bark with white lenticels and aromatic inner bark. *Leaves* alternate, lanceolate-oblong to oblong-ovate, blunt toothed, from 4–15 cm long, smooth and glossy green above, pale beneath with whitish brown hairs on the prominent midrib. *Flowers* in open racemes 5–15 cm long, with 5 sepals and 5 white petals, fragrant. The calyx persistent in fruit. *Fruit* globose, red to purple-black, bitter or sweetish. Flowers from spring to summer.

Habitat and cultivation

Native to North America in dry woods from Nova Scotia to North Dakota, south to Florida and Texas. Also grown elsewhere in any soil but dies if there is air pollution. Propagated from seed, hardwood cuttings or budding. Frost and drought resistant.

Parts used
The stem bark collected in the autumn. The bark exposed to the sun or tinged green is highest in active constituents.

Active constituents
1) Cyanogenic glycosides including (+)-mande-lonitrile glucoside (prunasin),[120] a derivative of amgydalin, which is hydrolysed by enzymes to hydrocyanic acid (0.075–0.16%) and benzaldehyde[44]
2) Coumarins including scopoletin, scopolin[121] and β-methylaesculetin
3) Phenolic acids including benzoic, trimethylgallic and p-coumaric acids
4) Tannins (non-hydrolysable) consisting of monomeric and polymeric units based on leucocyanidin[122]

Also contains volatile oil and resin.

Actions
1) Antitussive
2) Sedative
3) Astringent

Scientific information
Prunus has been an official medicine both in Britain and the USA[44] having been introduced to settlers in the latter country by the Native American Indians. It has not been much investigated overall.

In vitro—The herb suppresses cell growth and causes apoptosis of colorectal cancer cells.[123] It also has antibacterial activity against *Staphylococcus aureus* and *Bacillus subtilis* and antifungal activity against *Microsporum gypseum*.[124]

Medicinal uses
Respiratory tract
The herb is used in situations where coughing is serving no useful purpose and is causing exhaustion i.e. coughs due to:

- pertussis
- tracheitis
- cardiac failure
- dry mucous membranes (geriatric)

- injuries
- psychogenic
- lung cancer
- irritable/persistent bronchial cough

Gastro-intestinal tract
- nervous dyspepsia
- diarrhoea

Pharmacy
Three times daily

Infusion of powdered bark	– 0.5–2 g
Tincture BPC (1949)	– 2.0–4 ml
Fluid Extract (25%)	– 1.0–2 ml

In the treatment of irritable coughs the most effective preparation is a syrup.

Historical uses
Consumption; convalescence from febrile conditions; scrofula; urinary irritation; palpitations of febrile or dyspnoeic origin. Externally for ulcers and acute ophthalmia.

Rubus idaeus

Raspberry

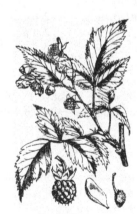

Family Rosaceae

Description
A suckering shrub with many stiff, erect, usually prickly, reddish stems growing up to 1–2 m high. *Leaves* pinnate with 3–7 oval, toothed, long-pointed

leaflets 5–12 cm, green above and densely white-hairy beneath. *Flowers* white, in dense clusters forming a compound inflorescence on lateral shoots. Petals about 5 mm, widely spaced, about as long as the sepals. Carpels red and opaque, hairy, on a conical receptacle. Flowers and fruits from spring to late summer.

Habitat and cultivation
Native to Europe in woods in mountainous regions with cold climates. Grown in gardens for their fruit, from suckers set out in rows. When the fruiting stems die, they should be cut out in winter to allow the previous year's growth to have room to fruit.

Parts used
The leaves.

Active constituents
1) Tannins (around 5%) being a complex mixture of monomeric glycosides of ellagic acid and oligomeric units—dimers of sanguiin H-6[125–127]
2) Flavonoids mainly kaempferol and quercetin[126,128,129]
3) Phenolic acids including p-coumaric, caffeic and gallic acids.[129] The phenolic content of the herb is generally good[129] but can be quite variable with geographical location.[130]

Also contains volatile oil.[131]

Nutritional constituents[132]
Vitamins: A, B-complex, C and E
Minerals: Iron, manganese, potassium, zinc, copper, calcium, magnesium and phosphorus

Actions
1) Astringent
2) Partus praeparator

Scientific information
Rubus has been an official medicine in the *British Pharmaceutical Codex* where it was indicated for use in menorrhagia as well as for those conditions for which it is still used in herbal medicine today.[44]

Although it has been a folklore medicine for over two thousand years, being particularly

valued in gynaecological applications, there is surprisingly little scientific investigation into its chemistry and pharmacology and much of what does exist was done in the first half of the 20th Century. The active constituents that may be responsible for the herb's actions on smooth muscle are not known[131] but it has been observed that at least two constituents seem to be responsible.[133]

The fruit is well characterised and due to its high phenolic content is being viewed as a potential source of medicines for the future.[131]

Gynaecological
In vivo—Although few clinical trials have been undertaken, when used by pregnant women in preparation for childbirth the limited information available indicates that it may have reduced premature deliveries or overdue deliveries, shortened labour (effect may be small) and decreased the need for medical intervention.[134,135]

Other
In vitro—All or parts of the phenolic constituents are likely to be responsible for much of its activity. To-date these include:-

- anti-oxidant activity[130,136]
- cytotoxicity to leukaemia cells including a line that has become resistant to chemotherapeutic drugs[129]
- inhibition of elastase[137]

The tannins would largely be responsible for the astringent actions of the herb. (See Appendix III for general pharmacology of tannins.)

Medicinal uses
Gastro-intestinal tract
- diarrhoea

Reproductive tract
Rubus is specifically used as a uterine tonic.

- leucorrhoea
- dysmenorrhoea
- facilitate parturition (*BHP* specific)

Externally

The tannins extracted into water (as a tea) can be used for:

- stomatitis
- tonsillitis
- bleeding gums
- conjunctivitis
- wounds
- burns

Pharmacy

Three times daily

Infusion of dried herb   – 4–8 g

Fluid Extract (25%)   – 4–8 ml

As a partus praeparator *Rubus* can be used prior to and throughout pregnancy. The studies on pregnant women concluded it is safe and has no deleterious effects on either mothers or their babies.[134,135]

Precautions and/or safety

The herb is not mutagenic or cytotoxic *in vitro* using standard tests but co-administered with mutagens it had variable effects in enhancing or negating their effects.[138]

Interactions

In vitro—The herb and the tannin fraction alter the permeability of some co-administered drugs like verapamil and ketoprofen.[138] Although there are no *in vivo* reports of interactions, tannin-rich herbs could theoretically alter the metabolism of other drugs taken at the same time.[138]

Historical uses

Cold infusion for laxity of the bowels; stomach complaints of children. In combination with *Ulmus rubra* to draw and clean wounds and burns and aid healing. The fruit was used medicinally in former times.

RUBIACEAE

The Rubiaceae or Madder family is a very large family (450–500 genera) of trees, shrubs, climbers and less commonly herbs. The leaves are opposite, simple, usually entire with stipules between the petioles or between the petiole and the axis, sometimes fused and sheathing, and other times leaf-like and forming a pseudo-whorl with the true leaves. Flowers usually form compound fascicles or panicles, but are sometimes solitary.

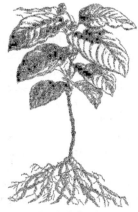

Family Rubiaceae

Cephaelis ipecacuanha

Ipecac

Description
A shrubby perennial with a fibrous root with stems to 45 cm. *Leaves* few, somewhat crowded at the top, opposite, oval and dark green with wavy edges. It produces terminal clusters of small mauve-white flowers in autumn, followed by small purple berries each containing 2 seeds.

Habitat and cultivation
Native to Brazil, Bolivia and Columbia. It grows under taller trees in rich loamy soil in hot, moist forests. It has also been cultivated in India but not very successfully.

Parts used
Roots or rhizomes collected from the wild any time in dry weather, generally in late summer.

Active constituents
1) Alkaloids (min. 2%) including emetine and cephaeline and their derivatives. The two alkaloids make up 90% of this fraction and occur in the ratio 2:1[1-3]

383

2) N-containing glucosides including ipecoside[2]
3) Iridoid glucosides[2]

C. acuminata is also used as a source of ipecac—C. ipecacuanha is known commercially as Brazil or Rio ipecac (Matto Grosso) whilst C. acuminata, grown in Central America, goes by the various names of Costa Rica, Nicaragua, Panama or Cartagena (Colombia) ipecac.[4] The different geographical regions produce ipecac with some variation in their alkaloid content. Brazilian ipecac has the highest emetine content and has been the preferred medicinal root.[5] The wide use of the herb has put a strain on its survival.[5]

Actions
1) Expectorant
2) Emetic
3) Diaphoretic
4) Antiprotozoal

Scientific information
Ipecac was first known in Europe in 1672. At this time Helvetius, a Dutch physician, used the herb (without disclosing its identity), to cure the Dauphin of amoebic dysentery. This secret ingredient was purchased from him by Louis XIV in 1688 for 1,000 louis d'or and its general use followed.[3]

It is an official medicine all over the world except in China.[4] Since the mid 20th century ipecac has been used as an emetic. It is still in use as a syrup for inducing emesis in the emergency treatment of ingested poisons, having saved many lives over the decades.[6] However it is now being recommended to treat rare cases only due to concern over its inappropriate use.[7,20]

The main alkaloids are central to the action of the herb. In larger doses they induce emesis in a two-fold manner, through irritation of the mucosal receptors in the stomach and by action on brainstem chemoreceptors. Used in smaller doses through gastric irritation the alkaloids appear, by reflex, to increase the fluid secretions of mucous glands in the respiratory tract.[8] Smaller doses were also used to achieve diaphoresis.

Recent investigation of the minor alkaloids of the herb found they have potential to inhibit HIV in vitro[9] and the whole herb has been used in vivo in a mix to improve chronic obstructive pulmonary disease (COPD)—i.e. emphysema and chronic bronchitis.[10]

Medicinal uses
Respiratory tract
• pertussis
• tracheitis
• croup
• laryngitis
• acute and chronic bronchitis
• COPD
• fever

Gastro-intestinal tract
• ingested poison by emesis
• amoebic dysentery

Precautions and/or safety
Properly used ipecac has a good safety and efficacy record.[3] Minor side-effects with normal doses are hyperemesis, diarrhoea and lethargy.[11] Excessive doses can lead to more serious adverse reactions such as Mallory-Weiss tears, gastrointestinal haemorrhage, weakness in both skeletal and cardiac muscle leading to mild tremors, convulsions, tachycardia, hypotension, arrhythmias, dyspnoea, myositis and myocardial damage. Fatalities due to excessive use of Cephaelis have been recorded.[12-14] Cardiomyopathy induced by ipecac may be reversible but it is not known at what point damage becomes permanent.[15,16]

Syrup of Ipecac has been generally available as it was seen as an advantage for the public to have access to a fast and safe home treatment for unintentional poisonings. This ease of access and relatively cheap cost has led to the preparation being abused, in particular as a purge by people with eating disorders. Regular use of the herb can lead to a reduced emetic response which then requires higher doses to produce the desired effect. Excretion of the alkaloids is relatively slow (they can be detected in urine up to 60 days after ingestion)[17-19] and continued abuse can lead to emetine, the alkaloid with the greatest toxicity, attaining high and possibly fatal levels.[20] There are some who question the wisdom of retaining the medicine for public sale.[17,20]

Interactions
The alkaloids of ipecac may interact with drugs using CYP2D6 and CYP3A4.[21]

Cinchona spp. [Restricted Herb]

Peruvian bark, Jesuits' bark

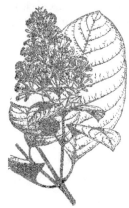

Family Rubiaceae

Description
A number of different species are used. All are evergreen trees and grow to 25 m. *Leaves* entire, ovate, with a prominent mid rib. Both petiole and lamina may be purplish-green when young or old. *Flowers* tubular, crimson, fragrant, growing in terminal clusters. *Fruit*, a capsule containing many flat and winged seeds.

Habitat and cultivation
Native to mountainous, tropical parts of South America, mainly in Peru. Now cultivated in plantations in India, Indonesia, and West Africa. Propagated from cuttings in late spring.

Parts used
Bark of trunk, branches and roots removed from trees 6–8 years old. Species/hybrids used include *C. ledgeriana* (cinchona flava), *C. succirubra* (cinchona rubra), *C. officinalis* and *C. calisaya* (cinchona flava).

Active constituents
1) Alkaloids—more than 30 have been identified comprising a maximum of 15%. 30–60% are of quinine type including quinine, quinidine, cinchonidine and cinchonine and their derivatives[22-24]
2) Tannins including cinchotannic acid
3) Phenolics including phenylpropanoids, procyanidin dimers of epicatechin and free acids
4) Triterpenes including quinovin derivatives

Also some volatile oil, resin and wax.

Quinine content is highest in *C. calisaya*. When these species have been cultivated out of their natural habitat they produce much lower levels of quinine except for *C. ledgeriana*.[25]

Actions
1) Febrifuge
2) Antiprotozoal
3) Bitter
4) Astringent
5) Orexigenic
6) Spasmolytic

Scientific information
Cinchona is a traditional medicine of the American Indians and was most likely introduced to Europe when the Jesuit priests took samples back from the Andes in the 1640s. It was known as *Pulvis cardinalis* or Jesuits' powder, and was used to successfully treat the "ague" including that suffered by King Charles II.[26] The herb can be found listed in the *London Pharmacopoeia* of 1677[27] and is represented still in pharmacopoeias worldwide in the form of its isolated alkaloids. Whilst it was not effective in the treatment of all fevers[28] it was successful in curing malaria which was endemic in parts of England at that time (known as "marsh fever" or "ague").

The demand for the drug in the west eventually out-stripped production and pressure on native trees in South America prompted European countries to try to cultivate the plant in their tropical colonies. This met with limited success.[25] Quinine was eventually isolated from cinchona bark in the 19th century and synthetic versions of it were successfully produced from 1930 onwards.[25]

All the main alkaloids of the bark are potentially antiplasmodial.[29] They appear to act by interfering with *Plasmodium*'s breakdown of haemoglobin during the blood stage of its life cycle. This in turn produces free radical metabolites that cannot be eliminated and so they cause toxic damage to the microbe.[30] Although as an antimalarial drug quinine was superseded by newer drugs, these have become less useful as the various *Plamasmodium* organisms have become resistant to them. Quinine is still used to treat some types of malaria.

Cinchona was also used to treat palpitations as early as the 1700s and was the first medicine used to treat cardiac arrhythmias.[31,32] The alkaloids are spasmolytic and are still used in medicine—quinine as a treatment for nocturnal leg cramps and quinidine in the treatment of arrhythmias.[31]

The bitter action is pronounced, causing stimulation of appetite and digestive secretions. This property is employed by the food and drink industry, for example in tonic water, and accounted for around 40% of the quinine production from cinchona bark in the late 1980s.[33]

More recent *in vitro* research has established that the herb has anti-microbial activity against some common pathogenic bacteria and *Candida albicans*;[34] cinchonine may help increase the effectiveness of chemotherapeutic agents in cancer cells that have become drug-resistant;[35-37] the alkaloids have a depressive affect on neutrophil function[38] and inhibit monoamine oxidase.[39]

It is a restricted herb.

Medicinal uses
The herb is used to treat:-

- malaria
- dyspepsia
- atonic dyspepsia
- splenomegaly
- anorexia
- rheumatism
- myalgia
- alcoholism
- hypochlorhydria
- muscular cramps
- influenza

Also used externally as a gargle for pharyngitis and in tooth powders.

CONTRAINDICATIONS—Pregnancy (quinine is oxytocic).

Precautions and/or safety
Can cause vomiting and with excessive use can lead to symptoms referred to as "cinchonism". This includes tinnitus, nausea, headache, visual disturbance, skin eruptions, gastroenteritis and possibly also coma and death. Quinine has also been associated with a number of side-effects including blood abnormalities, lupus anticoagulant, multi-organ failure and neurological abnormalities.[40,41] It can be the cause of quite severe allergic reactions.[27]

Galium aparine

Cleavers, goosegrass

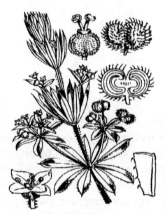

Family Rubiaceae

Description
A prostrate or scrambling annual with square, stout, branched stems to 2 m, densely clothed in retrorse, hooked, scabrid hairs on the sharply acute angles. *Leaves* and stipules sessile, in whorls of 5–8, 10–60 × 2–8 mm, linear-oblanceolate, often spatulate or obovate on exposed lateral shoots, margins flat but also densely clothed in similar hairs. *Flowers* generally 2, in axillary divaricating cymes with a whorl of leaf-like, scabrid bracts at the base of the pedicels. Corolla whitish, 1–2 mm wide. *Seeds* in pairs

2.5–4 mm in diameter, globose or sub-globose, one often smaller than the other or absent, densely covered with hooked bristles. Flowers from spring to autumn.

Habitat and cultivation
An annual weed of temperate Eurasia which self-sows freely and is naturalised elsewhere scrambling among tall grasses and other plants. Propagated also by seeds which hook onto passing animals to drop off in other places. Drought tender, frost resistant.

Parts used
The herb harvested from spring to summer when in flower and/or fruit.

Active constituents
1) Iridoid glucosides[42] including monotropein, asperuloside[43] and aucubin
2) Phenolic acids including hydroxybenzoic, p-coumaric, gallic and caffeic acids
3) Flavonoids including quercetin, hesperidin and luteolin
4) Coumarins
5) Tannins (about 5%) of the condensed type

Also contains fatty acids,[44,45] sterols,[44,46] anthraquinones,[47] alkaloids,[48,49] *n*-alkanes and some ascorbic acid.[50]

Actions
1) Diuretic
2) Astringent (mild)
3) Lymphatic alterative

Scientific information
In vitro—Galium has demonstrated antibacterial activity against *Staphylococcus aureus.*[51]

As can be seen from the above chemical analysis, this herb is poorly researched and much of the chemical investigation was undertaken decades ago. The iridoid glucosides are thought to be responsible for the diuretic effect and to have an action on the lymphatic system.

It is used as a diuretic with an alterative action and reduces lymphatic swelling though just how this occurs is not known.

Medicinal uses
Respiratory
• all lymphadenopathies including that associated with upper respiratory infections/inflammations

Urinary tract
• cystitis
• oedema
• dysuria

Skin
The other main use for this herb is in the treatment of chronic and other skin diseases:

• psoriasis
• eczema

Externally
• burns
• abrasions

Pharmacy
Three times daily
Infusion of dried herb   – 2–4 g
Expressed juice   – 5–15 ml
Tincture 1:5 (25%)   – 4–10 ml
Fluid extract (25%)   – 2–4 ml

Historical uses
As a broth for loosing weight; as a spring tonic; jaundice, scurvy; scrofula; stones and urinary obstructions; insomnia. Internally and externally for staunching bleeding; cancer. Externally for freckles; sunburn; healing old and "green" wounds; countering the bites of poisonous/venomous creatures. As an ointment applied to hard swellings in the throat. The juice for earache (drops).

Mitchella repens

Partridge berry

Description
A perennial, evergreen, mat-forming plant growing about 30 cm tall. *Leaves* sessile, opposite, rounded,

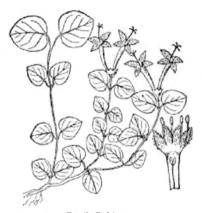

Family Rubiaceae

glossy green. *Flowers* tubular with 4 petals, white or pink, growing in terminal pairs. *Fruit* a single dry red berry per flower. Flowers from May–July in the Northern Hemisphere.

Odour—faint; taste—slightly bitter.

Habitat and cultivation
Native to North America growing in woods from Florida and Texas to Minnesota. It is sometimes cultivated as a ground cover.

Parts used
The whole herb including underground parts.

Active constituents
1) Saponin(s)
2) Tannins
3) Mucilage

Also alkaloids and a bitter principle. The details of constituents are unknown as the herb has not been studied in recent times. Available data is scant and some of it relates back to characterization carried out in the late 19th century.

Actions
1) Partus praeparator
2) Astringent
3) Antispasmodic/antidysmenorrhoeic

Also considered diuretic by the Eclectics.

Scientific information
The medicinal benefits of *Mitchella* were best appreciated in its native America, knowledge of it having been gathered by European settlers from the indigenous Indian communities. It was held in high regard by Eclectic herbalists, its action was seen as a gentle tonic specific for the uterus. Previously called by the name "Squaw vine" the name partridge berry is now preferred.[52]

Medicinal uses
Gastro-intestinal tract
As an astringent it has been indicated for:

• catarrhal colitis

Reproductive tract
As a uterine tonic is has been used for:

• dysmenorrhoea
• amenorrhoea
• facilitate childbirth

It was employed by the Eclectics to alleviate false labour pains and help prevent premature deliveries and miscarriages.[52]

Pharmacy
Three times daily
Infusion of dried herb   – 2–4 g
Liquid extract (25%)   – 2–4 ml

Historical uses
Hysteria; weak and feeble conditions of the uterus including prolapse; dropsy, urinary retention, bladder irritation; diarrhoea. Externally for sore nipples.

RUTACEAE

The Rutaceae or rue family consists of about 150 genera of mostly evergreen but sometimes deciduous, armed or unarmed trees and shrubs of temperate and tropical regions but they are rare in Europe.

- Leaves alternate or opposite, simple or compound and sometimes reduced to 1 leaflet, dotted with glands
- Flowers sometimes unisexual, mostly regular and in various inflorescences
- Sepals 3–5, petals 3–5, rarely absent; stamens 3–10 but sometimes 20–60 arising from a disc. Ovary 4–5-celled
- Fruit may be a capsule, a leathery-skinned berry, a drupe, a samara, a follicle or sometimes separating into sections

The best known members of the family are the *Citrus*.

Agathosma betulina
[Formerly *Barosma betulina*]

Short or round buchu

Description
A much-branched shrub. Leaves glabrous, dark green, oval more than 2 cm long, sharply serrate.

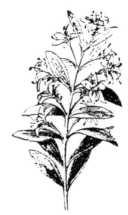

Family Rutaceae

Rich in oil glands. *Flowers* pink, 5-petaled, star-like, and solitary, growing at the end of short axillary branchlets. Filaments, hairy. *Fruit* a capsule with 5 carpels.

Habitat and cultivation
Native to South Africa, growing mainly in the Western Cape. Buchu is propagated by cuttings of the mature wood and is cultivated in other places with a similar climate. e.g. California. *A. crenulata* is also used.

Parts used
Leaves harvested and dried when the herb is in flower or is fruiting.

Active constituents
1) Volatile oil (up to 2.5%) predominantly menthone and isomenthone also limonene, diosphenol ('buchu camphor'), ψ-diosphenol and pulegone.[1] The composition of this fraction can be very variable
2) Flavonoids including diosmin (0.8%), rutin and hesperidin (0.12%)[2]

Also mucilage, resin and tannins.
There are other species of *Agathosma* that have been used in medicine but their volatile oil make-up is different. *A. betulina* has high levels of diosphenol and ψ-diosphenol whilst *A. crenulata* has a high content of pulegone.[3] Their pharmacology is also different.[3] The genus is subject to some hybridization however and the resulting morphological changes can make it harder to distinguish the preferred *A. betulina*.

Nutritional constituents
Vitamins: Some of B group and C
Minerals: Calcium, chromium, magnesium, phosphorus and potassium

Actions
1) Diuretic
2) Urinary antiseptic

Scientific information
Buchu is a traditional medicine in South Africa that was introduced to settlers by the indigenous people.[4] It was subsequently taken to Britain in 1790 when it became an official medicine appearing in the *British Pharmacopoeia* and *Codex* from 1821 to 1963. It was recommended as a urinary tract remedy, particularly for infections.[5] Although it was used in mainstream medicine there have not been any clinical trials conducted on it and there is not a great deal of current research into its pharmacology or chemistry.
Buchu oil is used as a flavouring in foods and in the perfume industry.[3]

In vitro—The herb has:

- a degree of inhibition of COX-2 but not COX-1[6]
- good anti-oxidant activity[6]
- no (extract)[3] or very low (essential oil)[6] antibacterial effect against a small test range of bacteria including *Escherichia coli* a common pathogen in cystitis.

The antimicrobial activity of buchu was actually increased by subjecting it to a simulated digestion process suggesting it may require this sort of transformation to become effective *in vivo*.[7]

Medicinal uses
Urinary tract
- cystitis
- urethritis
- prostatitis
- dysuria

Pharmacy
Three times daily
Infusion of dried herb   – 1–2 g
Tincture 1:5 (60%)   – 2–4 ml
Fluid Extract (90%)   – 0.3–1.2 ml
CONTRAINDICATIONS—Pregnancy.

Precautions and/or safety
Can cause gastro-intestinal disturbance.

Historical uses
Urinary gravel and calculus, stomach ache, nausea, vomiting, as a digestive tonic; fever, cholera, coughs and colds; prophylaxis of cancer; dysmenorrhoea. Topically for sprains, fractures, rheumatism and bruises.

Ruta graveolens

Rue

Description
A perennial semi-deciduous aromatic herb growing to 80 cm high. *Basal stem* woody and little branched.

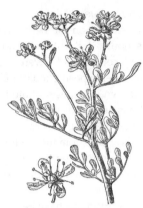

Family Rutaceae

Whole plant dotted with oil glands. *Leaves* glabrous, glaucous, blue-green, alternate and deeply divided into spatulate-oblong segments, 3–12 mm long. *Flowers* 1.5–2 cm in terminal corymbs; petals concave and incurved at the tips, yellowish-green, flowering in summer and early autumn. *Fruits* sub-cylindrical, brown-green capsules, 5.5 mm in diameter, rough, and 4–5-lobed at apex. *Seeds* black.

Odour—strong and characteristic; taste—pungent.

Habitat and cultivation
Native to Southern Europe growing on well drained, rocky soils. Cultivated worldwide, easily grown from seed or cuttings but hard to transplant. Does not like wet conditions.

Parts used
The herb gathered just prior to, or during, flowering. If handled in sunlight rue can cause photosensitivity—see Precautions.

Active constituents
1) Volatile oil (0.1–0.7%). 38 constituents have so far been identified mostly methyl and nonyl ketones of which the predominant ones are undecan-2-one and nonan-2-one, also terpenoids[8,9]
2) Flavonoids mainly rutin, also quercitin and isoflavones including fomononetin and biochanin A[10–13]
3) Furanocoumarins and coumarins (at least 34) including the methoxy-psoralens—bergapten (5-methoxypsoralen) and xanthotoxin—rutamarin (chalepin acetate), scopoletin and umbelliferone[9,13–17]
4) Alkaloids of quinoline and acridone type (at least 39 identified) including graveoline and chalepensin.[14,18–20] These have low solubility[9]

Also contains tannins, phenolic acids,[11] lignans[12] and a number of glycosides[12]

Actions
1) Spasmolytic
2) Emmenagogue
3) Antitussive

Scientific information
Ruta has had a long history of use as a medicinal herb in many cultures and with a reputation for treating a large range of conditions. It has fallen from popular use in modern phytotherapy but was known from the time of Hippocrates as an antidote to poison and by Galen and Pliny the Elder for its antifertility action.[21] Both the herb and its oil have been official medicines, the latter having been used as an antispasmodic, emmenagogue, local irritant and anthelmintic.[5] Rue was also used in the Mediterranean as a flavouring agent for food and drinks. There has been quite extensive examination of the herb's chemical constituents which are pharmacologically active but there are no relevant clinical studies reported using preparations of whole extracts of *Ruta*.

Antimicrobial
In vitro—The herb has antimicrobial activity against *Trichomonas vaginalis*[22] and a range of Gram-positive bacteria including *Staphylococcus aureus* and *S. epidemidis*, *Streptococcus pyogenes*, *Listeria monocytogenes*, *Pseudomonas aeruginosa*, *Bacillus subtilis* and *B. cereus*.[13,23–25] The coumarins do not seem to contribute greatly to this activity.[24]

Nervous system
In vitro—Due to the herb's historical use in the nervous system extracts have been screened and have shown:

• moderate inhibition of acetyl cholinesterase (raising acetylcholine levels may help with cognitive function)[26] possibly some binding affinity to $GABA_A$-benzodiazepine sites—not established in human models[17,27]

- blocking of ion channels particularly potassium—this may explain some of the action on the nervous system.[28] It has also suggested a theoretical use for the herb in the treatment of multiple sclerosis although no clinical trials have so far been undertaken.[29]

Other

The alkaloids have strong cytotoxicity for a number of different cancer cell lines[14,30] and the whole extract is anti-oxidant.[11]

Rutin is well known and utilised in orthodox preparations to strengthen capillaries and reduce oedema.[31]

Medicinal uses

Gastro-intestinal tract

Ruta is useful in this tract as a spasmolytic and because it is considered to increase circulation to the digestive organs:

- griping
- bowel tension
- flatulence

Nervous system

As a gentle sedative it may be used for:

- tension
- spasms
- nervous over-activity

Reproductive tract

Now used mainly in this context to bring on a delayed period:

- atonic amenorrhoea
- suppressed menstruation

Pharmacy

Three times daily

Infusion dried herb   – 0.5–1 g
Fluid Extract (25%)   – 0.5–1 ml

CONTRAINDICATIONS—Pregnancy.

Precautions and/or safety

In vitro safety studies on the herb have indicated that rutin is non-toxic[32] but the whole extract,[33] alkaloids[34] and coumarins[35,36] were mutagenic to test organisms after exposure to UV light.

Ruta is known to cause photodermatitis, a vesiculo-bullous dermatitis with erythema,[37–40] and in extreme cases topical contact can cause systemic reactions.[41] This results from the methoxypsoralens in contact with skin reacting to UV light. Psoralen derivatives are used in orthodox treatment for psoriasis.

Other adverse reactions have been attributed to *Ruta* although the occurrence appears to be rare. One isolated case of an elderly woman who used infusions of the herb in conjunction with a number of orthodox cardiac medications suffered reversible cardio-, hepato- and nephro-toxicity and increased prothrombin time.[42] A number of women have sustained multiple organ failure, in a few cases leading to death, after using the herb to terminate pregnancy. The causal link was complicated by the fact that the local name used in Uruguay, where the cases arose, can refer to species other than *R. graveolens* and that *Ruta* is often combined with other herbs for this purpose.[43]

Historical uses

As a diuretic; an antidote to all poisons (a main part in Mithridates antidote); treatment for the plague; "to abate venery and ability to procreate!" (anaphrodisiac?); for epilepsy and vertigo; used internally and externally for pains including of chest and breathing, sciatica, joints and to improve eyesight especially affected by overuse. As a prophylactic against fits from the ague and disease generally. For treating worms; dropsy; to staunch a bleeding nose. More recent uses for coughs, croup; palpitation; hysteria; nervous nightmares (expressed juice). Used in West Indies for infertility, amenorrhoea and childbirth. Externally applied to swollen testicles, wheals and pimples, warts, morphew, scabs, tetter, ringworm, sores, stinking ulcers; the juice used for earache; as an insecticide including for fleas; chronic bronchitis; headache (fresh leaves placed on temples).

Zanthoxylum americanum

Northern prickly ash

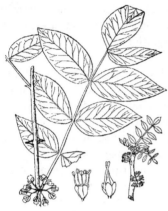

Family Rutaceae

Z. clava-herculis

Southern prickly ash

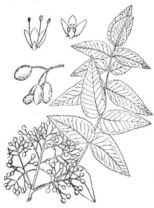

Family Rutaceae

Description

Z. americanum is a deciduous shrub or tree growing 7 × 3 m. Branches alternate, armed with strong, conical, brown prickles with a broad base, scattered irregularly, but most often occurring in pairs at the junction of branches. *Leaves* alternate and pinnate usually of 5 pairs with a terminal leaflet, ovate acute and downy beneath, lemon-scented when crushed. The common petiole is round and usually prickly on the back. *Flowers* small, greenish, aromatic, dioecious or polygamous, in small, dense, sessile umbels in the axils of young branches, appearing before the leaves. Sterile flowers have 5 oblong, erect sepals with 5 stamens; female flowers grow on separate trees and have a more compressed calyx and styles twisting into close contact at the top followed by red to green oval capsules covered with lemon-scented dots, 2-valved and 1-seeded. *Seeds* oval and black. Flowers April to May in USA.

Zanthoxylum clava-herculis is also a deciduous shrub or tree but may grow taller to 10 m, and the bark is covered with large, triangular, corky knobs and the petioles and branches with larger prickles. *Leaves* pinnate with 5–17 leaflets, ovate-lanceolate, shining and smooth on the upper surface with crenate-serrulate margins. *Flowers* plentiful, greenish, in terminal panicles, appearing before the leaves. Both species fruit August to October in USA.

Odour bark—slight, berries—aromatic; taste bark and berries—pungent and bitter.

Habitat and cultivation

Both are native to North America. Z. *americanum* grows in moist woods and thickets from Quebec to Florida, Okalahoma to Minnesota. Z. *clava-herculis* grows on light to medium, well-drained soils from Southern Virginia to Florida and west to Texas and Okalahoma. Both are frost resistant and drought tender.

Parts used

The berries and the bark.

Active constituents

1) Alkaloids including mostly chelerythrine and magnoflorine in Z. *clava-herculis*; nitidine and laurifoline in Z. *americanum*.[44-46] Also candicine and tembetarine

2) An isobutylamide, neoherculin (0.025%) in bark of Z. *clava-herculis*.[47,48] Berries of this species also contain neoherculin and an hydroxylated form of it.[49] The same isobutylamide is found in Z. *piperitum*, an oriental species, and is known as α-sanshool. It is identical to echinacein

3) Lignans (both species)—asarinin and sesamin[48,50]
4) Cinnamamide derivatives—herclavin (*Z. clava-herculis*),[51] a methylcinnamide (*Z. americanum*)[52]
5) Coumarins (*Z. americanum*):
   a) furanocoumarins in berries including 5-methoxypsoralen (bergapten) and 8-methoxypsoralen (xanthotoxin), imperatorin, psoralen and cnidillin.[53,54] Bark has low levels of these constituents[54]
   b) pyranocoumarins including alloxanthoxyletin, dipetaline and xanthoxyletin[50,55,56]

Also contains tannins, resins and a volatile oil, the latter being in higher concentration in the berries.

Actions
1) Circulatory stimulant
2) Diaphoretic
3) Sialagogue
4) Carminative
5) Antirheumatic

Scientific information
Many species of *Zanthoxylum* are used medicinally in their countries of origin, they contain a broad range of pharmacological constituents and activities. Indigenous American Indians valued this herb and used it more extensively than is the case in modern phytotherapy. Western herbal medicine uses both species interchangeably although *Z. clava-herculis* is considered the more active.[49] The bark and berries of both were official medicines in the United States and Britain up until the mid 20th century.

There has not been much recent evaluation and no *in vivo* studies have been reported.

In vitro—Studies have shown that:

- berries, root and stem bark of *Z. americanum* are cytotoxic to several cancer cell lines—(mainly furancoumarins and lignans)[50,53]
- various fractions of *Z. americanum* are antifungal to a broad range of organisms some of which are resistant to standard antifungals. Activity is increased by exposure to UV light

and berries are much more active than bark—(mainly furanocoumarins)[54]
- extracts from *Z. clava-herculis* have potential use as antimicrobials against methicillin-resistant *Staphylococcus aureus*—MRSA (chelerythrine)[44]

Neoherculin is insecticidal with effectiveness against the eggs of body lice.[49] The lignans are being widely studied and have potential as antioxidant, cytotoxic, anti-inflammatory, antimicrobial, hypocholesterolaemic, antiallergic, hepatoprotective and hypotensive agents.[57]

Furanocoumarins like psoralens intercalate with DNA and, in the presence of UV light, are genotoxic binding to DNA bases and preventing normal cell division (See Apiaceae). Different furancoumarins appear to have specificity for particular DNA base pairs.[58] Fungi have a predominance of adenine and thymine bases, compared to mammalian DNA, and they are susceptible to the specific action of 5-methoxypsoralen.[58] However as furanocoumarins have general genotoxic effects this may limit their use. Traditional preparations of bark are low in furanocoumarins and as this part of the herb had a reputation for treating skin infections other constituent(s) present, and as yet untested, are likely to contribute to this activity.[54]

8-methoxypsoralen has been used to increase melanin pigment in skin exposed to UV light for the purpose of treating vitiligo,[5] also used to treat psoriasis.

According to the *BHP* the berries are more active than the bark for circulatory disorders.

Medicinal uses
Cardiovascular system
As a circulatory stimulant where it is considered to improve arterial function:

- circulatory insufficiency
- intermittent claudication
- Buerger's disease
- Raynaud's phenomenon
- peripheral vascular disease
- fevers

Musculoskeletal
- arthritis
- rheumatism

Pharmacy
Three times daily

Bark
Decoction of dried bark   –   1–3 g
Tincture 1:5 (45%)   –   2–5 ml
Fluid Extract (45%)   –   1–3 ml

Berries
Decoction of dried berries   –   0.5–1.5 g
Fluid Extract (45%)   –   0.5–1.5 ml

Historical uses
Toothache (bark chewed); skin diseases; sores; colic; cholera; typhoid, sore throat, urogenital and upper respiratory infections. Externally for wounds, burns, indolent ulcers (powder).

SALICACEAE

The Salicaceae or willow family consists of 4 genera and about 500 species of dioecious and deciduous trees and shrubs distributed almost worldwide.

- Leaves alternate, simple, generally petioled.
- Flowers unisexual, in more or less silky-hairy catkins without a perianth. Stamens 1 or many, ovary 1-celled.
- Fruit a small capsule and seeds with tufts or hairs.

Salix (willow) and *Populus* (poplar) are the main medicinal genera.

exist and the various species may be interchangeable. There is however an enormous scope for the research and clinical assessment of the whole of this genus.

Other species of *Populus* not described here, which are traditionally used in medicine include:

Populus x *canadensis*	Canadian poplar
P. tremula	aspen
P. yunnanensis	Yunnan poplar
P. tremuloides	quaking aspen
P. deltoides	necklace poplar
P. nigra	Lombardy polar
P. trichocarpa	Western balsam poplar
P. x *canescens*	grey poplar

Populus spp.

There are a number of *Populus* species that have been traditionally used in medicine. They appear to have been used for their barks and/or their buds, but roots and leaves have also been used. Most of the current scientific information available is based on a much smaller number of species and is represented, in use, by *P. tremuloides* and *P. alba* bark, and *P.* x *gileadensis* buds. A degree of overlap must

Populus alba

White poplar

Description

A tall, spreading deciduous tree to 25 m high which suckers profusely. Bark smooth or shallowly fissured and grey. *Shoots* white-tomentose, buds white but not sticky or aromatic. *Leaves*, petiole 1.5–5 cm long, white tomentose; lamina

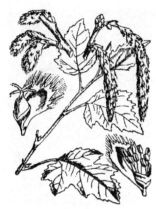

Family Salicaceae

on vegetative shoots 3–10 × 2–9.5 cm, more or less deltoid with 3–5 lobulate or toothed primary lobes; on adult shoots lamina is smaller, ovate to oblong, lobed or strongly toothed, always white and loosely tomentose beneath and glabrous green and shining on the upper surface; base truncate, rounded or sub-cordate, apex obtuse or rounded. *Catkins*, female, more or less pendant, 2–8 cm long, bracts membranous, shining and brown in upper part; cup shaped disc. *Capsules* containing dense, white cottony hairs which give the appearance of snow under the trees. Flowers in spring before leaves appear.

Habitat and cultivation
Native to Britain, South Central Europe and North Africa and naturalised elsewhere. Easily grown from cuttings, suckers or poles. Planted along roadsides, used as shelter belts and along streams. Frost resistant, drought tender.

Parts used
Dried bark, preferably collected in spring as the sap begins to rise.

Active constituents
1) Phenolic glycosides including salicin, populin and benzoyl salicoside (populoside)[1-3]
2) Tannins

Catechol and a small amount of α-tococopherol have been isolated from *P. tremuloides*.[4,5]

Actions
1) Antirheumatic
2) Antiseptic
3) Astringent
4) Cholagogue
5) Diuretic
6) Anodyne
7) Anti-inflammatory

Scientific information
The bark of all the *Populus* species are considered to be chemically similar and all contain salicortin, the precursor of salicin, as a main constituent.[3] The phenolic glycosides listed are derivatives of salicylic acid, a synthetic version of which is sold worldwide as aspirin (See *Salix alba*).

Pharmacological information on whole extracts of the above species is lacking and chemical investigations were carried out many years ago. There is very little current information, other than tests done on *P. tremula*, the European aspen.

In vitro—*P. tremula* is antioxidant[6] and antibacterial against *Streptococcus pneumoniae* and *Haemophilus influenzae*.[7]

A commercial preparation containing *Solidago virgaurea*, *Fraxinus excelsior* (common ash) and *P. tremula* exhibits strong anti-oxidant and anti-inflammatory activity.[8-11]

In vivo—The 3 herb combination above was shown in clinical trials to be an effective anti-inflammatory and analgesic for a variety of arthritides, the benefit apparently comparable to that of NSAIDs.[12,13]

In Canada traditional healers use the bark of *P. tremuloides* to treat digestive and gynaecological disorders.[14]

The properties of these species show many features in common with salicylate-containing willow bark (See *Salix alba*).

Medicinal uses
Respiratory tract
• colds with fever

Gastro-intestinal tract
• diarrhoea
• anorexia with stomach/liver disorders

Urinary tract
- cystitis
- infections of this tract

Musculoskeletal
The combined actions improve waste excretion and treat pain and inflammation.

- rheumatoid arthritis (*BHP* specific)
- arthritis
- muscular rheumatism

Pharmacy
Three times daily
Decoction of dried herb   – 1–4 g
Fluid Extract (25%)   – 1–4 ml
Potter's upper limit is 5 g and 5 ml.

Precautions and/or safety
The commercial preparation containing *P. tremula* was safe with few side-effects.[12,13,15] There have been recorded cases of contact allergy to the salicyl alcohol and salicylaldehyde in *P. tremula* bark.[16,17]

Historical uses
See the end of *P* x *gileadensis*.

Populus species used traditionally for their leaf buds include *P.* x *canadensis*, *P.* x *gileadensis*, *P. nigra*, *P. trichocarpa* and *P. yunnanensis*. The balsam poplar *P. tacamahaca*, which appears to be identical to *P. balsamifera*[18] is also used.

Populus x gileadensis

Balm of Gilead poplar

Description
Deciduous tree to about 60 m high, with a spreading habit and extensive suckers. Bark grey, fissured. *Buds* very viscid and glabrous; young leaves balsam scented. Petioles 3.5–7 cm long and glandular viscid. *Leaves* 6–23 × 5.5–20 cm, broad ovate, hairy on veins above and beneath, green above, greenish white beneath. Margins ciliate, crenate-serrate with gland-tipped teeth, without translucent border. Leaf base cordate or sub-cordate, sometimes

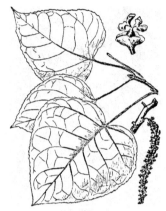

Family Salicaceae

rounded with 2 glands; apex cuspidate or acuminate. *Flowers* catkins female, pendulous 13–19 cm long at anthesis. Bracts 4–5 mm long excluding long filiform lobes, greenish white. Cup-shaped disc 1.5–3 mm deep, long, broad, ovoid, containing abundant long, white, silky hairs.

Habitat and cultivation
The origin of this species is unknown but it is thought to be a hybrid of the North American *P. deltoides* and *P. tacamahaca* and is only known as a female clone. Propagated by cuttings or suckers, forming large clumps. Planted for shelter in many countries. Drought and frost resistant.

Parts used
The leaf buds harvested in winter.

Active constituents
1) Flavonoids the nature and content of which varies for the particular species, but includes chrysin. They are major constituents in *P. nigra* and *P. candicans* but minor in *P. tacamahaca* which has mainly dihydrochalcones[19,20] *P. nigra*
2) Phenolic esters of caffeic and isoferulic acids[21,22]
3) Volatile oil (up to 0.5%) including mainly sesquiterpenes also monoterpenes and hemiterpenes[23] *P. tacamahaca*
4) Aromatic acids and esters of cinnamic and coumaric acids but little or no caffeic and isoferulic acids or esters[22]
5) Volatile oil—terpenoids (11–13%) mainly bisabolol and humulene[18]

Also oleoresin and in *P. balsamifera* prostaglandins E, F, A and B and arachidonic acid the content of which varies with the time of year.[24] (Arachidonic acid is believed to be a precursor for plant-based prostaglandins.) Phenolic glycosides populin, salicin and benzoyl salicoside as found in the bark, have also been reported.[20]

P. x candicans is less well characterised than the other two but is believed to be chemically similar to *P. tacamahaca*. It appears likely that misidentification of *P. x gileadensis* occurs and buds of the above species may be used interchangeably.[25]

Actions
1) Expectorant
2) Antiseptic
3) Anti-inflammatory
4) Counter-irritant

Scientific information
There has been a great deal more investigation of the chemistry of the bud exudates than the bark, however once again this information is old and no longer easily available. No pharmacological information is available. *German Commission E* has approved the use of buds for external problems like superficial skin injuries, haemorrhoids, frostbite and sunburn.

Propolis derived from bees visiting poplar trees has many constituents in common with the bud exudate.[26]

According to the *BHC* the lipophilic fraction of *P. nigra* buds has strong antibacterial, antifungal, anti-inflammatory and "capillary" activities. The caffeic acid derivatives and volatile oil fractions are antimicrobial and the latter is also expectorant.

Medicinal uses
Respiratory tract
Mainly used internally in this area to treat both acute and chronic problems:

- bronchitis
- coughs
- sore throats
- laryngitis with aphonia (*BHP* specific)

Externally
In ointment form for:

- myalgia
- arthritis
- gout
- muscle strain
- rheumatism
- haemorrhoids
- painful wounds

Also an infusion can be gargled to treat laryngitis.

Pharmacy
Three times daily

Infusion of dried herb	– 4 g
Tincture 1:5 (45%)	– 4–8 ml
Fluid Extract (90%)	– 4–8 ml
Topical use in ointment 20–30%	

Precautions and/or safety
Rarely allergy, systemic or contact—see above.

Historical uses
As a cleansing agent; for sciatica and strangury. Headaches. Juice of leaves applied locally for ear ache and the leaves used for epilepsy. The buds for "dull sight"; as a beauty aid and for external inflammations; water collected from the "hollow places of the tree for warts; pushes; wheals and breakings out of the body". The herb was used by *Culpeper* to dry up milk flow after weaning. Also used for gonorrhoea and gleet and as a substitute for Peruvian bark (*Cinchona*—quinine) in intermittent fevers, for coughs and 'flu. Bark used externally as styptic; with *Salix* spp. as ash for arthritic joints.

Salix spp.

There are 300–500 species of willow world-wide, including those below, containing salicin and used medicinally.

S. alba	willow, white willow
S. daphnoides	violet willow

S. fragilis	crack willow
S. pentandra	bay willow
S. purpurea	purple osier

Salix alba

Willow, white willow

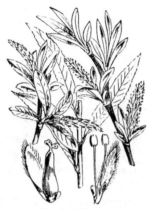

Family Salicaceae

Description
A deciduous tree up to 26 m tall with deeply fissured grey bark and ascending branches. *Leaves* alternate, shortly petiolate to 11 cm long, lanceolate with silky whitish hairs on both sides. *Flowers* appear at the same time as the leaves, growing in dense cylindrical catkins. Male catkins up to 5 cm long with 2 stamens and yellow anthers; female catkins up to 4 cm long. Blooms in spring.

Odour—slight; taste—astringent and bitter.

Habitat and cultivation
Native to Britain, Europe, Asia and North America growing in moist grassland, marshes and along streams. Widely naturalised elsewhere. Easily grown from cuttings in spring. Frost resistant, drought tender.

Parts used
The bark collected from young branches during the growing period. Salicin is highest in spring and summer, lowest in winter. This genus hybridizes easily.

Active constituents
1) Phenolic glycosides[27] (max. 11%) including salicylates as salicortin (an ester of salicin) and salicin. In *S. alba* the main form is salicortin up to a maximum of 1% also a low level of free salicin, 2'-acetylsalicortin and triandrin. *S. purpurea* (up to 8.5%) including salireposide and tremulacin. *S. daphnoides* (up to 8.4%) including triandrin, salicylic acid, picein and tremulacin.[28] *S. fragilis* (up to 10.2%)
2) Flavonoids (max. 4%) including prunin (naringenin 7-glucoside) and salipurposide in *S. purpurea* and *S. daphnoides*[27]
3) Tannins (8–20%) mainly of the condensed type

Also a lignan—sisymbrifolin (*S. alba*),[29] flavan-3-ols and oligomeric procyanidins (*S. purpurea*),[30] anthocyanins (variety of species)[31] and polysaccharides including arabinan (*S. alba*).[32]

Actions
1) Anti-inflammatory
2) Analgesic
3) Antipyretic
4) Astringent
5) Antirheumatic

Scientific information
The analgesic and antipyretic effects of *Salix* were known to the ancient Egyptians and Greeks and were commonly used through the ages from the early physicians like Hippocrates and Dioscorides to the present day. Modern re-evaluation of the herb is attributed to Edward Stone who in 1758 reported to his peers his successful use of the bark to treat the pain and fever of malaria.[33,34] "Salicine", the name given to the active constituent, also found in wintergreen oil and meadowsweet, was isolated in 1828. When limited supplies of bark failed to satisfy medical need a totally synthetic version was produced which, with refinement to acetylsalicylic acid or "aspirin", was produced in 1853. Acetylsalicylic acid did not however enter into common medical use until the end of the 19th century. The mechanism of its anti-inflammatory action through inhibition of prostaglandin synthesis was not elucidated

until 1971 and its use as an anti-coagulant was not established until 1988.[35] This form of salicylate replaced *Salix* use in conventional medicine.

Willow bark is still widely used in Germany, along with *Harpagophytum* in the treatment of joint inflammation.[36] It has been approved by *German Commission E* as an antirheumatic agent and to treat fever and headaches. Although analgesic, anti-inflammatory, antipyretic and lack of ulcerogenic effects have been demonstrated in animal models these effects in humans are largely deduced from empirical use.[37]

Anti-inflammatory
It has been assumed that the action of *Salix* is primarily due to its salicylic acid content. However although salicin is converted to salicylic acid *in vivo* its effective level is probably too low to be responsible for the type of anti-inflammatory effects observed with acetylsalicylic acid. It has been proposed that other constituents like the flavonoids or tannins must contribute or that the herb's mechanism of action is quite different to that of acetylsalicylic acid.[28–40] The mode of action of *Salix* is in fact considered to be much wider than that of standard NSAIDs[41] and it has been shown that it is much more effective as an anti-inflammatory than either salicin or salicylic acid at equivalent doses.[37]

In vitro—Apart from the strong anti-oxidant activity of *Salix* (related to the high level of phenolics),[42] and the effect this would have on inflammation, other mechanisms that may account for its anti-inflammatory action include:-

- inhibition of COX-1[55]
- inhibition of COX-2 (strong and selective action)[43,44]
- inhibition of LOX[36]
- modulation of cytokine release and prostaglandin production (weak)[43]—this mechanism has been questioned[45]
- inhibition of hyaluronidase (by flavonoids)[36]

However the complete mode of *Salix*'s activity is still not understood.

In vivo—Commercial willow bark extracts have been tested in clinical trials albeit of short duration.

In the treatment of low back pain these extracts have been shown to:-

- be as effective as the COX-2 inhibitor, rofecoxib, in subjective and objective measures of improvement[46]
- be cost effective as a treatment, reducing the need for additional conventional therapy[47,48]
- give dose-dependent improvement—stronger salicin containing extracts achieving better pain reduction.[47,48]

For the treatment of osteoarthritis two trials have been reported. In one the extract gave moderate improvement, measured both objectively and subjectively, in patients with osteoarthritis of hip and knee.[49] In contrast another trial found no significant reduction in pain levels when standardised extracts were used to treat either osteoarthritis or rheumatoid arthritis for a period of 6 weeks.[50] Again only short term studies have been conducted.

Reviews to-date conclude that the evidence of an anti-inflammatory effect in the treatment of osteoarthritis and/or low back pain is not consistent and this may relate to variations in doses used.[36] However there is moderate evidence in support of short-term improvement in pain level by these standardised preparations.[37,51]

Other
In vitro—The bark and all its main fractions inhibit the growth of lung and colon cancer cells.[52] *S. alba* protects fibroblasts from UVA light[53] and inhibits binding to specific 5-hydroxytryptamine receptors, a potential aid in the treatment of migraines.[54]

In vivo—A combination of *Tanacetum parthenium* and *Salix* in tablet form effectively reduced the severity, duration and frequency of migraine attacks.[54]

Salix extracts standardised on salicin (240 mg) inhibited platelet aggregation compared to placebo but this effect was about one fifth that of acetylsalicylic acid given at a dose of 100 mg.[55] (That would make *Salix* one-tenth as strong as aspirin in this effect.)

Medicinal uses
Respiratory tract
• influenza
• common cold
• fevers
• respiratory catarrh

Nervous system
• pain of varying origin
• mild headaches

Musculoskeletal
The analgesic and anti-inflammatory activities come together in the treatment of:

• gouty arthritis
• systemic connective tissue disorders marked by inflammation
• arthritis
• ankylosing spondylitis
• rheumatism, muscular and arthritic

Pharmacy
Three times daily
Decoction of dried herb   – 1–2 g
Tincture 1:5 (25%)   – 5–8 ml
Fluid Extract (25%)   – 1–2 ml
   Commercial preparations are likely to contain a mixture of species[28] and are standardised on salicin content. The daily doses used in trials were based on either 120 mg or 240 mg of salicin where 120 mg of salicin is equivalent to 393 mg of dried willow bark.

Pharmacokinetics
Studies have identified salicylic acid (86%) and its metabolites, gentisic (4%) and salicyluric acid (10%), in plasma after ingestion of willow bark tablets.[56] Salicin is metabolised before and/or during absorption. Salicylic acid is the first metabolite detected in plasma; it reaches a peak in less than 2 hours and appears to be absorbed through the mucosa of the stomach or upper digestive tract.[57] Its half life is around 2.5 hours, excretion is mainly as salicyluric acid in urine with 95% of urinary excretion being completed by 24 hours.[57] Peak serum levels of salicylic acid are very much lower than for synthetic salicylates (1.4 mg/L after 240 mg salicin compared to 35–50 mg/L after 500 mg of acetylsalicylic acid).[49,57]

Precautions and/or safety
In general clinical trials using standardised extracts found side effects were minimal being equivalent to, or lower than, that for placebo. The most frequently reported reactions were allergic reactions—pruritus and exanthema—and gastro-intestinal reactions, all of which were easily resolved.[47] *Salix* was considered safe and well tolerated.[48,49]
   Serious side effects recorded are an anaphylactic response to a commercial preparation, which contained willow bark as one of its ingredients, in an aspirin-sensitive person[58] and one case of a severe allergic reaction to standardised *Salix* amongst those patients taking part in the above clinical trials.[48]

Interactions
There is the potential for *Salix* to increase the effect of warfarin[59] although this interaction has not been reported to-date.

Historical uses
To staunch bleeding; to prevent vomiting. "It helpeth also to stay thin, hot, sharp distillations from the head upon the lungs, causing a consumption." The leaves to treat windy colic; both leaves and seeds used for "subduing lust". Urinary retention; spots and discolouration of the skin. Tonic for digestive tract and post acute illness; worms; chronic diarrhoea; dysentery. "Redness and dimness of sight; films that grow over the eyes." Leaves and/or bark for dandruff and scurf (topically).

SCROPHULARIACEAE

The Scrophulariaceae or Figwort family contains 4500 species throughout the world.

- They are perennial, biennial or annual herbs or small shrubs
- The stems are generally square
- The leaves are alternate, opposite or whorled, usually simple but sometimes dissected
- The flowers are usually bisexual and irregular, growing in cymes in the axils of the upper leaves or bracts, and sometimes forming terminal racemes or panicles, or occasionally solitary
- The calyx has five equal lobes, the sepals are connate
- The corolla usually consists of 5 connate petals, often 2-lipped but sometimes almost regular. 4 fertile stamens
- Fruit usually a capsule with numerous seeds

Medicinal plants in this family are:

Digitalis lanata	Scrophularia nodosa
Digitalis purpurea	Verbascum thapsus
Euphrasia spp.	Veronicastrum virginica
Hebe spp.	

Digitalis spp. [No longer used]

Foxglove

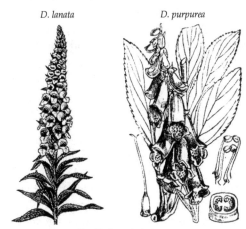

D. lanata   D. purpurea

Family Scrophulariaceae

Description
D. lanata, Grecian foxglove, may be biennial or perennial and grows over 1 m tall in flower. The flowering stem is glabrous below and white hairy above. *Basal leaves* in a rosette, stem leaves alternate, lanceolate, glabrous. *Flower*, whitish with

purple veins, in dense racemes. *Calyx*, shorter than bracts. *Corolla* as long as, or shorter than bracts. Middle lobe of lower lip longer than the others. Flowers in summer.

Digitalis purpurea, foxglove, is a biennial or short lived perennial. *Leaves* with long, winged petioles grow in a basal rosette the first year. Lamina lanceolate-elliptic, grey, hairy-tomentose above and soft to the touch. *Stem* leaves smaller with shorter petioles. Flowering stem simple, hairy, over 2.5 m tall in the second spring. *Flowers* in racemes. *Corolla*, campanulate, usually pinkish purple with dark purple white-ringed spots in the lower part. Sometimes corolla is white. *Fruit* a capsule.

Flowers from late spring to summer.

Habitat and cultivation
D. lanata is native to Greece and the Danube area, growing in thickets and rough ground. Naturalized in north-east North America and planted in gardens in other countries. Always grown from seed.

D. purpurea is native to Western Europe. Foxglove is naturalized in most countries and is grown from seed but self-sows readily especially along forest margins, stony river-beds and roadsides.

Parts used
Leaves harvested in summer.

Active constituents
1) Cardenolides, more than 50 have been identified.[1] They vary somewhat between the two species. *D. lanata* is the preferred species. It has primary glycosides—lanatosides A-C—that are converted within the leaf to secondary glycosides which are then converted to digoxin, digitoxin and gitoxin.[2,3] (Lanatoside C is the most important primary glycoside as it is converted to digoxin.[4])*D. purpurea* contains purpurea glycosides A and B and glucogitaloxin as primary glycosides that are transformed into digitoxin, gitoxin and gitaloxin, however glycoside content can vary greatly depending on geographical location[5–7]
2) Sterols[8]
3) Digitanol glycosides

Also triacylglycerols,[8] flavones,[9] phenylethanoid glycosides,[10] anthraquinones and organic acids.

Actions
1) Anti-arrhythmic
2) Cardiac tonic

Scientific information
Digitalis was used in the past as a medicine for external problems like old wounds and ulcers and internally as an expectorant and to treat epilepsy. It was described by *Culpeper* as "a gentle cleanser to purge the body both up and down—to open obstructions of spleen and liver".

Its main modern use in treating heart problems is attributed to William Withering who having used *D. purpurea* successfully wrote a monograph in the late 18th century describing its clinical effects. The herb subsequently became an official drug appearing in pharmacopoeias world-wide.[11]

Interestingly enough the cardiac glycosides are not easily synthesised and the manufacture of the main drug used today, digoxin, still relies on the extraction of the glycoside from *D. lanata* which is cultivated on a large scale in the Netherlands.[12] Digitoxin is the most important active constituent in *D. purpurea*, (gitoxin has low solubility)[5] but it is infrequently used today as it is less safe than digoxin.

The mode of action of the glycosides in aiding cardiovascular function is not fully elucidated but involves raising sodium and calcium levels in cardiac muscle cells with very little energy expenditure.[13] *Digitalis'* cardiac glycosides therefore:

a) increase the force of contraction of the heart, improving cardiac output, through improved heart muscle function
b) modulate the rhythm of heart both directly through the sodium pump and indirectly by reducing the sympathetic nervous system input to the heart's activity

Consequences of the improved force of heart contraction include reduced heart enlargement, reduced venous pressure and improved renal function resulting in increased diuresis.[11]

Recent research has found that cardiac glycosides very similar to those of *Digitalis* are produced endogenously by patients with heart failure.[14] Both species of *Digitalis* are also potential antitumour agents.[15,16]

Medicinal uses
Past cardiac uses of the herb include:

- heart failure
- atrial fibrillation
- arrhythmias

***Digitalis* is no longer used by medical herbalists. CONTRAINDICATIONS—Ventricular tachycardia**

Pharmacokinetics
Only about a fifth of the amount of digoxin ingested is absorbed. Digoxin has an elimination half life of 36 to 48 hours depending on renal function as this is the route of excretion.[13]

Precautions and/or safety
The cardiac glycosides have a narrow therapeutic index—they need to reach a high enough serum level to become effective but if that level rises too much higher they then become toxic. There are many reports of toxicity and fatalities have occurred.[17] Toxic effects recorded are nausea, vomiting, anorexia, diarrhoea, abdominal pain, visual disturbances, hypotension, syncope, cold sweats and arrhythmia.[13,18]

Euphrasia rostkoviana
[Formerly *E. officinalis*]

Eyebright

Description
A little, much-branched annual, variable in size and shape of leaves, and size and colour of the flowers, and semi-parasitic on the roots of grasses. It is usually from 15–25 cm high, glabrous or slightly downy. *Leaves* small, 6–10 mm, sessile, opposite, ovate and deeply toothed; teeth of lower leaves obtuse and upper ones finely pointed. *Stems* and leaves covered with downy hair. *Flowers* are in the axils of the

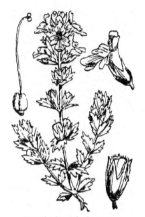

Family Scrophulariaceae

leaves in loose, terminal leafy spikes and are about 6–8 mm across. *Calyx* with 4–5 pointed teeth, with glandular hairs. *Corolla* white overall, with upper lip streaked with purple and with a yellow spot in the throat. The tube usually shorter than the spreading lobes. *Capsule* oblong. A very variable species. Flowers from mid-summer to autumn.

Habitat and cultivation
Native to pastures throughout Europe, Russia and Central Asia from the Mediterranean to the Arctic and in alpine pastures. Unable to be cultivated because of its semi-parasitic relationship with certain grasses, it is only gathered in the wild.

Parts used
The herb gathered as it comes into flower.

Active constituents
1) Tannins (0.56%)[19,20]
2) Iridoid glucosides including aucubin, catalpol, euphroside and eurostoside[21–23]
3) Flavonoids (0.38%)[24,25]
4) Phenolic acids including ferulic, vanillic and caffeic acids[25]

Also contains phenylpropanoid glycosides (eukovoside and leucosceptoside),[26] lignan glucosides,[27,28] sterols, coumarins, alkaloids, volatile oil and mucilage.[29]

Nutritional constituents
Vitamins: Rich in A and C,[30] also contains B complex, D and some E

Minerals: Iron, silicon, and a trace of iodine, copper and zinc

Actions
1) Anticatarrhal
2) Astringent
3) Anti-inflammatory
4) Antiseptic

Scientific information
The name *Euphrasia officinalis* may relate to a number of the medicinal species including *E. rostkoviana*, *E. stricta* and *E. brevipita*. The species appear to be very similar chemically and pharmacologically.[20,25] There is little current information available. In Persian medicine it is used to treat headaches (due to "warm humour"), type 2 diabetes and hayfever.

In vitro—It is a strong anti-oxidant due to the phenolic constituents possibly augmented by the iridoid fraction.[19]

Extracts are also cytotoxic.[31] For actions of aucubin see Appendix III.

No clinical trials have been conducted, however it has been valued and used by herbalists for many centuries.

Medicinal uses
Respiratory tract
The main application of the herb internally is to treat over-secretion of the mucous membranes of the upper respiratory tract. The combined actions of anti-catarrhal, anti-inflammatory and antiseptic having benefits for:

- sinusitis
- head colds
- ear congestion
- nasal catarrh especially very runny secretions

Gastro-intestinal tract
- gastritis

Externally
As the common name affirms this is the herb to treat all conditions of the eyes, being used as an eye wash or compress:

- conjunctivitis
- blepharitis
- styes
- eye strains
- eye inflammation

Pharmacy
Three times daily

Infusion of dried herb	– 2–4 g
Tincture 1:5 (45%)	– 2–6 ml
Fluid Extract (25%)	– 2–4 ml

As an external preparation for eye problems a standard infusion should be prepared and strained well before application. Discard infusion after 12 hours, and prepare fresh.

Historical uses
The herb has been known throughout history as a beneficial treatment for all eye problems including to restore lost sight in the elderly. It "strengthens a weak brain or memory".

Scrophularia nodosa

Figwort

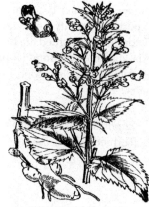

Family Scrophulariaceae

Description
A perennial, with nodules on the rhizomes, which dies back in winter. Flowering stems quadrangular, to 60 cm high. *Leaves* opposite with 4 cm petioles and the ovate to triangular, irregularly

serrate leaf blades are about 10 × 6 cm and hair-less; the base is broadly sub-cordate to cordate and the apex sharply acute. Colour, mid green, with prominent veins beneath. *Flowers* are in cymes in lax terminal and lateral panicles in the axils of mostly linear bracts and form a narrow, leafless, glandular-hairy inflorescence. Calyx 2–3 mm long, entire and with broad ovate lobes. Corolla 7–11 mm long, greenish, with a dark red-dish brown, erect upper lip with rounded lobes. Sterile stamen flap broader than long. *Capsule* about 6 mm long, broad-ovoid. Flowers from mid-summer to autumn.

Habitat and cultivation
Originally from temperate Eurasia, it can be grown elsewhere. Figwort is usually grown from seed and self-sows freely. Large clumps may also be divided. It prefers a dampish semi-shady to sunny situation. Frost resistant and drought tender.

Parts used
The flowering stems and leaves gathered when the flowers are open. *Culpeper* states the root is used in the same way as the aerial part of the herb.

Active constituents
1) Flavonoids including diosmin and hesperidin
2) Iridoid glycosides (around 5%) mostly aucu-bin, harpagide and harpagoside, also catalpol and its derivatives and scrophulosides A_{1-8}.[32-34] Highest in leaves and flowers[32]
3) Phenolic acids—vanillic, chlorogenic, caffeic and arenarioside[34,35]
4) Cardioactive glycosides
5) Saponins

A high level of ascorbic acid in the leaves.[36]

Actions
1) Depurative
2) Diuretic
3) Cardiostimulant
4) Dermatological agent

Scientific information
Iridoids generally are very active pharmacologi-cally. Both harpagide (found in *Harpagophytum*) and aucubin (found in *Plantago*) are anti-inflammatory. Arenarioside though present in low concentration also has many biological activities including anti-oxidant, antitumour and antibacterial.[37]

In vitro—The iridoids isolated from the seed pods stimulate fibroblast growth, this may explain the herb's historical use as a vulnerary.[38] Other spe-cies of *Scrophularia* with similar phenolic acids are antibacterial.[39]

Medicinal uses
Skin
Scrophularia is exclusively used in modern phyto-therapy for skin problems. While little is known about the pharmacological actions of the herb's particular constituents, it has all the actions neces-sary to resolve skin conditions:

- eczema
- psoriasis
- pruritus
- chronic skin conditions
- skin conditions with poor circulation

Externally
May be used as a poultice in the treatment of the above skin conditions.

Pharmacy
Three times daily

Infusion of dried herb	– 2–8 g
Tincture 1:10 (45%)	– 2–4 ml
Fluid Extract (25%)	– 2–8 ml

Precautions and/or safety
Should not be used by patients who have tachycardia.

Historical uses
Leprosy; internally and externally to dissolve blood clots derived from injury; hip pain; goi-tre; cancer and fistulae. Bruised leaves for burns, piles and swellings; as a fomentation for sprains;

inflammations; scrofulous sores and gangrene. Also used for removing redness, spots and freckles.

Verbascum thapsus

Mullein

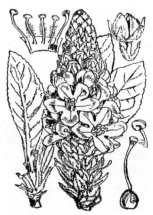

Family Scrophulariaceae

Description
A biennial with hairy stems growing to about 1 m tall in flower. *Basal leaves* 7–20 × 3.5–10 cm, short stemmed in a rosette; elliptic or obovate, white hairy, sometimes crenate or crenulate. Stem leaves sessile, narrower and longer. *Inflorescence* to 80 cm high, dense and woolly, usually single but some-times with 1–2 branches near the base. Bracts lanceolate, flowers with tiny stalks, 1 to several in each axil. Calyx 8–12 mm long, deeply lobed with triangular-acuminate lobes. Corolla 1.5–3 cm in diameter, yellow and hairy with rounded lobes. Stamens 5; 3 upper stamens with white-villous filaments, 2 lower stamens glabrous or nearly so. *Capsule* 8–10 mm long, broad ovoid and exserted from the calyx. Flowers from mid-summer to autumn.

Habitat and cultivation
Native to Europe and Western Asia and natura-lised elsewhere in open, dry, stony areas from sea level to about 1000 m. Grown only from seed and needs full sun. Drought and frost resistant.

Parts used
The flowers, leaves and stems are used. The herb is gathered just prior to, or at the start of, flowering.

Active constituents
1) Mucilage (3%) and gum[40]
2) Iridoid glycosides including aucubin and catalpol[23,40–43]
3) Flavonoids including hesperidin, verbascoside (a derivative of luteolin) and rutin[40,41,44]
4) Saponins including oleanane-type saikosa-ponins called mulleinsaponins[40–42,45]
5) Phenylethanoid glycosides including deriva-tives of ferulic and caffeic acids, leucoscepto-side and arenarioside[41,46]
6) Lignans[46]

Also contains resin, volatile oil,[42] sterones,[42] lipids and sterols including sitosterol[42] and α-spinasterol.[47] The iridoid glycosides harpagide and harpagoside have been identified in the roots of *V. thapsus*.[48]

Official preparations can be derived from *V. thapsiforme* and *V. phlomoides* too.[11]

Nutritional constituents
Vitamins: A, B complex and D
Minerals: High in iron, magnesium, potassium and sulphur

Actions
Internally
1) Expectorant
2) Demulcent
3) Diuretic (mild)

Externally
4) Emollient
5) Vulnerary

Scientific information
Both flowers and leaves have been official medi-cines in a number of European countries,[11] the herb including the root, having been used from ancient times particularly for respiratory tract ailments. *German Commission E* has approved the use of flowers in treating respiratory catarrh.

In vitro—Aqueous and alcohol extracts have antimicrobial activity inhibiting:-

- bacteria—*Klebsiella pneumoniae*,[49] *Staphylococcus aureus*,[49,50] *Escherichia coli*[50] and *Mycobacterium phlei*[50]
- viruses—HSV-1 and a variety of influenza viruses—(flower extracts)[40,51]
- fungi—*Microsporum cookerii* and *M. gypsum.*[52]

The herb also has some limited cytotoxicity to liver cancer cell lines[53] and a saponin from *V. thapsiforme* inhibits protein biosynthesis, possibly giving it use as an antitumour agent.[54]

In vivo—Clinical trials on a combination of *Allium sativa*, *Verbascum thapsus*, *Calendula officinalis*, *Hypericum perforatum*, lavender and vitamin E oil was as effective for the relief of otalgia associated with acute otitis media as a pharmaceutical anaesthetic preparation.[55,56]

Medicinal uses
Respiratory tract
The herb internally is considered to act as a mucous membrane tonic:

- bronchitis
- respiratory catarrh
- whooping cough
- haemoptysis
- coughs†
- tracheitis
- common colds
- tuberculosis
- pleurisy

BHP specific for bronchitis with hard cough and soreness. *Weiss* recommends *Verbascum flos.* for sub-acute and chronic respiratory problems rather than for acute use.

Externally
- earache
- wounds

---

†Especially hard, persistent ones.

Pharmacy
Three times daily
Infusion of dried herb   – 4–8 g
Fluid Extract (25%)   – 4–8 ml
    Preparations for eardrops can be made by steeping the flowers in good quality vegetable oil in a covered glass jar and leaving it on a window ledge for 6 weeks before straining.

Precautions and/or safety
There is one reported case of contact dermatitis and respiratory allergy to mullein from occupational handling of the herb.[57]

Historical uses
Roots—for lasks and fluxes of the belly; ruptures; cramps and convulsions; as gargle for toothache; as a diuretic. *Flowers* (oil)—for piles; frost bite; for gout; warts (externally); belly-ache and colic; tumours; swellings; inflammation of throat; externally—warts; eczema of outer ear; ear discharges; to draw thorns/splinters. *Leaves* (warmed)—applied to "blotch or boil" in the groin; ringworm; burns. *Leaves* (sun-dried)—for irritation of respiratory tract. *Seeds* as vermifuge.

Veronicastrum virginicum
[Formerly *Leptandra virginica*]

Culver's-root, black root

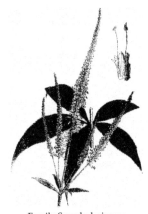

Family Scrophulariaceae

Description

A perennial plant with a single stem growing to 1.5 m from a horizontal, woody rootstock. *Stems* simple, erect and smooth. *Leaves* lanceolate, acuminate, and serrate in whorls of 3–7 around the stems. *Flowers* tiny in showy, terminal spikes up to 20 cm long. Calyx 4 or 5-parted. Corolla tube-shaped, white or purple with 2 projecting stamens. *Fruit* an oblong-ovate, flattened, many-seeded capsule.

Odour—when fresh is almond-like, taste—nauseous and bitter—this diminishes with drying.

Habitat and cultivation

Native to North America from New England to Minnesota and Kansas, growing in rich moist soils and sunny, sheltered situations. It is cultivated elsewhere and may be grown from seed or cuttings. It is frost resistant but drought tender.

Parts used

The dried root and rhizome harvested in autumn from second year plants.[58] The root may be kept indefinitely.

Active constituents

1) Volatile oil based on cinnamic acid
2) Bitter glycoside—leptandrin
3) Saponins
4) Tannins

Also includes a glycoside similar to senegin, sterols (verosterol) and resin. There are almost no available studies into the constituents of this herb and although the species has been found to contain iridoids[59] (aucubin), the level reported by one source was very low.[60]

Actions

1) Cholagogue
2) Mild cathartic
3) Diaphoretic
4) Spasmolytic

Scientific information

Although the root had been an official medicine in the USA (until 1955) and Britain little detail is known about its chemical and pharmacological characteristics. It was used by indigenous Americans and entered official medicine around 1852.

The fresh root is certainly more potent being cathartic and emetic, these properties diminish as it dries.

Medicinal uses

Gastro-intestinal tract

Mainly used for treating liver dysfunction:

* chronic constipation with hepatic disorders
* cholecystitis
* jaundice

BHP specific for constipation with symptoms of hepatic congestion.

Pharmacy

Three times daily

Decoction of dried herb	– 0.5–4 g
Tincture 1:5 (70%)	– 2.5–10 ml
Fluid Extract (70%)	– 0.5–4 ml

Precautions and/or safety

The fresh root, according to *Grieve*, may cause "bloody stools and possibly abortion".

Historical uses

Diarrhoea (stomachic); cholera infantum; chronic dysentery. As a diaphoretic it was used in intermittent fever; for leprosy; cachectic diseases and with cream of tartar for dropsy. Also used for tenderness or heavy pain around liver, intestinal atony and mental depression (Eclectics). *Grieve* states that mixed reports of the action of *Veronicastrum* may arise depending on whether the herb was used in the fresh or dried state.

SOLANACEAE

The Solanaceae is a worldwide family but with many members in the Southern Hemisphere and its greatest diversity in tropical Central and South America. Although it contains many useful food plants such as the potato, tomato, tamarillo, pepino, aubergine and all the capsicums, the Solanaceae often also contain powerful alkaloids some of which may be used in small quantities in drugs but many of which can be deadly poisons.

The family consists of herbaceous plants, shrubs, climbers and small trees. Some have prickles or produce unpleasant scents when bruised.

- The flowers are regular with usually 5 sepals and 5 joined petals
- There are usually 5 stamens the anthers of which often touch one another and form a cone around the pistil. They release pollen either through holes at the top or slits down the sides
- Many produce fleshy fruits containing numerous flat seeds, but some, such as tobacco, have capsules full of tiny seeds

There are native and naturalised species in other parts of the world. Medicinal plants of the Solanaceae include *Capsicum* and the poisonous:

Atropa belladonna	deadly nightshade
Datura stramonium	thorn apple
Hyoscyamus niger	henbane
Solanum dulcamara	bittersweet

Atropa belladonna [Restricted Herb]

Deadly nightshade

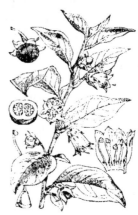

Family Solanaceae

Description

A stout, shrubby perennial, growing from whitish roots to 1–1.5 m tall. Lower leaves petioles over

411

7 cm, in upper leaves they are shorter. Lamina large, elliptic-ovate, with short, glandular hairs, mainly on veins and a pointed tip. *Flowers* solitary, pendulous, on recurved pedicels growing from the leaf axils. Calyx lobed to halfway up the corolla which is campanulate, brownish purple-mauve and tinged with green. *Fruit* a broad-ovoid, slightly flattened berry, glossy black with purple juice. Seeds numerous. Flowers late summer to autumn. N.B. All parts are poisonous but especially the fruit, which is juicy and sweet so tempting to children.

Habitat and cultivation

Native to Southern Europe and Western Asia, growing in woods, thickets and waste places. Naturalized in other countries and also cultivated for medicine since the 19th century.

Parts used

Dried aerial parts collected when the plant is in flower. The dried root is also used but it is higher in alkaloids and is used in much lower doses.

Active constituents

1) Alkaloids of tropane-type[1-3]—*herba* (min. 0.3%), *radix* (min. 0.4%), however the levels fluctuate with maturation of the plant as well as plant part.[4] Includes mainly hyoscyamine and its racemate, atropine, scopolamine (hyoscine), smaller amounts of atropamine and belladonnine and also calystegines (*herba*)[5]
2) Flavonoids mostly derived from kaempferol and quercetin
3) Volatile bases including nicotine
4) Coumarins including scopoletin

There are steroidal glycosides in the seeds.[6]

Actions

1) Spasmolytic
2) Anticholinergic
3) Anhidrotic
4) Anti-asthmatic

Scientific information

From ancient times *Atropa* was known to be potentially toxic and the name is supposedly derived from "Atropos" one of the three Fates who "cut the thread of life". In the 1830s its importance to the pharmaceutical world was established when atropine was isolated. Both root and leaf extracts were official medicines until relatively recent times.[7]

Atropine was shown over a century ago to inhibit vagal stimulation of the heart and it became a drug for use in bradycardia and to treat heart block after myocardial infarction. The mode of action of the alkaloids is through their competing with acetylcholine for muscarinic receptor sites in the central and autonomic nervous systems, the parasympathetic system is the one that uses mainly acetylcholine as a neurotransmitter.

Atropine, scopolamine and *Atropa* tincture at low dose reduce heart rate and increase respiratory sinus arrhythmia (vagotonic) but at higher doses they have the opposite effect and are described as vagolytic.[8] The anticholinergic activity of the herbal extract is greater than that of the alkaloids alone.[9]

Medicinal uses

Atropa is a restricted herb but where it is legal for herbalists to use it, it is used to treat:-

- colic/spasms within bowel, gall-bladder, urinary bladder and kidney
- prophylactically to prevent griping due to laxatives
- asthma and whooping cough
- enuresis
- parkinsonism—by reducing rigidity and tremor

Its action also reduces glandular secretions including saliva, hydrochloric acid, sweat and mucus. The root is used for external applications too as a counter-irritant and analgesic to treat:-

- lumbago
- rheumatism
- neuralgia
- painful haemorrhoids/colic (as suppositories)

Pharmacokinetics

Studies show that atropine has a short half-life and total plasma clearance of it occurs within 4 hours, excretion occurring in urine, either in its original form, or as a metabolite.[10]

Precautions and/or safety

There are many reports of intoxication by *Atropa* occurring mostly through accidental ingestion by children or from the incorrect identification of them as other species of edible berries.[11] The most common symptoms are difficulty speaking or dysarthria, tachycardia, mydriasis (excessive dilation of pupils), hallucinations, urinary retention, pyrexia and flushing and in more severe cases lethargy and coma, permanent consequences or fatalities are however uncommon.[12–15] Consumption of the berries, which are a rich source of alkaloids, can manifest as psychosis.[16] Side-effects may also be caused just by contact with the plant.[17]

Capsicum annuum

Cayenne pepper, chilli pepper

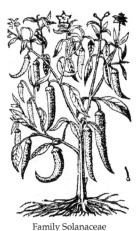

Family Solanaceae

Description

Shrubs of varying height, grown as annuals in cold climates and perennials in hot climates. Whole plant tender when young but perennials develop a woody trunk and are evergreen all year in hot areas. *Stem* erect, angular. Branches are brittle and split or break easily. *Leaves* stalked, entire, oval or elliptic, bright dark green. *Flowers* shortly stalked, and pendant, erect with a whitish corolla with 5 wide-spreading lobes. *Fruit* a very variable berry with thick rind and dry walls, usually oblong, conical and bright red. It contains small flat, white seeds.

Habitat and cultivation

Native of Central and tropical South America, *Capsicum annuum* is cultivated in hot climates worldwide. Cayenne peppers are grown from seed which may take about 3 weeks to germinate. They will grow where tomatoes grow but need a longer season, warmer conditions and high light intensity to fruit well. They need fertile but not over rich soil and should never be allowed to dry out. They may be grown in pots, inside or outside, but are susceptible to mites indoors. Drought and frost tender.

N.B. Some people may be "burned" just by handling peppers and contact with the inner walls and seeds of fresh hot peppers should be avoided. The burning is made worse by water and may be relieved by putting the hands in milk.

Parts used

The ripe fruits of a number of species have been used, the main ones are *C. annuum*, *C. frutescens*, *C. chinense*, *C. pendulum*, *C. pubescens* and *C. baccata*.[18] Within *C. annuum* there are a large number of sub-species and natural populations are heterogeneous.[24] The medicinal value of the herb is directly related to its pungency.[19]

Active constituents

1) Alkaloids called capsaicinoids (0.1–1.0%[20,21]) including capsaicin and dihydrocapsaicin (both can account for up to 90% of the herb's pungency), their glucosides[22] and up to 16 minor capsaicinoids.[23–29] The capasaicinoids are based on vanillylamine[20,25] and vary in type and content depending on species, state of maturity, nutritional and environmental conditions,[23] processing and storage.[24,30]

2) Flavonoids including derivatives of quercetin, luteolin and apigenin[31,32]

3) Carotenoid pigments including carotenes and xanthophylls predominantly capsanthin[24,33]

4) Diterpene glycosides called capsianosides[34-36]
5) Phenolics either as free acids or derivatives of sinapic, p-coumaric, ferulic and caffeic acids[31,32,36]

Also volatile oil, fatty acids[37] and steroidal saponins.[38]

In the seeds

6) Steroidal saponins—capsiciosides A-D[39]

Nutritional constituents
Vitamins: High in A, C and E,[40] also contains B complex
Minerals: Iron, calcium, potassium, magnesium, phosphorus and sulphur

Actions
Internally
1) Stimulant
2) Spasmolytic
3) Diaphoretic
4) Carminative

Externally
5) Rubefacient
6) Antiseptic
7) Counter-irritant

Scientific information
Records of *Capsicum's* use date back as far as 7000 BC. The pungent type of chilli pepper originated in Mexico and reached Europe first, in the 15th Century, before becoming established in Asia.[41]

The main active constituent, capsaicin, was identified in the mid 19th Century although its therapeutic potential was only fully recognised a century later.[18] The capsacinoid glucosides are much less pungent but still retain some of the beneficial biological activities of the alkaloids themselves.[22]

Capsicum has been an official medicine for both internal and external use in pharmacopoeias throughout Europe[7] and it is still employed as a food-flavouring, medicine and ingredient in the cosmetic industry worldwide.[42] Much of the scientifically identified action of the herb is due to pharmacological effects of capsaicin, mediated through the nervous system, however *Capsicum* does contain other significant constituents. It is approved by *German Commission E* for external use to treat painful muscle spasms.

Anti-oxidant
In vitro—Constituents with anti-oxidant activity include phenolics, vitamins, saponins and capsaicin.[29,32,43-46]

Nervous system
When capsaicin is applied to the skin it causes a triple response of itch and/or pain, flare and wheal. If contact is prolonged it produces a refractory period where nerves become desensitised not only to further exposure to capsaicin but also to other noxious stimuli.[18] This effect occurs through stimulation of vanilloid-1 receptors (now called transient receptor potential channels of the vanilloid 1 receptor class or TPRV1s) which are present in specific sensory neurons of the skin, called nociceptors. These receptors integrate pain stimuli, especially those associated with inflammation, as well as stimuli from noxious chemicals and heat.[18] They are not only found as sensors in skin (peripheral nerves) but also occur in the spinal cord and central nervous system where they perceive pain associated with internal tissues.

The neurological mechanism of action of capsaicin involves an increased influx of sodium and, most especially, calcium ions through non-selective ion channels. Depolarisation of nerve fibres follows this influx, with release and subsequent depletion of neurotransmitter peptides, including substance P and calcitonin-gene related peptide.[47] It can take several hours to build up neurotransmitter levels again and during this time nerve fibres are effectively anaesthetised.[48] The neurotransmitters are believed to be responsible for the signs of neurogenic inflammation namely plasma extravasation, vasodilation and leukocyte recruitment.[18] They may also cause degranulation of mast cells[49] and their action has been shown to involve increased levels of inflammatory mediators[50] but this does not include histamine release.[49] Capsaicin can also cause sensory loss by denervation of nerve fibres. This loss may be short-term as seen in epidermal and sub-epidermal layers of skin when it is applied under occlusive dressings[51] or more long term and possibly permanent when capsaicin is used at very high doses. TPRV1s are ubiquitous in the body being found in nerves innervating many other tissues as well as in non-neuronal tissues[47] and capsaicin can influence activity in a range of cells, at least in part, through altered levels of sodium and calcium ions.[52,53] The study of vanilloid receptors is relatively new and their biochemical complexity and significance is yet to be fully elucidated.

Apart from their role in the analgesia of painful conditions, the level of TPRV1s is increased in tissues associated with a number of pathological conditions like inflammatory bowel disease, vulvodynia and rectal hypersensitivity and this may give capsaicin a potential role in their treatment.[18,54] Its pungency is however a limiting factor to its usefulness as a systemic therapeutic agent.

In vivo—There are a number of clinical trials of *Capiscum* in topical preparations. It has been beneficial for:-

- chronic and acute low back pain[55,56] (quality of these trials has been questioned)[57,58]
- surgical pain—plasters applied at acupressure points[59,60]
- diabetic neuropathy[61]
- post-mastectomy pain syndrome[62]
- cluster headaches[63]
- post-herpetic neuralgia[64]
- pain due to osteoarthritis[65] and rheumatoid arthritis[66]
- reflex sympathetic dystrophy[67]

Gastro-intestinal system
In vitro—Permeability of gastro-intestinal epithelial cells to macromolecules is increased by contact with *Capsicum* an effect that may increase absorption of both nutrients and allergens *in vivo*.[68]

In vivo—Studies of *Capsicum's* effects on the gastro-intestinal tract found that it:-

- protects gastric mucosa (including from aspirin-induced ulceration)[69] and oesophageal mucosa—possibly by improving regional blood flow[70]

- improves oesophageal clearance without changing its motility[71]
- delays gastric emptying[72,73]
- speeds food transit through the small intestine[72,73]
- reduces the volume of food required to perceive distension and a sense of discomfort[74]
- reduces symptoms of functional dyspepsia including a sense of fullness, epigastric pain and nausea[48]
- raises threshold for rectal pain in men with irritable bowel syndrome[74]

Capsicum does not appear to increase oro-caecal transit time[72,74] or alter faecal output volume[71] but may increase bowel motion frequency slightly.[74]

Ingestion of large amounts of strong chilli can cause reflux,[75] however moderate dietary amounts do not worsen heartburn in sufferers of the condition (though it may hasten its onset)[70] nor do they increase reflux induced by a fatty meal.[76] Prolonged exposure to capsaicin may actually reduce the perceived discomfort associated with reflux due to nerve analgesia.[70]

Capsicum has been commonly contra-indicated in peptic ulceration, as it was believed to damage the gastric mucosa and increase acid production. However chilli consumption in normal Indian diets did not delay healing, or cause visible damage, to the gastric mucosa during standard treatment of duodenal ulcers[77] and may even have protected against ulcer development.[78]

Cancer
Studies relate predominantly to capsaicin. Those conducted using non-human models have shown capsaicin's potential as an antitumour and cancer-preventative agent is contradictory and that it can both protect against and promote cancer cell growth, a phenomenon that has yet to be explained.[79]

In vitro—*Capsicum* itself is cytotoxic to buccal mucosa fibroblasts in a dose-dependent manner[80] and greatly potentiates the anti-cancer activity of green tea.[81]

Capsaicin does not appear to have tumour promotion activity in human models.[82] On the contrary it has been shown to prevent promotion by known chemical carcinogens[83,84] (probably due in part to anti-oxidant and anti-inflammatory actions[82]) and also to biochemical changes which occur through increased levels of intracellular calcium.[85] Capsaicin does not appear to induce apopotosis in normal cells[86] but does so in cancer cells including neuroblastoma, leukaemia, prostate, melanoma, gastric, liver and breast cancer cells.[24,85-90] The cells vary in their sensitivity to capsaicin's cytotoxicity.[90] It also has anti-angiogenic activity and inhibits chemotactic motility, DNA and protein synthesis.[90,91]

Capsanthin too may have potential as an aid to cancer treatment as it enhances the effect of chemotherapeutic agents in cell lines that have become multi-drug resistant.[92]

In vivo—There are large numbers of people who consume chillies as part of their daily diet and have done so for generations. Epidemiological studies have produced contradictory data of the link between dietary chilli and the risk of developing cancers with some showing a positive risk[42] (stomach,[93] gall-bladder[94]) and others showing no correlation.[95]

Capsicum has been used to treat oral mucositis, a side-effect of cancer chemo- and radio-therapy, because capsaicin is readily "perceived" by superficial nerve sensors in mucous membranes producing a reduction in pain perception that allows patients to continue their treatment.[96] This analgesia is however of short duration.[97]

Circulatory system
In vitro—*Capsicum* inhibits platelet aggregation possibly through inhibition of phospholipase A_2[82] whilst capsaicin can dilate coronary arterial vessels.[98]

In vivo—*Capsicum* consumption transiently increased heart rate and blood pressure partly due to its pungency but also through some as yet undetermined mechanism.[108] A clinical trial found a chilli supplement was of some benefit to healthy men, increasing myocardial perfusion and reducing resting heart rate, but of no apparent benefit to women.[99] There were no significant changes in blood pressure or lipid profiles for either gender with its short-term use[99] but regular consumption

of chilli-containing food was protective against lipoprotein oxidation,[100] increased fat metabolism (oxidation) in women[101] and carbohydrate metabolism (oxidation) in men.[102]

Eating hot chillies does not worsen the symptoms associated with existing haemorrhoids.[103]

Endocrine system
In vitro—There is evidence that *Capsicum* could benefit diabetes treatment through activation of a control mechanism for lipid and glucose metabolism via peroxisome proliferator-activated receptors.[104]

In vivo—*Capsicum* and capsaicin stimulate the sympathetic nervous system which in turn may be responsible for its noted increase on metabolic energy expenditure or thermogenesis.[105,108] Increased thermogenesis has been demonstrated in non-obese people, although at very high levels the effect is blunted in this group (due to desensitization).[105] A blunted response to capsaicin-stimulated thermogenesis also occurs in obese people given doses that were effective for the non-obese.[106] Dietary use of *Capsicum* can increase resting metabolic rate,[107] raise body temperature,[108] increase heat loss,[108] increase carbohydrate metabolism[109] and at high enough doses can reduce dietary fat and protein intake as well as decreasing appetite.[105,110,111] Some of these effects have been achieved using the herb in an encapsulated form, so that the action does not seem to be mediated by oral sensation.[105] Both hypothalamus and brain stem appear to be involved in these processes being stimulated indirectly through nerve signals, by direct contact with circulating capsaicin[108] and by increased serum adrenalin and nor-adrenalin levels.[109]

Capsicum is used in Jamaica to treat diabetes with capsaicin identified as responsible for decreasing blood glucose levels. Postprandial insulin levels[112] and blood glucose[113] have been reported to be reduced by the herb although another study failed to find it altered basal metabolic rate, insulin or blood glucose levels.[99]

Administered with a glucose-load low dose capsaicin increased both the level of glucose absorbed and mobilisation of glycogen by glucagon, in healthy people, mediated through stimulation of capsaicin-sensitive afferent nerves.[114] It may increase glucose absorption through increased blood flow in the gastro-intestinal tract, it also increases subsequent glucose utilisation i.e. carbohydrate metabolism. *Capsicum* has been used in a number of weight loss supplements but its efficacy has not been tested in any clinical trials to-date.[115]

Antimicrobial

In vitro—Ground chilli was inactive in inhibiting the growth of *Candida* species[116] but one of its saponins has good activity against a number of fungi including *Candida albicans, Aspergillus fumigatus* and *Pneumocystis carinii*.[117,118]

The herb is active against cercaria (larvae) of the parasitic *Schistosoma mansoni*,[119] *Helicobacter pylori*,[120] *Streptococcus pyogenes* and some *Bacillus* and *Clostridium* species.[121] Capsaicin does not appear to have a role in the antimicrobial activity, having shown little antibacterial activity to a number of common pathogens.[121,122]

In vivo—*Capsicum, Phytolacca* and *Guaiacum* used together in the treatment of tonsillitis improved patients' ability to swallow and reduced earache, headache and fatigue.[123]

At high doses *Capsicum* does not appear to have any activity against *H. pylori*[124] (this lack of effect may be due to inappropriate research methodology).[125]

Other

In vitro—Capsaicin promotes a two-fold increase in the absorption of NSAIDs through skin tissue,[126] inhibits 5-LOX activity[127] and causes contraction of bronchial smooth muscle.[128]

In vivo—Due to its ability to desensitize nerves capsaicin preparations have been successfully and safely used intravesically in the treatment of overactive bladders.[41,129] Unfortunately its irritant nature makes its oral use difficult to tolerate.

Capsaicin is effective as a cream in the treatment of pruritus[50,130] and as a nasal spray for vasomotor rhinitis.[131]

Carotenoids are anti-oxidant and epidemiologically associated with a lowered risk for cardiovascular disease, cancer and macular degeneration.[132]

Medicinal uses
Cardiovascular system
* poor peripheral circulation

Gastro-intestinal tract
* flatulence
* colic
* dyspepsia
* ationic digestion especially in elderly (*BHP* specific)

Externally
* neuralgia
* rheumatic pain
* chilblains (*BHP* specific)
* lumbago (*BHP* specific)
* chronic laryngitis (gargle)

Pharmacy
Three times daily
Infusion of dried herb – 30–120 mg[†] (powdered)
Tincture 1:20 (60%)   – 30–1 ml
Tincture 1:3 (60%)   – 0.06–0.2 ml

Topical use of *Capsicum* can cause irritation of skin at concentrations above 1%. As a gargle 1.25–2.5 ml of 1:3 tincture or 0.5–1 g of powder to 500 ml of boiling water.

Chillies retain two thirds of their vitamin A and C content even after cooking.[41]

Precautions and/or safety
Chilli as a regular part of the diet may reduce iron absorption by up to 38%.[133]

There are a few reports of contact dermatitis from handling the herb including contact eczema,[134] urticaria[135] and Sweet's syndrome (characterised by erythema, papules, pustules and haemorrhagic bullae)[136] but this appears to be quite rare. Occupational exposure to inhaled chilli dust was not found to be associated with any pathology.[137]

Although considered safe at recommended doses,[42] *in vitro* and animal studies have produced

---

[†]2.5 ml ($^1/_2$ teaspoon) dried powder in a cup (250 ml) of boiling water. Use 15 ml diluted per dose.

contradictory results regarding *Capsicum* and capsaicin's potential for genotoxicity, mutagenicity and carcinogenicity—both toxic and protective effects have been demonstrated and the exact effect may be concentration dependent.[42] Capsaicin is mutagenic[21] (this effect was however moderated when whole *Capsicum* extract was used[138]), induces single strand breaks, albeit without damage, in DNA[90,139] and causes oxidative damage to DNA.[140] On the other hand it is also antigenotoxic,[141] did not act as a co-mutagen and was protective against damage by aflatoxin and tobacco mutagens.[21]

DNA single strand breaks are not significantly produced by normal levels of *Capsicum*[139] but there is concern that if capsaicin-containing preparations are over-used or applied over large areas the constituent's ability to pass through skin may cause its cellular levels to rise to concentrations near those capable of causing such breaks.[90] There may then be a potential for genotoxicity through imperfect strand repair,[90] inflammatory alterations in cell function and/or free radical release.[139] Although *in vivo* studies have not to-date indicated an increased cancer risk from using capsaicin topically it has been suggested that as skin irritation is associated with increased tumour incidence and capsaicin causes irritation it may become a risk factor.[42]

Pepper spray prepared from *Capsicum* relies on the irritant nature of capsaicin which when sprayed into eyes causes increased tear production, inflammation, burning pain, blepharospasm and swelling.[142] Although the eyes do not appear to sustain permanent damage this spray can stop the blink reflex for up to 5 days.[143,144] It can also cause nasal irritation, broncho-constriction, shortness of breath, severe coughing and sneezing. In excessive amounts capsaicin can be a strong irritant to receptors involved in circulatory and respiratory reflexes,[145] it may permanently damage sensory nerves and could possibly cause death.

Historical uses

To drive cold from the body; ward off disease, coughs, gastric ulcers, appetite stimulation, hair growth, rheumatism, gout, bronchitis, bronchial catarrh, toothache; to help with delirium tremens. Externally as a cataplasm; for relaxed uvula,

cutaneous allergies, rhinitis, post-herpetic neuralgia, cluster headache.

Datura stramonium [Restricted Herb]

Thorn apple, Jimson weed

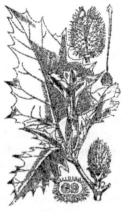

Family Solanaceae

Description

A foetid annual growing over 1 m. *Stems* light green, glabrous, and larger branches are U-shaped with 2 equal rounded forks. Petiole over 8 cm; lamina large, over 20 cm. *Leaves* pointed, coarsely lobed or sharp toothed. *Flowers* solitary, axillary and short stalked. Calyx 4–5 cm long, ribbed and reflexing at fruiting. Corolla greenish white, funnelform 6–8 cm long, lobes pointed and twisted in the bud. *Fruit* erect, ovoid, 4–5 cm with numerous slender spines over 1 cm long, splitting into 4 when seeds ripen. *Seeds* reniform and black when ripe. Flowers from late spring to late summer.

There are four varieties of *D. stramonium* identified according to geographical location and varying in colour and smoothness of the capsule. Genetically purple flowers are dominant to white flowers and spines are dominant to smooth capsules.[146]

Habitat and cultivation

Native to tropical and subtropical America, naturalized in similar climates world-wide, growing along roadsides, in waste places and cultivated ground.

Parts used
Dried leaves and flowering tops.

Active constituents
1) Alkaloids at least 25 have been identified[146,147] (comprising 0.2–0.45%).[148] Active alkaloids are of the tropane-type[2,149] including mainly L-hyoscyamine and scopolamine (hyoscine) in ratio 2:1,[148] also atropine. Content varies with geographical location,[146] plant part (highest in tender stems) and state of maturation (higher in younger plants).[148]
2) Flavonoids including derivatives of quercetin and kaempferol

Also contains withanolides, coumarins, tannins and glycoprotein (lectin).[150]

Actions
1) Spasmolytic
2) Anti-asthmatic
3) Mucolytic

Scientific information
Datura was introduced to Europe by the Romany gypsies around the 16th Century, the name, *Datura*, being derived from the Indian word "dhat" meaning a poison. The herb has been an official medicine in India and Britain, used in the treatment of parkinsonism.[7] Its alkaloids and actions are like those of *Atropa*.

Datura has recently been shown to be anti-mutagenic in standard tests[151] and to have anti-bacterial activity against some gram-positive bacteria.[152] The lectin can bind to brain cancer cells, *in vitro*, inducing them to differentiate.[153]

Medicinal uses
Datura is a restricted herb and due to its high alkaloid level is used infrequently and in very small doses to treat:-

* parkinsonism, specifically muscular spasm and excessive salivation
* asthma
* pertussis

The medicinal effects of *Datura* can be achieved through its ingestion as well as by using it as a smoke inhalation. In this latter form it reduces airway resistance in asthmatics[154] and at one time was available in a proprietary preparation to aid asthma treatment.[155]

Hyoscyamine is identifiable in the urine of people intoxicated by *Datura*.[156,168]

Precautions and/or safety
There are many reports in the literature of intoxication from this herb.[157–163] Symptoms of toxicity are similar to those for *Atropa* and due to the anticholinergic activity of the alkaloids. They include hallucination, tachycardia, agitation, mydriasis and confusion. Toxicity can occur as early as 5–15 minutes after consumption of the herb, persist for 24–48 hours and the resultant depression and short-term memory loss can last for several weeks.[159] Eye contact with the herb may be sufficient to cause mydriasis.[164]

The annual incidence of poisoning by *Datura* does not appear to be high[165,166] although numbers may be increasing due to its free and easy availability. *Datura*, seeds especially, can occur as a food contaminant causing accidental poisoning[167] but many cases of intoxication are intentional being induced by young people using it for its hallucinogenic action.[157] Toxicity from *Datura* occurs at lower levels than other members of this family.[159] As the lethal dose is close to that required to produce hallucinations severe cases of toxicity are not uncommon.[160] Its use can lead to coma and around 5% of reported poisonings are fatal.[160] Deaths have been recorded both in animals and humans.[159,168] Injestion of just 10 flowers can be fatal to humans.

Hyoscyamus niger [Restricted Herb]

Henbane

Description
A densely hairy, viscid annual or biennial with 30–60 cm tall flower-stems. Basal stemmed leaves in a rosette, stem leaves clasping, sessile. Lamina 15–20 cm oblong coarsely dentate or with lobes. *Flowers*, subsessile, dull yellow strongly netted with

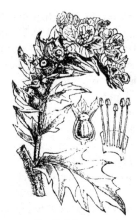

Family Solanaceae

purple veins, clustered at the top of the stem, in 2 rows in the axils of the leaf-like bracts. Filaments white, anthers and style purple. *Fruit* a more or less globose capsule containing many seeds. Flowers from spring to winter. Whole plant smells nauseating.

Habitat and cultivation
Native to Europe, West Asia and North Africa henbane is naturalized in many countries, growing in waste places along roadsides and in sandy areas by the sea. It is always grown from seed.

Parts used
Dried leaves with or without flower heads.

Active constituents
1) Alkaloids of tropane-type (0.05–0.15%) predominantly L-hyoscyamine[169] and scopolamine (hyoscine) in ratio 1.2:1, also atropine and other alkaloids including calystegines.[170] Levels of alkaloids vary with geographical location.
2) Flavonoids including derivatives of quercetin and kaempferol[171]

Also contains volatile amines. The seeds of the herb are used in Chinese traditional medicine and their constituents include lignanamides, withanolides, phenolic acids and sterols.[172,173]

Actions
1) Antispasmodic
2) Sedative

Scientific information
The medicinal value of henbane has been known for thousands of years. It was used as an analgesic (both internally and topically), as a smoke inhalation[174,176] and as eye drops.[175] Apart from its therapeutic value, it was also used in "witchcraft" because of its hallucinatory properties and as a poison, featuring in some notorious crimes like that of Dr. Crippen who used it to murder his wife.[176]

Although not much used now *Hyoscyamus* featured in many pharmacopoeias until the latter part of last century.[7] In modern medicine the isolated alkaloids have been used, the demand for scopolamine having been higher than for hyoscyamine and atropine[177] as its effect is one of sedation whereas the latter alkaloids are cerebral stimulants/hallucinogens.[7] The alkaloids decrease secretions including those of mucous membranes, stomach, salivary and sweat glands. *Hyoscyamus* is considered a milder herb than the related *Atropa belladonna*.

Recent research has found that the seeds have a range of antimicrobial activity.[178]

Medicinal uses
Hyoscyamus is a restricted herb that is used to treat:-

- urinary tract spasms/colic
- griping due to laxatives
- asthma
- pertussis
- travel sickness
- tremors

Precautions and/or safety
As for the other tropane alkaloid-containing herbs in the Solanaceae, there are a number of reports of henbane intoxication, either accidental or through people seeking "highs", although it use does not appear to result in many fatalities.[179–184] Symptoms of poisoning are as for other anticholinergic agents—mydriasis, tachycardia, arrhythmia, agitation, convulsion and possibly coma.[185] Eye contact with the herb may be sufficient to cause mydriasis.[186]

TILIACEAE

The Tiliaceae or Linden family consists of about 50 genera of trees, shrubs or rarely herbs distributed widely throughout the world. The leaves are usually alternate and simple. Flowers are regular and usually bisexual and mostly in cymes in leaf axils or in cymose panicles. Peduncle united for about half its length to a large ligulate bract. Sepals and petals usually 5 but sometimes fewer, or flowers may be without petals altogether. Stamens are many and fruit a capsule or drupe. *Tilia* is the main medicinal genus.

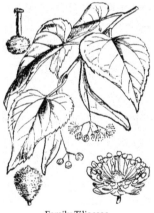

Family Tiliaceae

Tilia spp. [Tilia x europaea, T. platyphyllos and T. cordata]

Lime, linden

Description
Tilia x *europaea*, the common or European lime, is a large deciduous tree to 40 × 5 m with an erect, branching trunk and reddish bark and buds. *Leaves* alternate, broadly ovate to 10 cm long, obliquely cordate or truncate, sharply serrate, dull green above with axillary tufts beneath. *Flowers* yellowish, fragrant, in drooping cymes of 5–10, staminodes present. Peduncle linked for about half its length to a large pale, ligulate bract. *Fruit* globose, 1–3 seeded, faintly 5-ribbed. *T. platyphyllos*, the large-leaved lime, is similar but with larger leaves, and branches and leaves pubescent. Cymes generally 3, or rarely 4–6 flowered. *T. cordata*, the small-leaved lime, grows to about 30 m and has nearly orbicular leaves, broader than long, finely serrate. Cymes 5–7 flowered, staminodes lacking. Flowers in mid-summer.

421

Habitat and cultivation

These 3 species are native to Europe up to latitude 65°N. Planted in cooler climates elsewhere. Grown from seed, cuttings, layers or grafting, in cool, deep soils in open, sunny places. Frost resistant but drought tender.

Parts used

The flowers with their bracts harvested in early summer when the flowers are fully open.[1]

Active constituents

1) Volatile oil (up to 0.1%) including limonene, p-cymene, careen, germacrene-D, anethole and farnesol[2,3]
2) Flavonoids (about 1%) including derivatives of quercetin—quercitrin, rutin and hyperoside—and kaempferol—tiliroside and astragalin[4,5]
3) Phenolic acids including ferulic, chlorogenic, p-coumaric, caffeic and derivatives of cinnamic acid[6]
4) Mucilage (3–10%)[7]
5) Tannins (around 2%) of condensed type

It also contains saponins including scopoletin.[8]

Nutritional constituents

Minerals: Calcium, potassium, selenium, zinc and chromium[9,10]

Actions

1) Diaphoretic
2) Hypotensive
3) Sedative
4) Spasmolytic
5) Diuretic
6) Mild astringent

Scientific information

An official medicine in many countries, *Tilia* spp. have been valued as medicines in folklore.[1] The flowers are approved by *German Commission E* for the treatment of colds and cold-related coughs. Very little current research of any sort has been conducted into the herb in spite of its widespread uses in many parts of the world.

A number of the active constituents have been examined in isolation and some research was undertaken in the past.

In vitro—Constituents including the flavonoids and scopoletin are hepatoprotective, anti-oxidant, inhibitory to the growth of some cancer cells[11,12] and may, along with the herb itself, have immunomodulatory activity—stimulating T-cell proliferation. To date this has only be shown in animal models.[13]

The flavonoids from *Tilia* interact with benzodiazepine receptors in brain tissue of animals—this may indicate part of the mechanism for its relaxing effect.[14]

Human lymphocytes themselves have benzodiazepine receptors that influence immune function again this may explain the reputation that *Tilia* has in benefiting fevers, colds and influenza.[15]

Other studies report that the herb does not appear to have a strong anti-oxidant activity (its phenolic content is moderate).[16] As an infusion it showed no mutagenic activity, acting instead as a desmutagen.[17]

In vivo—An epidemiological study on the drinking of herbal teas, including lime flower, found the practice was associated with a reduced incidence of breast cancer.[18]

Weiss quotes a study in which lime flower tea was used to treat children with influenza and this, with bed rest, was superior to antibiotic treatment.

Medicinal uses

Cardiovascular system

The actions of *Tilia*, including diuresis, give it an important place in the treatment of circulatory problems but added to this is the traditional reputation the species has in the prophylactic treatment of arteriosclerosis:

• hypertension
• varicose veins
• phlebitis

Respiratory tract
It may be used in the treatment of:

- fevers
- influenza
- common cold
- upper respiratory catarrh
- irritable coughs

Nervous system
As a relaxant it is used to help in the treatment of any condition of nervous tension.

- migraine
- restlessness
- insomnia
- hysteria
- headaches

Externally
Tilia may be used topically to treat skin conditions.

Pharmacy
Three times daily
Infusion of dried herb   –   2–4 g
Tincture 1:5 (25%)   –   4–10 ml
Fluid Extract (25%)   –   2–4 ml
    For diaphoresis a hot infusion is the most effective dosage form.

Precautions and/or safety
The herb has no known toxicity[19] but *Tilia* pollen has been reported as a significant inhaled allergen[20] and there are cases of contact dermatitis and respiratory allergy to the flowers.[21-23]
    Lime flower tea reduced iron absorption from a simple meal by 52%, and may be best drunk between meals.[24]

Historical uses
Apoplexy; epilepsy; vertigo; indigestion; nervous vomiting; palpitations. As a bath for treatment of hysteria. Externally for burns and sores.

TURNERACEAE

This is a family of herbs, shrubs and trees of tropical and subtropical regions. The leaves are alternate, simple and stalked. Flowers regular in parts of 5, occurring in the axils of the upper leaves. The fruit is a many-seeded capsule.

Turnera diffusa
[Formerly known as *Turnera aphrodisiaca*]

Damiana

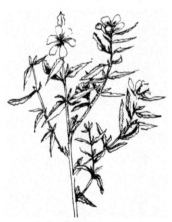

Family Turneraceae

Description
An aromatic shrubby perennial up to 60 cm tall. *Leaves* alternate, obovate, simple, petiolate, and pale green to 2.5 cm long. *Flowers* in axils of the upper leaves, small, yellow, appearing early to late summer. *Fruit* a small globular capsule.

Habitat and cultivation
Native to Western Mexico, Southern California and Texas on dry, sandy or rocky soils in full sun. Propagation is from seed sown in spring, division in autumn or cuttings rooted in summer.

Parts used
The stem and leaves.

Active constituents[1]
1) Volatile oil (around 0.5%)[2]—at least 50 individual constituents have been isolated. They include mainly caryophyllene and its oxide, 1,8-cineol, δ-cadinene, elemene, α- and β-pinene, thymol and myrtenal. The composition varies between fresh and dried herb and with geographical location[3-6]
2) Benzoquinone—arbutin (up to 0.7%)[5]
3) Cyanogenic glycosides—tetraphyllin B[7]

424

4) Bitter—damianin[2]
5) Flavonoids including derivatives of luteolin, quercitrin, apigenin and chrysoeriol[8]

Also contains phenolic acids,[1] sitosterol,[1] resins, gums, tannins and alkaloids.

Nutritional constituents
Vitamins: β-carotene and C
Minerals: Manganese, iron, copper, zinc, calcium and potassium[9,10]

Actions
1) Antidepressant
2) Thymoleptic
3) Stomachic
4) Mild laxative
5) Mild diuretic
6) Aphrodisiac

The herb has a strong reputation as an aphrodisiac in its countries of origin.[11]

Scientific information
Damiana was an official medicine in the *United States Formulary* from 1888–1947. In spite of its wide ranging uses it has been poorly researched pharmacologically.

In vitro—It has progestin-receptor binding activity.[12] The essential oils are better characterised than most of the constituents and are believed to contribute to the herb's long-standing reputation as an aphrodisiac.[3,4] As part of the nonpolar fraction, they are probably also responsible for this fraction's range of antibacterial activity to both Gram-positive and Gram-negative organisms, the whole extract itself has very little activity however.[13]

In vivo—There is some research into products which contain the herb. One of these is a preparation containing nutritional supplements with *Turnera*, *Ginkgo* and *Panax ginseng* which in clinical trials increased sexual satisfaction in women, including reducing vaginal dryness in peri-menopausal women.[14,15] As the preparation did not demonstrate oestrogen activity *in vitro*,[16] its mode of action may occur through circulatory and/or nerve function changes.[15] The same combination was also reported to improve erectile function in men.[15,17]

A combination of *Turnera*, *Ilex paraguayensis* (yerba) and *Paulina cupana* (guarana) used by obese, but otherwise healthy people, slowed their gastric emptying resulting in the perception of fullness occurring earlier and leading to weight loss over a period of weeks.[18] Weight loss ceased on maintenance therapy but weight gain did not occur.

Medicinal uses
Gastro-intestinal tract
- atonic constipation
- nervous dyspepsia

Urinary tract
- urinary tract infections

Nervous system
Its action is a tonic, with a slightly euphoric, anti-depressant action:

- depression
- neuralgia
- exhaustion
- herpes especially HSV-2

Reproductive tract
- impotence
- low sexual interest
- sexual inadequacies of psychological and/or emotional origin *BHP* specific for anxiety neurosis with a predominant sexual factor.

Pharmacy
Three times daily
Infusion of dried herb   – 2–4 g
Fluid Extract (60%)   – 3–6 ml

Historical uses
Giddiness; loss of balance; dysmenorrhoea, dyspepsia, diarrhoea, headache, enuresis, stomach ache; gonorrhoea, diabetes.

ULMACEAE

The *Ulmaceae* or Elm family consist of 15 genera of usually deciduous trees and shrubs of the Northern Hemisphere.

- Leaves are alternate and simple, often asymmetrical at base and stalked
- Flowers are small and inconspicuous, grow in clusters or racemes, with a 3–9 parted calyx but no petals
- Fruit a samara, nut or drupe

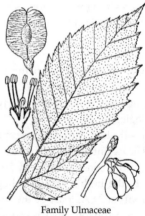

Family Ulmaceae

Ulmus rubra
[Formerly *U. fulva*]

Slippery elm (from the feel of the moistened inner bark)

Description
A small to medium sized deciduous tree to 20 × 5 m tall, with a broad, open crown and spreading branches; branchlets pubescent. *Trunk* erect and branching, bark dark brown, aromatic, rough and furrowed. *Leaves* alternate, large, 15–20 cm long, dark green turning dull yellow in autumn, simple, rough above, pubescent below to 12 cm long, ovate to oblong, acuminate, with serrate margins. *Flowers* small, inconspicuous growing in dense, axillary clusters in spring, followed by flat, conspicuous one-seeded samara.

Odour—slight; taste—mucilaginous.

Habitat and cultivation
Native to North America from Southern Canada to Florida growing in poor soils in moist woodlands and along streams, rarely in dry places. Grown from seed in spring. Collected in the wild, not usually cultivated. Frost resistant, drought tender.

Parts used
The inner bark collected in spring.

Active constituents
1) Mucilage consisting of branched polysaccharides based on galactose, rhamnose and galacturonic acid units[1-3]
2) Tannins (small amount)

Also contains starch and a small amount of calcium oxalate.[5]

Nutritional constituents
Vitamins: E, K and P
Minerals: Iron, sodium, calcium, selenium, iodine, copper, zinc, some potassium and phosphorus

Actions
1) Demulcent
2) Emollient
3) Nutritive
4) Antitussive

Scientific information
Originating from the indigenous North American Indian tradition, *Ulmus* has been an official medicine in the pharmacopoeias of Britain[4] and the United States.[5] The species name *rubra* refers to the colour of the buds whilst *fulva* indicates the "yellow" colour of the bark.

Very little research has been conducted into the pharmacology of the herb although a related species, *Ulmus davidiana*, has been the subject of some study in its country of origin, Korea.

Cancer
In vitro—*Ulmus* has antitumour and anti-oxidant activities[6,7] and the latter action may contribute to an anti-inflammatory effect.[6]

Slippery elm is one of the original four constituents in the *Essiac* formula used as a supportive treatment for cancer. *Essiac*-type preparations have anti-oxidant[12] and antiproliferative activity,[8] some antimutagenic activity[9] and also encourage cancer cell differentiation.[10] The levels required to produce these effects may however be difficult to attain *in vivo*.[8,11]

Results from *in vitro* and *in vivo* studies of *Essiac's* benefits as an anticancer therapy are still controversial.[11,12] Anecdotal evidence exists but to-date there is a paucity of clinical trials to support them. Hospital studies undertaken by the *Canadian Breast Cancer Research Initiative 1996* were inconclusive[8,13] and one other reported trial failed to find positive effects.[14]

Gastro-intestinal tract
In vivo—No formal trials have evaluated the benefit of slippery elm in inflammatory bowel conditions however data gathered from patients with the condition show that it is one of the herbs commonly used by them.[6,15]

Other
In vivo—Slippery elm was part of a diet-controlled treatment used in a small group of patients with chronic psoriasis which produced encouraging results.[16]

There is an anecdotal report of *Ulmus* relieving an intractable cough associated with lung cancer where many much stronger pharmaceuticals failed to have any effect.[17]

Medicinal uses
The primary action of this herb is through its high mucilage content. It soothes the digestive tract and it may be used as an adjunct in the treatment of respiratory and urinary tract problems. (See "Mucilages" in Appendix III.)

The mucilage and starch in the herb added to its nutritional constituents make it a nutritious food that is easily assimilated. It is a useful aid in convalescence.

Gastro-intestinal tract
• oesophagitis
• gastritis
• colitis
• diarrhoea
• peptic ulcers

Externally
The herb is also used externally to draw and soothe:

- boils
- abscesses
- burns
- wounds

Pharmacy
As often as required
internally.

Powdered bark	–	5–20 ml in about ten times the volume of water[†]
	–	4 g in 500 ml as a nutritious gruel
Fluid Extract (60%)	–	5 ml

The mucilage is best extracted in water and hot or cold infusions may be made from the powdered bark or a decoction from the coarser material. Tinctures of the bark are made but the herb is mostly used in the form of powder or tablets.[†]

To soothe the digestive tract may be used as often as required.

Externally the powder or coarse bark is made into a poultice by adding boiling water and applying as hot as is bearable without damaging the skin.

Historical uses
Pleurisy; bronchitis; haemoptysis; TB; typhoid fever; cystitis; irritation of urinary tract; worms. Externally for gangrene (in combinations); rheumatism; gout; synovitis; toothache; dental caries.

[†]N.B. Mix powder with a little water to a smooth consistency before adding the rest of the water, stirring all the time to prevent it becoming lumpy.

URTICACEAE

The Urticaceae contain 45 genera and about 1000 species. They are annual or perennial herbs, shrubs and soft wooded trees but rarely climbers. They often have stinging hairs. Leaves may be opposite or alternate and flowers are usually unisexual, in cymes. Among the medicinal plants of this family are *Urtica* and *Parietaria*.

Parietaria diffusa [Also known as *P. officinalis*]

Pellitory-of-the-Wall

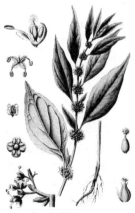

Family Urticaceae

Description

An upright perennial with round, pale green-reddish stems growing about 40 cm high. *Leaves* alternate, 5–7 cm long, lanceolate-ovate, slightly glossy green, softly hairy and brittle. Those on flowering stems often become yellow with brown blotches in autumn. *Flowers* tiny, greenish, usually unisexual, arranged in terminal and axillary cymes. Female flowers have a tubular perianth with 4 teeth, male flowers have a perianth of 4 parts surrounded by an involucre of 1 bract and 2 bracteoles. The *fruit* is enclosed by the perianth. Blooms mid summer into autumn.

Habitat and cultivation

Native to Britain and parts of Europe, pellitory grows along dry hedge banks in rocky places and in stone walls. Hence its common name. It can be grown in gardens and also in pots.

Parts used

The dried aerial parts of the herb harvested during or just prior to flowering.

Active constituents

1) Flavonoids including derivatives of quercetin, kaempferol and isorhamnetin[1]

2) Phenolic acids including p-coumaric, ferulic, isoferulic acids and other carboxylic acids[2]
3) Glucoproteins[3]

Also contains a bitter, tannins, mucilage[4] and reasonable quantities of fatty acids.[5]

Nutritional constituents
Minerals: Sulphur, potassium and calcium

Actions
1) Diuretic
2) Demulcent

Scientific information
Parietaria once enjoyed more recognition and a much broader use than in recent times. It was an official medicine but does not appear in pharmacopoeias in the latter part of the 20th Century.[2]

Much research has been undertaken into the constituents of the pollens of this family, which are glycoproteins, as they are apparently responsible for many respiratory allergies suffered by people in the Mediterranean area.[3]

The older herbalists valued the herb as the best treatment for lithiasis of bladder and kidneys. In Italy its primary use has been, and is, for sprains and contusions, its use in the urinary tract being secondary.[6] It has also been used there to treat herpes infections, the fresh plant being applied topically.[7]

In vitro—Using an animal model of a viral infection akin to HIV it showed good inhibitory activity.[7]

Medicinal uses
Urinary tract
As a demulcent and litholitic herb its main use has been in the treatment of:-

- cystitis
- dysuria
- pyelitis
- urinary gravel or calculus
- oedema of renal origin
- oliguria

Pharmacy
Three times daily

Infusion of herb	– 1.0–5 g
Tincture 1:5 (45%)	– 2.0–10 ml
Fluid extract (25%)	– 2.5–5 ml

Historical uses
Old or dry coughs, shortness of breath; wheezing; to ease pain of childbirth, to "bring down women's courses" (an emmenagogue); obstructions of liver and spleen; dropsy. Externally for stings and insect bites; as a gargle for sore throats; toothache; skin blemishes including sunburn; ear drops for earache and "noise"; tumours; inflammation and infections of skin including ulcers; to stop hair loss; to heal fistulas; muscle or tendon injuries and/or bruises; piles.

Urtica dioica

Stinging nettle

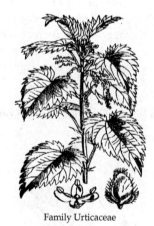

Family Urticaceae

Description
An erect, square-stemmed, rhizomatous perennial, usually dioecious but sometimes with a few flowers of the other sex. Sparsely to densely hairy with short-stalked stinging hairs as well. *Stems* up to 1.5 m tall in flower, rarely branched. *Leaves* opposite, dark green, acute to acuminate, usually cordate at base and coarsely serrate; ovate in subspecies

dioica, 6–16 cm long; narrowly to broadly lanceolate in subspecies *gracilis*, 10–20 cm long. *Flowers* tiny, in unisexual racemes 2–5 cm long in subspecies *dioica* up to 9 cm long in subspecies *gracilis*. *Perianth* green and 4-partite; female flowers have unequal perianth segments, the 2 larger segments enclosing the achene; male flowers have 4 equal segments. Flowers from summer to autumn. *U. urens* is also used medicinally.

Habitat and cultivation

Native to Britain, Northern Europe and Asia and found wild in temperate zones worldwide. Grown from seed or division of rhizomes and thrives in moist soils. Frost resistant, drought tender.

Parts used

The herb collected just prior to, or during flowering (gloves should be worn). The root or rhizomes are also a recognised medicine, these parts are usually harvested in spring or autumn.

Active constituents

Aerial parts:

1) Flavonoids including derivatives of quercetin, rutin, kaempferol and isorhamnetin[8–10]
2) Amines including histamine,[11] acetylcholine[11,12] and serotonin (5-hydroxytryptamine), mainly in stinging hairs[13]
3) Phenolic constituents[8] including vanillic, ferulic, chlorogenic and caffeoylmalic acids[14] and vanillin[8,15]
4) Sterols including β-sitosterol[16]

Also contains the triterpenoid ursolic acid,[8] tannins, coumarins (scopoletin),[8] oleoresin,[17] lignans,[27] omega-3 fatty acids (highest in young leaves),[18] carboxylic acids and leukotrienes (*U. urens*).[19]

Root/rhizomes:

5) Sterols including β-sitosterol[20]
6) Coumarins including scopoletin[20]
7) Lectins (up to 0.42%) referred to as *Urtica dioica* agglutinin (UDA), these are dipeptide units and exist in 4 different forms or isolectins[21]

Also contains oleoresin, fatty acids,[18] lignans,[22] triterpenoids (oleanolic and ursolic acids), phenolic constituents and polysaccharides[23]

Nutritional constituents

Vitamins: A, B_2, C, E, carotenoids (chlorophyll, lutein and beta-carotene) and K. Fresh extracts contain B_1 too[17,18]

Minerals: Calcium (significant amount), magnesium, potassium, silicic acid, iron, selenium, zinc, manganese and copper.[24–26] Mineral content of herb is around 2G%, leaves 1–5%.[27]

Actions

1) Antihaemorrhagic
2) Nutritive
3) Diuretic

Scientific information

Nettles have been used for thousands of years as a traditional medicine as well as for their food value and until quite recently for making fabric, rope and bowstrings. They are commonly used throughout the world and have been employed in the treatment of a wide variety of problems some of these uses being quite different to that known to modern western herbalists. In Turkey, for example, the herb is used for 26 different applications including cancer, respiratory, circulatory and gastro-intestinal problems and as a vulnerary.[28,29]

In recent years in Germany *Urtica* has been officially accepted as safe and effective for specific applications including benign prostatic hyperplasia[30] and as supportive therapy for lower urinary tract infections[31] and rheumatic conditions.[32] *German Commission E* also approves use of the herb to prevent and treat renal gravel and the root to treat dysuria due to benign prostatic hyperplasia stages 1 and 2.

The use of the roots in phytotherapy is not new, roots and herb having been sometimes used interchangeably in the past; however their chemical make-up is different.

Anti-oxidant

In vitro—The flavonoids contribute to the herb's anti-oxidant capacity[9] however there are a number of other phenolic constituents to augment this action.[33-36] Water extracts are strongly anti-oxidant and may have metal chelating ability.[37]

The roots do not have significant activity but some of their constituents may be converted *in vivo* to increase this potential.[33]

Prostate/urinary function

In recent times the root has attracted attention in relation to the treatment of benign prostatic hyperplasia (BPH). This use is not based on tradition.

In vitro—The mechanism of action in treating prostatic problems is not completely understood but appears to involve nettle root's ability to:-

- inhibit binding of Sex Hormone Binding Globulin (SHBG) to prostatic receptor sites[38,39]—lignans, their metabolites and fatty acids also have this activity[22,40]
- possibly displace free circulating steroid hormones from SHBG sites[38]
- inhibit sodium/potassium pump in the prostate membrane—this may inhibit prostatic cell metabolism[41]
- inhibit aromatase conversion of testosterone to oestrogens (equivalent in effect to synthetic drugs but much higher concentrations of *Urtica* are required)[38,42]
- inhibit epidermal growth factor (UDA)[38]
- act as an anti-inflammatory—see below

The level of β-sitosterol is considered too low to be able to contribute significantly to this action but the lignans and triterpenoids are likely to do so. The inhibition of aromatase is increased when *Serenoa* or *Pygeum* and *Urtica radix* are used together.[38]

In vivo—A number of clinical trials have been conducted beginning around 1950, using *Urtica radix* alone or with other herbs. To date these trials have shown:-

- improvement in symptoms and quality of life with modest decrease in prostate size using *Urtica radix* alone[43,44]
- *Serenoa* and *Urtica radix* were effective in treating/inhibiting the progression of moderate to severe BPH[45] and reduced symptoms.[46-49] They

were well-tolerated over the long-term[50] and were as effective as the standard drug therapies currently available namely tamsulosin[51] and finasteride,[52] with fewer side effects[53]
- *Pygeum africanum* and *Urtica* did not show significant improvement in objective or subjective symptoms[54] in one study but did in another[55]

The root decreased levels of SHBG in healthy men but the effects on serum hormone levels and prostate cell growth have been less clear.[38]

Due to perceived short-comings in most of the trials conducted to-date phytotherapy is still considered by some to require more rigorous testing before being accepted as a proven treatment for BPH.[56-58] However it has been estimated that in Europe herbal treatment comprises 80% of all BPH treatment officially used and an estimated 40,000 men have so far been treated with *Urtica* root.[38,59]

Urtica herba was used as a bladder wash, in combination with other herbs, after prostate surgery to effectively reduce infection and bleeding.[60]

Antimicrobial

In vitro—The herb has activity against various bacteria including *Staphylococcus aureus*,[37,61] *S. epidermis*,[37,61] *Streptococcus pyogenes*,[61] *S. pneumoniae*[37] and *Escherichia coli*.[37,61] (A similar test carried out using *U. urens* found it was inactive).[62,63] It is also active against *Mycobacterium tuberculosis*[64] and has antifungal activity against *Candida albicans*.[37]

Aqueous leaf extracts inhibit a protease enzyme responsible for the neurotoxicity of *Clostridium botulinum*.[65]

UDA has antifungal activity[66] and good antiviral activity[67] including against the transmission of HIV[68,69] and cytomegalovirus.[70] It appears to make HIV more vulnerable to immune system destruction through changes to the viral envelope.[71] It also selectively stimulates a subset of T-cell lymphocytes.[72] However even though UDA is water-soluble its bioavailability is uncertain.

In addition to the above antimicrobial activity extracts have significant immunomodulatory effects, the *herba* increases neutrophil activity (flavonoids)[10] and the *radix* stimulates lymphocyte proliferation (polysaccharides).[23]

In vivo—Very few clinical trials have been undertaken. A mouthwash consisting of yarrow, juniper and nettles did not reduce gingivitis or plaque growth or inhibit the bacteria responsible[73] but a much earlier study found *Urtica* may be helpful in the treatment of tuberculosis patients with hepatic pathology.[74]

Analgesic/anti-inflammatory

The use of nettle stings to reduce the pain of inflamed joints has been known for hundreds of years and skin applications were also used by Roman soldiers to warm them during their stay in the cold climate of Britain.

In vitro—The *herba* alters cytokines and immune function related to inflammation including that associated with pathological changes in rheumatoid arthritis.[32,75–80] An extract partially inhibited 5-LOX and did inhibit COX activity.[81]

In vivo—*Urtica* has been approved for use in the treatment of rheumatic disease in Germany. Older studies used the *herba* to treat both osteo- and rheumatoid arthritis with encouraging results.[27,31] More recently there are anecdotal reports of nettle leaf stings being used to successfully relieve joint pain[82,83] and a clinical trial showing the sting reduced osteoarthritic pain.[84]

Endocrine

In vitro—The herb is a strong activator of receptors involved in the control of glucose and lipid metabolism–peroxisome proliferator-activated receptors.[85] It can also inhibit α-glucosidase.[86]

In vivo—Nettles have been used in various countries as a traditional treatment for diabetes.[87,88] A clinical trial using a combination of *Anethum graveolens* (dill), ginkgo and nettles in the treatment of type 2 diabetics significantly reduced blood sugar levels.[89]

Other

In vitro—*Urtica* (especially fresh herb) has good antiplatelet activity, including that induced by adrenalin,[90] an action that is possibly due to modulation of arachidonic acid metabolism at the cell membrane.[91,92] Platelets are involved in the manifestation of a variety of diseases including atherosclerosis, allergic and non-allergic inflammation and tumour progression. This together with the presence of acetylcholine, a biochemical involved in many cellular processes as well as neurotransmission,[93] may be significant to the herb's broad range of actions.

As a traditional antihypertensive, nettle roots have been shown in animal experiments to have a vaso-relaxant effect. Although no direct studies have confirmed this in humans the herb has proven to be diuretic and this may also help reduce blood pressure.[27,94]

Tests have been conducted into the *herba's* reputation as a therapeutic agent in the treatment of cancer. *Urtica* itself has no cytotoxicity in cancer cell lines suggesting that any efficacy it has in treating malignancy is likely to occur through immune modulation (demonstrated in animal models).[95] In addition extracts inhibit the metabolism of DNA in prostate cancer cells[96] and protect against cancer development by inhibiting inflammatory cytokines.[97] The root inhibits the growth of prostate epithelial cancer cells but not stromal cells, again without cytotoxicity.[98] This activity also occurs with the isolated polysaccharide fraction.[99]

In vivo—The herb reduces the symptoms of allergic rhinitis although only one clinical study has been carried out to-date.[100] Possible mechanisms are through anti-inflammatory and immunomodulatory activities.

The list of nutritive constituents may explain the traditional use of *Urtica* as a spring tonic.

Medicinal uses

Respiratory tract
- haemoptysis
- epistaxis

Gastro-intestinal tract
- melaena
- haemorrhoids
- stomach haemorrhage

Genitourinary tract
- increase lactation
- benign prostatic hyperplasia (*radix*)
- chronic cystitis (*radix* and *herba*)
- menorrhagia

Musculoskeletal
- gout
- osteoarthritis
- rheumatoid arthritis

Skin
- cutaneous eruptions
- eczema, infantile and nervous (psychogenic)

Externally
- skin ulcers
- wounds

Pharmacy
Three times daily

Infusion of dried herb	–	3–6 g
Tincture 1:5 (25%)	–	2–6 ml
Fluid Extract (25%)	–	2–4 ml
Fresh juice	–	5–10 ml

Root preparations for treating *BPH* were effective at doses of 4–6 g of fresh root per day as an infusion or as an extract equivalent to 300–600 mg dried root.

It takes about 10 minutes to effectively extract minerals from the herb by infusion.[24] Mineral content can vary with time of year gathered (P and K highest in spring, Ca, Mg and S highest in late summer) and year of harvest. Content does not appear to differ according to habitat or whether the herb is fresh or dried.[101]

Dry, powdered nettles can be used as snuff for epistaxis or on bleeding wounds. The young tops can be cooked and eaten as a nutritious vegetable.

Precautions and/or safety
The herb is not cytotoxic or mutagenic in standard tests.[61] A slight genotoxic effect on a standard test has been attributed to the testing regime used.[102]

Clinical trials using both root and herb showed they were well tolerated, without serious side-effects.[27,43,44,59] Mild gastro-intestinal discomfort and rare systemic allergic reactions are listed as potential side-effects.[27] The sting of fresh nettle is unpleasant and causes a weal with erythema and itching. The hairs are brittle at their tips, due to the high level of silica, and if broken off for example by touching them, bulbs at their bases which contain histamine, acetylcholine, serotonin and leukotrienes are injected into the skin. The skin reacts within 3–5 minutes and a stinging paraesthesia can persist for 12 hours.[103,104] This is not an allergic reaction but a chemical reaction that occurs in everyone. The nettle cannot sting after drying or cooking.

There is one report of an actual allergic reaction to the herb.[105] Although the pollen of *Parietaria* spp. are commonly implicated in causing respiratory allergies *U. dioica* seems to have a much lower allergenic potential,[106] that may however be underestimated.[107]

Historical uses
Sting used in Roman times to treat arthritis and also sciatica; neuralgia; lumbago and tendonitis. Internally to treat asthma; bronchitis; coughs; dyspnoea; pertussis; tuberculosis; bladder and kidney stones; scurvy; worms in children; mad dog bites; lethargy (externally too); nose bleeds; nasal polyps; hemlock and henbane poisoning antidote; impotence–seeds. Externally for burns; stings and bites; hair rinse for stimulating growth and treating dandruff; "leprosy, morphew and discolourings"; itch (as a wash).

VALERIANACEAE

The valerian family consists of about 10 genera of perennial herbs, rarely shrubs, native mostly to the northern hemisphere. Leaves opposite, simple, pinnatifid or compound. Flowers small, often in cymes. Calyx obsolete, or variously toothed or involuted in the flower, and becoming pappus-like in the fruit.

Valeriana officinalis

Valerian

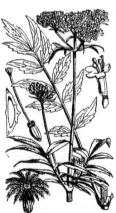

Family Valerianaceae

Description
A robust perennial growing from 0.5–1 m tall in flower and dying back in winter. *Leaves* very variable, compound, pinnate, soft green; basal leaves to about 20 cm long, stalked, with large oval or lance-shaped leaflets, entire or strongly and unevenly toothed. Upper leaves opposite, sessile and smaller. New spring growth reddish brown. *Flowers* grow in dense, branched, flat-topped clusters at the top of hollow, grooved stems. The calyx forms a pappus in fruit. Corolla is 4–5 mm across, pale pink, funnel-shaped, somewhat swollen at the base of the tube, with 5 unequal, spreading lobes. The tube is 4–5 mm long. *Fruit* is 4 mm long, hairless and oblong-oval. Flowers in summer.

Odour—characteristic; taste—sweetish at first then camphoraceous and bitter.

Habitat and cultivation
Native to Britain and Europe in damp, sunny or semi-shady places. Grows from seed and will self-sow, or from root division in autumn or spring while dormant. Frost resistant but drought tender.

Parts used
The roots and rhizomes harvested in autumn.

435

Active constituents

1) Volatile oil (around 1%), at least 64 constituents have been isolated from this fraction.
The composition is very variable depending
on subspecies, age, geographical location,
genetic make-up (see below) and method of
extraction.[1-13] Composed of:
   a) sesquiterpenes based on and including
   kessane, valeranone and valerenic acids—
   mainly valerenal, also valerianol, kessanyl
   acetate and hydroxyvalerenic acids
   b) monoterpenes (31%) including mainly
   bornyl acetate and borneol also α-pinene,
   β-caryophyllene and camphene
   c) esters (16%)
2) Alkaloids (up to 0.1%) including actinidine[14]
3) Iridoid epoxy-esters (valepotriates) around
0.3–1.7% including valtrate, isovaltrate (making up about 90%) and acevaltrate[2,15,16]
4) Flavonoids including hesperidin, 6-methylapi-
genin[17] and linarin[18]
5) Lignans (around 0.55%) many based on
pinoresinol, also an olivil derivative[19,20]

Also contains choline (3%), phenolic acids
including chlorogenic, ferulic and p-coumaric
acids,[21,22] sterols—clionasterol glycosides,[23] tannins, polysaccharides,[24] resins and gums, amino
acids (rich in glutamine) and fixed oil. Although
γ-aminobutyric acid (GABA)[25] has been reported,
its presence is controversial.

Valerian displays polyploidy and occurs as diploid, tetraploid and octaploid types.[9]

There are a few other main species used medicinally in the west such as *V. edulis* and *V. wallichii*
however the presence of valerenic acid, with ace-
toxyvalerenic acid and valerenal, only occurs in
V. officinalis.[26,27]

The valepotriates present in all medicinal species are lowest in *V. officinalis*. They are unstable and
degrade on storage or processing to iridoid aldehydes
and acids, mainly baldrinal and homobaldrinal[90] but
also isovaleric acid which is responsible for the familiar, and to some unpleasant, smell of the herb.

Nutritional constituents
Minerals: Magnesium, copper, calcium, chromium,
iron, potassium and zinc[28-30]

Actions

1) Spasmolytic
2) Carminative
3) Sedative/relaxant
4) Hypotensive
5) Anodyne (mild)

Scientific information
Valeriana has been known as a calming agent since
early Roman and Greek times, Dioscorides describing it as a mild sedative. Some other species of this
genus, numbering over 200, have formed part of
the traditional medicine in their countries of origin,
having been used in much the same way. *V. officinalis* has been listed in pharmacopoeias around the
world[31] and has been approved by *German Commission E* for the treatment of restlessness and insomnia due to nervous conditions.

Apart from being one of the top selling medicinal herbs its constituents are used in cosmetics and
as flavourings.[1]

Anti-oxidant
In vitro—Valerian has anti-oxidant activity.[22,32]

Nervous system
In modern times valerian has been used mainly
to modify mood, through improved sleep, and to
reduce anxiety.[33] As a frequently used herb it has
attracted a great deal of scientific interest. In spite
of all the research that has been undertaken the
mechanism of action and constituent(s) responsible remain uncertain.[34]

In vitro—At one time the valepotriates were
considered responsible for the action of valerian
however it is now accepted they cannot account for
all of the observed effects and other constituents
are likely to contribute. Evidence so far suggests
the mode of action may be due to:-

• modulation of GABA$_A$ receptors. GABA is an
inhibitor of neural transmission in the brain, its
receptors being modulated by drugs like benzodiazepines, barbiturates, anaesthetics and
also by sesquiterpenes particularly valerenic
acid,[34] borneol and its derivatives.[35] There are
indications that valerian may effectively raise

levels of GABA by preventing its re-uptake and may also facilitate its transport in the brain.[35] Plant derived GABA, if present, would not be expected to contribute greatly as it cannot cross the blood-brain barrier.[36] Glutamine on the other hand can cross into the brain and can be metabolised to GABA.[25] Research done on GABA receptors in the past used very high concentrations in order to show effects, as its binding capacity is low, so this mechanism would not seem likely to be wholly responsible for the herb's actions[40]

- modulation of A_1 adenosine receptors.[19] Adenosine is a neuro-modulator in the central nervous system and the A_1 adenosine receptor is a main subtype found in the brain. It may be one of the most important biochemicals involved in inducing sleep—its agonists induce sedation whilst antagonists like caffeine are stimulatory.[19] Agonists of adenosine A_1 receptors appear to be not only sedative but also anti-convulsive, analgesic, anti-diuretic, anti-arrhythmic and negatively inotropic. Whilst hydrophilic constituents of the herb are able to act as partial agonists at these sites,[37] a lipophilic constituent—isovaltrate—is an inverse agonist and therefore a stimulant.[38] There is also some indication that methanol but not ethanol extracts have agonist activity[39]
- interaction at serotonin receptors—the herb is a partial agonist at 5-hydroxytryptamine$_{5a}$ receptor sites[40]
- interaction at benzodiazepine receptor sites not directly related to GABA$_A$ receptors[41]—some of the flavonoids have sleep enhancing and sedative properties and they may interact with these receptor sites[42]
- affinity for melatonin receptors[43]

The action of valerian may occur through any one or a combination of constituents at all or some of the above receptor sites or the action may rely on synergism amongst them.[18]

Sleep

In vivo—Clinical studies into the effectiveness of valerian as a sleep aid have not been consistent. In some studies it gave a modest improvement to sleep,[44] in some no improvement compared to placebo in sleep disturbed volunteers[45-47] and yet others found it was as effective as benzodiazepine sedatives.[48,49]

Valerian on its own has been shown to:-

- reduce sleep latency (time to fall asleep)[50-53]
- reduce time spent awake before going back to asleep[52]
- improve subjective perception of sleep[50]
- improve the quantity of slow-wave or deep sleep[53,54]

Partial extracts have also been of some benefit in sleep disorders—the valepotriates helped insomniacs who had withdrawn from long term use of benzodiazepines[55] and a sesquiterpene fraction improved sleep quality in poor sleepers.[56]

Most studies into the efficacy of *Valeriana* for sleep used it in combination with one or more other herbs:

- *Valeriana* and *Humulus*—this combination was effective in reducing sleep latency and improving slow wave sleep and subjective well being,[39,57] (*Valeriana* alone was no better than placebo[39]), being at least as effective as the antihistamine diphenylhydramine in treating mild insomnia[58] and as benzodiazepines in non-chronic, non-psychiatric sleep disorder.[59] The combination also acted indirectly, via adenosine receptors, to reduce the stimulant effect of caffeine in healthy volunteers[60]
- *Valeriana* and *Melissa*—this combination was effective in reducing dyssomnia and general motor restlessness (as occurs in ADHD) in children under 12 years old.[61] It also improved sleep quality in healthy non-insomniacs[61,62] as well as those with sleep disorders.[61]
- *Valeriana* and *Piper*—each of these herbs was equally effective in reducing stress related to insomnia and the combination significantly improved sleep in terms of reduced latency, hours slept and waking mood[63,64]
- *Valeriana* used in a more complex formula gave improved sleep quality associated with menopausal disturbances[65]

There are many reviews of the clinical trials to-date on the effectiveness of valerian alone or in combination as an aid to insomnia with varying conclusions ranging from positive through inconclusive to negative.[66-71]

It has been suggested that valerian supports the readiness to fall asleep[72] and the sedative effect may indeed be mild.

Other CNS effects
Valerian was tested as one-off doses to see if it was a potential risk for users through impaired cognitive or psychomotor performance or altered mood. Comparative tests with acute doses of the benzodiazepines, diazepam and triazolam, or diphenhydramine, found that these pharmaceuticals did impair cognitive function whereas valerian's effect even at the highest dose tested (1800 mg) was no different to placebo.[73-76] No deterioration in performance was measurable either after 2 weeks continuous intake.[76]

Some studies have reported a minimal impact on cognitive function with a change in electrical brain activity occurring after the intake of a valerian-hops preparation, which may last some hours[77,78] and also with valerian syrup.[78] Function was normal the following day, there being no residual sedative or hang-over effects, in fact there was a subjective feeling of being more alert/active and feeling better perhaps due to an improved perception of sleep quality.[78] Valerian and lemon balm whilst reducing laboratory-induced anxiety also slightly lowered some aspects of cognitive performance.[79] At the highest dose tested, which was three times that recommended, stress was reported to have increased slightly suggesting a biphasic response to the combination.[79]

In a laboratory setting the herb reduced stress-induced rises in systolic blood pressure and heart rate as well as subjective awareness of stress without impairing cognitive performance.[80]

A clinical study of people suffering depression with anxiety disorder showed the response was better when both *Hypericum* and *Valeriana* were used than when *Hypericum* was used on its own.[81] Valerian on its own may not improve the symptoms of anxiety[82] but a preparation containing valepotriates reduced the objective assessment of anxiety in patients with generalised anxiety disorder.[83]

Valerian has had a reputation in Europe as a treatment for epilepsy and was an especially favoured treatment in the 18th and 19th centuries. The first anecdotal reports of its benefits for epilepsy, particularly childhood epilepsy, had been reported around the 16th century.[84] Isovaleric acid and chemically related substances have anticonvulsant activity[84] and constituents with adenosine A_1 agonist activity would also be expected to be active but no modern investigations have been undertaken.

Other
In vitro—Extracts are:-

- anti-inflammatory, may also be neuroprotective[85]
- antimicrobial (some cultivars only)—antibacterial including against *Aspergillus niger*, *Escherichia coli* and *Staphylococcus aureus*[4] and antiviral through inhibition of HIV-1 replication (valtrate)[86]
- able to act as a cancer preventative[87] and are desmutagenic in standard tests[88]

Uses of valerian beyond those specific to the nervous system still relies largely on tradition.

Medicinal uses
Cardiovascular system
- hypertension (especially related to stress)

Gastro-intestinal tract
- irritable bowel syndrome
- intestinal cramps
- colitis
- dyspepsia

Nervous system
The fact that the herb can quieten or tranquillise without the sedation associated with its pharmaceutical equivalent, makes it particularly valuable in the treatment of:

- anxiety
- hysteria

- restlessness
- migraine
- hypochondriasis
- tension
- stress
- nervousness
- epilepsy
- insomnia/disturbed sleep patterns

Pharmacy
Three times daily
Infusion of dried root   – 1–3 g
Tincture 1:5 (70%)   – 3–5 ml
Fluid Extract (60%)   – 0.3–1 ml

For insomnia a single dose may be used half an hour before retiring. It may take 2 weeks for the effects of valerian to become manifest.[26]

Preparations of the herb may differ markedly from one another not only due to the great variability of the crude plant but also the processing used in its manufacture. According to the *American Herbal Pharmacopoeia* extraction of valepotriates requires 70% alcohol whereas extraction of valerenic acids occurs with a minimum of 30% alcohol.[67]

A comparison of aqueous and ethanol extracts found the valerenic acids extracted were similar in both but that the aqueous extract lacked valepotriates.[2] However another analysis on processed valerian products reported that whilst valepotriates were present at low levels in aqueous extracts they were undetectable in all other preparations tested including tablets, capsules and liquids other than teas.[89] In ethanol extracts containing even a small amount of water the valepotriates degrade by 90% within a few weeks so that the freshness of the extract may be a critical factor[90] to their presence. However any residual valepotriates present in preparations are probably metabolised by gut flora to baldrinal and homobaldrinal.[26]

Pharmacokinetics
Studies are not extensive. After oral dosing with valerian, valerenic acid reached maximum serum levels within 1–2 hours, was still detectable after 5 hours and had a half life of around 1 hour.[91]

Through the counter-effect to caffeine it was found that the combined extract of valerian and hops reached adenosine receptors in the brain within 60 minutes of administration.[60] This gives a time frame for administering the herb as a sleep aid.

Precautions and/or safety
In vitro—At doses 2 to 3 orders of magnitude greater than recommended, valerian was cytotoxic to hepatoma cells, but it was concluded unlikely that the herb can be considered hepatotoxic based on this study.[92]

Toxicity studies link dichloromethane extracts of *Valeriana* at high doses to DNA damage, but not lower doses, and the herb is not cytotoxic.[93] Valepotriates have been a main safety concern as they are reported to be cytotoxic, genotoxic[94] and to inhibit DNA synthesis which would make their presence in extracts undesirable.[95] However in most preparations their level is low to begin with due to their instability and furthermore they are likely to be degraded in the gut prior to absorption. Their toxicity in humans has not been established.[15]

In vivo—The combined valerian and hops preparation did not cause rebound insomnia when it was withdrawn.[58,59] Clinical trials using valerian alone or in combination reported no serious adverse effects in any age group.[44,50,57,61,62,81] Haematological and biochemical parameters including liver function tests were reported unchanged after 1 month's treatment.[62] Reviews conclude there are no safety issues regarding its use,[67] side-effects are rare and usually minor—see below. Even use of the isolated valepotriates[83] and sesquiterpene fraction[56] were without adverse reactions.

Valerian increased the number of normal sperm produced (though not necessarily increasing fertility) and did not damage male fertility even at 3 times the normal dose.[96] An epidemiological study determined there were no apparent adverse effects on foetal development through maternal use of the herb in pregnancy.[97]

Given the popularity of the herb it has been well trialled, anecdotally, with very few reported side effects. Possible minor effects include vivid dreams,[63] mild tiredness, sleep disturbance,[62] nausea,[98] agitation,[98] drowsiness[98] and headache.[99]

Even an overdose of valerian (20 times the recommended dose) produced only mild symptoms.[100]

Serious side-effects that have been attributed to it include a case of acute cholestatic hepatitis in a patient with Epstein-Barr virus who also used paracetamol and ibuprofen;[101] an anaphylactic reaction[98] and sedation.[98] Also an isolated report of psychotic changes in an alcoholic who used valerian and ginkgo—no causal link determined[102] and a case of cardiac complications and delirium in a person on multiple drugs who withdrew from using the herb.[103]

Interactions
In vitro—Studies have indicated a potential for valerian to interact with the p-glycoprotein transport system and drugs metabolised by CYP1A2, CYP3A4, CYP2C19 and CYP2D6, approximately 25% use the latter. The level required to cause such inhibition may not however be reached *in vivo*.[104-107]

Valerian and valerenic acid both inhibit liver-microsome glucuronidation, an activity that is associated with drug and endogenous metabolite handling.[108]

In vivo—Valerian did not interfere with test drugs metabolised by the above cytochrome P450 isozymes or with those using CYP2E1.[109,110] There is in fact only one report of suspected interaction between valerian and lorazepam, the herb apparently enhancing the sedative effect of the benzodiazepine.[111]

Historical uses
It was used in the First World War to treat people with shattered nerves caused by air raids. Coughs; croup; the plague; as a diuretic; St Vitus' dance; cholera; to strengthen eyesight; an antidote to bites and stings; flatulence. Internally and externally to heal sores. Externally as a drawing agent.

VERBENACEAE

The Verbenaceae consists of herbs, shrubs or trees, with square stems and opposite or rarely alternate leaves. The flowers are similar to those of the Lamiaceae except that the ovary is entire, with the style proceeding from the top, and the flowers are in racemes or cymes rather than in verticils. The fruit is dry or succulent usually shorter than the persistent calyx, 2- or 4-celled with one seed in each cell.

Vitex agnus-castus and *Verbena officinalis* are medicinal plants of the Verbenaceae.

Verbena officinalis

Vervain

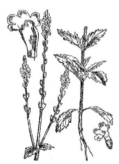

Family Verbenaceae

Description

An annual or short-lived erect perennial, nearly glabrous, with square stemmed, spreading, wiry branches which may grow to 80 cm tall. *Basal leaves* stalked, obovate or oblong, dark green and deeply toothed, upper leaves opposite, few, often sessile and lanceolate. *Flowers* very small, pale blue, in long, slender spikes, the lower ones becoming distant as the spike lengthens, each one sessile in the axil of a small bract. Flowers from summer to autumn.

Habitat and cultivation

Native to Europe, North Africa and West Asia, in damp, sunny situations and widely naturalised. Grows from seed and is better shown fresh each year. Old plants become straggly and less productive. Drought tender, frost resistant.

Parts used

The herb gathered at, or just prior to, flowering. In Germany the roots are also used.[1]

Active constituents

1) Iridoids—mainly verbenalin (cornin) around 0.1–0.3% highest during flowering and in mature plants.[2-7] Also hastatoside and aucubin

441

2) Phenylpropanoids (up to 5%) including verbascoside and its isomer eukovoside and their
   derivatives[2,5,6]
3) Flavonoids including those based on luteolin,
   apigenin, kaempferol, quercetin, diosmetin and
   wogonin[2,3,5,6,8,9]
4) Volatile oil including citral, limolene, cineol
   and β-myrcene[10]

Also contains mucilage, tannins, sterols including
daucosterol[11] and β-sitosterol,[12] triterpenes including ursolic and oleanolic acids[13,14] and fatty acids.[15]

Nutritional constituents
Vitamins: C[16] and β-carotene[17]
Minerals: Rich in minerals especially calcium and
magnesium, also sodium, potassium, iron, copper,
zinc and manganese[18]

Actions
1) Nervine
2) Thymoleptic
3) Diaphoretic
4) Sedative
5) Spasmolytic

Also reputedly a galactagogue.

Scientific information
Verbena is a medicinal herb that enjoyed a great
reputation in the past, being used for a wide
range of health conditions.[19] Although the active
constituents have been investigated in recent
times the pharmacological activity has not and
the herb appears to have lost some of its former
esteem.

Verbena has been part of the medical tradition
of both the East and the West. In Spain the herb
has been used as a topical anti-inflammatory,[20] in
Sicily as a treatment for psoriasis,[21] in Morocco for
hypertension[22] and in China for malaria.

In vitro—Studies that have been conducted
indicate:-

- the essential oil has good anti-oxidant activity[23]
- the herb can moderately inhibit COX-1
  activity.[24] (Animal studies indicate the

herb and/or isolated constituents have
anti-inflammatory activity[12,20] and that the herb
has potential as a neuroprotective agent for
example against Alzheimer's disease.[25])
- the flavonoids have antibacterial activity
  against *Staphylococcus aureus*, *Bacillus subtilis*
  and *Escherichia coli*[26]
- the herb has strong oestrogen and progester-
  one-receptor binding capacity[27] (an early study
  had shown it to be androgenic[1])
- citral, at concentrations equivalent to that
  found in infusions, is apoptotic in several hae-
  mopoietic cancer cell lines[28]

In vivo—An epidemiological study found that
drinking herbal teas, *Verbena* being one commonly
consumed, was inversely related to the incidence
of breast cancer possibly due to the polyphenol
(flavonoids and phenylpropanoids) and/or essential oil content.[29]

Medicinal uses
Cardiovascular system
- fevers (in early stages)
- colds
- influenza

Gastro-intestinal tract
- cholecystalgia
- jaundice

Nervous system
- depression
- melancholia
- epilepsy
- migraine
- hysteria
- convalescence

Reproductive tract
- increase lactation

Pharmacy
Three times daily

Infusion	– 2–4 g
Tincture 1:5 (40%)	– 5–10 ml
Fluid Extract (25%)	– 2–4 ml

Precautions and/or safety

Verbena infusions inhibited iron absorption in an *in vitro* model[30] and an *in vivo* test with a single food source has estimated inhibition of iron up-take to be around 59%.[31] Iron absorption is inhibited by polyphenols but the effect is less than occurs with black tea. The actual inhibition may be altered when taken with complex meals, as occurs in real life.

There is a report of contact dermatitis to the herb.[32]

Historical uses

Abscesses; tumours; sores/wounds—styptic and vulnerary; as an antidote to poisons, haemorrhoids; facial neuralgia; calculus; "cold complaints of the womb", infertility; aphrodisiac; headaches (poultice); rheumatism (external); worms; the plague; mouth ulcers, acute dysentery, enteritis. As a wash for freckles and morphews; to clear eyesight and strengthen it.

Vitex agnus-castus

Chaste tree, agnus-castus

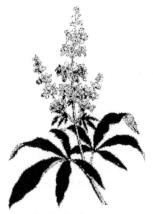

Family Verabenaceae

Description

An aromatic, deciduous shrub or small tree, growing 1–4 × 2 m high with branches that divide frequently at the top. Branches are felted with dense white hairs. *Leaves* are long-stalked, palmate with 5–7 lance-shaped leaflets, green above and felted beneath. *Flowers* grow in long, terminal, interrupted spikes and are small and usually lavender coloured, rarely rose-pink. Corolla 6–9 mm, almost two-lipped, hairy outside. Stamens longer and projecting. Calyx hairy. *Fruits* fleshy and reddish black. Flowers mid to late summer.

Habitat and cultivation

Native to Southern Europe and Western Asia growing in moist, well-drained soil in sheltered, sunny places. Grown from stratified seed or cuttings. Frost resistant, drought tender.

Parts used

The berries harvested when ripe in autumn.

Active constituents

1) Iridoid glycosides including agnuside, aucubin and eurostoside[33]
2) Flavonoids—mainly the tetramethoxyflavone, casticin, also orientin, eupatorin, apigenin, luteolin and penduletin[34-36]
3) Essential oil
   a) monoterpenes—sabinene, 1,8-cineole, β-caryophyllene and farnesene[37]
   b) diterpenes including those of labdane type—vitexlactam, rotundifuran, vitetrifolin B, C and D—and clerodane type[38-41]
   c) sesquiterpenes—spathulenol[35]

Also contains fatty acids including linoleic acid.[42]

Nutritional constituents

Vitamins: C and carotene

Actions

1) Hormone regulator
2) Galactagogue

Vitex has been documented as having emmenagogue, vulnerary, carminative, anthelmintic and anti-inflammatory properties but scientific corroboration of these is lacking.

Scientific information

Various parts of chaste tree have been used medicinally for thousands of years. The fruits in particular, besides being used as a food spice by the monks (hence the name monk's pepper), were believed to ensure celibacy and chastity which would have been an added advantage to them. Unlike *Verbena* the reputation of this herb seems to have grown in recent times making it one of the most commonly used herbs employed for hormonal imbalance. Its primary use today, for menstrual disorders, was however known from ancient Greek times.[43]

There have been a number of studies into its action over the last fifty years and clinical efficacy has resulted in *German Commission E* approving the herb for premenstrual syndrome (PMS), mastalgia and irregular menstruation.

Hormonal
In vitro—The chemistry and pharmacology of *Vitex* is complex but mechanisms thought to contribute to its action include:-

- interaction at dopamine D_2-receptors in the anterior pituitary gland which reduces prolactin levels, is due at least in part to the diterpenes, and is presumed to be the mechanism by which the herb helps with breast discomfort, referred to as mastalgia or mastodynia.[38,44,45] Dopamine agonists have been found empirically to reduce breast pain and heaviness and mood disturbances associated with PMS. (Prolactin is elevated in 70% of women who suffer breast discomfort premenstrually[50])
- interaction with oestrogen receptor (ER) sites[46]—the action appears complex. The whole extract had no binding affinity for ERα[47] although its constituent linoleic acid bound to both ERα and ERβ sites.[42] On the other hand the flavonoids, apigenin and penduletin, have affinity for ERβ receptors—these receptors are involved in fat tissue regulation, prevention of malignant proliferation and may counter ERα activity[38,48]
- may interact at cholinergic receptor sites[49]
- interaction/agonist activity at μ-opiate and possibly other opiate receptor sites.[45] The μ-opiate receptor is mainly activated by β-endorphin, an endogenous peptide, which

helps regulate the menstrual cycle via the hypothalamic- pituitary-adrenal (HPA) axis. The opiate system is also involved in pain perception, mood and appetite regulation and the level of β-endorphin is inversely proportional to the severity of PMS symptoms like abdominal discomfort, anxiety and food cravings.[49]

In vivo–At least 30% of women are considered to experience pre-menstrual problems and according to one set of criteria for about 2.5–3.0% of all women of reproductive age symptoms are severe whilst in 40% they are moderate. The aetiology of PMS symptoms is proposed to be due to one or several of the following factors[50]:-

- low progesterone levels in the luteal phase
- disturbance of aldosterone activity (fluid retention)
- imbalance in HPA axis activity with reduced adrenal hormones
- disturbances in neurotransmitters
- prostaglandin deficiency
- raised levels of prolactin
- nutritional factors e.g. low calcium and magnesium levels, vitamin deficiencies, food intolerance
- stress

Clinical trials into the effects of *Vitex* for hormonally-related problems have so far shown benefit for:-

- moderate to severe PMS[51]
- the majority of symptoms associated with PMS including psychological (anger, irritability, mood alteration, negative feelings) and physical (bloating, headache, breast fullness, pain, fluid retention)[52–55]
- PMDD—Premenstrual dysphoric disorder— effects comparable to fluoxetine, the SSRI being specifically better for psychological symptoms and *Vitex* for physical ones[56]
- cyclical mastalgia[54,57,58]—prolactin level reduction comparable to bromocriptine
- luteal phase defects due to latent hyperprolactinaemia—it reduced prolactin level,

normalised length of the luteal phase and progesterone production[57,59]

- pathologically raised prolactin levels[57]
- infertility—due to secondary amenorrhoea or
luteal insufficiency[60]—*Vitex* raised progesterone levels, lengthened duration of raised basal
temperature in the luteal-phase and normalised the length of both long and short cycles[61]
- menopausal hot flushes and night sweats—
Vitex was one herb in a combination. There
were no adverse changes to hormone levels,
vaginal tissues or liver function[62]

A number of clinical trials conducted some decades
ago reported that *Vitex* benefited acne vulgaris,[63,64]
premenstrual fluid retention,[65] amenorrhoea[66] and
increased lactation.[67] There are also anecdotal
reports of the herb reducing prolactin levels caused
by pituitary micro-adenomas.[68,69]

Based on measurements in healthy men it
seems that the dose of *Vitex* used can vary the
response of prolactin secretion (biphasic)—levels
were increased slightly at low doses of *Vitex* but
decreased slightly at higher doses.[70] Furthemore
these changes were larger the higher the base level
of prolactin prior to dosing.[70]

Other
In vitro—Both water and ethanol extracts of *Vitex*
are significantly anti-oxidant, the flavonoids were
not considered to be wholly responsible for this
activity.[35,71]

Extracts have antitumour and antiproliferative
activity in a number of fast growing or cancer cell
lines including gastric,[72] prostate,[73] breast,[74] ovary,[75]
colon[75] and lung.[75] This action does not seem to be
specific for cancer cells however,[75] affecting other
relatively fast growing cell lines and indicating a
potential use of the herb in the treatment of benign
prostatic hyperplasia.[73]

In vivo—Melatonin levels were increased in
healthy men in a dose-dependent manner by *Vitex*
although the actual circadian rhythm of secretion
was unaffected.[76]

Sprays made from the berries had good insecticide properties against fleas, mosquitoes, flies and
ticks.[77]

Medicinal uses
Reproductive tract
Vitex is used almost exclusively in women as a hor-
mone balancer for:

- amenorrhoea, secondary
- metrorrhagia
- oligomenorrhoea
- infertility
- menopausal symptoms
- menorrhagia
- polymenorrhoea
- cyclical mastalgia
- premenstrual syndrome
- to help regulate menstrual cycle on cessation of
contraceptive pill

Its indications include any condition that subsided
in pregnancy and returned at the cessation of breast
feeding or any premenstrual aggravation.

Skin
- acne (70% improvement in 3 months)

This effect may be due to an anti-androgenic action.
It is useful for teenage acne in both sexes.

Pharmacy
Three times daily
Decoction   – 0.2–2 g
    The daily dose that follows may be effectively
taken as a single dose before breakfast.
    Tincture 1:5 (25%)–1–3 ml (20–60 drops).
    Alternatively the weekly dose may be given in
equal doses, three times a day.
    Vitex used in the above trials were standardised
on casticin and represented the equivalent of
120–480 mg of herb daily.
    The study on prolactin changes in men used a
low dose of 120 mg and high dose of 480 mg.

Precautions and/or safety
All the above clinical trials report good tolerance to
the herb. Although most trials on PMS measured
improvements after 3 cycles, these can be expected
to occur sooner than that. In the one study that

used a 3 cycle treatment protocol with follow-up carried out 3 cycles after cessation of *Vitex*, symptoms had returned to around 22% below where they were before *Vitex* was used.[53]

In spite of the herb's ability to reduce prolactin levels it is not contra-indicated in lactation and in fact studies have supported its use for improving milk flow, a process governed by prolactin. The biphasic response to *Vitex* may explain this anomaly or it may be due to mechanism(s) not yet understood.

Side-effects that have been reported include nausea, headache, itching, erythema, gastro-intestinal disturbances, depression, fatigue, breast pain, menstrual disorders and acne.[51,78] They are however infrequent, mild and reversible. Large doses should be avoided although no toxicity due to overdose has been reported.

There is one report of mild ovarian hyperstimulation syndrome attributed to the use of *Vitex* in a woman undergoing unstimulated *in-vitro* fertilisation treatment[79] and one of arteriospasm.[78]

Interactions

No interactions have been reported in the extensive testing that has been done to-date although a theoretical interaction has been suggested between *Vitex* and dopaminergic antagonists.[78]

Some of the clinical trials on PMS included women using contraceptive pills (unspecified type) as the latter do not always improve these symptoms. No interactions have been reported from using the two concomitantly.[52,53]

Historical uses

To curb sexual desire; inflammation, injuries; animal bites, an enlarged spleen; inflamed uterus. Paralysis; pains in the limbs; weakness.

VIOLACEAE

This family contains herbs, shrubs and trees which usually have alternate, simple and stipulate leaves.

- The flowers are solitary, axillary or in racemes
- There are five free sepals, and five free petals, equal or unequal, the lowest sometimes spurred
- There are 5 stamens, united at the base into a ring
- The ovary consists of 3 fused carpels
- The fruit is a capsule dehiscing by 3 valves, or an indehiscent berry

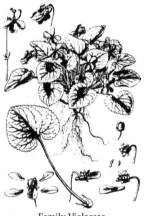

Family Violaceae

Viola odorata

Sweet violet

Description

A rhizomatous perennial forming a rosette of dark green, long stemmed, finely hairy, ovate-cordate leaves, with up to 15 crenations each side. Leaf stems may be from less than 5 to more than 10 cm long. *Flowers* sweetly fragrant, 1.5–2.5 mm across with 5 violet, blue, white or pink petals longer than the sepals, with a spur 3–5 mm long. Sepals green, narrowly oblong. *Capsule* globose, hairy, about 1 cm long. Flowers from spring to autumn.

Habitat and cultivation

Native to Europe, Asia Minor and North West Africa and grown worldwide from seed or rooted stolons. Prefers winter sun and summer shade growing well under deciduous trees in slightly acid soils. Removing stolons encourages flowers. Frost resistant, drought tender.

Parts used

Leaves and flowers harvested at, or just prior to, flowering.

Active constituents

1) Saponins
2) Phenolic glycosides including methyl salicylate
3) Alkaloids including odoratine
4) Essential oil consisting largely of aliphatic hydrocarbons[1]
5) Flavonoids including rutin

Also β-nitroproprionic acid,[2] mucilage[3] and cyclotides of which at least 13 have been isolated and sequenced. Cyclotides are cyclic peptides containing between 28–37 amino acids with a peptide backbone and residues of cysteine which cross-link to create a cystine knot, their make-up varies seasonally.[4-6] Cyclotides have been found in members of the Violiaceae family as well as in the Rubiaceae and Curcubitaceae.

Nutritional constituents

Vitamins: A and C

Actions

1) Laxative
2) Expectorant
3) Antineoplastic

Scientific information

Although a medicinal plant of long standing there is very little current research into the herb apart from the discovery of the cyclotides. Sweet violet has had a reputation as an anticancer herb, particularly recommended for breast and gastrointestinal cancers, and may also have some protection against metastases (*BHP*). It was used both internally and externally to treat malignancies.

In vitro—The herb has good activity against *Trichomonas vaginalis*,[7] *Staphylococcus aureus*, *Pseudomonas aeruginosa*, *Shigella flexeri*, *Salmonella typhimurium*, *S.typhi* and *Escherichia coli*.[8]

The cyclotides are currently attracting interest as they have a variety of pharmacological activities[5,9] including:-

- cytotoxicity to a range of cancer cell lines
- antimicrobial including against HIV
- insecticidal
- haemolytic

Unlike other peptides they are stable to chemical, heat and enzyme degradation and therefore have great medicinal potential however the extent to which they contribute to the activity of *V. odorata in vivo* is still to be established.

In vivo—*V. odorata* oil was an effective insect repellent and feeding deterrent to mosquitoes.[10]

Medicinal uses

Respiratory tract

- bronchitis
- pulmonary congestion
- dry coughs
- chronic nasopharyngeal catarrh

Pharmacy

Three times daily

Infusion of dried herb	– 2–4 g
Tincture 1:5 (25%)	– 2–5 ml (suggested guidelines)
Fluid Extract (25%)	– 2–4 ml

Historical uses

To moderate anger; insomnia; to comfort and strengthen the heart; gout; laxative; epilepsy; ague; inflammation of eyes and female reproductive tract; pleurisy; jaundice; quinsy; TB; headache due to insomnia/tiredness; epilepsy; kidney and bladder problems; all conditions of head. Internally and externally for cancer; pain in throat cancer; tongue cancer. Externally for swellings; inflammations; piles; bruises.

Viola tricolor

Heartsease, wild pansy

Description

An annual growing from a short-lived rosette. *Stems* erect or ascending to 7–30 cm tall, angular, soft and branching, short haired or glabrous. *Leaves* 2–4 cm

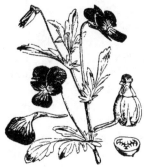

Family Violaceae

long with 3–7 crenations or blunt teeth each side. Basal leaves alternate, broadly ovate, narrowed to a long petiole, with short, linear lobed stipules. Stem leaves becoming narrow-elliptic with uppermost leaves wedge-shaped. *Flowers* solitary in leaf axils, 1.5–2.5 cm wide. Petals violet, blue and/or yellow and cream, spur 3–4 mm long. Sepals narrowly triangular, 5–8 mm long. *Capsule* ellipsoid, glabrous, 5–10 mm long. Flowers and fruits from spring to autumn.

Habitat and cultivation
Native to Eurasia, naturalised elsewhere. Grows from seed and self-sows in a light soil and sunny places. Disappears in hot weather and reappears with autumn rain and cooler temperatures. It transplants easily. Frost resistant, drought tender.

Parts used
The aerial parts harvested at, or just prior to, flowering.

Active constituents
1) Flavonoids including the derivative of apigenin—violanthin also violaquercitrin and rutin[11]
2) Saponins[11]
3) Alkaloids
4) Mucilage (10%)[11]
5) Phenolic acids[12] including salicylates (0.3%)[11]

Also cyclotides similar to *V. odorata*,[13] carotenoids including violaxanthin,[14-16] anthocyanins,[17,18] tannins[11] and coumarins.[11]

Nutritional constituents
Vitamins: C and E[11]

Actions
1) Anti-inflammatory
2) Expectorant
3) Diuretic
4) Antirheumatic
5) Laxative

Scientific information
The medicinal uses of heartsease were much broader in the past than they are today and the herb was at one time an official medicine in the *United States Pharmacopoeia*. Various European traditions have also used *V. tricolor* for the treatment of cancer,[19] atherosclerosis[20] and psoriasis.[21]

Like *V. odorata* there has not been much modern research other than interest in the cyclic peptides, the cyclotides.

In vitro—It has antimicrobial activity against a range of Gram-positive and Gram-negative bacteria, with good activity against *Staphylococcus aureus*, *S. epidermidis*, *Bacillus cereus* and also against the fungal pathogen *Candida albicans*.[12] The constituents of the herb act synergistically to give the whole extract a better antimicrobial action than isolated fractions.[12] Extracts also have significant anti-inflammatory (comparable to diclofenac)[22] and anti-oxidant activity.[23]

The cyclotides are structurally like those of *V. odorata* and they also display cytotoxicity and a strong activity against myeloma and lymphoma cancer cell lines.[13] Cyclotides have other pharmacological actions[24]—see *V. odorata*.

In vivo—an ointment containing *Mahonia aquifolium*, *Centella asiatica* and *V. tricolor* was used to treat adult atopic eczema without a clear benefit.[25]

Medicinal uses
Cardiovascular system
The flavonoids must contribute to its use for:

- capillary fragility

Respiratory tract
- acute bronchitis
- pertussis

Urinary tract
- dysuria
- polyuria
- cystitis

Musculoskeletal
- rheumatism

Skin
It has proved beneficial used both internally and externally (as a compress) for:

- eczema
- cradle cap
- tuberculous skin conditions
- cutaneous eruptions especially in children

Pharmacy
Three times daily
Infusion   – 2–4 g
Tincture 1:5 (25%)   – 2–5   ml   (suggested guidelines)
Fluid Extract (25%)   – 2–4 ml

Precautions and/or safety
Large doses can apparently cause nausea and/or vomiting.[11] There is a documented case of an infant with a glucose-6-phosphate-dehydrogenase deficiency developing haemolysis after been given a tea made from the herb.[26]

Historical uses
Convulsions and fits of epilepsy; insomnia; asthma; inflammations of lungs and breast; pleurisy; scabs; itch; French-pox; heart diseases; ague.

ZINGIBERACEAE

The Zingiberaceae or Ginger family are monocotyledons. The family consists of about 40 genera of rhizomatous herbs growing throughout the tropics.

- Stems are usually erect or cane-like, growing in clumps
- Leaves are elongate, entire, with parallel or pinnate veins, with the base partly or completely sheathing the stem
- Inflorescence is a head, spike or panicle either on a separate stalk or terminating a leafy stem
- Flowers are irregular, calyx and corolla tubular, each 3-lobed, and 1 fertile stamen enfolding the style

Medicinal and culinary plants of the Zingiberaceae include the genera *Alpinia, Amomum, Curcuma, Elettaria* and *Zingiber*.

Zingiber officinale

Ginger

Description
A herbaceous perennial monocotyledon, ginger grows to about 1 m rising from a coarse, irregular,

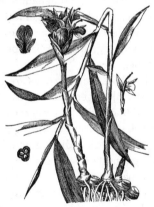

Family Zingiberaceae

tuberous rhizome. *Stems* are smooth and reed-like with alternate light green leaves, 20 × 2 cm sheathing the stem. *Flowers* are borne in spikes on shorter leafless stems about 30 cm tall. The spike consists of numerous greenish-yellow imbricated bracts from behind which the flowers are produced. They are not numerous, and are yellow speckled with purplish dots and generally have a purple lip. *Fruit* is an oblong capsule which breaks open irregularly.

Odour—characteristic and aromatic; taste—pungent and aromatic.

451

Habitat and cultivation

Native of tropical Asia and widely cultivated in other tropical areas. Grown from division of the rhizomes in rich, moist soil and semi-shade. Drought and frost tender.

Parts used

The rhizome is harvested after the plant dies back and used fresh or dried. There are a number of main cultivars of *Z. officinale* used medicinally and 2 other morphologically similar species, *Z. zerumbet* and *Z. cassumunar*, that are sometimes used as "adulterants" of *Z. officinale*.[1]

Active constituents

1) Volatile oil (1–4%). At least 54 constituents have been identified comprising mono- and sesquiterpenes. Although the composition can vary its main constituents usually include α-zingiberene, ar-curcumene, β-sesquiphellandrene, β-phellandrene, β-bisabolene, camphene and geranial.[2-7] These are responsible for the aroma of the herb[4]

2) Phenolics which give the herb its pungency[8,9] and include:

   a) arylalkanones the main ones are gingerols of which [6]-gingerol is the most abundant (around 6%)[10] with [8]-gingerol and [10]-gingerol, shogaols[11,12] including [6]-shogaol also paradols, gingediols, gingediacetates, gingerdiones, gingerenones and zingerones[11-17]

   b) phenylpropanoids including diarylheptanoids of which at least 26 have been identified[18,19]

   c) phenolic acids including syringic, gallic, cinnamic, vanillic and ferulic acids[20,21]

Zingiber's oleoresin accounts for between 4–8% of the crude herb and is made up of approximately 25% volatile oil, 33% phenolics,[22] fats and waxes.

Also contains proteases including zingibain,[23,24] steroids,[9] starch,[25] indolic compounds (melatonin, tryptamine and serotonin),[26,27] flavonoids,[28] saponins, alkaloids, lipids (9%)[29] and small amounts of salicylate.[30]

Cultivars may differ in their relative content of active constituents[31] and geographical origin, method of processing, analytical procedure and freshness of starting material can affect the final chemical make-up.[4,32-35] Although the quantitative chemistry of constituents within the species varies with genetic origin the qualitative make-up is apparently quite consistent.[8,36,37] On the other hand the different species are qualitatively different and therefore distinguishable.[36]

Fresh and dried ginger—The essential oil content does not differ very markedly between dried and fresh ginger[38] and the gingerols are still the predominant pungent constituents in the dried form.[16] The shogaols are produced from dehydration of their corresponding gingerols as *Zingiber* is dried, heat-processed or stored long-term, [6]-shogaol forms from [6]-gingerol and so on through the series.[12,39] Shogaols are not present to any extent in the fresh material[37] but their level increases in dried ginger as the level of gingerols decrease.[11] Once extracted both constituents are relatively stable by avoiding high temperatures. *In vitro* models found that in conditions that reflect the pH and temperature found in the stomach [6]-shogaol may be substantially converted back to [6]-gingerol.[39]

On storage the content of ar-curcumene increases whilst zingiberene and β-sesquiphellandrene decrease.[22]

Nutritional constituents

Vitamins: A, B-complex and C
Minerals: Calcium, iron, phosphorus, sodium, potassium and magnesium[40]

Actions

1) Carminative
2) Anti-emetic
3) Spasmolytic
4) Peripheral circulatory stimulant
5) Anti-inflammatory
6) Diaphoretic

Scientific information

Ginger has been used for over 2500 years as a medicine and spice and the demand for it today is high as it is not only valued for these purposes but is also used in the cosmetic industry. It is one of the most widely used food spices in the world and is a frequent constituent of Chinese and Ayurvedic formulations. The name ginger derives from the Sanskrit word *"sringavera"* (relating to the shape of the root) which was transformed to the English name "ginger".[41]

It has been and is still an official preparation in a number of pharmacopoeias worldwide[42] and is approved in Germany by *Commission E* for the treatment of dyspepsia and to prevent motion sickness. Much of the research into the herb has been conducted over the last 50 years.

[6]-gingerol, as ginger's main constituent, has been particularly well studied, however at least 400 constituents have been characterised from the extract, many of them are pharmacologically active and no doubt they also have synergistic actions that contribute to the herb's overall actions.[43]

About 80% of the world production of ginger comes from China.

Anti-oxidant

In vitro—The herb as well as more than 50 of its individual constituents[44] have very good anti-oxidant and radical scavenging activity[17,18,45-52] including against nitric oxide[53] and lipid peroxidation.[44,54-57] It appears likely that after absorption through the gastro-intestinal tract this antioxidant activity is retained though possibly at a reduced level.[58]

Zingiber has displayed cell protecting activity for a range of different cell types and this may be due, wholly or in part, to its anti-oxidant potential. Although most studies used animal models[51] it did also protect human red blood cells from the toxic effect of parabens (p-hydroxybenzoic acid).[59]

Anti-inflammatory

In vitro—The gingerols, shogaols and paradols have been credited with many of ginger's anti-inflammatory properties[60] although the full extent of actions and constituents responsible still remain to be uncovered. It is very likely that the constituents act synergistically to produce this activity.[36]

Mechanisms behind the anti-inflammatory action are likely to include:-

- strong inhibition of COX-1 and COX-2 enzymes with reduced production of prostaglandins and thromboxanes from arachidonic acid.[16,60-63] Ginger and to a lesser extent individual phenolic constituents reduce COX-2 synthesis in addition to inhibiting its activity[64]
- inhibition of 5-LOX and the metabolism of arachidonic acid to leucotrienes[63,65]
- antioxidant—oxidation may help fuel inflammatory reactions[71]
- blocking of various inducers of genes coding for pro-inflammatory cytokines—this was demonstrated in synoviocytes from osteoarthritic joints.[66,67] (The action of the herb on some cytokine production may be complex, in one study it was biphasic—augmenting cytokine production at low concentration, inhibiting it at higher levels. In addition augmentation increased over time, after initial ginger exposure)[68]
- agonist action at vanilloid receptor sites TRPV1 (see *Capsicum*)—some of the gingerols and shogaols, particularly [6]- and [8]-gingerol, have a vanillyl moiety that behaves like capsaicin (See *Capsicum*) although they are less potent[69,70]

(Dual inhibition of COX and LOX reduces the potential for side-effects and should make the anti-inflammatory activity more effective[71,72]).

Ginger combined with galangal (*Alpinia galangal*) inhibits gene-induced inflammatory cytokine production in cells similar to microglial cells, suggesting a possible protective effect against inflammation-induced neurodegenerative diseases.[73]

[6]-gingerol can permeate through epidermal tissue to some extent.[74] It inhibits UVB-induced COX-2 activity (so may be photo-protective)[75] and increases anti-inflammatory enzyme activity in prostate cells.[76]

In vivo—There are not many clinical trials assessing the anti-inflammatory effects of ginger. Early studies on its use to treat arthritis, both osteo- and rheumatoid, had found it was beneficial in reducing pain and swelling being especially useful for discomfort in muscles.[71,77] More recently it improved arthritis of the knee joint (gonarthritis) after 6 months use.[78]

Other reported trials have used *Zingiber* in combination with various herbs. Combinations with *A. galangal*[79] and with *Withania somnifera, Boswellia serrata* and *Curcuma longa*[80] both produced symptomatic improvement in osteoarthritis of the knee. The ginger/galangal combination used for a three week period to treat osteoarthritis of hip or knee though beneficial was less effective than ibuprofen.[81]

Anti-emetic

Although the anti-emetic property of ginger was used traditionally and is one of the modern uses to be officially endorsed in Germany,[82] the mechanisms behind this action are not fully understood. The active constituents for anti-emesis appear to be the main gingerols and [6]-shogaol and probably some of the other more minor arylalkanones.[83,84] Proposed mechanisms are largely based on investigations using animal models and include[83]:-

- a central mechanism—this does not seem very likely as ginger has no effect on vestibular optokinetic nystagmus[85] and it does not cause drowsiness like other centrally-acting anti-emetics[86]
- inhibition of neurotransmitters known to induce nausea—serotonin,[83,87] neurokinin,[83] acetylcholine and/or histamine.[88] 5-HT$_3$ receptors are involved in acute nausea/vomiting and neurokinin receptors are involved in delayed and acute nausea/vomiting, chemotherapy induces both neurotransmitters[89]
- by increasing gastro-intestinal motility and reducing feedback to central chemo-receptors—motion sickness slows gastric emptying and alters gastric motility.[90] *In vivo* ginger has been shown to increase gastro-duodenal motility in a fasting state and after a meal[91] but does not increase the rate of gastric emptying[90,92]

- prevention of gastric dysrhythmia and raised levels of vasopressin[93]—both events occur in motion sickness.[88]

In vivo—Ginger has been used in clinical trials to treat nausea of varying origin.

It has been well tested for alleviating nausea in early pregnancy as at this stage it is possible to avoid progression to hyperemesis gravidarum.[94] It was effective to varying degrees for the treatment of both nausea and vomiting in early pregnancy[95–98] being as good as, or better than vitamin B6[99–101] and as effective as dimenhydrinate with fewer side effects.[102] It was also an effective treatment for hyperemesis gravidarum.[103]

In post-operative nausea and vomiting it gave inconsistent results with some studies showing a positive benefit[104–109] and others showing no improvement compared to placebo.[110–114,124]

For nausea due to chemotherapy ginger was effective as a prophylactic[115] with fewer side-effects than conventional anti-emetics.[116]

In assessing ginger's efficacy in treating motion sickness (kinetosis), most studies used a simulator to induce the condition. *Zingiber* preparations gave a range of results from lack of effect[90,117] to effects superior to dimenhydrinate[118] and placebo.[93] It reduced nausea, prolonged time to its onset and shortened recovery time after motion ceased.[93] In actual sea travel it was beneficial as a prophylactic.[119,120]

In artificial stimulation of the vestibular system ginger reduced the symptoms of vertigo but it did not prevent nystagmus.[85,121]

Across these anti-emetic studies of varying aetiology results have been somewhat variable, but reviewers have, in the main, concluded that ginger is both effective and safe.[122–128]

Cancer

Anti-oxidant and anti-inflammatory agents are believed to help prevent the development of cancer and ginger has shown good activity in both of these areas.[49,51,76]

In vitro—In addition ginger and/or its constituents inhibit the growth of a number of cancer cell lines including some that have become drug-resistant (DR). Those found to be susceptible include ovary,[129] colorectal,[130] prostate,[131] breast,[132,133] gastric,[134] laryngeal,[135] liver (DR),[136] pancreas (DR),[137] leukaemia,[51,138,139] oral squamous[140] and lung.[141]

The mechanism of direct anticancer activity is multi-factorial, occurring through a variety of biochemical pathways, and includes enhanced apoptosis,[132–135,138,140,141] cell cycle arrest[130,133,134,137,142] and chemoprevention.[131,143–146] The extract and/or constituents may also have some benefit in halting metastatic spread of the disease by modulating angiogenesis[129,142,147] and reducing cell motility and adhesion.[133]

[6]-gingerol increases the uptake of chemotherapeutic agents in cancer cells which have become drug resistant by increasing their transport into cells using P-glycoprotein.[148]

In vivo—There are no trials using ginger in cancer treatment however a diet rich in phenolics is linked epidemiologically with a lower risk of cancer development and ginger contains a high proportion of these constituents.[149]

Circulation

Although ginger is a traditional herb for stimulating circulation there is an absence of relevant research in humans into possible mechanisms.

In vitro—*Zingiber* protected endothelial cells from monocyte adhesion, a process involved in inflammation and atheroma formation.[150] Many of the arylalkanone constituents and ginger itself have strong antiplatelet activity through inhibition of arachidonic acid metabolism to thromboxane, prostaglandin and prostaglandin-endoperoxides in platelets.[61,151,152,220]

In vivo—Heart disease is related to arterial inflammation which occurs via arachidonic acid metabolism and ginger could therefore be beneficial.[153]

Studies have been mainly concerned with the effect of the herb on platelet activity and they have not been conclusive. Concomitant consumption of fat and 5 g of ginger in normal healthy people countered the decreased fibrinolytic activity which occurred with fat intake alone[154,155] and a single dose of 10 g[156] or 5 g ginger daily for a week[157] inhibited platelet aggregation. There is also an

anecdotal account of a patient with a high platelet count being given ginger powder with beneficial results.[158]

However, regular daily ginger at a lower dose (4 g), taken over three months, did not affect platelet aggregation, fibrinolytic activity, fibrinogen or lipid levels in coronary artery disease patients[156] and in young healthy adults 15 g raw or 40 g of cooked ginger daily for 2 weeks did not significantly change their thromboxane levels.[159]

Although the herb has a traditional use in the Indian sub-continent for the treatment of hypertension there are no studies reporting the effect of ginger on blood pressure.

Antimicrobial

In vitro—A range of antimicrobial activity has been shown for the extract and/or the essential oil including:-

- virucidal for HSV-1,[160] HSV-2,[161] rhinovirus 1B[162] and hepatitis C virus[163]
- antibacterial to *Staphylococcus aureus, Bacillus cereus, B.subtilis, Listeria monocytogenes, Proteus mirabilis, Vibrio parahaemolyticus, Pseudomonas aeruginosa, Escherichia coli, Salmonella typhimurium, Streptococcus pyogenes, S. pneumoniae, Haemophilus influenzae, Campylobacter jejuni*[164–172] and as many as 19 strains of *Helicobacter pylori*.[21,173–177] In addition ginger and [10]-gingerol can act synergistically with some antibiotics against resistant strains of bacteria[166,173,178]
- antimycobacterial including against *Mycobacterium tuberculosis*[179]
- antifungal including against *Candida albicans, Aspergillus niger, Cryptococcus neoformans* and *Trichophyton mentagrophytes*[170,180,181]
- antiparasitic against *Schistosoma mansoni* (although the *in vivo* activity is uncertain)[182,183] and against the larvae of the fish borne nematode *Anisakis*[184]
- molluscicidal against the snail vector of *Schistosoma* transmission[183]

Other
In vitro—Other activities that have been established for ginger and/or its constituents include:

- a unique specificity of the proteases which are more effective than papain[23]
- good inhibition of the enzyme aldose reductase which may play a part in the tissue damage caused by diabetes[185]
- protection of neurones from the effect of β-amyloid, the protein implicated in Alzheimer's disease[186]
- some phyto-oestrogenic activity[187]
- stimulation of TRPA1 receptors which perceive a burning sensation and are activated by the inflammatory peptide bradykinin[188]
- immuno-suppressive activity reducing lymphocyte proliferation via decreased production of cytokines but the significance of this *in vivo* is uncertain[189]
- potential as a protective agent against ulcers, gastritis and gastric cancer associated with bacterial infection[177]

In vivo—Zingerone appears to be a nerve irritant that on repeated exposure causes desensitization to oral trigeminal nerve chemoreceptors, a pattern of perception that is qualitatively similar to but milder than capsaicin.[190,191]

Zingiber reduces artificially-induced stress responses in healthy volunteers as measured by ACTH and cortisol levels.[192] Other *in vivo* studies have shown:-

- in spite of its reputation as an antidiabetic herb in some traditions ginger taken daily for 3 months did not reduce blood sugar in patients with coronary artery disease.[156] However GI dysrhythmia in healthy volunteers due to hyperglycaemia was reduced by it, through reduced endogenous prostaglandin synthesis, and the herb may therefore reduce gastro-intestinal discomfort normally experienced by diabetics[193]
- a combined preparation of feverfew and ginger was an effective treatment for migraine headaches when taken in the mild phase[194]

- ginger, as part of a Japanese herbal combination, reduced levels of Immunoglobulin E in the sera of sufferers of refractory atopic dermatitis[195,196]
- a herbal combination which included *Zingiber* as well as gallic acid was ineffective in reducing body weight and food intake in healthy overweight people.[197,198] Unlike *Capsicum*, *Zingiber* has not been shown to increase postprandial metabolic rate[198]

Inconsistencies in pharmacological activity and clinical outcomes of ginger could be attributed to variability in both manufactured and raw ginger products,[12,43] dosage/dosage-regime differences and lack of a standardised test product. Gingerol content for example was found to vary widely amongst manufactured ginger products.[12,199] Standardisation of ginger however would present problems as there are so many active constituents.

Medicinal uses
Cardiovascular system
- cold extremities
- poor peripheral circulation

Respiratory tract
Some of the volatile oil components appear to be excreted through the lungs and would have an effect on:

- bronchitis
- common cold

Gastro-intestinal tract
- nausea and vomiting
- flatulence
- colic
- anorexia
- atonic dyspepsia especially in the elderly

Taken prophylactically it may help nausea induced by chemotherapy.

Reproductive tract
- dysmenorrhoea
- amenorrhoea

Musculoskeletal
- arthritis
- rheumatism

Pharmacy
Three times daily
Infusion of dried powdered – 0.25–1 g
rhizome
Infusion of fresh herb (grated) – 0.3–3 g
Weak Tincture BP (1973)   – 1.5–3 ml
Strong Tincture BP (1973)   – 0.25–0.5 ml

The 1:5 tincture is referred to as "Weak" and the 1:2 as "Strong" ginger tincture. 70% ethanol content has been determined as the most effective extracting medium.[200]

As an anti-emetic effective doses have ranged from the equivalent of 1–6 g powdered rhizome daily. In the study on prevention of seasickness 500 mg gave 4 hours of protection.[119]

Precautions and/or safety
Safety data on the herb indicate that it is safe to use in pregnancy.[95,98,201] In general ginger appears to be safe even at doses of up to 6 g daily.[124] Some studies have monitored the effects of its continuous use over 2.5 years and found no serious side effects.[77]

Standard *in vitro* assays showed ginger is not genotoxic[202] and actually protects DNA from damage by known carcinogens.[203,204] However there are contradictory reports on both its mutagenic and anti-mutagenic potential.[205-208]

Reported side-effects are rare and minor and include mild gastro-intestinal symptoms—heartburn, nausea, flatulence, mild diarrhoea—and also sleepiness.[81,124] Although uncommon it is possible some people may develop contact dermatitis from handling ginger[209,210] or asthma from inhalation of its dust.[211]

Ginger is assumed to increase bleeding due to its antiplatelet activity. *In vivo* doses of up to 4 g of the herb taken daily for 3 months did not alter any of the factors associated with platelet function.[156,212]

Consumption of more than 6 g of ginger as a single dose may be associated with increased sloughing of gastric epithelial cells.[213]

Interactions
In vitro—The increased uptake of chemotherapeutic drugs and their reduced transport out of cancer cells by P-glycoprotein has raised the possibility of a potential interaction between ginger and drugs transported in this way.[148]

The ginger/galangal combination modulates the expression of CYP1A2 and CYP3A4 and the transporter protein MDR1.[214]

In vivo—[6]-gingerol was estimated to be two- to four-fold less active than aspirin in terms of its effect on inhibiting platelet aggregation.[215] An increased risk of bleeding in patients who use ginger whilst taking warfarin is generally expected[216] however a study of healthy subjects taking a single dose of warfarin and ginger together found no interaction in terms of pharmacokinetics (metabolism) or pharmacodynamics (physiological effects).[217,218] A literature search failed to find evidence of interactions.[219]

Ginger (1 gm daily) used with **nifedipine** in normal and hypertensive patients synergistically inhibited platelet aggregation in a manner similar to low dose aspirin (75 mg daily).[220]

There is one report in the literature of an interaction between **phenprocoumon** and ginger in an elderly patient resulting in a raised INR and epistaxis.[221]

Historical uses
The herb has a long history of use in China. The fresh rhizome is used to treat vomiting; coughs; abdominal distension and pyrexia. The dried rhizome for abdominal pain; lumbago and diarrhoea. Also used for alcoholic gastritis; diarrhoea due to relaxed bowel. Hot infusion for restarting menstruation halted due to cold. Also for cataracts, toothache, insomnia, baldness, haemorrhoids and to increase longevity.

Abortifacient: an agent which causes expulsion of the foetus

Acetylcholinesterase: the enzyme that metabolises acetylcholine a neurotransmitter responsible for many biochemical activities. A deficit of the transmitter can reduce memory function and inhibiting its enzymic breakdown is one approach used to treat Alzheimer's disease

Adaptogen: an agent which helps the body accommodate to stress or change from any source

Aglycone: molecule after the glycoside or sugar group has been removed

Alterative: an agent used to improve elimination of metabolic waste and in so doing restores normal body functions

Analgesic: an agent used to relieve pain, it can be administered orally or topically

Anaphrodisiac: an agent used to lessen sexual function and desire

Angiogenesis: the growth of new blood vessels, apart from its natural occurrence as part of maturation it also occurs during wound healing and metastatic tumour growth

Anhidrotic: an agent that reduces sweating

Anodyne: an agent used to soothe or ease pain

Antacid: an agent used to neutralise acid in the stomach

Anthelmintic: an agent used to expel or destroy parasitic worms in the gastro-intestinal tract

Anti-arthritic: an agent used to relieve and heal arthritic conditions

Anticancer: an agent that reduces the viability of cancer cells

Anticarcinogenic: an agent that reduces the frequency of occurrence of spontaneous or induced cancers

Anticatarrhal: an agent which reduces catarrh or excessive mucus secretion

Anticoagulant: an agent which slows or prevents clotting of blood

Antidote: an agent which counteracts or neutralises poison

Antilithic: an agent used to prevent the formation of calculi (stones) or gravel which can occur in the urinary system or gall bladder

Antimitotic: an agent which inhibits the division of cells i.e. mitosis

Antineoplastic: an agent that inhibits or destroys tumours

Antipyretic: an agent which prevents or reduces fevers

Antiscorbutic: an agent which prevents or cures scurvy

Antioxidant: an agent that prevents oxidation a process believed to be the initiating factor in the development of many disease conditions such as cancer and heart disease

Antiproliferative: an agent that inhibits cell or tissue growth

Antiseptic: an agent used to prevent, resist and counteract infection

Antispasmodic: an agent used to reduce or prevent excessive involuntary muscular contractions or spasms

Antisudorific: an agent which stops or prevents sweating

Antitussive: an agent which relieves or reduces coughing

Aperient: an agent which acts as a mild laxative

Aphrodisiac: an agent used to stimulate sexual interest

Apoptosis: a process of programmed cell death that occurs naturally. If defective it can lead to disease conditions i.e. its failure to occur is associated with the development of cancer whereas if it occurs excessively it can cause hypotrophy

Aquaretic: an agent that increases urine output by increasing renal blood flow and glomerular filtration without the accompanying loss of electrolytes

Astringent: an agent that contracts tissue, making them firmer and reducing their discharges

Asthenospermia: loss of or reduced sperm motility

Bacteriostatic: an agent that inhibits the growth or proliferation of bacteria without necessarily killing them

Bitter: an agent that has a bitter taste but also promotes digestive function and improves appetite

Bronchodilator: an agent which increases the diameter of the respiratory airways

Cardio-active: an agent which acts on the heart

Cardiotonic: an agent which has a beneficial action on the heart

Carminative: an agent which improves digestion and relieves the discomfort of flatulence and/or colic

Cathartic: an agent which causes evacuation of the bowels

Cholagogue: an agent which stimulates or aids the release of bile from the gall bladder

Choleretic: an agent which stimulates the production of bile in the liver

Co-mutagen: an agent that is not mutagenic itself but may become so in conjunction with other agents

Counter-irritant: an agent which when applied topically increases local circulation. It is used for the temporary relief of a deep seated painful irritation

Creatine kinase: an enzyme involved in regulation of energy in cells, it uses creatine to store energy from ATP. Levels may be elevated in pathologies like cancer due to increased energy demand so that its inhibition may constitute a therapeutic approach to disease

Cytotoxic: an agent that is toxic to cells causing their death

Demulcent: an agent that is used internally to sooth and protect irritated tissues and surfaces

De-obstruent: an agent that removes obstructions from the body by improving the normal channels of elimination

Depurative: an agent which promotes the natural channels of elimination

Desmutagen: an agent that reduces the damage caused to DNA by a mutagen

Diaphoretic: an agent that increases perspiration and elimination through the skin, often used to reduce temperature in fevers

Diuretic: an agent that increases the production and flow of urine

Dyssomnia: sleep disorder affecting the ability to go to sleep or stay asleep

Dysthymia: defined as a chronic mood disorder, manifesting as depression alternating with feeling normal

Emetic: an agent that induces vomiting

Enterotoxin: an agent that is toxic in the gastrointestinal tract and may cause vomiting, abdominal pain and/or diarrhoea

Elastase: the enzyme responsible for breaking down elastic fibres, it is implicated in tissue damage associated with chronic inflammation

Emmenagogue: an agent that promotes menstruation

Emollient: an agent that softens, soothes and protects the skin

Enterohepatic cycling: the process in which metabolites that are initially absorbed from the intestine, pass to the liver for subsequent excretion in bile and are then re-absorbed for a second time from the gastro-intestinal tract. Such a process results in plasma levels for that substance showing two peaks separated by a time interval. It occurs regularly with respect to bile salts and can occur with extraneous metabolites

Expectorant: an agent which promotes the removal of excess mucus from the lungs and air passages

Febrifuge: an agent that reduces fever (antipyretic)

Fibronectin: an adhesive molecule, synthesised in fibroblasts, which binds collagen to the cell

Functional dyspepsia: persistent or recurrent pain or discomfort centred in the upper abdomen present for at least 12 weeks in the preceding 12 months

Galactagogue: an agent which increases or promotes the flow of breast milk

Glucosidase or α-glucosidase: enzyme that cleaves disaccharides and allows the ready absorption of glucose from the gastro-intestinal tract

Glutathione: a tripeptide containing sulphur and derived from cysteine that acts as an anti-oxidant, protecting cells from free radical damage

Glycation: non-enzyme addition of sugar units to proteins or lipids, a process that occurs in diabetes and old age, resulting in damage to these molecules and changes in their normal function

Haemorrheology: the various aspects of blood flow and blood cell behaviour measured in haematology

Haemostatic: an agent which reduces or stops bleeding

Hepatic: an agent used to strengthen, tone and stimulate bile secretions, improving liver function

Hirsutism: excessive hairiness

Hypolipidaemic: an agent that lowers blood lipid levels

Hypotensive: an agent that lowers blood pressure

Hypnotic: an agent that induces sleep

Menometrorrhagia: A cycle where bleeding occurs with both a short interval and heavy flow

Mutagen: an agent that alters the integrity of DNA

Mydriasis: excessive or prolonged dilation of pupil

Nervine: an agent that tones and strengthens the nervous system

Nitric oxide: a gas able to influence a great many biological functions. It is generated *in vivo* where it has a signalling function that can be positive e.g. dilation of blood vessels or negative e.g. escalation of inflammatory processes, depending on its site of production, level and duration

Nutritive: an agent that nourishes the body

Osteoclastogenesis: the production of osteoclasts, the cells responsible for the resorption and remodelling of bone

Oxytocic: an agent that stimulates uterine contraction i.e. has the same action as oxytocin

Parasiticide: an agent which destroys parasites

Parturient: an agent used to facilitate childbirth

Pectoral: an agent that strengthens and improves the function of the respiratory tract

Phenolic: an aromatic ring bearing an hydroxyl group. Within the context of plant constituents can include simple phenolics, phenolic acids, flavonoids, stilbenes, coumarins, tannins and lignans. They are epidemiologically associated with positive health benefits

Phospholipases: a class of enzymes responsible for metabolising phospholipids. There are 4 major groups which vary in their point of cleavage. Intracellular phospholipase A2 is involved in cell signalling and inflammatory processes by producing arachidonic acid from phospholipids

Pleurodynia: Severe paroxysms of intercostal pain believed to be of rheumatic origin

Properidin: a serum protein capable of inactivating bacteria and viruses

Refrigerant: an agent which has cooling properties, lowers body temperature and relieves thirst

Roehmheld's syndrome: a rose-coloured rash associated with some diseases

Rubefacient: an agent that, when applied locally, stimulates capillary dilation and causes reddening of the skin, thus relieves congestion and inflammation of deeper tissues

Sedative: an agent that relaxes and reduces nerve conduction

Sialagogue: an agent that promotes the secretion and flow of saliva

Soporific: an agent that promotes sleep

Spasmolytic: an agent that counteracts or relieves convulsions or spasmodic pains

Sternutatory: an agent which promotes sneezing by irritating the mucous membrane in the nasal passages

Stimulant: an agent that increases functional activity and energy in the body

Stomachic: an agent that relieves stomach pain

Styptic: an agent that stops external bleeding when applied topically

Sudorific: an agent which induces sweating

Superoxide dismutase: an enzyme present in nearly all cells, in mitochondria and extracellularly. It converts superoxides into oxygen and hydrogen peroxide and in doing so protects biochemicals from damage by reactive oxygen species

Tachyphylaxis: a fall off in effectiveness of a therapeutic agent with its continuous or frequently repeated use

Thromboxane: thromboxane A_2 is produced from arachidonic acid via cyclo-oxygenase activity. In platelets it is responsible for blood clot formation via platelet aggregation and vasoconstriction. It is degraded to thromboxane B_2

Thymoleptic: an agent that acts as a tonic or restorative to the nervous system and at the same time is stimulating, engendering a feeling of well-being

Topoisomerase I and II: enzymes involved in making breaks and links in DNA strands, used in the process of cell replication, transcription or viral insinuation

Tonic: an agent that improves function, energises and tones the body or particular tissues or organs

Tyrosinase: the enzyme that catalyses the production of the skin pigment melanin, its inhibition may represent a treatment approach for hyperpigmentation disorders

Vasoconstrictor: an agent that causes constriction of blood vessels

Vasodilator: an agent that causes dilation of blood vessels

Vermifuge: an agent which expels or destroys worms

Vulnerary: an agent used to hasten the healing of wounds

Xanthine oxidase: the enzyme responsible for converting purines to uric acid. Excessive uric acid can result in gout and kidney stones

AIDS: Acquired Immune Deficiency Syndrome a condition in which the normal immune response becomes defective. The disease is spread by contact with body fluids of carriers of the Human Immunodeficiency Virus (HIV)

COX: cyclo-oxygenase enzymes involved in production of prostanoids from arachidonic acid metabolism. The prostanoids consist of prostaglandins, prostacyclin and thromboxane, metabolites involved in inflammation and immune stimulation

COX-1: cycloxygenase-1 an enzyme involved in arachidonic acid metabolism and prostanoid synthesis it is mainly concerned with maintaining homeostasis but is also expressed at sites of inflammation. It is found in most cells and plays a role in gastric cytoprotection, renal blood flow and platelet function but may also be involved in tumourigenesis

COX-2: cycloxygenase-2 is an isozyme of COX-1 but it is induced rather than being constitutively present in most cells. It is induced primarily by inflammation

CYP: Cytochrome P450 isozymes, a very large group of related enzymes involved at the membrane of mitochondria or endoplasmic reticulum of various tissues where they metabolise a range of endogenous and exogenous chemicals. They may also contribute to the synthesis of hormones, cholesterol and vitamin D in different tissues. The hepatic enzymes are the main ones of interest in herb/drug interactions where the interaction may result in either decreasing or increasing the activity of the drug or herb

DNA: deoxyribonucleic acid

ESCOP: European Scientific Cooperative on Phytotherapy, an umbrella body established in 1989 representing phytotherapists across Europe for consultations on medicine regulation

GABA: gamma-amino butyric acid, the main inhibitory neurotransmitter in mammalian cells, its action being to relax, and reduce muscle tone. There are different neuronal receptor sites of GABA that act as channels for ion flow their composition being complex. $GABA_A$ receptors can bind benzodiazepines, barbiturates and alcohol for example. Binding by benzodiazepine increases the affinity of GABA to $GABA_A$ potentiating the effect of this inhibitory transmitter leading to sedation and reduced anxiety

HDL: High density lipoprotein

HIV: Human immuno-deficiency virus, a group of viruses responsible for causing Acquired Immune Deficiency Syndrome or AIDS

HRT: Hormone Replacement Therapy, commonly refers to the use of synthetic or extraneous hormone intake by women either as oestrogens or progestogens or a combination of the two

HSV-I: Herpes simplex virus type I, the virus associated with cold sores, ocular herpes and some genital herpes

HSV-II: Herpes simplex virus type II, the virus associated with genital herpes and viral meningitis

INR: International normalised ratio, a measure of blood coagulability, the higher the INR value the slower blood is to coagulate. INR is regularly monitored for patients on strong anticoagulants like warfarin

LDL: low density lipoprotein

LOX (5-LOX): lipoxygenase. Lipoxygenases are enzymes found in animal as well as plant cells where they convert fatty acids to their hydroperoxides. In humans they produce leukotrienes, metabolites involved in immune and inflammatory activities. The enzymes have different specificities for their chemical action—mammalian LOX enzymes consist of 5-LOX, 8-LOX, 12-LOX and 15-LOX

MAO: Monoamine oxidase, an enzyme that catalyses the oxidative deamination of monoamines. Monoamines are neurotransmitters e.g. serotonin, adrenalin, nor-adrenalin and dopamine which are deactivated by this enzyme and so inhibitors (**MAOI**) are used to prevent this happening as a treatment strategy in depression

MRSA: Methicillin Resistant *Staphylococcus aureus*

NF-kB: Nuclear factor kappa B, a transcription factor involved in cellular processes in response to such stimuli as stress, cytokine release, microbial antigens, free radicals and oxidised LDL. Its improper control is associated with disease conditions like cancer, septic shock and immune dysfunction including autoimmune conditions

NSAIDs: Non-steroidal anti-inflammatory drugs e.g. aspirin

PABA: para-amino benzoic acid, a precursor molecule for folic acid synthesis in bacteria only. It is essential for human amino acid metabolism and may have benefits in therapeutic doses although it is not considered an essential nutrient or vitamin. It has been used commercially in sunscreens as a UV filter but it associated with damage to DNA and may contribute to the development of skin cancer

RNA: ribonucleic acid

PAF: Platelet Activating Factor a glycerophospholipid that is a signalling molecule acting on leucocytes to cause vasodilation, platelet aggregation, inflammation and allergic responses like anaphylaxis and bronchoconstriction

SARS: Severe acute respiratory syndrome caused by a coronavirus and potentially fatal

SPP.: species, used in taxonomy

TNF-α: Tumour necrosis factor alpha, a cytokine involved in regulation of immune function, cell growth and systemic inflammation. Its excess is related to the development of disease conditions including cancer

TSH: Thyroid Stimulating Hormone

UGT: UDP-glucuronosyltransferase isozymes are involved in glucuronidation of endogenous biochemicals and drugs in a variety of tissues as part of their metabolism.

Acetoside: see **verbascoside**.

Amentoflavone: a biflavone with numerous biological actions including anti-angiogenic, antimicrobial, antitumourigenic, anti-inflammatory, antiulcerogenic, antidepressant, antioxidant and analgesic.

Anethole: (also called isoestragole) an aromatic terpenoid ether occurring in the essential oil of members of the Apiaceae imparting the characteristic "aniseed" taste to them. It has sedative, anticonvulsant, carminative and mild expectorant properties and its dimers are oestrogenic.

Apigenin: a trihydroxyflavone with anti-inflammatory, antibacterial, spasmolytic, neuroprotective, antitumorigenic, immuno-modulating and anti-allergy properties. It is also showing potential in improving trans-membrane conduction, as an aid to standard cancer therapy and may be weakly progestogenic.

Arenarioside: a phenylpropanoid, its actions include anti-oxidant, antitumour, anti-inflammatory and antibacterial.

Asparagine: an amino acid important for nervous system function and in liver transaminase reactions. It was first isolated from asparagus and is responsible for the characteristic smell eating the vegetable imparts to urine.

Aucubin: an iridoid that is anti-inflammatory, hepatoprotective, antitumour, antibacterial and a stimulant to collagen synthesis.

Azulenes: e.g. chamazulene, matricin and achillin. They are sesquiterpenes found in essential oils and have potential anti-inflammatory, antiallergic, anti-ulcer, anti-spasmodic activities and are strongly antioxidant.

Berberine: an alkaloid with antiproliferative, antimicrobial, anti-inflammatory, antihaemorrhagic, anticholinergic and anti-arrhythmic activities.

Bergapten: a psoralen also known as 5-methoxypsoralen and originally derived from bergamot oil. Apart from having activities common to other psoralens it is used in perfumery and as a constituent of sun screen lotions where it protects skin and enhances tanning.

Betulin: a saponin with anti-oxidant; cytoprotective; anti-viral and anti-inflammatory activities.

Betulinic acid: a saponin with anti-inflammatory, anti-viral, anti-malarial and anti-oxidant activities it is also showing promise as an antitumourigenic.

Bitters: refers specifically to substances that not only taste bitter but produce certain pharmacological effects mediated through the taste receptors on the tongue. They increase digestive secretions including saliva and those produced in stomach, liver and pancreas and also enhance appetite and the process of digestion. Bitters also help to improve the effectiveness of peristalsis and therefore reduce griping and indigestion.

β-sitosterol: a plant-based sterol with a broad range of possible pharmacological activities. They include immuno-modulation including support for the immune system brought about by physical stress, anti-inflammatory, anticancer, antimicrobial and possibly also enhancement of insulin release. It may be especially useful in chronic inflammatory and auto-immune conditions and in benign prostatic hyperplasia. It competes with cholesterol for uptake in the digestive tract and therefore has the effect of lowering serum cholesterol. It has poor solubility.

Borneol: is a monoterpene with rubefacient and expectorant actions. Internally it modulates GABA receptors and has been used as a sedative, analgesic and anxiolytic.

Caffeic acid: a phenolic acid derived from benzoic acid and found commonly in plants. It is an intermediate in tannin synthesis. Like chlorogenic acid it is a strong anti-oxidant and has anti-cancer and anti-inflammatory properties.

Camphor: a monoterpene that is locally rubefacient and slightly anaesthetic, refrigerant, antipruritic and antiseptic. Internally it stimulates digestive secretions, peristalsis and relaxes sphincters. It also stimulates the central nervous system and the circulation. At the same time it causes peripheral and coronary dilation. It is diaphoretic and lowers body temperature. Inhaled, it promotes a more fluid mucus flow.

Carnosol: a diterpene with anti-inflammatory and anti-proliferative activities that may also reduce blood glucose and lipid levels.

Carvacrol: a monoterpene, the isomer of thymol. It is has strong antibacterial properties, is spasmolytic, anti-oxidant, antimutagenic and a stimulant of mucus secretion.

Carvone: a monoterpene which exists as isomers with differing odours. It has antiseptic, relaxant, carminative and anticancer properties.

Caryophyllene: a bicyclic sesquiterpene present as a constituent of many essential oils including clove oil and cannabis. One of its isomers, it has 4, is α-humulene. It has weak antibacterial activity and is anti-inflammatory, antioxiant and locally anaesthetic. It may also potentiate the activity of chemotherapeutic agents.

Chlorogenic acid: a phenolic constituent which is chemically related to caffeic acid. It is widespread in plant foods and has strong anti-oxidant, antimicrobial and astringent properties and may also help to regulate blood glucose levels and protect DNA from damage.

Choline: a naturally occurring metabolite. It is used in the synthesis of lecithin and for membrane lipids and fat metabolism in the liver. It is also used in the synthesis of acetylcholine the neurotransmitter used by parasympathetic nerves and at neuromuscular junctions. It is involved in lipid transport in the body and is essential to human life. It is not however classed as a vitamin as it can be synthesised in the body.

Cineol or cineole: also known as eucalyptol. Chemically an ether with anti-inflammatory, anti-oxidant, expectorant and antimicrobial properties it also increases the rate of ciliary movement and reduces the production of mucous. Externally it is rubefacient and expectorant through an irritant action on skin and mucous membranes although its irritant effect is less than that of eucalyptus oil.

Citral: a monoterpene with a citrus-like smell. It calms the central nervous system and is a strong antiseptic, anti-inflammatory, anti-cancer agent and insecticide. It is a mixture of isomers known also as geranial and neral. It is soluble in alcohol but only slightly so in water.

Citronellal: a monoterpene with a citrus-like smell. It is calming to the central nervous system, antifungal, antibacterial and insecticidal.

Diosmin: a flavonoid that reduces capillary fragility, and is considered stronger than rutin in this regard. It is also strongly anti-proliferative, venotonic, a stimulant of lymphatic circulation and protective of blood vessels.

Diosgenin: a steroidal saponin that has been used as a chemical building block to synthesise hormones including the contraceptive pill and corticosteroids, it also has anticancer activity, inhibits the invasiveness of tumours, induces differentiation in some cancer cells, may affect neuronal activity through altered membrane conductance, is neuro-protective, anti-inflammatory and inhibits osteoclastogenesis.

Elemene: sesquiterpene found at low levels in the volatile oil of a number of different species, it has a number of isomers. B-elemene has a broad range of anticancer activity as well as being an antioxidant.

Eugenol: a phenolic derivative that is anaesthetic, carminative and a powerful antiseptic. It is also a digestive stimulant, a rubefacient, an antiparasitic and it inhibits COX-2.

Estragole: see **methyl chavicol**.

Flavonoids: a group with variable pharmacological actions they are antioxidant. Their occurrence is widespread in plants and each may have additional and specific actions such as antispasmodic, diuretic and circulatory stimulants. The particular actions, if known, appears with the pharmacology of that herb. The bioflavonoids, rutin and hesperidin, are well known as strengthening agents for blood vessels.

Geraniol: a monoterpene with good antiseptic, antioxidant and anticancer properties. It is insecticidal and is calming to the central nervous system.

Glycoside: a sugar-containing chemical. These are greatly variable and abundant in plants and animals.

Helenalin: a sesquiterpene lactone of the pseudoguaianolide type found in the Asteraceae family. It has good anti-inflammatory, anti-platelet, anticancer, anti-trypanosomal, antibacterial and anti-malarial activity and may inhibit steroid synthesis.

Hydrastine: an alkaloid that is a peripheral vasoconstrictor, emmenogogue and astringent.

Hydroxyanthracene glycosides: These include the anthraquinones emodin and aloe-emodin which are polycyclic phenolic compounds. Apart from their laxative effects they are anticancer, antibacterial, antiviral, anti-mutagenic

and inhibit angiogenesis. However they may also be genotoxic.

Inositol: a cyclic alcohol molecule which occurs widely in nature and, in combination with phospholipids forms the basis of a wide range of important chemical messengers affecting cellular function. In combination with six phosphate molecules it forms phytic acid which can hinder calcium and iron absorption. It is not a vitamin as it can be synthesised *in vivo* but it was at one time considered a B vitamin.

Inulin: a fructan polymer, soluble in hot water but not in alcohol, made up of varying number of repeating units. It is non-digestible and reaches the large colon intact where it supports beneficial bacterial flora, helps improve bowel function, reduces serum lipid glucose levels, increases calcium absorption, supports immune function and has local anti-inflammatory activity. It may also be protective against the development of cancer and help reduce food intake.

Juglone: a naphthoquinone with strong anti-oxidant, cytotoxic, antibacterial, antifungal, antiviral and antiparasitic activities.

Lignans: polyphenolics derived from phenylalanine, they have anti-oxidant, cytotoxic, anti-inflammatory, antimicrobial, hypocholesterolaemic, anti-allergic, hepatoprotective and hypotensive activities and are weakly oestrogenic and anti-oestrogenic, blocking receptor sites on hormone sensitive cells.

Limonene: a monoterpene found in essential oils, it is calming to the central nervous system and is also antiseptic, chemopreventative, anticancer and antiviral.

Linalool: a monoterpene and major constituent of lavender oil with strong antimicrobial activity. It has relaxing effects on the nervous system and applied topically can reduce systolic blood pressure. It is also much used for its insecticidal properties.

Marrubiin: a diterpene derived from premarrubiin during extraction, it is expectorant, stimulates secretion from the mucous membrane, is antiviral and antibacterial and has bitter properties. Studies suggest it may also be analgesic, may prevent the development of oedema through an anti-inflammatory action and may be vasorelaxant. It has been found to normalise heart rhythm by inhibiting extra-systolic impulses.

Menthol: a monoterpene with strong anti-inflammatory, antimicrobial, antiparasitic, neuroprotective and antipruritic actions. It relaxes muscles of the gastro-intestinal tract and is carminative, externally it is cooling and numbing whilst at the same time acts as a rubefacient. It dries up catarrhal secretions and can be irritating to mucous membranes.

Methyl chavicol: (also called **estragole**) an aromatic terpenoid ether related to anethone (isoestragole) found in a number of different culinary herbs and used as a food flavouring. It has been found to be an hepato-carcinogen in rodents. It has antimicrobial, antioxidant, sedative, anticonvulsant and local anaesthetic activities.

Mucilage: chemically polysaccharides, physically they are slimy or jelly-like. They are known to soothe the tissues they come in contact with, on ingestion this occurs in the digestive tract. If used externally on the skin the action would be termed emollient. They are considered able to soothe tissues of the respiratory and urinary tract when taken orally.

Oleanolic acid: a widespread triterpenoid in the plant kingdom. It has good anti-oxidant, anti-inflammatory, antihyperlipidaemic, hypoglycaemic, antiulcerogenic, antibacterial and anticancer activity. It may also be involved in cellular signalling, may be neuroprotective and immunomodulatory with benefits for the cardiovascular system. In therapeutic doses it is hepatoprotective but can be toxic to liver. It has low water solubility.

PABA: para-amino benzoic acid a naturally occurring chemical which is an intermediate in folate synthesis. It is essential for bacterial health but not for humans as they are able to synthesise it. It is used in protein metabolism and erythrocyte synthesis. Was used as a UV filter in sunscreens but is associated with genotoxicity and may increase the risk of skin cancer.

Perillyl alcohol: a monoterpene found in volatile oil that is showing very good anticancer properties both *in vitro* and *in vivo*.

Phellandrene: a cyclic monoterpene with two isomeric forms found in many plant families. It has antifungal, antibacterial, serotoninergic and expectorant properties and is used commercially in the perfume industry for its fragrance.

Phenylpropanoids: organic molecules based on the amino acid phenylalanine which is converted to cinnamic acid, from which many important plant constituents arise. They include the simple phenolic acids through to the ubiquitous flavonoids, coumarins and lignans and display a wide range of pharmacological activities including antimicrobial, anti-inflammatory, analgesic, antispasmodic, anticancer, antiplatelet and antioxidant.

Pinene: a bicyclic monoterpene which exists in isomeric form and is found in the essential oils of many species. It has antibacterial, antiviral, anticancer, anti-inflammatory, antioxidant, acetylcholinesterase inhibiting and expectorant properties. Probably used by plants to interact with their environment e.g. by attracting insects.

Polysaccharides: long chain saccharides associated in a number of herbs with an immunostimulatory activity. They are however unlikely to be readily absorbed and systemically active but may still exert this action on tissues in which they do come in contact such as Peyer's patches in the gastro-intestinal tract.

Psoralens: chemically furanocoumarins or furocoumarins, used in orthodox medicine to treat psoriasis and vitiligo as they are toxic when applied to cells that are then exposed to UV light. They also have anticancer properties and are insecticidal.

Quercetin: a flavonol, the aglycone of rutin (sugar = rutinose) and quercetrin (sugar = rhamnose). It has anti-allergic, anti-inflammatory, anti-oxidant, anti-tumorgenic, antiviral, vasodilatory and hepatoprotective properties.

Rosmarinic acid: a phenolic acid with good anti-oxidant, anti-inflammatory, antibacterial, antiviral, astringent and antimutagenic activity.

Rutin: a flavonoid based on quercetin in combination with the disaccharide rutinose. It strengthens capillaries, improves circulation, chelates metals and is anti-inflammatory and strongly anti-oxidant.

Salicylic acid and salicylates: they aid healing of epithelial tissues and are antipyretic, promote peripheral circulation, sweat and bile production; increase catabolism and urinary output i.e. they are diuretic, antimicrobial; analgesic; anti-inflammatory and hypoglycaemic. Methyl salicylate is a rubefacient and is used topically as a liniment. The natural salicylates exhibit many of the same actions known for the pharmaceutically related compound Aspirin (acetyl salicylate) as can be seen above, but do not have aspirin's anti-platelet activity, or cause side-effects like gastric erosion. Those with allergies to salicylates may react to these derivatives found in plants.

Sanguinarine: an alkaloid with expectorant, anti-microbial, anti-oxidant, anti-inflammatory, anti-platelet and anticancer properties that inhibits DNA transcription.

Saponins: generally, a class of chemicals occurring naturally and recognisable by their tendency to froth when in solution (Sapo = soap). These constituents can stimulate a more fluid mucus in the respiratory tract and aid expectoration. They also can aid digestion and absorption of nutrients.

Scopoletin: a coumarin with blood pressure regulating, hepatoprotective, antioxidant and spasmolytic activity. It is also antimicrobial, anticancer and anti-inflammatory and may help reduce lipid levels.

Sparteine: an alkaloid acting on the autonomic ganglia and potentiating adrenaline's action in raising blood pressure. It is an anti-arrhythmic agent, reducing the irritability of the myocardium, depresses respiration and stimulates uterine contractions.

Tannins: a widely occurring group of natural polyphenol chemicals. Generally their action is based on their ability to precipitate protein or their astringency—they reduce secretions, stop bleeding; are antimicrobial as they precipitate the protein structures of pathogens; they form protective eschars or scars over abraded surfaces and they reduce peristaltic activity due to irritation/inflammation of the mucosa. They also extend the effectiveness of volatile oils when used in combination with them. Due to their action on proteins they may inhibit enzymic digestion in the GI tract and can cause constipation in the long term. There are two types of tannins—condensed and hydrolysable.

Thujone: a monoterpene with two isomers α- and β-thujone. They have antibacterial, antifungal, carminative, emmenagogue and vermifuge properties. A-thujone, the more toxic of the two, is a $GABA_A$ antagonist, has analgesic, insecticidal and anthelmintic properties. It can inhibit lactation and it is contraindicated in breast feeding. It has a relaxing and restorative effect mentally in moderate doses but is neurotoxic as an isolate.

Thymol: a potent anti-fungal and anti-bacterial, having expectorant, spasmolytic and anthelmintic properties. It is also a local rubefacient and inhibits platelet aggregation. Thymol has been tested against phenol, the standard medical antiseptic, and found to be twenty times stronger. It can enhance the sensitivity of $GABA_A$ receptors. It can cause irritation to the mucous membranes if used in large quantities.

Ursolic acid: is a triterpenoid with very similar properties to oleanolic acid.

Verbascoside: (also known as **acetoside**) a phenylethanoid that has hypotensive, anti-inflammatory, anti-oxidant, anticancer and cytoprotective activity.

Volatile oils: generally speaking are carminative; antimicrobial; expectorant; can stimulate circulation and are externally rubefacient; they are able to influence the central nervous system, sometimes being stimulant, as in the case of camphor, often causing relaxation as in citronellal. They are complex but are characterised by the fact that they evaporate easily (without leaving an oily stain) and have a strong odour.

Achene: a one-seeded fruit.

Adpressed: pressed flat to a surface; commonly used of flattened hairs.

Adventitious: arising in an unusual position.

Amplexicaul: clasping the stem.

Annual: a plant completing its life and seeding in one year or less.

Anther: the part of the stamen containing the pollen grains.

Anterior: on the side away from the axis so appearing in front.

Apetiolate: without a petiole.

Apex, apical: topmost point or structure.

Aristate: with a stiff awn or seta.

Auriculate: an ear-like flap at the base of a leaf-blade.

Awl-shaped: broad-based and tapering to a sharp point.

Axil, axillary: the angle between the leaf and the stem.

Axis: the central column of an inflorescence.

Barbs, barbate, barbellate: retrorse projections on hairs.

Biennial: a plant which grows in its first year and flowers and seeds in its second year.

Bifid, bilobed: cleft in two no further than to the middle.

Bilabiate: two lipped.

Bipinnate: twice cut, used of leaves cut into distinct segments which are themselves cut into distinct segments.

Blade: the flattened part of the leaf.

Bract: a little leaf or scale-like structure from the axil of which a flower often arises.

Bracteole: a secondary bract usually borne on the same axis as the flower; or in the Apiaceae, one of the bract-like structures of the secondary umbels.

Bulbil: a small bulb or tuber arising from the axil of the leaf or among the flowers and reproducing the plant e.g. garlic.

Calyx, calices: the collective name for the sepals; often joined together in a tube.

Campanulate: bell-shaped.

Capitulum: a head of small stalkless flowers crowded together at the end of a stem as in the Asteraceae.

Capsule: a dry fruit or seed pod which splits open when ripe.

Catkin: a crowded spike of tiny flowers usually hanging down like a tassel.

Caudex: a stem with subsidiary organs.

Cauline: belonging to the stem, especially the upper part.

Ciliate: fringed with hairs along the margin.

Clavate: club-shaped, thickened towards the apex.

Connate: joined together, especially of like parts e.g. stamens.

Cordate: heart-shaped.

Corm: a swollen underground stem surrounded by scales, and replaced annually by a new corm.

Corolla: the collective name for all the petals, often joined together in a tube.

Corona: structure or appendages which stand out from the petals and together form a ring round the centre of the flower, as in *Passiflora*.

Corymb: a flat or convex-topped inflorescence with outer flowers opening first.

Crenate: having shallow round teeth.

Cucullate: hooded or hood-shaped.

Cuneate: wedge-shaped cyathium.

Cyathium: a cup-like structure, especially the perianth-like involucre surrounding flowers in *Euphorbia*.

Cyme, cymose: a broad, more or less flat-topped simple or compound flower cluster, with the central flowers opening first.

Deciduous: plants whose leaves fall off in autumn.

Decussate: opposite; used of leaves which are in opposite pairs with each successive pair lying at right angles to the next—hence the leaves are in four ranks e.g. Lamiaceae.

Dentate: toothed.

Dichotomous: divided into two equal forks and often forked again and again e.g. *Viscum*.

Didynamous: with 4 stamens, one pair long, one pair short.

Digitate: leaflets arranged as in the fingers of a hand e.g. *Vitex*.

Dioecious: having fertile male and female flowers on different plants; plants one-sexed.

Disc: a fleshy part of the receptacle which surrounds or surmounts the ovary.

Disc-florets: the tube-like flowers at the centre of flower heads of some members of the Asteraceae.

Divaricate: spreading at a very wide angle.

Elliptic: rounded at both ends and widest in the middle.

Endosperm: nutritive tissue outside the embryo in a seed.

Entire: with a continuous margin completely lacking in teeth.

Filaments: the slender stalk of the stamen which bears the anthers.

Fimbriate: with hairs forming part of a fringe.

Glabrate: almost glabrous.

Glabrous: not hairy, therefore smooth.

Glaucous: covered or whitened with a bloom which is often waxy, giving the organ a bluish or greyish colour.

Globose, globular: globe-shaped or spherical.

Glume: a chaff-like bract, often the bracts at the base of spikelets of Poaceae.

Gynobasic: of a style appearing to be inserted at the base of an ovary.

Gynostegium: the column formed by the fusion of stamens, style and stigma.

Herbaceous: non-woody, soft and leafy.

Hermaphrodite: with fertile stamens and ovaries present in the same flower.

Hilum: the scar on the seed marking the place where it was attached.

Hispid: with coarse, stiff, rough hairs.

Hybrid: a plant resulting from the cross-breeding of two different species and possessing some of the characters of both. Hybrids are often infertile.

Imbricated: overlapping.

Indehiscent: not splitting to release seeds, as in *Linum*.

Inflorescence: a stem or branch of flowers.

Involucral: a collection of bracts or leafy structures surrounding a flower head, groups of flowers or a single flower, e.g. many members of the Lamiaceae have involucral bracts.

Keel: a lower petal of flowers of the Fabaceae resembling the keel of a boat.

Lamina: the leaf blade.

Lanate: clad in woolly, usually intertwined hairs.

Lateral: borne on the side of a branch etc.

Lax: loose and spreading.

Latex: milky juice in some members of the Asteraceae and other plants.

Lemma: the lower and outer of two fertile glumes of the floret of grasses.

Lenticels: a corky spot forming on young bark functioning as a pore.

Ligule: the small projection at the junction of the blade of a leaf with its sheath.

Ligulate: florets with strap-shaped corollas in the flower heads of the Asteraceae.

Linear: long and narrow with parallel sides.

Lyrate: shaped like a lyre, deeply cut with an enlarged terminal lobe and smaller lateral lobes.

Mealy: looking as though dusted with flour.

Membranous: paper-like, thin, dry and flexible.

Mericarp: a one-seeded part split off at maturity from an ovary of two or more fused carpels e.g. seeds of members of the Apiaceae.

Mucronate: with a short narrow point.

Naturalised: an introduced plant growing wild where it is not native.

Node: a point on a stem where one or more leaves arise.

Opposite: arising at the same level on opposite sides of the stem.

Orbicular: rounded in outline with length and breadth about the same.

Ovary: the part of the flower containing the ovules and later the seeds, usually with one or more styles or stigmas.

Ovule: a structure containing the egg which, after fertilisation, becomes the seed.

Palea: the upper and inner, and usually less robust of two fertile glumes of the floret of grasses.

Palmate: lobed or divided in a palm- or hand-like manner.

Panicle: a branched, racemose inflorescence of stalked flowers.

Pappus: hairs or bristles on the fruits of some Asteraceae which replace the calyx, as in *Silybum*.

Pedicel: the stalk of an individual flower.

Peduncle: a common leafless axil bearing several flowers.

Pellucid: clear, almost transparent.

Pendulous: drooping, or hanging down.

Perennial: living for more than two years and usually flowering every year.

Perfoliate: of a sessile leaf or bract completely encircling the stem looking as though the stem passes through it.

Perianth: the outer non-sexual parts of the flower, (sepals, petals), usually composed of two whorls; especially used when the corolla and calyx are not well differentiated or when either one is absent.

Petal: a unit of the corolla when completely free, usually coloured other than green.

Petiole: the stalk of a leaf.

Pilose: bearing soft, shaggy hairs.

Pinnate: the regular arrangement of leaflets in two rows on either side of the stalk or rachis.

Pinnatifid, pinnatisect: divided or dissected to varying degrees in a pinnate fashion, but not compound.

Pistil: the gynoecium, comprising the ovary, style and stigma.

Pollen: small grains contained in the anthers which contain the male reproductive cells.

Posterior: on the side nearest the axis therefore appearing at the back.

Puberulent: covered with exceedingly fine, short, dense hairs.

Pubescent: covered in short soft hairs.

Quadrangular: square or rectangular.

Raceme: an unbranched, (simple), elongated inflorescence with stalked flowers opening from the base.

Rachis: the stalk of a compound leaf.

Radical: used of leaves which arise from the root stock, as in *Taraxacum*.

Raphides: bundles of crystals of calcium oxalate.

Ray florets: the florets with strap-like corollas found in members of the Asteraceae.

Reflexed: bent abruptly backwards or downwards.

Regular: of flowers; radially symmetric.

Reniform: kidney-shaped.

Resin, resinous: a sticky substance which hardens when exposed to the air and is excreted by many plants, often in ducts or canals.

Retrorse: bent backwards or downwards.

Revolute: rolled outwards or to the lower side of the leaf.

Rhizome: an underground stem usually spreading horizontally, as in *Urtica*.

Root crown: the part of the stem at the ground surface.

Rootstock: a short, erect, underground stem, a stem with roots.

Rosette: a group of leaves radiating outwards from a centre, overlapping and often spreading over the ground.

Rugose: wrinkled.

Runcinate: pinnately and rather sharply lobed, with lobes more or less directed backwards.

Scabrid: rough to the touch because of minute, harsh projections.

Scape: a leafless, elongated peduncle arising from the crown of a plant and topped with a single flower, as in *Taraxacum*.

Scarious: very thin and dry and more or less translucent.

Scorpioid: a coiled cymose inflorescence, as in *Symphytum*.

Sepal: one separate part of a calyx of free members.

Septum: a partition or cross-wall as in the seedpod of *Capsella*.

Sericeous: silky.

Serrate: sharply toothed, with teeth pointing forward.

Sessile: without a stalk.

Sheath: a more or less tubular structure surrounding another as in the lower part of leaves.

Silique: a capsule with two valves falling away from a frame, (septum), bearing the seeds, as in *Capsella*.

Simple: not divided into segments, the opposite of compound.

Sinuate: with shallow, broad waves to the margin.

Spathe: a large bract enclosing a flower head as in *Allium*.

Spike: a slender, elongated cluster of more or less stalkless flowers, as in *Lavandula*.

Spine: a sharp-pointed, narrow projection, often hard, woody and piercing, as in *Crataegus*.

Stamen: the pollen-bearing organ consisting of the anther and the filament.

Staminodes: an infertile or rudimentary stamen without pollen.

Stigma: the part of the carpel which receives the pollen, usually found near the tip of the style.

Stipule: one of a pair of scale-like or leaf-like appendages at the base of a petiole.

Stolon: a horizontal stem spreading above or below ground, which roots at the tip to form a new plant.

Striate: with fine, longitudinal lines, grooves or ridges.

Strobilus: a cone-like structure containing reproductive organs as in *Humulus*.

Style: the elongated part of the carpel between the ovary and the stigma.

Subtend: to stand below, but usually close to another organ e.g. a bract below a flower.

Subulate: awl-shaped.

Superior: situated above another part.

Tendril: a slender, clasping twining organ.

Tepal: an individual member of the perianth.

Terete: circular in cross section.

Terminal: borne at the end of a stem.

Ternate: compound with parts arranged in threes.

Throat: the opening of a tubular or funnel-shaped corolla.

Tomentum: a dense matted covering of soft hairs, hence **tomentose** as of *Verbascum thapsus*.

Trifoliate: having three leaflets.

Truncate: appearing as though cut squarely across.

Umbel: a cluster of flowers whose spreading stalks arise from the apex of the stem as in *Foeniculum*.

Undulate: waved in a plane at right angles to the surface.

Venation: the arrangement of veins in a leaf etc.

Verticils: a whorl of flowers or leaves, in the Lamiaceae a false whorl of flowers that are in cymes.

Whorl: an arrangement of three or more parts or organs at the same level around an axis.

There is not always consistency across phytotherapy texts as to which herbs are contraindicated or best avoided for particular health conditions. The *BHP, Potters'* and *Martindale* for example record fewer contraindications than either *German Commission E* or the *BHC*. The same source may have been used by several authors for contraindication information often without an apparent reason.

Warnings may be based on the theoretical action(s) of a herb, or on the activity of its constituent(s) e.g. some contraindications for *Ephedra* are the same as those for ephedrine which only constitutes a small percentage of the whole herb (*Martindale*). Some are based on the view that no herb should be used in children, pregnancy or lactation until they are proved to be safe. Tradition is based on empirical use over many decades but may have failed to note contraindications for lack of stringent monitoring. The contraindications of a herb is therefore likely to change as new information emerges requiring additional caution or removing a previously held one.

I have included contraindications with their source (if available) and/or possible reasons for inclusion, although some appear to be unnecessary or over-stated. It is nonetheless the object of the medical herbalist to practice safely and it is therefore prudent to err on the side of caution until further evidence emerges to clarify these inconsistencies.

Pregnancy

Botanical Name	Common Name	Sources—Reason if Given
Anemone pulsatilla	pasque flower	BHC—protoanemonin causes abortion/teratogenic effects in livestock
Aloe barbadensis	aloe latex	BHC
Apium graveolens	celery seed	BHC
Arctostaphylos uva-ursi	bearberry	BHC, GCE
Barosma betulina	buchu	BHC
Berberis vulgaris	barberry	BHP (in early pregnancy), PNC, BHC
Cassia spp.	senna	BHC—recommends used only under medical supervision
Caulophyllum thalictroides	blue cohosh	recent anecdotal reports, even though PNC and BHP recommend for threatened miscarriage—see monograph
Cinchona spp.	cinchona	BHP, PNC—oxytocic (quinine) in large doses
Cytisus scoparius	broom	BHP, Mart, PNC—oxytocic (sparteine)
Fucus vesiculosus	bladderwrack	BHC
Fumaria officinalis	fumitory	BHC
Glycyrrhiza glabra	liquorice	BHC—no reason, avoid if prone to premature delivery (see monograph)
Hydrastis canadensis	golden seal	BHP, BHC
Inula helenium	elecampane	BHC
Juniperus communis	juniper	BHP, PNC, Mart—uterine stimulant
Leonurus cardiaca	motherwort	BHC—note BHP recommends for false labour pains!
Panax ginseng	Korean ginseng	BHC
Piscidia erythrina	Jamaica dogwood	BHC
Rhamnus purshiana	cascara	BHC
Rheum spp.	rhubarb	BHC
Ruta graveolens	rue	PNC—uterine stimulant
Salvia officinalis	sage	GCE
Tanacetum parthenium	feverfew	BHC
Tanacetum vulgare	tansy	BHP, PNC—an emmenagogue, thujone causes uterine contractions
Thuja occidentalis	thuja	BHP, PNC—an emmenagogue, thujone causes uterine contractions
Zanthoxylum spp.	prickly ash	BHC

Lactation

Stimulating laxative* use has been contraindicated in the past for lactating women and this may account for their appearance in this list but research has shown the levels of this type of herb that is secreted in breast milk is too low to affect the baby—see under relevant monograph.

Botanical Name	Common Name	Sources—Reason if Given
Aloe barbadensis*	aloe latex	BHC
Anemone pulsatilla	pasque flower	BHC
Arctostaphylos uva-ursi	bearberry	GCE
Cassia spp.*	senna	BHC—recommends used only under medical supervision
Fucus vesiculosus	bladderwrack	BHC
Inula helenium	elecampane	BHC
Rhamnus purshiana*	cascara	BHC
Rheum spp.*	rhubarb	BHC
Salvia officinalis	sage	No source—however BHP recommends for galactorrhoea

General conditions

Condition	Botanical Name	Common Name	Sources
Abdominal pain (unknown origin)	Aloe barbadensis	aloe latex	Mart
	Cassia spp.	senna	BHC, GCE, Mart
	Rhamnus purshiana	cascara	GCE, Mart
	Rheum spp.	rhubarb	Mart
Acute illness/infections	Panax ginseng	Korean ginseng	BHC, TCM
Appendicitis	All purgatives		Mart
	Aloe barbadensis	aloe	
	Cassia spp.	senna	BHC, GCE
	Rhamnus purshiana	cascara	GCE
Anxiety	Ephedra sinica	ephedra, ma huang	GCE
Bradycardia	Piscidia erythrina	Jamaica dogwood	BHC
Biliary obstruction	Cynara scolymus	artichoke	GCE
	Peumus boldo	boldo	GCE
	Taraxacum officinale	dandelion leaf/root	BHC, GCE (also indicated for gallstones!)
Cardiac disease	Fucus vesiculosus	bladderwrack	BHC
	Gelsemium sempervirens	yellow jasmine	BHP
Cardiac insufficiency	Piscidia erythrina	Jamaica dogwood	BHC
Cerebral circulation impairment	Ephedra sinica	ephedra/ma huang	GCE
Cholestatic liver disorders	Glycyrrhiza glabra	liquorice	GCE
Colitis	Menyanthes trifoliata	bogbean	BHC, BHP

Condition	Botanical Name	Common Name	Sources
Coronary thrombosis	Ephedra sinica	ephedra/ma huang	BHP
Depression	Humulus lupulus	hops	BHC, BHP
	Piper methysticum	kava	GCE
Diabetes	Plantago psyllium	psyllium hulls	BHC, GCE—if insulin control poor
Diarrhoea	Berberis vulgaris	barberry	BHP
	Menyanthes trifoliata	bogbean	BHC, BHP
Difficulty swallowing	Plantago psyllium	psyllium	See monograph
Dysentery	Menyanthes trifoliata	bogbean	BHC, BHP
Epistaxis	Panax ginseng	Korean ginseng	TCM
Gall-bladder empyema	Taraxacum officinale	dandelion root	BHC, GCE
	Taraxacum officinale	dandelion leaf	GCE
Glaucoma	Ephedra sinica	ephedra/ma huang	GCE
Haemorrhoids	Aloe barbadensis	aloe latex	BHC
Hypertension	Cytisus scoparius	broom	BHP
	Ephedra sinica	ephedra/ma huang	BHP, GCE, PNC
	Glycyrrhiza glabra	liquorice	BHC, PNC, Mart
	Hydrastis canadensis	golden seal	BHP
	Panax ginseng	Korean ginseng	BHC, GCE, TCM
Hyperthyroidism	Fucus vesiculosus	bladderwrack	BHC
Hypertonia	Glycyrrhiza glabra	liquorice	GCE
Hypokalaemia	Aloe barbadensis	aloe latex	Mart—with excessive use
	Cassia spp.	senna	Mart—with excessive use
	Glycyrrhiza glabra	liquorice	BHC, GCE, BHP, Mart
	Rhamnus purshiana	cascara	BHP, Mart—with excessive use
	Urginea maritima	squills	BHC
Hypotension	Gelsemium sempervirens	yellow jasmine	BHP
Hypothyroidism	Armoracia rusticana	horseradish	See monograph
Inflammation of GIT	Cassia spp.	senna	BHC, GCE
	Rhamnus purshiana	cascara	GCE
Intestinal obstruction	Aloe barbadensis	aloe latex	Mart
	Linum usitatissimum	linseed	GCE
	Plantago psyllium	psyllium hulls	BHC, GCE
	Rhamnus purshiana	cascara	BHC, GCE, Mart
	Rheum spp.	rhubarb	BHC, Mart

Condition	Botanical Name	Common Name	Sources
	Taraxacum officinale	dandelion leaf/root	GCE
Irritable bowel conditions	Aloe barbadensis	aloe latex	BHC
Liver cirrhosis	Glycyrrhiza glabra	liquorice	BHC, GCE
Liver disease	Peumus boldo	boldo	GCE
Menorrhagia	Panax ginseng	Korean ginseng	TCM
Myasthenia gravis	Gelsemium sempervirens	yellow jasmine	BHP
Peptic ulcers	Armoracia rusticana	horseradish	GCE
	Gentiana lutea	gentian	BHC, GCE
	Harpagophytum	devils claw	BHC, GCE
Phaeochromocytoma	Ephedra sinica	ephedra/ma huang	GCE
Prostatic enlargement	Ephedra sinica	ephedra/ma huang	GCE
Renal disorders	Aloe barbadensis	aloe latex	BHC, Mart
	Apium graveolens	celery seed	BHC
	Arctostaphylos uva-ursi	bearberry	BHC
	Armoracia rusticana	horseradish	GCE
	Capsella bursa-pastoris	shepherd's purse	GCE
	Glycyrrhiza glabra	liquorice	GCE
	Juniperus communis	juniper	BHP, Mart, GCE
	Rheum spp.	rhubarb	BHC (use in China for renal disease)
	Urginea maritima	white squill	Mart
Restlessness	Ephedra sinica	ephedra/ma huang	GCE
Stenosis of GIT	Plantago psyllium	psyllium hulls	BHC, GCE

BHC—British Herbal Compendium
BHP—British Herbal Pharmacopoeia
GCE—German Commission E Monographs
PNC—Potter's New Cyclopaedia of Botanical Drugs and Preparations
Mart—Martindale
TCM—Traditional Chinese Medicine

APPENDIX V INTERACTIONS

Actually reported in vivo *(mainly anecdotal cases)*

Alprazolam—*Hypericum, Piper*	**Amitriptyline**—*Hypericum*	**Antibiotics**—*Panax*
Anti-retrovirals (indinavir, nevirapine)—*Hypericum*	**Aspirin**—*Linum*	**Cardiac glycosides**—*Glycyrrhiza, Hypericum, Cassia* (chronic use)
Chemotherapeutic drugs (imatinib, irinotecan)—*Hypericum*	**Chlorzoxazone**—*Allium* (increase effect)	**Cilostazol**—*Ginkgo* (increase effect)
Clomipramine—haloperidol—*Panax*	**Contraceptive pill**—*Hypericum*	**Corticosteroids**—*Glycyrrhiza*
Cyclosporin—*Hypericum*	**Cytochrome P450-3A4**—*Hydrastis* (probe drugs only)	**Cytochrome P450-3A5**—*Hydrastis* (probe drugs only)
Cytochrome P450-2D6—*Hydrastis* (probe drugs only)	**Digoxin**—see **Cardiac glycosides**	**Diuretics**—*Glycyrrhiza, Cassia* (chronic use)
Ergot alkaloids—*Ephedra*	**Fexofenadine**—*Hypericum*	**Fluindione**—*Allium*
Furosemide—*Rosmarinus* (minimal)	**Guanethidine**—*Ephedra*	**Halothane**—*Ephedra*
Ibuprofen—*Ginkgo*	**Levodopa**—*Piper*	**Lithium**—*Psyllium* (reduced absorption)
Lorazepam—*Valeriana*	**Methadone**—*Hypericum*	**Nifedipine**—*Zingiber*
Omeprazole—*Hypericum*	**Oxytocin**—*Ephedra*	**Phenalzine MAOI**—*Panax, Ephedra*
Phenprocoumon—*Hypericum, Zingiber*	**Quazepam**—*Hypericum*	**Ritonavir**—*Allium* (caused GI toxicity when used together)
Saquinavir—*Allium* (decrease drug), *Hypericum*	**Sevoflurane**—*Aloe*	**Simvastin**—*Hypericum*

SSRIs e.g. sertaline, paroxetine—*Hypericum*	Tacrolimus—*Hypericum*	Theophylline—*Hypericum*
Trazodone—*Ginkgo*	Verapamil—*Hypericum*	Voriconazole—*Hypericum*
Warfarin—*Allium, Commiphora* (1 case), *Harpagophytum* (1 case), *Hypericum*		

Potential (based on in vitro *studies or by extrapolation)*

Anti-arrhythmics—*Aloe* latex (chronic use), *Cassia* (chronic use), *Rhamnus* (over dosing)	Anti-coagulant drugs—*Juniperus* (decrease effect)	Antidiabetics—*Plantago psyllium* may reduce blood sugar levels
Anti-retrovirals (amprenavir, lopinavir, atazanavir)—*Hypericum* (possibly)	Anti-thrombotics—*Vaccinium*—increase effect	Cardiac glycosides—*Aloe* latex (chronic use), *Cassia* (chronic use), *Convallaria, Rhamnus* (over dosing), *Urginea*
Ciprofloxacin (antibiotic)—Bergapten-containing herbs e.g. in Apiaceae and Rutaceae families	Cisplatin (chemotherapeutic drug)—*Allium*	Corticosteroids—*Cassia* (chronic use), *Aloe* latex (chronic use)
Diuretics—*Cassia* (chronic use), *Aloe* latex (chronic use)	Docetaxel—*Hypericum*	Drugs absorbed using organic anion-transporting polypeptide-B—*Cimicifuga, Vaccinium*
Erythromycin—*Hypericum*	Etoposide amsacrine—*Hypericum*	Hypoglycaemics—*Aloe*
Monoamine Oxidase Inhibitors (MAOI)—*Passiflora*	Nifedipine—*Ginkgo*	Omeprazole—*Ginkgo*
Paclitaxel—*Hypericum*	Ritonavir—*Hypericum*	P-glycoprotein transporter carried drugs—*Allium, Piper*
Warfarin—*Passiflora, Peumus, Salix*		

Any drug with which it is co-administered:-
Aloe—absorption may be reduced due to decrease transit time.
Althaea—mucilage may delay absorption.
Cassia—absorption may be reduced due to decrease transit time.
Plantago psyllium—fibre can alter absorption.
Rhamnus—absorption may be reduced due to decrease transit time.
Rheum—absorption may be reduced due to decrease transit time.
Tannin containing herbs e.g. *Rubus*—may alter absorption

Isozyme	Substrate	Inhibitor	Inducer	Herb Interaction
1A1				*Humulus*
1A2	clozapine, cyclobenzaprine, imipramine, mexiletine, naproxen, riluzole, tacrine, theophylline	cimetidine, fluoroquinolones, fluvoxamine, ticlopidine	tobacco	*Echinacea, Humulus, Matricaria, Piper, Salvia, Valeriana*
1B1				*Humulus*
2A6				*Allium*
2B6	bupropion, cyclophosphamide, efavirenz, ifosfamide, *methadone*	thiotepa, ticlopidine	phenobarbital, phenytoin, rifampin	
2C8		gemfibrozi, montelukast		*Hydrastis*
2C9	**NSAIDs:** diclofenac, ibuprofen, piroxicam **Oral Hypoglycemic Agents:** tolbutamide, glipizide **Angiotensin II Blockers:** irbesartan, losartan NOT candesartan, valsartan **Others:** celecoxib, fluvastatin, naproxen, phenytoin, sulfamethoxazole, tamoxifen, tolbutamide, torsemide, warfarin	amiodarone, fluconazole, isoniazid	rifampin, secobarbital	*Hydrastis, Matricaria, Thymus*

---

†Reference: http://medicine.iupui.edu/flockhart/table.htm.

480

Isozyme	Substrate	Inhibitor	Inducer	Herb Interaction
2C9*1				*Allium*
2C19	**Proton Pump Inhibitors:** omeprazole, lansoprazole, pantoprazole, rabeprazole **Anti-epileptics:** diazepam, phenytoin, phenobarbitone **Others:** amitriptyline, clomipramine, clopidogrel, cyclophosphamide, progesterone	fluoxetine, fluvoxamine, ketoconazole, lansoprazole, omeprazole, ticlopidine	N/A	*Allium, Hydrastis, Thymus, Valeriana*
2D6	**Beta Blockers:** S-metoprolol, propafenone, timolol **Antidepressants:** amitriptyline, clomipramine, desipramine, imipramine, paroxetine **Antipsychotics:** haloperidol, risperidone, thioridazine **Others:** aripiprazole, codeine, dextromethorphan, duloxetine, flecainide, mexiletine, ondansetron, tamoxifen, tramadol, venlafaxine	amiodarone, buproprion, chlorpheniramine, cimetidine, clomipramine, duloxetine, fluoxetine, haloperidol, methadone, mibefradil, paroxetine, quinidine, ritonavir	N/A	*Cephaelis, Hydrastis, Matricaria, Salvia, Thymus, Valeriana*
2E1	acetaminophen, chlorzoxazone, ethanol	disulfiram	ethanol, isoniazid	*Hypericum*
3A				*Echinacea*
3A4,5,7	**Macrolide antibiotics:** clarithromycin, erythromycin, NOT azithromycin, telithromycin **Anti-arrhythmics:** quinidine **Benzodiazepines:** alprazolam diazepam, midazolam triazolam **Immune Modulators:** cyclosporine, tacrolimus, (FK506) **HIV Protease Inhibitors:** indinavir, ritonavir, saquinavir **Prokinetic:** cisapride **Antihistamines:** astemizole, chlorpheniramine **Calcium Channel Blockers:** amlodipine, diltiazem felodipine, nifedipine, nisoldipine, nitrendipine, verapamil **HMG CoA Reductase Inhibitors:** atorvastatin, cerivastatin, lovastatin, NOT pravastatin, simvastatin	**HIV Protease Inhibitors:** indinavir, nelfinavir, ritonavir **Others:** amiodarone NOT azithromycin, cimetidine, clarithromycin, diltiazem erythromycin, fluvoxamine, grapefruit juice, itraconazole, ketoconazole, mibefradil, nefazodone, troleandomycin, verapamil	carbamazepine, phenobarbital, phenytoin, rifabutin, rifampin, troglitazone	3A4,5,7—*Allium* 3A4—*Cephaelis, Cimicifuga, Glycyrrhiza, Hydrastis, Hypericum, Matricaria, Trifolium, Salvia, Scutellaria, Thymus, Valeriana*

Isozyme	Substrate	Inhibitor	Inducer	Herb Interaction
	Others: aripiprazole, buspirone, gleevec, haloperidol (in part), methadone, pimozide, quinine NOT osuvastatin sildenafil tamoxifen trazodone vincristine			

REFERENCES

Apiaceae

1. Pasqua G et al. Eur J Histochem. 2003;47(1):87–90.
2. Lopes D et al. Chem Biodivers. 2004 Dec;1(12):1880–7.
3. Eeva M et al. Phytochem Anal. 2004 May–Jun;15(3):167–74.
4. Muller M et al. Acta Pharm. 2004 Dec;54(4):277–85.
5. Hensel A et al. Planta Med. 2007 Feb;73(2):142–50.
6. Ojala T et al. Planta Med. 1999 Dec;65(8):715–8.
7. Sigurdsson S, Gudbjarnason S. Z Naturforsch [C]. 2007 Sep–Oct;62(9–10):689–93.
8. Sigurdsson S et al. Anticancer Res. 2005 May–Jun;25(3B): 1877–80.
9. Sigurdsson S et al. Z Naturforsch [C]. 2004 Jul–Aug; 59(7–8):523–7.
10. Schempp H et al. Phytomedicine. 2006 Nov;13 Suppl 1: 36–44.
11. Wegener T, Wagner H. Phytomedicine. 2006 Nov 24; 13 Suppl 1:20–35.
12. Sarker SD, Nahar L. Curr Med Chem. 2004 Jun;11(11): 1479–500.
13. Schemann M et al. Phytomedicine. 2006 Nov 24;13 Suppl 1: 90–9.
14. Witchl M. Stuttgart:Medpharm Gmbh Scientific Publishers, 1994.
15. Kitajima K et al. Phytochemistry. 2003 Nov;64(5):1003–11.
16. Momin RA et al. J Agric Food Chem. 2000 Sep;48(9):3785–8.
17. Wei A, Shibamoto T. J Agric Food Chem. 2007 Mar 7; 55(5):1737–42.
18. Momin RA, Nair MG. Phytomedicine. 2002 May;9(4):312–8.
19. Momin RA, Nair MG. J Agric Food Chem. 2001 Jan;49(1): 142–5.
20. Destaillats F, Angers P. Lipids. 2002 May;37(5):527–32.
21. Lin LZ et al. J Agric Food Chem. 2007 Feb 21;55(4):1321–6.
22. Martindale, The Extra Pharmacopoeia 26th Ed. Pharmceutical Press London March 1973.
23. Tuetun B et al. Ann Trop Med Parasitol. 2004 Jun;98(4): 407–17.
24. Beattie PE et al. J Am Acad Dermatol. 2007 Jan;56(1):84–7.
25. Boumeester HJ et al. Plant Physiol. 1998 Jul;117(3):901–12.
26. Richter J, Schellenberg I. Anal Bioanal Chem. 2007 Mar; 387(6):2207–17.
27. Iacobellis NS et al. J Agric Food Chem. 2005 Jan 12; 53(1):57–61.
28. Zheng GQ et al. Planta Med. 1992 Aug;58(4):338–41.
29. Matsumura T et al. Phytochemistry. 2002 Oct;61(4):455–9.
30. Kunzemann J, Herrmann K. Lebensm Unters Forsch. 1977 Jul 29;164(3):194–200.
31. Nakano Y et al. Biol Pharm Bull. 1998 Mar;21(3):257–61.
32. Al-Bataina BA et al. Trace Elem Med Biol. 2003;17(2):85–90.
33. Satyanarayana S et al. J Herb Pharmcother. 2003;4(2):1–10.
34. Mazaki M et al. J Med Invest. 2006 Feb;53(1–2):123–33.
35. Wattenberg LW. Proc Nutr Soc. 1990 Jul;49(2):173–83.
36. Ripple GH et al. Clin Cancer Res. 1998 May;4(5):1159–64.
37. Vigushin DM et al. Cancer Chemother Pharmacol. 1998; 42(2):111–7.
38. Mahady G et al. Phytother Res. 2005 Nov;19(11):988–91.
39. Schempp H et al. Arzneimittelforschung. 2004;54(7):389–95.
40. Lado C et al. Fitoterapia. 2005 Mar;76(2):166–72.
41. Thompson Coon J, Ernst E. Aliment Pharmacocol Ther. 2002 Oct;16(10):1689–99.
42. Madisch A et al. Digestion. 2004;69(1):45–52.
43. Madisch A et al. Z Gastroenterol. 2001 Jul;39(7):511–7.
44. Holtmann G et al. Phytomedicine. 2003;10 Suppl 4:56–7.
45. May B et al. Aliment Pharmacol Ther. 2003 Apr 1;17(7): 975–6.
46. Goerg KJ, Spilker T. Phytother Res. 2003 Feb;17(2):135–40.
47. Micklefield G et al. Aliment Pharmacol Ther. 2003 Feb;17(3):445–51.
48. Garcia-Gonzalez JJ et al. Ann Allergy Asthma Immunol. 2002 May;88(5):518–22.

49. Niinimaki A et al. Allergy. 1981 Oct;36(7):487–93.
50. Wuthrich B, Dietschi R. Schweiz Med Wochenschr. 1985 Mar 16;115(11):258–64.
51. Schaneberg BT et al. Pharmazie. 2003 Jun;58(6):381–4.
52. Zhang FL et al. Biomed Chromatogr. 2007 Aug 17; 22(2):119–24.
53. Kartnig T. Herbs, spices & medicinal plants: Eds Craker LE, Simon JE Vol 3. Phoenix, AZ, Oryx Press. 1988:145–173.
54. Grimaldi R et al. J Ethnopharmacol. 1990 Feb;28(2):235–41.
55. Zheng CJ, Qin LP. Zhong Xi Yi Jie He Xue Bao. 2007 May; 5(3):348–51.
56. Satake T et al. Biol Pharm Bull. 2007 May;30(5):935–40.
57. Bhandari P et al. J Sep Sci. 2007 Aug;30(13):2092–6.
58. Wang XS et al. Carbohydr Res. 2003 Oct 31;338(22): 2393–402.
59. Siddiqui BS et al. J Asian Nat Prod Res. 2007 Jun;9(4): 407–14.
60. Govindan G et al. Planta Med. 2007 Jun;73(6):597–9.
61. Lu L et al. Int J Dermatol. 2004 Nov;43(11):801–7.
62. Lu L et al. Br J Dermatol. 2004 Sep;151(3):571–8.
63. Maquart FX et al. Connect Tissue Res. 1990;24(2):107–20.
64. Bonte F et al. Planta Med. 1994;60:133–135.
65. Lee J et al. Planta Med. 2006 Mar;72(4):324–8.
66. Coldren CD et al. Planta Med. 2003 Aug;69(8):725–32.
67. Tenni R et al. Ital J Biochem. 1998 Mar–Apr;37(2):69–77.
68. Sampson JH et al. Phytomedicine. 2001 May;8(3):230–5.
69. Bosse JP et al. Ann Plast Surg. 1979 Jul;3(1):13–21.
70. Widgerow AD et al. Aesthetic Plast Surg. 2000 May–Jun; 24(3):227–34.
71. Morisset R et al. Phytotherapy Res. 1987;1:117–21.
72. Young GL, Jewell D. Cochrane Database Syst Rev. 2000;(2): CD000066.
73. Gravel JA. Laval Medicine. 1965;36:413–415.
74. Guseva NG et al. Ter Arkh. 1998;70(5):58–61.
75. Inaloz HS et al. Int J Dermatol. 2003 Jul;42(7):558–60.
76. Incandela L et al. Angiology. 2001 Oct;52 Suppl 2:S61–7.
77. De Sanctis MT et al. Angiology. 2001 Oct;52 Suppl 2:S55–9.
78. Incandela et al. Angiology. 2001 Oct;52 Suppl 2:S45–8.
79. Cesarone MR et al. Angiology. 2001 Oct;52 Suppl 2:S15–18.
80. Cesarone MR et al. Minerva Cardioangiol. 1994 Jun;24(6): 299–304.
81. Incandela L et al. Angiology. 2001 Oct;52 Suppl 2:S9–13.
82. Pointel JP et al. Angiology. 1987 Jan;38(1):46–50.
83. Incandela L et al. Angiology. 2001 Oct;Suppl 2:S69–73.
84. Cesarone MR et al. Angiology. 2001 Oct;52 Suppl 2:S19–25.
85. Cesarone MR et al. Angiology. 2001 Oct;52 Suppl 2:S49–54.
86. Incandela L et al. Angiology. 2001 Oct;52 Suppl 2:S27–31.
87. Cesarone MR et al. Angiology. 2001 Oct;52 Suppl 2:S33–7.
88. Montecchio GP et al. Haematologica. 1991 May–Jun; 76(3):256–9.
89. MacKay D. Altern Med Rev. 2001 Apr;6(2):126–40.
90. Arpaia MR et al. Int J Clin Pharmacol Res. 1990;10(4): 229–33.
91. Cataldi A et al. Minerva Cardioangiol. 2001 Apr;49(2): 159–63.
92. Soumyanath A et al. J Pharm Pharmacol. 2005 Dec;57(9): 1221–9.
93. Mukherjee PK et al. Phytother Res. 2007 Dec;21(12):1142–5.
94. Wattanathorn J et al. J Ethnopharmacol. 2008 Mar 5; 116(2):325–32.
95. Bradwejn J et al. J Clin Psychopharmacol. 2000 Dec;20(6): 680–4.

96. Yoosook C et al. Phytomedicine. 2000 Jan;6(6):411–9.
97. Zheng MS. J Tradit Chin Med. 1989 Jun;9(2):113–6.
98. Qureshi S et al. Hindustan Antibiot Bull. 1997 Feb–Nov;39(1–4):56–60.
99. Mamtha B et al. Ind J Pharmacol. 2004;36(1):41–2.
100. Punturee K et al. Asian Pac J Cancer Prev. 2005 Jul–Sep;6(3):396–400.
101. Chakrabarty T, Deshmukh S. Sci Cult. 1976;42:573.
102. Chaudhuri S et al. J Indian Med Assoc. 1978;70:177–80.
103. Babu TD et al. J Ethnopharmacol. 1995 Aug 11;48(1):53–7.
104. Yoshida M et al. Biol Pharm Bull. 2005 Jan;28(1):173–5.
105. Park BC et al. Cancer Lett. 2005 Jan 31;218(1):81–90.
106. Siddique YH et al. Toxicol In Vitro. 2008 Feb;22(1):10–7.
107. Darnis F et al. Sem Hosp Paris. 1979 Nov 8–15;55:1749–50.
108. Shin HS et al. Korean J Gastroenterol. 1982;14:49–56.
109. Sastravaha G et al. J Int Acad Periodontol. 2005 Jul;7(3): 70–9.
110. WHO Monographs on Selected Medicinal Plants—Vol 1. WHO Geneva 1999.
111. Gonzalo Garijo MA et al. Allergol Immunopathol (Madr). 1996 May–Jun;24(3):132–4.
112. Chopra RN et al. Indigenous drugs of India, 2nd Ed. UN Dur and Sons Ltd. Calcutta 1958.
113. Hausen BM. Contact Dermatitis. 1993;29:175–9.
114. Jorge OA, Jorge AD. Rev Esp Enferm Dig. 2005 Feb; 97(2):115–24.
115. Mimica-Dukic N et al. Phytother Res. 2003 Apr;17(4):368–71.
116. Lee HS. J Agric Food Chem. 2004 May 19;52(10):2887–9.
117. Diaz-Maroto MC et al. J Agric Food Chem. 2005 Jun 29; 53(13):5385–9.
118. Lo Cantore P et al. J Agric Food Chem. 2004 Dec 29; 52(26):7862–6.
119. Strehle MA et al. Biopolymers. 2005 Jan;77(1):44–52.
120. Zaidi SF et al. J Agric Food Chem. 2007 Dec 12; 55(25):10162–7.
121. Dhalwal K et al. J Sep Sci. 2007 Aug;30(13):2053–8.
122. Bilia AR et al. J Agric Food Chem. 2000 Oct;48(10):4734–8.
123. Parejo I et al. J Agric Food Chem. 2004 Apr 7;52(7):1890–7.
124. Topal U et al. Int J Food Sci Nutr. 2007 Sep 18;[epub ahead of print].
125. De Marino S et al. Phytochemistry. 2007 Jul;68(13): 1805–12.
126. Barazani O et al. Planta Med. 1999 Jun;65(5):486–9.
127. Diaz-Maroto MC et al. J Agric Food Chem. 2006 Sep 6; 54(18):6814–8.
128. Fyfe K et al. Int J Antimicrob Agents. 1997 Jan;9(3):195–9.
129. Dadalioglu I, Evrendilek GA. J Agric Food Chem. 2004 Dec 29;52(26):8255–60.
130. Singh G et al. Phytother Res. 2002 Nov;16(7):680–2.
131. Khaldun AO. Zh Mikrobiol Epidemiol Immunobiol. 2006 May–Jun;(3):92–3.
132. Baliga MS et al. Nahrung. 2003 Aug;47(4):261–4.
133. Toda S. Phytother Res. 2003 May;17(5):546–8.
134. Stashenko EE et al. Anal Bioanal Chem. 2002 May; 373(1–2):70–4.
135. Ruberto G et al. Planta Med. 2000 Dec;66(8):687–93.
136. Satyanarayana S et al. J Herb Pharmacother. 2004;4(2): 1–10.
137. Howes MJ et al. J Pharm Pharmacol. 2002 Nov;54(11): 1521–8.
138. Liu Z et al. Wei Sheng Yan Jiu. 2004 Jul;33(4):458–60.

139. Albert-Puleo M. J Ethnopharmacol. 1980 Dec;2(4):337–44.
140. Javidnia K et al. Phytomedicine. 2003;10(6–7):455–8.
141. Namavar Jahromi B et al. Int J Gynaecol Obstet. 2003 Feb; 80(2):153–7.
142. Modaress Nejad V, Asadipour M. East Mediterr Health J. 2006 May–Jul;12(3–4):423–7.
143. Alexandrovich I et al. Atern Ther Health Med. 2003 Jul–Aug;9(4):58–61.
144. Savino F et al. Phytother Res. 2005 Apr;19(4):335–40.
145. Chakurski I et al. Vutr Boles. 1981;20(6):51–4.
146. Kim SI et al. Pest Manag Sci. 2004 Nov;60(11):1125–30.
147. Stager J et al. Allergy. 1991;46(6):475–8.
148. Iten F, Saller R. Forsch Komp. Klass Nat. 2004 Apr;11(2):104–8.
149. Subehan et al. J Ethnopharmacol. 2006 May 24;105(3): 449–55.
150. Zhu M et al. J Pharm Pharmacol. 1999 Dec;51(12):1391–6.
151. Moore M. Medicinal Plants of the Pacific West. Red Crane Publications Santa Fe, 1993.
152. Van Wagenen BC et al. J Nat Prod. 1988 Jan–Feb; 51(1):136–41.
153. Alstat E. Proc NHAA Int Conf. 1995 Mar;116–120.
154. McCutcheon AR et al. J Ethnopharmacol. 1995 Dec 1; 49(2):101–10.
155. Lee TT et al. Bioorg Med Chem. Oct;2(10):1051–6.
156. Van Wagenen BC. Diss Abstr Int. 1991 (B);51(12):5879.
157. Bergener P. Medical Herbalism. 2001;10(4):16.
158. Moerman D. Portland. Oregon:Timber Press, 1998.
159. Rodrigues VM et al. J Agric Food Chem. 2003 Mar 12; 51(6):1518–23.
160. Burkhardt G et al. Pharm Weekbl Sci. 1986 Jun 20;8(3):190–3.
161. Strehle KR et al. J Agric Food Chem. 2006 Sep 20; 54(19):7020–6.
162. Tabanca N et al. J Chromatogr A. 2006 Jun 9; 1117(2):194–205.
163. Fujimatu E et al. Phytochemistry. 2003 Jul;63(5):609–16.
164. Ishikawa T et al. Chem Pharm Bull (Tokyo). 2002 Nov; 50(11):1460–6.
165. Marero LM et al. J Nutr Sci Vitaminol (Tokyo). 1986 Feb;32(1):131–6.
166. Al-Bataina BA et al. J Trace Elem Med Biol. 2003;17(2): 85–90.
167. Chaudry NM, Tariq P. Pak J Pharm Sci. 2006 Jul;19(3): 214–8.
168. Prabuseenivasan S et al. BMC Complement Altern Med. 2006 Nov 30;6:39.
169. Kosalec I et al. Acta Pharm. 2005 Dec;55(4):377–85.
170. Lee HS. Planta Med. 2004 Mar;70(3):279–81.
171. Erler F et al. Fitoterapia. 2006 Dec;77(7–8):491–4.
172. Prajapati V et al. Bioresour Technol. 2005 Nov;96(16):1749–57.
173. Mumcuoglu KY et al. Isr Med Assoc J. 2002 Oct;4(10):790–3.
174. Veal L. Complement Ther Nurs Midwifery. 1996 Aug;2(4):97–101.
175. Kassi E et al. J Agric Food Chem. 2004 Nov 17; 52(23):6956–61.
176. Buechi S et al. Forsch Komplementarmed Klass Naturheilkd. 2005 Dec;12(6):328–32.
177. Fraj J et al. Allergy. 1996 May;51(5):337–9.
178. Stricker WE et al. J Allergy Clin Immunol. 1986 Mar;77(3):516–9.
179. Gazquez Garcia V et al. J Investig Allergol Clin Immunol. 2007;17(6):406–8.
180. Moreno-Ancillo A et al. Allergol Immunopathol (Madr). 2005 Sep–Oct;33(5):288–90.

Apocynaceae

1. Ognyanov I et al. Tetrahedron. 1968;24(13):4641–48.
2. Banerji A, Chakrabarty M. Phytochemistry. 1974;13(10): 2309–12.
3. Banerji A, Chakrabarty M. Phytochemistry. 1977;16(7): 1124–25.
4. Mukhopadhyay G et al. Phytochemistry. 1991;30(7):2447–9.
5. Atta-Ur-Rahaman et al. Phytochemistry. 1995;38(4):1057–61.
6. Farnsworth NR et al. J Pharm Sci. 1962 Mar;51(3):217–24.
7. Sakushima A, Nishibe S. Phytochemistry. 1988;27(3):915–19.
8. Mokry J et al. Experientia. 1961 Aug 15;17:354.
9. Sturdikova M et al. Pharmazie. 1986 Apr;41(4):270–2.
10. Mokry J et al. Experientia. 1962 Dec 15;18:564–5.
11. Mokry H et al. Experientia. 1963 Jun 15;19:311.
12. Grossmann E, Pavol E. Phytochemistry. 1973;12(8):2058.
13. Plat M et al. Ann Pharm Fr. 1962 Dec;20:899–906.
14. Proksa B et al. Planta Med. 1988 Jun;54(3):214–8.
15. Szostak H, Kowalweski Z. Pol J Pharmacol Pharm. 1975 Nov–Dec;27(6):657–63.
16. Garnier J et al. Phytochemistry. 1975 Jun;14(5–6):1385–7.
17. Le Men J, Pourrat H. Ann Pharm Fr. 1952 May;10(5): 349–51.
18. Hammouda Y, Le Men J. Ann Pharm Fr. 1956 May;14(5): 344–7.
19. Szatmari SZ, Whitehouse PJ. Cochrane Database Syst Rev. 2003(1):CD003119.
20. Kidd PM. Altern Med Rev. 1999 Jun;4(3):144–61.
21. Karpati E et al. Acta Pharm Hung. 2002;72(1):25–36.
22. Ravina A. Presse Med. 1966 Feb 26;74(11):525–7.
23. Dekoninck WJ et al. Arzneimittelforschung. 1978;28(9): 1654–7.

Araceae

1. Sugimoto N et al. Biol Pharm Bull. 1999 May;22(5):481–5.
2. Marongiu B et al. J Agric Food Chem. 2005 Oct 5; 53(20):7939–43.
3. Wu LJ et al. Yakugaku Zasshi. 1994 Mar;114(3):182–5.
4. Oprean R et al. J Pharm Biomed Anal. 2001 Mar; 24(5–6):1163–8.
5. Mukherjee PK et al. Planta Med. 2007 Mar;73(3):283–5.
6. Wojdylo A et al. Food Chem. 2007 Jan;105(3):940–9.
7. Belanger A et al. Agriculture and Agri-food Canada 2004 Research Summary. 1999–2000;27:50.
8. Martindale, The Extra Pharmacopoeia 26th Ed. Pharmaceutical Press London March 1973 p. 324.
9. Mehrotra S et al. Int Immunopharmacol. 2003 Jan;3(1): 53–61.
10. Acuna UM et al. Phytother Res. 2002 Feb;16(1):63–5.
11. Prabuseenivasan S et al. BMC Complement Altern Med. 2006 Nov;6(1):39.
12. Ahmad I, Aqil F. Microbiol Res. 2007 Jul;162(3):264–75.
13. Aqil F et al. Biotechnol J. 2006 Oct;1(10):1093–102.
14. Gautam R et al. J Ethnopharmacol. 2007 Mar;110(2): 200–34.

15. Thirach S et al. Acta Hortic. 2003;597:217–221.
16. Rau O et al. Pharmazie. 2006 Nov;61(11):952–6.
17. Oh MH et al. Phytomedicine. 2004 Sep;11(6):544–8.
18. Sugimoto N et al. Biol Pharm Bull. 1995 Apr;18(4):605–9.
19. Hanson KM et al. Electrophoresis. 2005 Feb;26(4–5):943–6.
20. Oprean R et al. J Pharm Biomed Anal. 1998 Oct;18(1–2): 227–34.

Araliaceae

1. WHO Monographs on Selected Medicinal Plants—Vol 2. WHO Geneva 2004 p. 83–96.
2. Tolonen A et al. Phytochem Anal. 2002 Nov–Dec;13(6):316–28.
3. Zgorka G, Kawka S. J Pharm Biomed Anal. 2001 Mar; 24(5–6):1065–72.
4. Li XC et al. Planta Med. 2001 Nov;67(8):776–8.
5. Schmolz MW et al. Phytother Res. 2001 May;15(3):268–70.
6. Wagner H et al. Arnzneimittelforschung. 1985;35(7):1069–75.
7. Bohn B et al. Arnzneimittelforschung. 1987 Oct;37(10): 1193–6.
8. Williams M. Br J Phyto. 1993/4;3(1):32–7.
9. Steinmann GG et al. Arzneimittelforschung. 2001 Jan;51(1): 76–83.
10. Amaryan G et al. Phytomedicine. 2003 May;10(4):271–85.
11. Kormosh N et al. Phytother Res. 2006 May;20(5):424–5.
12. Narimanian M et al. Phytomedicine. 2005 Aug;12(8): 539–47.
13. Panossian A et al. Phytomedicine. 2002 Oct;9(7):598–600.
14. Yu CY et al. Toxicol in Vitro. 2003 Apr;17(2):229–36.
15. Glatthaar-Saalmuller B et al. Antiviral Res. 2001 Jun;50(3): 223–8.
16. Wildfeuer A, Mayerhofer D. Arzneimittelforschung. 1994 Mar;44(3):361–6.
17. Narimanian M et al. Phytomedicine. 2005 Nov;12(10):723–9.
18. Ben-Hur E, Fulder S. Am J Chin Med. 1981 Spring;9(1): 48–56.
19. Chen Z et al. Zhonghua Nen Ke Xue. 2007 Mar;13(1):21–3.
20. Cicero AF et al. Arch Geron Geriatr Suppl. 2004;(9):69–73.
21. Asano K et al. Planta Med. 1986 Jun;(3):175–7.
22. Nasolodin VV et al. Gig Sanit. 2006 Mar–Apr;(2):44–7.
23. Eschbach LF et al. Int J Sport Exerc Metab. 2000 Dec;10(4): 444–51.
24. Dowling EA et al. Med Sci Sports Exerc. 1996 Apr;28(4): 482–9.
25. Goulet ED, Dionne IJ. Int J Sports Nutr Exerc Metab. 2005 Feb;15(1):75–83.
26. Kaloeva ZD. Farmakol Toksikol. 1986 Sep–Oct;49(5):73.
27. Sosnova T. Vestnk Oftalmol. 1969;5:59–61.
28. Collison RJ. Br J Phyto. 1991;2(2):61–71.
29. Tseitlin GJ et al. Paediatria. 1981;5:25–7.
30. Szolomicki J et al. Phytother Res. 2000 Feb;14(1):30–5.
31. Gaffney BT et al. Med Hypotheses. 2001 May;56(5):567–72.
32. Gaffney BT et al. Life Sci. 2001 Dec 14;70(4):431–42.
33. Panossian A, Wagner H. Phytother Res. 2005 Oct;19(10): 723–9.
34. Golikov AP. Lekarstvennye Sredstva Dal'nego Vostoka. 1966;7:63–65.
35. Mikunis RI et al. Lekarstvennye Sredstva Dal'nego Vostoka. 1966;7:227–230.
36. Donovan JL et al. Drug Metab Dispos. 2003 May;31(5): 519–22.
37. McCrae S. Can Med Assoc J. 1996;155:293–5.
38. Wang Y et al. Phytochem Anal. 2006 Nov;17(6):424–30.
39. Abd El-Aty AM et al. Biomed Chromatogr. 2008 May;22(5): 556–62.
40. Wang JY et al. Zhongguo Zhong Yao Za Zhi. 1993 Feb;18(2): 105–7.
41. Samukawa D et al. Yalugaku Zasshi. 1995 Mar;115(3):241–9.
42. Yip TT et al. Am J Chin Med. 1985;13(1–4):77–88.
43. Richter R et al. Phytochemistry. 2005 Dec;66(23):2708–13.
44. Lee SW et al. Planta Med. 2004 Mar;70(3):197–200.
45. Rho MC et al. J Agric Food Chem. 2005 Feb 23;53(4):919–22.
46. Tomoda M et al. Biol Pharm Bull. 1993 Nov;16(11):1087–90.
47. Ng TB, Wang H. Life Sci. 2001 Jan 5;68(7):739–49.
48. Zhang D et al. Free Radic Biol Med. 1996;20(1):145–50.
49. Liu ZQ et al. Biochem Biophys Acta. 2002 Aug 15;1572(1): 58–66.
50. Chang MS et al. Phytother Res. 1999 Dec;13(8):641–4.
51. Liu ZQ et al. J Agric Food Chem. 2003 Apr 23;51(9):2555–8.
52. Kim YH et al. J Biol Chem. 1996 Oct 4;271(40):24539–43.
53. Gillis CN. Biochem Pharmacol. 1997 Jul 1;54(1):1–8.
54. Wilasrusmee C et al. Am Surg. 2002 Oct;68(10):860–4.
55. Tong LS, Chao CY. Am J Chin Med. 1980 Autumn;8(3): 254–67.
56. Liu J et al. Mech Ageing Dev. 1995 Aug 31;83(1):43–53.
57. Cho JY et al. Planta Med. 2002 Jun;68(8):497–500.
58. See DM et al. Immunopharmacology. 1997 Jan;35(3):229–35.
59. Larsen MW et al. APMIS. 2004 Jun;112(6):369–73.
60. Jin J et al. Zhongguo Zhong Xi Yi Jie He Za Zhi. 2000 Sep; 20(9):673–6.
61. Takei M et al. Biochem Pharmacol. 2004 Aug 1;68(3):441–52.
62. Cho JY et al. Planta Med. 2001 Apr;67(3):213–8.
63. Bae EA et al. Arch Pharm Res. 2004 Jan;27(1):61–7.
64. Lim DS et al. J Infect. 2002 Jul;45(1):32–8.
65. Lee JH et al. Planta Med. 2004 Jun;70(6):556–8.
66. Solo'veva TF et al. Antibiot Khimioter. 1989 Oct;34(10): 755–60.
67. Sonoda Y et al. Immunopharmacology. 1998 Jan;38(3): 287–94.
68. Ma L et al. Zhongguo Zhong Xi Yi Jie He Za Zhi. 1995 Jul; 15(7):411–3.
69. Scaglione F et al. Drugs Exp Clin Res. 1990;16(10):537–42.
70. Srisurapanon S et al. J Med Assoc Thai. 1997 Sep;80 Suppl 1: S81–5.
71. Scaglione F et al. Drugs Exp Clin Res. 1996;22(2):65–72.
72. Helms S. Atlern Med Rev. 2004 Sep;9(3):259–74.
73. Lee TK et al. Mutat Res. 2004 Jan 10;557(1):75–84.
74. Ben-Hur E, Fulder S. Am J Chin Med. 1981 Spring;9(1): 48–56.
75. Kim YS, Jin SH. Arch Pharm Res. 2004 Aug;27(8):834–9.
76. Fei XF et al. Acta Pharmacol Sin. 2002 Apr;23(4):315–22.
77. Moon J et al. Biochem Pharmacol. 2000 May 1;59(9):1109–16.
78. Park JA et al. Cancer Lett. 1997 Dec 16;121(1):73–81.
79. Oh SH et al. Arch Pharm Res. 2004 Apr;27(4):402–6.
80. Popovich DG, Kitts DD. J Biochem Mol Toxicol. 2004;18(3): 143–9.
81. Wang Y et at. Zhongguo Shi Yan Xue Ye Xue Za Zhi. 2004 Jun;12(3):315–20.
82. Lee SJ et al. Biochem Pharmacol. 2000 Sep 1;60(5):677–85.
83. Choi HH et al. Int J Oncol. 2003 Oct;23(4):1087–93.
84. Liu WK et al. Life Sci. 2000 Aug 4;67(11):1297–306.
85. Sohn J et al. Exp Mol Med. 1998 Mar 31;30(1):47–51.
86. Matsunaga H et al. Cancer Chemother Pharmacol. 1995;35(4):291–6.

87. Oh M et al. Int J Oncol. 1999 May;14(5):869–75.
88. Loo WT et al. Life Sci. 2004 Nov 26;76(2):191–200.
89. Wang M et al. Zhongguo Zhong Yao Za Zhi. 1992 Feb; 17(2):110–2.
90. Gao R et al. Zhongguo Zhong Xi Yi Jie He Za Zhi. 1999 Jan; 19(1):17–9.
91. Matsunaga H et al. Biol Pharm Bull. 1994 May;17(5):635–9.
92. Gao R et al. Zhongguo Zhong Xi Yi Jie He Za Zhi. 1999 Jan; 19(1):17–9.
93. Yu Y et al. Cancer. 2007 Jun 1;109(11):2374–82.
94. Lee BH et al. Planta Med. 1998 Aug;64(6):500–3.
95. Matsunaga H et al. Chem Pharm Bull (Tokyo). 1990 Dec; 38(12):3480–2.
96. Zeng XL, Tu ZG. Ai Zheng. 2004 Aug;23(8):879–84.
97. Kim YS et al. Int J Biochem Cell Biol. 1998 Mar;30(3): 327–38.
98. Chang YS et al. Integ Cancer Ther. 2003 Mar;2(1):13–33.
99. Xie FY et al. Zhongguo Zhong Xi Yi Jie He Za Zhi. 2001 May;21(5):332–4.
100. Yun TK. Mutat Res. 2003 Feb–Mar;523–524:63–74.
101. Yun TK et al. J Korean Med Sci. 2001 Dec;16 Suppl: S28–37.
102. Yun TK, Choi SY. Int J Epidemiol. 1998 Jun;27(3):359–64.
103. Yun TK, Choi SY. Int J Epidemiol. 1990 Dec;19(4):871–6.
104. Cui Y et al. Am J Epidemiol. 2006 Apr 1;163(7):645–53.
105. Yun TK, Choi SY. Cancer Epidemiol Biomarkers Prev. 1995 Jun;4(4):401–8.
106. Kakizoe T. Eur J Cancer. 2000 Jun;36(10):1303–9.
107. Kwon BM et al. Bioorg Med Chem Lett. 1999 May 17;9(10): 1375–8.
108. Dou DQ et al. Planta Med. 2001 Feb;67(1):19–23.
109. Kim Yu A et al. Membr Cell Biol. 2000;14(2):237–51.
110. Jiang Y et al. Zhongguo Zhong Yao Za Zhi. 1992 Mar; 17(3):172–5.
111. Niu YP et al. Zhongguo Zhong Xi Yi Jie He Za Zhi. 2004 Feb;24(2):127–9.
112. Chen D et al. Zhongguo Zhong Xi Yi Jie He Za Zhi. 2003 Nov;23(11):845–7.
113. Gao RL et al. Zhongguo Zhong Xi Yi Jie He Za Zhi. 1992 May;12(5):285–7.
114. Niu YP et al. Zhongguo Shi Yan Xue Ye Xue Za Zhi. 2001 Jun;9(2):178–80.
115. Park HJ et al. J Ethnopharmacol. 1995 Dec 15;49(3):157–62.
116. Teng CM et al. Biochim Biophys Acta. 1989 Mar 24;990(3): 315–20.
117. Yuan J et al. J Tradit Chin Med. 1997 Mar;17(1):14–7.
118. Long MZ et al. Zhongguo Zhong Xi Yi Jie He Za Zhi. 2003 Nov;23(11):808–10.
119. Dai X et al. Zhongguo Zhong Xi Yi Jie He Za Zhi. 1999 Jan;19(1):17–9.
120. Zhan Y et al. Zhonghua Yi Xue Za Zhi. 1994 Oct;74(10): 626–8.
121. Kim SH, Park KS. Pharmacol Res. 2003 Nov;48(5):511–3.
122. Caron MF et al. Ann Pharmacother. 2002 May;36(5):758–63.
123. Kiesewetter H et al. Int J Pharmacol Ther Toxicol. 1992 Mar;30(3):97–102.
124. Tamaoki J et al. Br J Pharmacol. 2000 Aug;130(8):1859–64.
125. Yagi A et al. Planta Med. 1996 Apr;62(2):115–8.
126. Yoo HH et al. Am J Chin Med. 2006;34(1):137–46.
127. Gross D et al. Monaldi Arch Chest Dis. 2002 Oct–Dec; 57(5–6):242–6.

128. Wang W, Niu RJ. Zhongguo Zhong Xi Yi Jie He Za Zhi. 1993 Feb;13(2):91–3.
129. Lee JH et al. Planta Med. 2004 Jul;70(7):615–9.
130. Ohya T et al. Paediatr Int. 2004 Feb;46(1):72–6.
131. Zuin M et al. J Int Med Res. 1987 Sep–Oct;15(5):276–81.
132. Lee FC et al. Clin Exp Pharmacol Physiol. 1987 Jun;14(6): 543–6.
133. Tohda C et al. Jpn J Pharmacol. 2002 Nov;90(3):254–62.
134. Lee JY et al. Life Sci. 2004 Aug 13;75(13):1621–34.
135. Rudakewich M et al. Planta Med. 2001 Aug;67(6):533–7.
136. Choi K et al. Neurosci Lett. 2007 Jun 21;421(1):37–41.
137. Park H et al. Neurol Res. 2007;29 Suppl 1:S78–87.
138. Siddique MS et al. Acta Neurochir Suppl. 2000;76:87–90.
139. Zhang YW et al. Planta Med. 2001 Jul;67(5):417–22.
140. Lewis R et al. Phytother Res. 1999 Feb;13(1):59–64.
141. Coleman CI et al. J Clin Pharm Ther. 2003 Feb;28(1):5–15.
142. Wesnes KA et al. Psychopharmacology. 2000 Nov; 152(4):353–61.
143. Persson J et al. Psychopharmacology. 2004 Apr;172(4):430–4.
144. Wesnes KA et al. Psychompharmacol Bull. 1997;33(4): 677–83.
145. Kennedy DO et al. Pharmacol Biochem Behav. 2003 Jun; 75(3):701–9.
146. Scholey AB, Kennedy DO. Hum Psychopharmacol. 2002 Jan;17(1):35–44.
147. Kennedy DO et al. Physiol Behav. 2002 Apr 15;75(5): 739–51.
148. D'Angelo L et al. J Ethnopharmacol. 1986 Apr–May;16(1): 15–22.
149. Ziemba AW et al. Int J Sport Nutr. 1999 Dec;9(4):371–7.
150. Kennedy DO et al. Nutri Neurosci. 2001;4(4):295–310.
151. Kennedy DO et al. Pharmacol Biochem Behav. 2004 Nov; 79(3):401–11.
152. Bentler SE et al. J Clin Psychiatry. 2005 May;66(5):625–32.
153. Caso Marasco A et al. Drugs Exp Clin Res.1996;22(6):323–9.
154. Hallstrom C et al. Comp Med East West. 1982;6:277–82.
155. Cardinal BJ, Engels HJ. J Am Diet Assoc. 2001 Jun;101(6): 655–60.
156. Ellis JM, Reddy P. Ann Pharmacother. 2002 Mar;36(3):375–9.
157. Thommessen B, Laake K. Tidsskr Nor Laegeforen. 1997 Oct 30;117(26):3839–41.
158. Thommessen B, Laake K. Aging (Milano). 1996 Dec;8(6): 417–20.
159. Lee Y et al. J Steroid Biochem Mol Biol. 2003 Mar;84(4): 463–8.
160. Lee Y et al. Arch Pharm Res. 2003 Jan;26(1):58–63.
161. Cho J et al. J Endocinol Metab. 2004 Jul;89(7):3510–5.
162. Polan ML et al. J Womens Health. 2004 May;13(4):427–30.
163. Liu J et al. J Agric Food Chem. 2001 May;49(5):2472–9.
164. Amato P et al. Menopause. 2002 Mar–Apr;9(2):145–50.
165. Gray SL et al. Exp Biol Med. 2004 Jun;229(6):560–8.
166. Bae EA et al. Biol Pharm Bull. 2005 Oct;28(10):1903–8.
167. Ling C et al. Gen Comp Endocrinol. 2005 Feb;140(3): 203–9.
168. Chong SK et al. Int Arch Allergy Appl Immunol. 1984;73(3):216–20.
169. Pearce PT et al. Endocrinol Jpn. 1982 Oct;29(5):567–73.
170. Onomura M et al. Am J Chin Med. 1999;27(3–4):347–54.
171. Bae JW, Lee MH. J Ethnopharmacol. 2004 Mar;91(1):72–6.
172. Hartley DE et al. Nutr Neurosci. 2004 Oct–Dec;7(5–6): 325–33.

173. Huntley AL, Ernst E. Menopause. 2003 Sep–Oct;10(5): 465–76.
174. Wiklund IK et al. Int J Clin Pharmacol Res. 1999;19(3): 89–99.
175. Zhang WY et al. Zhonghua Yi Xue Za Zhi. 1994 Oct;74(10): 608–10.
176. Mkrtchyan A et al. Phytomedicine. 2005 Jun;12(6–7): 403–9.
177. Salvati G et al. Panminerva Med. 1996 Dec;38(4):249–54.
178. Choi HK et al. Int J Impot Res. 1999 Oct;11(5):261–4.
179. Sievenpiper JL et al. J Am Coll Nutr. 2004 Jun;23(3):248–58.
180. Reay JL et al. J Psychopharmacol. 2005 Jul;19(4):357–65.
181. Reay JL et al. Br J Nutr. 2006 Oct;96(4):639–42.
182. Choi S. Arch Pharm Res. 2002 Feb;25(1):71–6.
183. Lu ZQ, Dice JF. Biochem Biophys Res Commun. 1985 Jan 16;126(1):636–40.
184. Lee J et al. J Ethnopharmacol. 2007 Jan 3;109(1):29–34.
185. Oliveira DP et al. J Ethnopharmacol. 2005 Feb 28;97(2): 211–4.
186. Pieralisi G et al. Clinical Ther. 1991;13:373–82.
187. Forgo I et al. Notabene Med. 1982;12:721–7.
188. Forgo I et al. Arz Prax. 1981;33:1784–6.
189. Forgo I. Munch Med Woch. 1983;125:822–4.
190. Forgo I, Schimert G. Notabene Med. 1985;15:636–40.
191. Engels HJ et al. Med Sci Sports Exerc. 2003 Apr;35(4): 690–6.
192. Gaffney BT et al. Life Sci. 2001 Dec 14;70(4):431–42.
193. Engels HJ et al. J Strength Cond Res. 2001 Aug;15(3): 290–5.
194. Allen JD et al. J Am Coll Nutr. 1998 Oct;17(5):462–6.
195. Morris AC et al. Int J Sport Nutr. 1996 Sep;6(3):263–71.
196. Youl Kang H et al. J Strength Cond Res. 2002 May;16(2): 179–83.
197. Kim SH et al. J Sports Med Phys Fitness. 2005 Jun;45(2): 178–82.
198. Bucci LR. Am J Clin Nutr. 2000 Aug;72(2 Suppl):624–36.
199. Sheng ZL et al. Zhongguo Zhong Xi Yi Jie He Za Zhi. 1994 May;14(5):268–70.
200. Zhao XZ. Zhong Xi Yi He Za Zhi. 1990 Oct;10(10):586–9.
201. Hasegawa H et al. Planta Med. 1997 Oct;63(5):436–40.
202. Cui JF et al. J Chromatogr B Biomed Sci Appl. 1997 Feb 21;689(2):349–55.
203. Coon JT, Ernst E. Drug Saf. 2002;25(5):323–44.
204. Siegel RK. JAMA. 1979;241:1614–15.
205. Ang-Lee MK et al. JAMA. 2001 Jul 11;286(2):208–16.
206. Kabalak AA et al. J Womens Health. 2004 Sep;13(7): 830–3.
207. Hopkins MP et al. Am J Obstet Gynaecol. 1988 Nov; 159(5):1121–2.
208. Palanisamy A et al. J Toxicol Clin Toxicol. 2003;41(6): 865–7.
209. Ryu SJ, Chien YY. Neurology. 1995 Apr;45(4):829–30.
210. Lou BY et al. Yan Ke Xue Bao. 1989 Dec;5(3–4):96–7.
211. Shader RI, Greenblatt DJ. J Clin Psychopharmacol. 1985 Feb;5(2):65.
212. Jones BD, Runikis AM. J Clin Psychopharmacol. 1987 Jun;7(3):201–2.
213. Vazquez I, Aguera-Ortiz LF. Acta Psychia Scand. 2002 Jan;105(1):76–7.
214. Faleni R, Soldati F. The Lancet. 1996 Jul 27;348(9022):267.
215. Yuan CS et al. Ann Int Med. Jul 6;141:23–27.

216. Jiang X et al. Br J Clin Pharmacol. 2004 May;57(5):592–9.
217. Jiang X et al. J Clin Pharmacol. 2006 Nov;46(11):1370–8.
218. Sparreboom A et al. J Clin Oncol. 2004 Jun 15;22(12): 2489–503.
219. Gurley BJ et al. Drugs Aging. 2005;22(6):525–39.
220. Anderson GS et al. J Clin Pharmacol. 2003 Jun;43(6): 643–8.
221. Gurley BJ et al. Clin Pharmacol Ther. 2002 Sep;72(3):276–87.
222. Dasgupta A et al. Am J Clin Path. 2003 Feb;119(2):298–303.
223. Chow L et al. J Clin Lab Anal. 2003;17(1):22–7.

Areceae

1. *The United States Pharmacopoeia 24: National Formulary 19* Rockville, MD, United States Pharmacopeial Convention, 1999.
2. Iguchi K et al. Prostate. 2001 Apr 1;47(1):59–65.
3. Buck AC. J Urol. 2004 Nov;172(5):1792–9.
4. Habib FK, Wyllie MG. Prostate Cancer Prostatic Dis. 2004; 7(3):195–200.
5. Hiracek J et al. Steroids. 2007 Apr;72(4):375–80.
6. Drsata J. Cas Lek Cesk. 2002 Oct 11;141(20):630–5.
7. Vela Navarrete R et al. Actas Urol Esp. 2002 Mar;26(3): 163–73.
8. Schilcher H. Wien Med Wochenschr. 1999;149(8–10):236–40.
9. Raynaud JP et al. J Steroid Biochem Mol Biol. 2002 Oct; 82(2–3):233–9.
10. Iehle C et al. J Steroid Biochem Mol Biol. 1995 Sep;54(5–6): 273–9.
11. Bayne CW et al. Prostate. 1999 Sep 1;40(4):232–41.
12. Vacherot F et al. Prostate. 2000 Nov 1;45(3):259–66.
13. Bayne CW et al. J Urol. 2000 Sep;164(3):876–81.
14. Ravenna L et al. Prostate. 1996 Oct;29(4):219–30.
15. Sultan C et al. J Steroid Biochem. 1984 Jan;20(1):515–9.
16. Plosker GL, Brogden RN. Drugs Aging. 1996 Nov;9(5): 379–95.
17. Di Silverio F et al. Eur Urol. 1992;21(4):309–14.
18. Di Silverio F et al. Prostate. 1998 Oct 1;37(2):77–83.
19. Fong YK et al. Curr Opin Urol. 2005 Jan;15(1):45–8.
20. Boyle P et al. BJU Int. 2004 Apr;93(6):751–6.
21. Al-Shukri SH et al. Prostate Cancer Prostatic Dis. 2000 Nov; 3(3):195–9.
22. Aliaev IUG et al. Urologia. 2002 Jan–Feb;(1):23–5.
23. Boyle P et al. Urology. 2000 Apr;55(4):533–9.
24. Debruyne F et al. Prog Urol. 2004 Jun;14(3):326–31.
25. Pytel YA et al. Adv Ther. 2002 Nov–Dec;19(6):297–306.
26. Casarosa C et al. Clin Ther. 1988;10(5):585–8.
27. Vela Navarrete R et al. J Urol. 2005 Feb;173(2):507–10.
28. Wilde MI, Goa KL. Drugs. 1999 Apr;57(4):557–81.
29. Debruyne F et al. Prog Urol. 2002 Jun;12(3):384–92.
30. Buck AC. J Urol. 2004 Nov;172(5pt1):1792–9.
31. Dvorkin L, Song KY. Ann Pharmcother. 2002 Sep;36(9): 1443–52.
32. Wilt T et al. Cochrane Database Syst Rev. 2002;(3): CD0011423.
33. Wilt TJ et al. Public Health Nutr. 2000 Dec;3(4A):459–72.
34. Wilt T et al. Cochrane Database Syst Rev. 2000;(2):CD001423.
35. Sokeland J. BJU Int. 2000 Sep;86(4):439–42.
36. Wilt TJ et al. JAMA. 1998 Nov 11;280(18):1604–9.

37. Hill B et al. Prostate. 2004 Sep 15;61(1):73–80.
38. Willetts KE et al. BJU Int. 2003 Aug;93(3):267–70.
39. Djavan B. Urology. 2003 Sep;62(3):6–14.
40. Glemain P et al. Prog Urol. 2002 Jun;12(3):395–403.
41. Pecoraro S et al. Minerva Urol Nefrol. 2004 Mar;56(1):73–8.
42. Shoskes DA. Curr Urol Rep. 2002 Aug;3(4):330–4.
43. Loran OB et al. Urologica. 2003 Nov–Dec;(6):30–2.
44. Wu T. Zhonghua Nan Ke Xue. 2004 May;10(5):337–9.
45. Paubert-Braquet M et al. Eur Urol. 1998;33(3):340–7.
46. Ishii K et al. Biol Pharm Bull. 2001 Feb;24(2):188–90.
47. Shimada H et al. J Nat Prod. 1997 Apr;60(4):417–8.
48. Delos S. J Steroid Biochem Mol Biol. 1995 Dec;55(3–4): 375–83.
49. Breu W et al. Arzneimittelforschung. 1992 Apr;42(4):547–51.
50. Paubert-Braquet M et al. Prostaglandins Leukot Essen Fatty Acids. 1997 Sep;57(3):299–304.
51. Wagner H et al. Arzneimittelforschung. 1985;35(7):1069–75.
52. Vela Navarrete R et al. Eur Urol. 2003 Nov;44(5):549–55.
53. el-Sheikh MM et al. Acta Obstets Gynecol Scand. 1988; 67(5):397–9.
54. Prager N et al. J Altern Complement Med. 2002 Apr;8(2): 143–52.
55. Habib FK et al. Int J Cancer. 2005 Mar 20;114(2):190–4.
56. Giannakopoulos X et al. Adv Ther. 2002 Nov–Dec; 19(6):285–96.
57. Stepanov VN et al. Adv Ther. 1999 Sep–Oct;16(5):231–41.
58. Gurley BJ et al. Clin Pharmacol Ther. 2004 Nov;76(5): 428–40.
59. Markowitz JS et al. Clin Pharmacol Ther. 2003 Dec;74(6): 536–42.

Asclepiadaceae

1. Abe F, Yamauchi T. Chem Pharm Bull (Tokyo). 2000 Jul; 48(7):991–3.
2. Abe F, Yamauchi T. Chem Pharm Bull (Tokyo). 2000 Jul; 48(7):1017–22.
3. Claus EP. Pharmacognosy 4th Ed. Henry Kimpton. London 1961 p. 166.

Asteraceae

1. De Jong NW et al. Allergy. 1998 Feb;53(2):204–9.
2. Paulsen E et al. Contact Dermatitis 2001 Oct;45(4):197–204.
3. Hausen BM. Am J Contact Dermat. 1996 Jun;7(2):94–9.
4. Paulsen E et al. Contact Dermatitis. 1993 Jul;29(1):6–10.
5. Hausen BM, Oestmann G. Derm Beruf Umwelt. 1988 Jul–Aug;36(4):117–24.
6. Hausen BM, Osmundsen PE. Acta Derm Venereol. 1983; 63(4):308–14.
7. Jovanovic M et al. Med Pregl. 2004 May–Jun;57(5–6): 209–18.
8. Fernandez C et al. J Allergy Clin Immunol. 1993 Nov;92(5): 660–7.
9. Hausen BM. Am J Contact Derm. 1996 Jun;7(2):94–9.
10. Guo YP et al. New Phytol. 2005 Apr;166(1):273–90.
11. Agnihotri VK et al. Planta Med. 2005 Mar;71(3):280–3.
12. Rohloff J et al. J Agric Food Chem. 2000 Dec;48(12):6205–9.
13. Cornu A et al. J Agric Food Chem. 2001 Jan;49(1):203–9.
14. Orth M et al. Pharmazie. 2000 Jun;55(6):203–9.
15. British Herbal Compendium. British Herbal Medicine Association 1992.
16. Gherase F et al. Rev Med Chir Soc Med Nat Iasi. 2003 Jan–Mar;107(1):188–91.
17. Candan F et al. J Ethnopharmacol. 2003 Aug;87(2–3):215–20.
18. Glasl S et al. Pharmazie. 2003 Jul;58(7):487–90.
19. Hausen BM et al. Contact Dermatitis. 1991 Apr;24(4): 274–80.
20. Rucker G et al. Arch Pharm (Weinheim). 1991 Dec; 324(12):979–81.
21. Rucker G et al. Pharmazie. 1994 Feb–Mar;49(2–3):167–9.
22. Tozyo T et al. Chem Pharm Bull (Tokyo). 1994 May;42(5): 1096–100.
23. Glasl S et al. Z Naturforsch [C]. 2002 Nov–Dec;57(11–12): 976–82.
24. Gherase F et al. Rev Med Chir Soc Med Nat Iasis. 2004 Jan–Mar;108(1):177–80.
25. Falk AJ et al. J Pharm Sci. 1975 Nov;64(11):19-1838-42.
26. Chandler RF et al. J Pharm Sci. 1982 Jun;71(6):690–3.
27. Holetz FB et al. Mem Inst Oswaldo Cruz. 2002 Oct;97(7): 1027–31.
28. Lin LT et al. Phytother Res. 2002 Aug;16(5):440–4.
29. Shapira MY et al. J Am Acad Dermatol. 2005 Apr; 52(4):691–3.
30. No Authors listed. Int J Toxicol. 2001;20 Suppl 2:79–84.
31. Kardosova A et al. Int J Biol Macromol. 2003 Nov;33(1–3): 135–40.
32. Kato Y, Watanabe T. Bisosci Biotechnol Biochem. 1993 Sep;57(9):1591–2.
33. Washino T. Agric Biol Chem. 1986;50:263–69.
34. Washino T et al. Nipp Nogeik Kaishi. 1985;59:389–95.
35. Uchiyama Y et al. Biochem Biophys Acta. 2005 Oct 10;1725(3):298–304.
36. Liu S et al. Phytochem Anal. 2005 Mar–Apr;16(2):86–9.
37. Sun WJ et al. Yao Xue Xue Ba. 1992;27(7):549–51.
38. Wang X et al. J Chromatogr A. 2005 Jan 21; 1063(1–2):247–51.
39. Wang Hy, Yang JS. Yao Xue Xue Bao. 1993;28(12):911–7.
40. Umehara K et al. Chem Pharm Bull (Tokyo). 1996 Dec;44(12):2300–4.
41. Cai Y et al. Life Sci. 2004 Mar 12;74(17):2157–84.
42. Martindale, The Extra Pharmacopoeia 26th Ed. Pharmaceutical Press London March 1973.
43. Lin CC et al. Am J Chin Med. 1996;24(2):127–37.
44. Cho MK et al. Int Immunopharmacol. 2004 Oct;4(10–11): 1419–29.
45. Morita K et al. Mutat Res. 1984 Oct;129(1):25–31.
46. Kasai H et al. Food Chem Toxicol. 2000 May;38(5):467–71.
47. Chen FA et al. Food Chemistry. 2004 Aug;86(4):479–484.
48. Holetz FB et al. Mem Inst Oswaldo Cruz. 2002 Oct;97(7): 1027–31.
49. Eich E et al. J Med Chem. 1996 Jan 5;39(1):86–95.
50. Koshimizu K et al. Cancer Lett. 1988 Apr;39(3):247–57.
51. Xie LH et al. Chem Pharm Bull (Tokyo). 2003 Apr;51(4): 378–84.
52. Kaur N, Gupta AK. J Biosci. 2002 Dec;27(7):703–14.
53. Pool-Zobel BL. Br J Nutr. 2005 Apr;93 Suppl 1:573–90.
54. Welters CF et al. Dis Colon Rectum. 2002 May;45(5):621–7.
55. Rodriguez P et al. Contact Dermatitis. 1995 Aug;33(2): 134–5.
56. Fletcher GF, Cantwell JD. JAMA. 1978 Oct 6;240(15):1586.

57. Bryson PD et al. JAMA. 1978;239:2157.
58. Cicero AF. Acta Diabetol. 2004 Sep;41(3):91–8.
59. Wagner S et al. Planta Med. 2004 Oct;70(10):897–903.
60. Bilia AR et al. J Pharm Biomed Anal. 2002 Sep 5;30(2): 321–30.
61. Douglas JA et al. Planta Med. 2004 Feb;70(2):166–70.
62. Schmidt TJ et al. Planta Med. 2004 Oct;70(10):967–77.
63. Vanhaelen M. Planta Med. 1973 Jun;23(4):308–11.
64. Merfort I. Forsch Kompl Klass Naturheilkd. 2003 Apr; 10 Suppl 1:45–8.
65. Klaas C et al. Planta Med. 2002 May;68(5):385–91.
66. Lyss G et al. Biol Chem. 1997 Sep;378(9):951–61.
67. Schroder H et al. Thromb Res. 1990 Mar;15;57(6):839–45.
68. Kucera M et al. Arnzneimettelforschung. 2003; 53(12):850–6.
69. Alonso D et al. Dermatol Surg. 2002 Aug;28(8):686–8.
70. Knuesel O et al. Adv Ther. 2002 Sep–Oct;19(5):209–18.
71. Jeffrey SL, Belcher HJ. Altern Ther Health Med. 2002 Mar–Apr;8(2):66–8.
72. Francois G, Passreiter CM. Phytother Res. 2004 Feb; 18(2):184–6.
73. Schmidt TJ et al. Planta Med. 2002 Aug;68(8):750–1.
74. Iauk L et al. Phytother Res. 2003 Jun;17(6):599–604.
75. Wagner H et al. Boll Chim Farm. 1987 Nov;126(11):458–61.
76. Wagner H, Jurcic K. Arzneimettelforschung. 1991 Oct;41(10):1072–6.
77. Puhlmann J et al. Phyotchemistry. 1991;30(4):1141–5.
78. Woerdenbag HJ et al. Planta Med. 1994 Oct;60(5):434–7.
79. Paulsen E. Contact Dermatitis. 2002 Oct;47(4):189–98.
80. Spettoli E et al. Am J Contact Dermat. 1998 Mar;9(1): 49–50.
81. Hausen BM. Hautarzt. 1980 Jan;31(1):10–7.
82. Bergonzi MC et al. Pharmazie. 2005 Jan;60(1):36–8.
83. Reider N et al. Contact Dermatitis. 2001 Nov;45(5):269–72.
84. No authors listed. Int J Toxicol. 2001;20 Suppl 2:1–11.
85. Kordali S et al. J Agric Food Chem. 2005 Mar 9;53(5): 1408–16.
86. Bertelli J, Crabtree J. Tetrahedron. 1968;24(5):2079–89.
87. Blagojevic P et al. J Agric Food Chem. 2006 Jun 28;54(13): 4780–9.
88. Juteau F et al. Planta Med. 2003 Feb;69(2):158–61.
89. Karp F, Croteau R. Arch Biochem Biophys. 1982 Jul; 216(2):616–24.
90. Beauhaire J et al. Tetrahedron Lett. 1984;25(26):2751–4.
91. Rucker G et al. Phytochemistry. 1991 Jan;31(1):340–2.
92. Raynaud J et al. Aller Immunol. 1987 Jun;19(6):255–6.
93. Kaul VK et al. Indian J Pharm. 1976;36(3):117–25.
94. Kordali S et al. J Agric Food Chem. 2005 Nov;53(24): 9452–8.
95. Omer B et al. Phytomedicine. 2007 Feb 19;14(2–3):87–95.
96. Scotti MT et al. Bioorg Med Chem. 2007 Apr 15;15(8): 2927–34.
97. Guarrera M et al. J Eur Acad Dermatol Venereol. 2001 Sep;15(5):486–7.
98. Wake G et al. J Ethnopharmacol. 2000 Feb;69(2):105–14.
99. de Freitas MV et al. Toxicol In Vitro. 2008 Feb;22(1): 219–24.
100. Meschler JP, Howlett AC. Pharmacol Biochem Behav. 1999 Mar;62(3):473–80.
101. Padosch SA et al. Subst Abuse Treat Prev Policy. 2006 May;10;1(1):14.
102. Dettling A et al. J Stud Alcohol. 2004 Sep;65(5):573–81.
103. Baumann IC et al. Z Allgemeinmed. 1975 Jun 20;51(17): 784–91.
104. Quinlan MB et al. J Ethnopharmacol. 2002 Apr;80(1): 75–83.
105. Guarrera PM. J Ethnopharmacol. 1999 Dec;15;68(1–3): 183–92.
106. Lachenmeier DW et al. Forensic Sci Int. 2006 Apr; 20158(1):1–8.
107. Arnold WN. JAMA. 1988 Nov 25;260(20):3042–4.
108. Barney JN et al. J Chem Ecol. 2005 Feb;31(2):247–65.
109. Thao N et al. JEOR. 2004 Jul/Aug;16(4):358.
110. Geissman TA, Ellestad GA. J Org Chem. 1962;27:1855–9.
111. Tigno XT et al. Clin Hemorheol Microcirc. 2000;23(2–4): 167–75.
112. Fraisse D et al. Ann Pharm Fr. 2003 Jul;61(4):265–8.
113. Carnat A et al. Fitoterapia. 2000 Sep;71(5):587–9.
114. Marco J et al. Phytochemistry. 1991 Jan;30(7):2403–4.
115. Mizushina Y et al. J Biochem (Tokyo). 1999 Aug;126(2): 430–6.
116. Drake D, Lam J. Phytochemistry. 1974 Feb;13(2):455–57.
117. Wallnofer B et al. Phytochemistry. 1989;28(10):2687–91.
118. Kundu S et al. Tetrahedron Lett. 1966;7(10):1043–7.
119. Geissman TA, Lee KH. Phytochemistry. 1971 Mar;10(3): 663–4.
120. Hiramatsu N et al. Biofactors. 2004;22(1–4):123–5.
121. Xiufen W et al. Biofactors. 2004;21(1–4):281–4.
122. Nguyen MT et al. Biol Pharm Bull. 2004 Sep;27(9): 1414–21.
123. Hatsukari I et al. Anticancer Res. 2002 Sep–Oct;22(5): 2777–82.
124. Chen CP et al. J Ethnopharmacol. 1989 Dec;27(3):285–95.
125. Davidov MI et al. Urol Nfrol (Mosk). 1995 Sep–Oct;(5): 19–20.
126. Ukiya M et al. J Nat Prod. 2006 Dec;69(12):1692–6.
127. Neukirch H et al. Phytochem Anal. 2004 Jan–Feb;15(1): 30–5.
128. Hamburger M et al. Fitoterapia. 2003 Jun;74(4):328–38.
129. Della Loggia R et al. Planta Med. 1994 Dec;60(6):56–20.
130. Zitterl-Eglseer K et al. J Ethnopharmacol. 1997 Jul;57(2): 139–44.
131. Akihisa T et al. Phytochemistry. 1996 Dec;43(6):1255–60.
132. Zitterl-Eglseer K et al. Phytochem Anal. 2001 May–Jun; 12(3):199–201.
133. Yoshikawa M et al. Chem Pharm Bull (Tokyo). 2001 Jul;49(7):863–70.
134. Bako E et al. J Biochem Biophys Methods. 2002 Oct–Nov;53(1–3):241–50.
135. Kishimoto S et al. Biosci Biotechnol Biochem. 2005;69(11): 2122–8.
136. Toom M et al. J Eur Pharm Sci. 2007 Sep;32(1 Suppl 1):S25.
137. Marukami T et al. Chem Pharm Bull (Tokyo). 2001 Aug;49(8):974–8.
138. Wagner H et al. Arzneimittelforschung. 1985;35(7): 1069–75.
139. Janssen AM et al. Pharmaceutisch Weekblad. 1986;8:289–92.
140. WHO Monographs on Selected Medicinal Plants—Vol 2. WHO Geneva 2004 p. 35–44.
141. Iauk L et al. Phytother Res. 2003 Jun;17(6):599–604.
142. Krazhan IA, Garazha NN. Stomatologiia (Mosk). 2001;80(5):11–13.

143. Modesto A et al. J Clin Pediatr Dent. 2000 Spring;24(3): 237–43.
144. Tarle D, Dvorzak I. Farmacevtski Vestnik. 1989;40:117–20.
145. Samochowiec E et al. Wiad Parazytol. 1979;25(1):77–81.
146. Kalvatchev Z et al. Biomed Pharmacother. 1997;51(4): 176–80.
147. Amirghofran Z et al. J Ethnopharmacol. 2000 Sep;72(1–2): 167–72.
148. Jimenez-Medina E et al. BMC Cancer. 2006;6(1):119.
149. Corina P et al. Oftalmologia. 1999;46(1):55–7.
150. Bezakova L et al. Pharmazie. 1996 Feb;51(2):126–7.
151. Chakurski I et al. Vutr Boles. 1981;20(6):51–4.
152. Fuchs SM et al. Skin Pharmacol Physiol. 2005 Jul–Aug;18(4): 195–200.
153. Pommier P et al. J Clin Oncol. 2004 Apr 15;22(8):1447–53.
154. Lievre M et al. Clin Trials Metaanal. 1992;28:9–12.
155. Cordova CA et al. Redox Rep. 2002;7(2):95–102.
156. Gordana S et al. Food Res Int. 2004 Aug;37(7):643–50.
157. Wagner H et al. Arzneimittelforschung. 1984;34(6):659–61.
158. Reider N et al. Contact Dermatitis. Nov;45(5):269–72.
159. No authors. Int J Toxicol. 2001;20 Suppl 2:13–20.
160. Ramos A et al. J Ethnopharmacol. 1998 May;61(1):49–55.
161. Elias R et al. Mutagenesis. 1990 Jul;5(4):327–31.
162. Bakkali F et al. Mutat Res. 2005 Aug;1:585(1–2):1–13.
163. de Kraker JW et al. Plant Physiology. 1998 Aug;117(4): 1381–92.
164. Mares D et al. Mycopathologia. 2005 Aug;160(1):85–91.
165. Kisiel W, Zielinska K. Phytochemistry. 2001 Jun;57(4): 523–7.
166. de Kraker JW et al. Plant Physiol. 2002 May;129(1):257–68.
167. Du H et al. Zhongguo Zhong Yao Za Zhi. 1998 Nov; 23(11):682–3.
168. Roberfroid MB. Br J Nutr. 2005 Apr;93 Suppl 1:S13–25.
169. Malarz J et al. Plant Cell Rep. 2005 Jun;24(4):246–9.
170. HeY et al. Zhongguo Yao Za Zhi. 2002 Mar;27(3):209–10.
171. Schaffer S et al. J Physiol Pharmacol. 2005 Mar;56 Suppl 1:115–24.
172. El SN, Karakaya S. Int J Food Sci Nutr. 2004 Feb;55(1): 67–74.
173. Kim TW, Yang KS. Arch Pharm Res. 2001 Oct;24(5):431–6.
174. Pool-Zobel BL. Br J Nutr. 2005 Apr;93 Suppl 1:S73–90.
175. Menne E et al. J Nutr. 2000 May;130(5):1197–9.
176. Roberfroid MB et al. J Nutr. 1998;128(1):11–9.
177. Kleessen B et al. Am J Clin Nutr. 1997;65:1397–1402.
178. Delzenne NM et al. Br J Nutr. 2005 Apr;93 Suppl 1:S157–61.
179. Rollinger JM et al. Curr Drug Discov Technol. 2005 Sep;2(3):185–93.
180. Cavin C et al. Biochem Biophys Res Commun. 2005 Feb 18;327(3):742–9.
181. Lee KT et al. Biol Pharm Bull. 2000 Aug;23(8):1005–7.
182. Bischoff TA. J Ethnopharmacol. 2004 Dec;95(2–3):455–7.
183. Rani P, Khullar N. Phytother Res. 2004 Aug;18(8):670–3.
184. Aqil F, Ahmad I. Methods Find Exp Clin Pharmacol. 2007 Mar;29(2):79–92.
185. Guevara JM et al. Rev Gastroenterol Peru. 1994 Jan–Apr;14(1):27–31.
186. Van Loo J et al. Br J Nutr. 2005 Apr;93 Suppl 1:S91–8.
187. Kolhapure SA, Mitra SK. Med Update. 2004;12(2):51–61.
188. Fallah Huseini H et al. Phytomedicine. 2005 Sep;15;12(9):619–24.
189. Cadot P et al. Clin Exp Allergy. 1996 Aug;26(8):940–4.
190. Cadot P et al. Int Arch Allergy Immunol. 2003 May;131(1): 19–24.
191. Shimoda H et al. Bioorg Med Chem Lett. 2003 Jan;20; 13(2):223–8.
192. Wittemer SM et al. Phytomedicine. 2005 Jan;12(1–2): 28–38.
193. Zhu X et al. J Agric Food Chem. 2004 Dec 1;52(24):7272–8.
194. Schutz K et al. J Agric Food Chem. 2004 Jun 30;52(13): 4090–6.
195. Hinou J et al. Ann Pharm Fr. 1989;47(2):95–8.
196. Schutz K et al. J Agric Food Chem. 2006 Nov;15;54(23): 8812–7.
197. Wang M et al. J Agric Food Chem. 2003 Jan 29;51(3):601–8.
198. Betancor-Fernandez A et al. J Pharm Pharmacol. 2003 Jul;55(7):981–6.
199. Zapolska-Downar D et al. Life Sci. 2002 Nov 1;71(24): 2897–2908.
200. Li H et al. J Pharmacol Exp Ther. 2004 Sep;310(3):926–32.
201. Fintelmann V. Zeit Allg Med. 1996;72(Suppl 2):3–19.
202. Englisch W et al. Arzneimittelforschung. 2000;50:260–5.
203. Lupattelli G et al. Life Sci. 2004 Dec 31;76(7):775–82.
204. Dorn M. Br J Phytotherapy. 1995;4(1):21–26.
205. Heckers H et al. Atherosclerosis. 1977 Feb;26(2):249–53.
206. Thompson Coon JS, Ernst E. J Fam Pract. 2003 Jun;52(6): 468–78.
207. Pittler MH et al. Cochrane Library. 2002;(3):CD003335.
208. Wegener T. Wien Med Wochenschr. 2002;152(15–16): 412–7.
209. Speroni E et al. J Ethnopharmacol. 2003 Jun;86(2–3): 203–11.
210. Kirchoff R et al. Phytomedicine. 1994;1(2):107–15.
211. Kraft K. Phytomedicine. 1997;4(4):369–78.
212. Bundy R et al. J Altern Complement Med. 2004 Aug;10(4): 667–9.
213. Holtmann G et al. Aliment Pharmacol Ther. 2003 Dec;18(11–12):1099–1105.
214. Wegener T, Fintelmann V. Wien Med Wochenschr. 1999;149(8–10):241–7.
215. Zhu XF et al. Fitoterapia. 2005 Jan;76(1):108–11.
216. Ruppelt BM et al. Mem Inst Oswald Cruz. 1991;86 (Suppl 2):203–5.
217. Pittler MH et al. CMAJ. 2003 Dec 9;169(12):1269–73.
218. Rocchietta S. Minerva Med. 1959;50:612–8.
219. Wittemer SM et al. Phytomedicine. 2005 Jan;12(1–2): 28–38.
220. Quirce S et al. J Allergy Clin Immunol. 1996 Feb;97(2):710–1.
221. Miralles JC et al. Ann Allergy Asthma Immunol. 2003 Jul;91(1):92–5.
222. Franck P et al. Int Arch Allergy Immunol. 2005 Feb;136(2): 155–8.
223. Still DW et al. Ann Bot (Lond). 2005 Sep;96(3):467–77.
224. Nieri P et al. Planta Med. 2003 Jul;69(7):685–6.
225. WHO Monographs on Selected Medicinal Plants—Vol 1. WHO Geneva 1999 p. 125–144.
226. Chen Y et al. J Nat Prod. 2005 May;68(5):773–6.
227. Pellati F et al. Phytochem Anal. 2005 Mar–Apr; 16(2):77–85.
228. Perry NB et al. J Agric Food Chem. 2001 Apr;49(4):1702–6.
229. Pellati F et al. J Pharm Biomed Anal. 2004 Apr;16;35(2): 289–301.
230. Speroni E et al. J Ethnopharmacol. 2002 Feb;79(2):265–72.

231. Sloley BD et al. J Pharm Pharmacol. 2001 Jun; 53(6):849–57.
232. Cheminat A et al. Phytochemistry. 1988;27(9):2787–94.
233. Mazza G, Cottrell T. J Agric Food Chem. 1999 Aug; 47(8):3081–5.
234. Lii JR et al. Zhongguo Zhong Yao Za Zhi. 2002 Jan; 27(1):40–2.
235. Thude S, Classen B. Phytochemistry. 2005 May;66(9): 1026–32.
236. Classen B et al. Planta Med. 2005 Jan;71(1):59–66.
237. McKenna et al. The Desk Reference for Major Herbal Supplements. New York; Haworth Herbal Press, 2002.
238. Razic S et al. J Pharm Biomed Anal. 2003 Nov; 24;33(4):845–50.
239. Hostettmann K. Forsch Komplement Klass Naturheilkd. 2003 Apr;10 Suppl 1:9–12.
240. Claus EP. Pharmacognosy 4th Ed. Henry Kimpton. London 1961 p. 74–5.
241. Crowe S, Lyons B. Paediatr Anaesth. 2004 Nov;14(11): 916–9.
242. Bruno JJ, Elliss JJ. Harv Health Lett. 2005 Feb;30(4):6.
243. Dy GK et al. J Clin Oncol. 2004 Dec 1;22(23):4810–5.
244. Grabe DW, Garrison GD. Ann Pharmacother. 2004 Jul–Aug;38(7–8):1169–72.
245. Caruso TJ, Gwaltney JM Jr. Clin Infect Dis. 2005 Mar 15;40(6):807–10.
246. Hu C, Kitts DD. J Agric Food Chem. 2000 May;48(5): 1466–72.
247. Matthias A et al. J Clin Pharm Ther. 2004 Feb;29(1):7–13.
248. Bauer R. Wien Med Wochenschr. 2002;152(15–16):407–11.
249. Gan XH et al. Int Immunopharmacol. 2003 Jun;3(6): 811–24.
250. Bauer R. Z Arztl Fortbild (Jena). 1996 Apr;90(2):111–5.
251. Alban S et al. Planta Med. 2002 Dec;68(12):1118–24.
252. Barrett B. Phytomedicine. 2003 Jan;10(1):66–86.
253. Borchers AT et al. Am J Clin Nutr. 2000 Aug;72(2): 339–347.
254. Kim LS et al. Altern Med Rev. 2002 Apr;7(2):138–49.
255. Randolph RK et al. Exp Biol Med (Maywood). 2003 Oct;228(9):1052–6.
256. Sharma M et al. Phytother Res. 2006 Dec;20(12):1074–9.
257. Zwickey H et al. Phytother Res. 2007 Nov;21(11):1109–12.
258. Gertsch J et al. FEBS Lett. 2004 Nov 19;577(3):563–9.
259. Clifford LJ et al. Phytomedicine. 2002 Apr;9(3):249–53.
260. Rininger JA et al. J Leukoc Biol. 2000 Oct;68(4):503–10.
261. Cech NB et al. Planta Med. 2006 Dec;72(15):1372–7.
262. See DM et al. Immunopharmacology. 1997 Jan;35(3): 229–35.
263. Agnew LL et al. J Clin Pharm Ther. 2005 Aug;30(4):363–9.
264. Schwarz E et al. J Immunother. 2002 Sep/Oct;25(5): 413–20.
265. Melchart D et al. J Altern Complement Med. 1995 Summer;1(2):145–60.
266. Neri PG et al. J Ocul Pharmacol Ther. 2006 Dec;22(6):431–6.
267. Melchart D et al. Phytother Res. 2002 Mar;16(2):138–42.
268. Binns SE et al. Planta Med. 2000 Apr;66(3):241–4.
269. Binns SE et al. Planta Med. 2002 Sep;68(9):780–3.
270. Reinke RA et al. Virology. 2004 Sep;1;326(2):203–19.
271. Cohen HA et al. Arch Pediatr Adolesc Med. 2004 Mar;158(3):217–21.
272. Heinen-Kammerer T et al. Gesundheitswesen. 2005 Apr; 67(4):296–301.
273. Kohler G et al. Wien Med Wochenschr. 2002;152(15–16): 393–7.
274. Schulten B et al. Arzneimittelforschung. 2001;51(7):563–8.
275. Lindenmuth GF, Lindenmuth EB. J Atlern Complement Med. 2000 Aug;6(4):327–34.
276. Henneicke-von Zepelin H et al. Curr Med Res Opin. 1999;15(3):214–27.
277. Goel V et al. J Clin Pharm Ther. 2004 Feb;29(1):75–83.
278. Schoop R et al. Adv Ther. 2006 Sep–Oct;23(5):823–33.
279. Saunders P et al. Can J Physiol Pharmacol. 2007 Nov; 85(11):1195–9.
280. Shah SA et al. Lancet Infect Dis. 2007 Jul;7(7):473–80.
281. Sperber SJ et al. Clin Infect Dis. 2004 May 15;38(10): 1367–71.
282. Melchart D et al. Arch Fam Med. 1998 Nov–Dec;7(6): 541–5.
283. Taylor JA et al. JAMA. 2003 Dec 3;290(21):2824–30.
284. Turner RB et al. Antimicrob Agents Chemother. 2000 Jun;44(6):1708–9.
285. Barrett BP et al. Ann Intern Med. 2002 17 Dec;137(12): 939–46.
286. Turner RB et al. N Engl J Med. 2005 Jul 28;353(4):341–8.
287. Yale SH, Liu K. Arch Intern Med. 2004 Jun 14;164(11): 1237–41.
288. Kligler B. Am Fam Physician. 2003 Jan 1;67(1):77–80.
289. Osowski S et al. Forsch Komplementarmed Klass Naturheilkd. 2000 Dec;7(6):294–300.
290. Islam J, Carter R. South Med J. 2005 Mar;98(3):311–18.
291. Linde K et al. Cochrane Database Syst Rev. 2006 Jan 25;(1):CD000530.
292. Percival SS. Biochem Pharmacol. 2000 Jul1;5;60(2):155–8.
293. Giles JT et al. Pharmacotherapy. 2000 Jun;29(6):690–7.
294. Melchart D et al. Cochrane Database Syst Rev. 2000;(2): CD000530.
295. Vonau B et al. Int J STD AIDS. 2001 Mar;12(3):154–8.
296. Speroni E et al. J Ethnopharmacol. 2002 Feb;79(2):265–72.
297. Chicca A et al. Br J Pharmacol. 2008 Mar;153(5):379–85.
298. Huntimer ED et al. Chem Biodivers. 2006 Jun;3(6): 695–703.
299. Hinz B et al. Biochem Biophys Res Commun. 2007 Aug 24;360(2):441–6.
300. Potii VV. Klin Khir. 2000 Oct;(10):15–6.
301. Krochmal R et al. Evid Based Complement Alternat Med. 2004 Dec;1(3):305–313.
302. Nordeng H, Havnen GC. Pharmcoepidemiol Drug Saf. 2004 Jun;13(6):371–80.
303. Gallo M et al. Arch Intern Med. 2000 Nov 13;160(20): 3141–3.
304. Matthias A et al. Life Sci. 2005 Sep;277(16):2018–29.
305. Woelkart K et al. J Clin Pharmacol. 2005 Jun;45(6):683–9.
306. Huntley AL et al. Drug Saf. 2005;28(5):387–400.
307. Mullins RJ, Heddle R. Ann Allergy Asthma Immunol. 2002 Jan;88(1):42–51.
308. Yang S et al. J Herb Pharmacother. 2002;2(3):1–11.
309. Fraunfelder FW. Am J Ophthalmol. 2004 Oct;138(4): 639–47.
310. Soon SL, Crawford RI. J Am Acad Dermatol. 2001 Feb;44(2):298–9.
311. Kocaman O et al. Eur J Intern Med. 2008 Mar;19(2):148.
312. Lee AN, Werth VP. Arch Dermatol. 2004 Jun;140(6):723–7.
313. Neff GW et al. Liver Transpl. 2004 Jul;10(7):881–5.
314. Budzinski JW et al. Phytomedicine. 2000 Jul;7(4):273–82.

315. Yale SH, Glurich I. J Altern Complement Med. 2005 Jun; 11(3):433–9.

316. Raner GM et al. Food Chem Toxicol. 2007 Dec;45(12): 2359–65.

317. Gorski JC et al. Clin Pharmacol Ther. 2004 Jan;75(1): 89–100.

318. Gurley BJ et al. Clin Pharmacol Ther. 2004 Nov;76(5): 428–40.

319. Gurley BJ et al. Mol Nutr Food Res. 2008 Jan 23 [Epub ahead of print].

320. Gurley BJ et al. Mol Nutr Food Res. 2008 Jan 23 [Epub ahead of print].

321. Izzo AA, Ernst E. Drugs. 2001;61(15):2163–75.

322. Paolini J et al. J Chromatogr A. 2005 May 27;1076(1–2): 170–8.

323. Flamini G et al. JEOR. 2003 Mar/Apr 15:127–9.

324. Rucker G et al. Nat Toxins. 1997;5(6):223–7.

325. Elema ET et al. Pharm Weekbl Sci. 1989 Oct 20;11(5): 161–4.

326. Hendriks H et al. Pharm Weekbl Sci. 1983 Dec 16;5(6): 281–6.

327. Woerdenbag HJ et al. Biochem Pharmacol. 1989 Jul 15;38(14):2279–83.

328. Wagner H et al. Arzneimittelforschung. 1984;34(6):659–61.

329. Edgar J et al. Am J of Chinese Med. 1992;20(3–4):281–8.

330. Pieroni A et al. J Ethnopharmacol. 2004 Apr;91(2–3): 331–44.

331. Herz W et al. J Org Chem. 1977 Jun 24;42(13):2264–71.

332. Habtemariam S, Macpherson AM. Phytother Res. 2000 Nov;14(7):575–7.

333. Claus EP. Pharmacognosy 4th Ed. Henry Kimpton. London 1961 p. 165–6.

334. Kupchan SM, Knox JR, Udayamurthy MS. J Pharm Sci. 1965 Jun;54(6):929–30.

335. Wagner H et al. Arzneimittelforschung. 1985;35(7): 1069–75.

336. Vollmar A et al. Phytochemistry. 1986 Jan;25(2):377–81.

337. Habtemariam S. Phytother Res. 2001 Dec;15(8):687–90.

338. Habtemariam S. Phytother Res. 1998 12;422–6.

339. Habtemariam S. Planta Med. 1998 Dec;64(8):683–5.

340. Kreutzer S et al. Planta Med. 1990 Aug;56(4):392–4.

341. British Pharmaceutical Codex 1911. The Pharmaceutical Press. 72 Great Russell St.WC.

342. Timmermann B et al. Phytochemistry. 1985;24(5):1031–4.

343. Hoffmann J et al. Phytochemistry. 1988;27(2):493–6.

344. The Dispensatory of the United States of America. Ed. J. Remington et al. Twentieth Ed. 1918.

345. McLaughlin S. Biomass. 1988;16(3):151–60.

346. Stojakowska A et al. Z Naturforsch. 2004 Jul–Aug; 59(7–8):606–8.

347. Stojakowska A et al. Phytochem Anal. 2006 May;17(3): 157–61.

348. Konishi T et al. Biol Pharm Bull. 2002 Oct;25(10):1370–2.

349. Bohlmann F et al. Phytochemistry. 1978;17(7):1165–72.

350. Yosioka I, Yamada Y. Yakugaku Zasshi. 1963 Aug;83: 801–2.

351. Picman AK. Biochem Syst Ecol. 1986 May 12;14(3):255–81.

352. Spriridonov NA et al. Phytother Res. 2005 May;(5): 428–32.

353. Dirsch VM et al. Planta Med. 2001 Aug;67(6):557–9.

354. Dorn DC et al. Phytother Res. 2006 Nov;20(11):970–80.

355. Cantrell CL et al. Planta Med. 1999 May;65(4):351–5.

356. Kowalewski Z et al. Arch Immunol Ther Exp (Warz). 1976;24(1):121–5.

357. El Garhy MF, Mahmoud LH. J Egypt Soc Parasitol. 2002 Dec;32(3):893–900.

358. Paulsen E et al. Contact Dermatitis. 2001 Oct;45(4): 197–204.

359. Al-Gammal SY. Bull Indian Inst Hist Med Hyderabad. 1998 Jan;28(1):7–11.

360. Carle R, Gomaa K. Br J Phytotherapy. 1991/2;2(4):147–53.

361. Maday E et al. Eur J Drug Metab Pharmacokinet. 1999 Oct–Dec;24(4):303–8.

362. Povh N et al. J Supercritical Fluids. 2001 Nov;21(3): 245–256.

363. Baranska M et al. Analyst. 2004 Oct;129(10):926–30.

364. WHO Monographs on Selected Medicinal Plants—Vol 1. WHO Geneva 1999 p. 86–94.

365. Svehlikova V et al. Phytochemistry. 2004 Aug;65(16): 2323–32.

366. Yamamoto A et al. Chem Pharm Bull (Tokyo). 2002 Jan;50(1):47–52.

367. Bottcher H et al. Postharvest Biol Technol. 2001 Mar; 22(1):39–51.

368. Eliasova A et al. Z Naturforsch. 2004 Jul–Aug;59(7–8): 543–8.

369. Wang Y et al. Planta Med. 2004 Mar;70(3):250–5.

370. Basgel S, Erdemoglu SB. Sci Total Environ. 2006 Apr 15; 359(1–3):82–9.

371. Safayhi H et al. Planta Med. 1994 Oct;60(5):410–3.

372. Calzado MA et al. Biochim Biophys Acta. 2005 Jun 30;1729(2):88–93.

373. Gerritsen ME et al. Am J Pathol. 1995 Aug;147(2):278–92.

374. Miliauskas G et al. Food Chemistry. 2004 Apr;85(2): 231–7.

375. Lee KG, Shibamoto T. J Agric Food Chem. 2002 Aug 14;50(17):4947–52.

376. Rekka EA et al. Res Commun Mol Pathol Pharmacol. 1996 Jun;92(3):361–4.

377. Mazokopakis EE et al. Phytomedicine. 2005 Jan; 12(1–2):25–7.

378. Carl W, Emrich LS. J Pros Dentistry. 1991;66:361–9.

379. Fidler P et al. Cancer. 1996 Feb 1;77(3):522–5.

380. Charuluxananan S et al. J Med Assoc Thai. 2004 Sep; 87 Suppl 2:S185–9.

381. Paladini AC et al. J Pharm Pharmacol. 1999 May;51(5): 519–26.

382. Viola H et al. Planta Med. 1995 Jun;61(3):213–6.

383. Haggag EG et al. J Herb Pharmacother. 2003;3(4):41–45.

384. Fokina GI et al. Vopr Virusol. 1991 Jan–Feb;36(1):18–21.

385. Musci I et al. Acta Microbiol Hung. 1992;39(2):137–47.

386. Trovato A et al. Boll Chim Farm. 2000 Sep–Oct;139(5): 225–7.

387. Uteshev BS et al. Eksp Klin Farmakol. 1999 Nov–Dec; 62(6):52–5.

388. Macchioni F et al. Med Vet Entomol. 2004 Jun;18(2):205–7.

389. Pampiglione S et al. Parassitologia. 2001 Sep;43(3):113–5.

390. Wang Y et al. J Agric Food Chem. 2005 Jan 26;53(2):191–6.

391. Kassi E et al. J Agric Food Chem. 2004 Nov 17;52(23): 6956–61.

392. Illek B, Fischer H. Am J Physiol. 1998 Nov;275(5): L902–L910.

393. Rosenberg RS et al. Biochem Biophy Res Commun. 1998 Jul 30;248(3):935–9.

394. Lepley DM et al. Carcinogenesis. 1996 Nov;17(11): 2367–75.

395. Lepley DM, Pelling JC. Mol Carcinog. 1997 Jun;19(2):74–82.

396. Wang C, Kurzer MS. Nutr Cancer. 1998;31(2):90–100.

397. van Rijn J, van den Berg J. Clin Cancer Res. 1997 Oct;3(10):1775–9.

398. Ogasawara H et al. J Allergy Clin Immunol. 1986 Aug;78(2):321–8.

399. Madisch A et al. Z Gastroenterol. 2001 Jul;39(7):511–7.

400. Schempp H et al. Arzneimittelforschung. 2004;54(7): 389–95.

401. De la Motte S et al. Arzneimittelforschung. 1997 Nov;47(11):1247–9.

402. Kupfersztain C et al. Clin Exp Obstet Gynecol. 2003;30(4):203–6.

403. Hertog MG et al. Lancet. 1993 Oct 23;342(8878):1007–11.

404. Merfort I et al. Pharmazie. 1994 Jul;49(7):509–11.

405. Glowania HJ et al. Z Hautkr. 1987 Sep 1;62(17):1267–71.

406. Nissen HP et al. Z Hautkr. 1998 Mar;21;63(3):184–90.

407. Patzelt-Wenczler R, Ponce-Poschl E. Eur J Med Res. 2000 Apr 19;5(4):171–5.

408. Aertgeets P et al. Z Hautkr. 1985 Feb 1;60(3):270–7.

409. Brandao MG et al. Cad Saude Publica. 1998 Jul–Sep;14(3):613–6.

410. Martins HM et al. Int J Food Microbiol. 2001 Aug 15; 68(1–2):149–53.

411. Momcilovic B et al. Arh Hig Rada Toksikol. 1999 Jun;50(2):201–10.

412. Hurrell RF et al. Br J Nutr. 1999 Apr;81(4):289–95.

413. Gomes-Carneiro MR et al. Mutat Res. 2005 Aug 1; 585(1–2):105–12.

414. Czeczot H, Kusztelak J. Acta Biochim Pol. 1993;40(4): 549–54.

415. Reider N et al. Clin Exp Allergy. 2000 Oct;30(10):1436–43.

416. Subiza J et al. J Allergy Clin Immunol. 1989 Sep;84(3):353–8.

417. de la Torre Morin F et al. J Investig Allergol Clin Immunol. 2001;11(2):118–22.

418. Subiza J et al. Ann Allergy. 1990 Aug;65(2):127–32.

419. Ganzera M et al. Life Sci. 2006 Jan 18;78(8):856–61.

420. Budzinski JW et al. Phytomedicine. 2000 Jul;7(4):273–82.

421. Janssen K et al. Am J Clin Nutr. 1998 Feb;67(2):255–62.

422. Heck AM et al. Am J Health Syst Pharm. 2000 Jul 1;57(13):1221–7.

423. Lev-Yadun S. J Theor Biol. 2003 Oct 21;224(4):483–9.

424. WHO Monographs on Selected Medicinal Plants—Vol. 2. WHO Geneva 2004 p. 300–316.

425. Davis-Searles PR et al. Cancer Res. 2005 May 15;65(10): 4448–57.

426. Kim NC et al. Org Biomol Chem. 2003 May 21;1(10): 1684–9.

427. Takemoto T et al. Yakugaku Zasshi 1975 Aug; 95(8):1017–21.

428. Wallace SN et al. Phytochem Anal. 2005 Jan–Feb; 16(1):7–16.

429. Schulte K et al. Arch Pharm. 1970 Jan;303(6):7–17.

430. Flora K et al. Am J Gastroenterol. 1998 Feb;93(2):139–43.

431. Varga Z et al. Phytother Res. 2001 Nov;15(7):608–12.

432. Skottova N et al. Phytother Res. 1999 Sep;13(6):535–7.

433. Varga Z et al. Phytomedicine. 2004 Feb;11(2–3):206–12.

434. Soliman KF, Mazzio EA. Proc Soc Exp Biol Med. 1998 Sep;218(4):390–7.

435. Dehmlow C et al. Life Sci. 1996;58(18):1591–1600.

436. Manna SK et al. J Immunol. 1999 Dec 15;163(12):6800–9.

437. Hruby K et al. Hum Toxicol. 1983;2:183–195.

438. Siddiqui U et al. J Clin Gastroenterol. 2004 Aug; 38(7):605–10.

439. Laekeman G et al. J Pharm Belg. 2003;58(1):28–31.

440. Bean P. Am Clin Lab. 2002 May;21(4):19–21.

441. Giese LA. Gastroenterol Nurs. 2001 Mar–Apr;24(4):95–7.

442. Dvorak Z et al. Toxicol Lett. 2003 Feb 3;137(3):201–12.

443. Saller R et al. Drugs. 2001;61(14):2035–63.

444. Mulrow C et al. Evid Rep Technol Assess (Summ). 2000;(21):1–3.

445. Rambaldi A et al. Cochrane Database Syst Rev. 2005 Apr 18;(2):CD003620.

446. Jacobs BP et al. Am J Med. 2002 Oct 15;113(6):506–15.

447. Tanamly MD et al. Dig Liver Dis. 2004 Nov;36(11):752–9.

448. Hoofnagle JH. Hepatology. 2005 Jul;42(1):4.

449. Zi X, Agarwal R. Proc Natl Acad Sci USA. 1999 Jun; 96(13):7490–5.

450. Thelen P et al. Planta Med. 2004 May;70(5):397–400.

451. Zi X et al. Cancer Res. 2000 Oct 15;60(20):5617–20.

452. Zi X et al. Cancer Res. 1998 May 1;58(9):1920–9.

453. Bhatia N et al. Cancer Lett. 1999 Dec 1;147(1–2):77–84.

454. Tyagi A et al. Carcinogenesis. 2004 Sep;25(9):1711–20.

455. Tyagi AK et al. Biochem Biophys Res Commun. 2003 Dec 26;312(4):1178–84.

456. Zi X et al. Clin Cancer Res. 1998 Apr;4(4):1055–64.

457. Kang SN et al. Biochem Pharmacol. 2001 Jun 15;61(12): 1487–95.

458. Gazak R et al. Curr Med Chem. 2007;14(3):315–38.

459. Thelen P et al. J Urol. 2004 May;171(5):1934–8.

460. Singh RP, Agarwal R. Mutat Res. 2004 Nov 2;555(1–2): 21–32.

461. Yoo HG et al. Int J Mol Med. 2004 Jan;13(1):81–6.

462. Singh RP, Agarwal R. Curr Cancer Drug Targets. 2004 Feb;4(1):1–11.

463. Chu SC et al. Mol Carcinog. 2004 Jul;40(3):143–9.

464. Dhanalakshmi S et al. Int J Cancer. 2003 Sep 20;106(5): 699–705.

465. Tyagi AK et al. Oncol Rep. 2004 Feb;11(2):493–9.

466. Lee DG et al. Arch Pharm Res. 2003 Aug;26(8):597–600.

467. Stermitz FR et al. J Nat Prod. 2000 Aug;63(8):1146–9.

468. Wilasrusmee C et al. Am Surg. 2002 Oct;68(10):860–4.

469. Amirghofran Z et al. J Ethnopharmacol. 2000 Sep;72(1–2): 167–72.

470. Kalmar L et al. Agents Actions. 1990 Mar;29(3–4):239–46.

471. Katiyar SK. Int J Oncol. 2005 Jan;26(1):169–76.

472. Zhou B et al. Biol Pharm Bull. 2004 Jul;27(7):1031–6.

473. Meroni PL et al. Int J Tissue React. 1988;10(3):177–81.

474. Tager M et al. Free Radic Res. 2001 Feb;34(2):137–51.

475. Hernandez V. STEP Perspect. 1995 Summer;7(2):13–5.

476. Gil'miiarova FN et al. Vopr Pitan. 2001;70(5):29–34.

477. Skottova N, Krecman V. Physiol Res. 1998;47(1):1–7.

478. Huseini HF et al. Phytother Res. 2006 Dec;20(12):1036–9.

479. Wallace SN et al. Phytochem Anal. 2005 Jan–Feb; 16(1):7–16.

480. Duan L et al. Appl Biochem Biotechnol. 2004 Spring; 113–6:559–68.

481. Wallace SN et al. Appl Biochem Biotechnol. 2003 Spring; 105–8:891–903.

482. Campodonico A et al. Drug Dev Ind Pharm. 2001;27(3): 261–5.
483. Schandalik R et al. Arzneimittelforschung. 1992;42:964–8.
484. Adverse Drug Reaction Committee. Med J Aust. 1999 Mar;1;170(5):218–9.
485. Boerth J, Strong KM. Herb Pharmacother. 2002;2(2):11–7.
486. Venkataramanan R et al. Drug Metab Dispos. 2000 Nov;28(11):1270–3.
487. Sridar C et al. Drug Metab Dispos. 2004 Jun;32(6):587–94.
488. Beckmann-Knopp S et al. Pharmacol Toxicol. 2000 Jun;86(6):250–6.
489. Zuber R et al. Phytother Res. 2002 Nov;16(7):632–8.
490. Patel J et al. Am J Ther. 2004 Jul–Aug;11(4):262–77.
491. Mills E et al. Eur J Clin Pharmacol. 2005 Mar;61(1):1–7.
492. DiCenzo R et al. Pharmacother. 2003 Jul;23(7):866–70.
493. Piscitelli SC et al. Pharmcother. 2002 May;22(5):551–6.
494. Gurley BJ et al. Clin Pharmacol Ther. 2004 Nov;76(5): 428–40.
495. Van Erp et al. J Clin Oncology. 2005;23(16S):2096.
496. Miyase T et al. Chem Pharm Bull (Tokyo). 1994 Mar;42(3): 617–24.
497. Bader G et al. Phytochemistry. 1992 Feb;31(2):621–3.
498. Bader G et al. Planta Med. 1995 Apr;61(2):158–61.
499. Choi SZ et al. Arch Pharm Res. 2004 Feb;27(2):164–8.
500. Sung JH et al. Arch Pharm Res. 1999 Dec;22(6):633–7.
501. Fotsch G et al. Pharmazie. 1989 Aug;44(8):555–8.
502. Choi SZ et al. Arch Pharm Res. 2005 Jan;28(1):49–54.
503. Reznicek G et al. Phytochemistry. 1991;30(5):1629–33.
504. Reznicek G et al. Planta Med. 1992 Feb;58(1):94–8.
505. Chaturvedula VS et al. Bioorg Med Chem. 2004 Dec 1; 12(23):6271–5.
506. Apati P et al. J Pharm Biomed Anal. 2003 Aug;8;32(4–5): 1045–53.
507. Prosser I et al. Arch Biochem Biophys. 2004 Dec 15;432(2): 136–44.
508. Prosser I et al. Phytochemistry. 2002 Aug;60(7):691–702.
509. Schmidt CO et al. Arch Biochem Biophys. 1999 Apr 15;364(2):167–77.
510. Kabal AA et al. Phytochemistry. 2002 Apr;59(8):805–10.
511. Gross SC et al. Nutr Cancer. 2002;43(1):76–81.
512. Borchert VE et al. Naunyn Schmiedebergs Arch Pharmacol. 2004 Mar;369(3):281–6.
513. Thiem B, Goslinska O. Fitoterapia. 2002 Oct;73(6):514–6.
514. Bader G et al. Pharmazie. 1990 Jul;45(8):618–20.
515. Bader G et al. Pharmazie. 2000 Jan;55(1):72–4.
516. Plohmann B et al. Pharmazie. 1997 Dec;52(12):953–7.
517. Meyer B et al. Arzneimittelforschung. 1995 Feb;45(2): 174–6.
518. Strehl E et al. Arzneimittelforschung. 1995 Feb;45(2): 172–3.
519. Rohnert U et al. Z Naturforsch. 1998 Mar–Apr;53(3–4): 233–40.
520. Von Kruedener S et al. Arzneimittelforschung. 1995 Feb;45(2):169–71.
521. Klein-Galczinsky C. Wien Med Wochenschr. 1999;149(8–10):248–53.
522. Zielinska M et al. Acta Biochim Pol. 2001;48(1):183–9.
523. Meyer-Buchtela E. Tee-Rezepturen—Ein Handbuch fr Apotheker und frzte. Stuttgart Deutscher Apotheker Verlag.
524. Bongartz Z, Hesse A. J Chromatogr B Biomed Appl. 1995 Nov 17;673(2):223–30.
525. Melzig MF. Wien Med Wochenschr. 2004 Nov;154(21–22): 523–7.
526. Groenewegen WA et al. J Pharm Pharmacol. 1986 Sep; 38(9):709–12.
527. WHO Monographs on Selected Medicinal Plants—Vol. 2. WHO Geneva 2004 p. 317–328.
528. Heptinstall S et al. J Pharm Pharmacol. 1992 May;44(5): 391–5.
529. Fonseca JM et al. J Plant Physiol. 2005 May;162(5):485–94.
530. Cutlan AR et al. Planta Med. 2000 Oct;66(7):612–7.
531. Christensen LP et al. Arch Deramtol Res. 1999 Jul–Aug; 291(7–8):425–31.
532. Williams CA et al. Phytochemistry. 1999 Jun;51(3):417–23.
533. Long C et al. Phytochemistry. 2003 Sep;64(2):567–9.
534. Murch SJ et al. Lancet. 1997 Nov 29;350(9091):1598–9.
535. Makheja AN, Bailey JM. Prostaglandins Leukot Med. 1982 Jun;8(6):653–60.
536. Jain MK, Jahagirdar DV. Biochim Biophys Acta. 1985 Apr 11;814(2):319–26.
537. Loesche W et al. Biomed Biochim Acta. 1988;47(10–11): S241–3.
538. Hwang D et al. Biochem Biophys Res Commun. 1996 Sep 24;226(3):810–8.
539. Li-Weber M et al. Eur J Immunol. 2002 Dec;32(12): 3587–97.
540. Kwok BH et al. Chem Biol. 2001 Aug;8(8):759–66.
541. Piela-Smith TH, Liu X. Cell Immunol. 2001 May 1; 209(2):89–96.
542. Heptinstall S et al. Lancet. 1985 May 11;1(8437):1071–4.
543. Groenewegen WA, Heptinstall S. J Pharm Pharmacol. 1990 Aug;42(8):553–7.
544. Loesche W et al. Thromb Res. 1987 Dec 1;48(5):511–8.
545. Heptinstall S et al. J Pharm Pharmacol. 1987 Jun;39(6): 459–65.
546. Krause S et al. Arzneimittelforschung. 1990 Jun;40(6): 689–92.
547. Fukuda K et al. Biochem Pharmacol. 2000 Aug 15;60(4): 595–600.
548. Sumner H et al. Biochem Pharmacol. 1992 Jun 9;43(11): 2313–20.
549. Patrick M et al. Ann Rheum Dis. 1989 Jul;48(7):547–9.
550. Maizels M et al. Headache. 2004 Oct;44(9):885–90.
551. Pittler MH, Ernst E. Cochrane Database Syst Rev. 2004;(1): CD002286.
552. Pittler MH et al. Cochrane Database Syst Rev. 2000;(3): CD002286.
553. Vogler BK et al. Cephalalgia. 1998 Dec;18(10):704–8.
554. Prusinski A et al. Neurol Neurochir Pol. 1999;33 Suppl 5:89–95.
555. Murphy JJ et al. Lancet. 1988 Jul 23;2(8604):189–92.
556. Johnson ES et al. Br Med J (Clin Res Ed). 1985 Aug 31; 291(6495):569–73.
557. Diener HC et al. Cephalagia. 2005 Nov;25(11):1031–41.
558. Rios J, Passe MM. J Am Acad Nurse Pract. 2004 Jun;16(6): 251–6.
559. Ernst E, Pittler MH. Public Health Nutr. 2000 Dec;3(4a): 509–14.
560. Cady RK et al. Med Sci Monit. 2005 Sep;11(9):PI65–9.
561. Pfaffenrath V et al. Cephalalgia. 2002 Sep;22(7):523–32.
562. Cottrell K. CMAJ. 1996 Jul 15;155(2):216–9.
563. Miglietta A et al. Chem Biol Interact. 2004 Oct 15; 149(2–3):165–73.

564. Ross JJ et al. Planta Med. 1999 Mar;65(2):126–9.
565. Yip-Schneider MT et al. Mol Cancer Ther. 2005 Apr;4(4):587–94.
566. Zhang S et al. Cancer Lett. 2004 Aug 10;211(2):175–88.
567. Zhang S et al. Cancer Lett. 2004 May 28;208(2):143–53.
568. Guzman ML, Jordan CT. Expert Opin Biol Ther. 2005 Sep;5(9):1147–52.
569. Kang SN et al. Br J Pharmacol. 2002 Mar;135(5):1235–44.
570. Patel NM et al. Oncogene. 2000 Aug 24;19(36):4159–69.
571. Zhang S et al. Carcinogenesis. 2004 Nov;25(11):2191–9.
572. O'Neill LA et al. Br J Clin Pharmacol. 1987 Jan;23(1):31–3.
573. Pozarowski P et al. Cell Cycle. 2003 Jul–Aug;2(4):377–83.
574. Tiuman TS et al. Antimcrob Agents Chemother. 2005 Jan;49(1):176–82.
575. Fischer HN et al. Phytochemistry. 1998 Sep;49(2):559–62.
576. Kalodera Z et al. Pharmazie. 1996 Dec;51(12):995–6.
577. Hwang DR et al. Bioorg Med Chem. 2006 Jan 1;14(1):83–91.
578. Li-Weber M et al. Cell Death Differ. 2002 Nov;9(11):1256–65.
579. Gromek D et al. Pol J Pharmacol Pharm. 1991 May–Jun;43(3):213–7.
580. Brown AM et al. J Pharm Pharmacol. 1997 May;49(5):558–61.
581. Bailey NJ et al. Planta Med. 2002 Aug;68(8):734–8.
582. Nelson MH et al. Am J Health Syst Pharm. 2002 Aug 15;59(16):1527–31.
583. Anderson D et al. Hum Toxicol. 1988 Mar;7(2):145–52.
584. Curry EA et al. Invest New Drugs. 2004 Aug;22(3):299–305.
585. Jovanovic M, Polijacki M. Med Pregl. 2003 Jan–Feb;56(1–2):43–9.
586. Lamminpaa A et al. Contact Dermatitis. 1996 May;34(5):330–5.
587. Mensing H et al. Hautarzt. 1985 Jul;36(7):398–402.
588. Hausen BM. Derm Beruf Umwelt. 1981;29(1):18–21.
589. Fernandez de Corres L. Contact Dermatitis. 1984 Aug;11(2):74–9.
590. Paulsen E et al. Contact Dermatitis. 2002 Jul;47(1):14–8.
591. Goulden V, Wilkinson SM. Br J Dermatol. 1998 Jun;138(6):1018–21.
592. Heck AM et al. Am J Health Syst Pharm. 2000 Jul 1;57(13):1221–7.
593. Abebe W. J Clin Pharm Ther. 2002 Dec;27(6):391–401.
594. Biggs MJ et al. Lancet. 1982 Oct 2;320(8301):776.
595. Miller LG. Arch Intern Med. 1999 May 24;159(10):1142–3.
596. Tetenyi P et al. Phytochemistry. 1975 Jul;14(7):1539–44.
597. Judzentiene A, Mockute D. Biochem Sys Ecol. 2005 May;33(5):487–98.
598. Dragland S et al. J Agric Food Chem. 2005 Jun 15;53(12):4946–53.
599. Keskitalo M et al. Biochem Syst Ecol. 2001 Mar;29(3):267–85.
600. Rohloff J et al. J Agric Food Chem. 2004 Mar 24;52(6):1742–8.
601. Croteau R, Shaskus J. Arch Biochem Biophys. 1985 Feb 1;236(2):535–43.
602. Hethelyi P et al. Phytochemistry. 1981;20(8):1847–50.
603. Tournier H et al. J Pharm Pharmacol. 1999 Feb;51(2):215–9.
604. Umlauf D et al. Phytochemistry. 2004 Sep;65(17):2463–70.

605. Appendino G et al. Phytochemistry. 1982 Jun;21(5):1099–1102.
606. Uchio Y. Tetrahedron. 1978;34(19):2893–99.
607. Appendino G et al. Phytochemistry. 1984;23(11):2545–51.
608. Appendino G et al. Phytochemistry. 1983;22(2):509–12.
609. Chandra A et al. Phytochemistry. 1987;26(11):3077–8.
610. Ognyanov M et al. Phytochemistry. 1983;22(8):1775–7.
611. Schinella GR et al. J Pharm Pharmcol. 1998 Sep;50(9):1069–74.
612. Chandler RF et al. Lipids. 1982 Feb;17(2):102–6.
613. Wilkomirski B, Kucharska E. Phytochemistry. 1992;31(11):3915–6.
614. Vislobokov AI et al. Bull Exp Biol Med. 2004 Oct;138(4):390–2.
615. Polle AY et al. Biochemistry (Mosc). 2002 Dec;67(12):1371–6.
616. Chiasson H et al. J Econ Entomol. 2001 Feb;94(1):167–71.
617. Bandonien D et al. Food Res Int. 2000;33(9):785–91.
618. Brown AMG et al. Phytother Res. 1997 Nov;11(7):479–84.
619. Xie G et al. Int Immunopharmacol. 2007 Dec 15;7(13):1639–50.
620. Mark KA et al. Arch Dermatol. 1999 Jan;135(1):67–70.
621. Burkhard PR et al. J Neurol. 1999 Aug;246(8):667–70.
622. Vijverberg K et al. Theor Appl Genet. 2004 Feb;108(4):725–32.
623. Van Baarlen P et al. Genome. 2000 Oct;43(5):827–35.
624. Keane B et al. Environ Monit Assess. 2005 Jun;105(1–3):341–57.
625. Kashiwada Y et al. J Asian Nat Prod Res. 2001;3(3):191–7.
626. Kisiel W, Barszcz B. Fitoterapia. 2000 Jun;71(3):269–73.
627. Hansel R et al. Phytochemistry. 1980;19(5):857–61.
628. Rauwald HW, Huang JT. Phytochemistry. 1985;24(7):1557–9.
629. Schutz K et al. Rapid Comun Mass Spectrom. 2005;19(2):179–86.
630. Williams CA et al. Phytochemistry. 1996 May;42(1):121–7.
631. Su Q et al. Eur J Clin Nutr. 2002 Nov;56(11):1149–54.
632. Simandi B et al. J Supercritical Fluids. 2002 Jun;23(2):135–42.
633. Hannemann K et al. Lipids. 1989 Apr;24(4):296–8.
634. Cicero AF et al. Acta Diabetol. 2004 Sep;41(3):91–8.
635. Onal S et al. Prep Biochem Biotechnol. 2005;35(1):29–36.
636. Trojanova I et al. Fitoterapia. 2004 Dec;75(7–8):760–3.
637. Koo HN et al. Life Sci. 2004 Jan 16;74(9):1149–57.
638. Baba K et al. Yakugaku Zasshi. 1981 Jun;101(6):538–43.
639. Takasaki M et al. Biol Pharm Bull. 1999 Jun;22(6):606–10.
640. Chakurski I et al. Vutr Boles. 1981;20(6):51–4.
641. Hu C, Kitts DD. Phytomedicine. 2005 Aug;12(8):588–97.
642. Hu C, Kitts DD. Mol Cel Biochem. 2004 Oct;265(1–2):107–13.
643. Pichtel J et al. Environ Pollut. 2000 Oct;110(1):171–8.
644. Jovanovic M, Poljacki M. Med Pregl. 2003 Jan–Feb;56(1–2):43–9.
645. Mark KA et al. Arch Dermatol. 1999 Jan;135(1):67–70.
646. Lovell CR, Rowan M. Contact Dermatitis. 1991 Sep;25(3):185–8.
647. Jovanovic M et al. Contact Dermatitis. 2004 Sep;51(3):101–10.
648. Wakelin SH et al. Br J Dermatol. 1997 Aug;137(2):289–91.
649. Guin JD, Skidmore G. Arch Dermatol. 1987 Apr;123(4):500–2.

650. Paulsen E et al. Contact Dermatitis. 2001 Oct;45(4): 197–204.
651. Jovanovic M et al. Contact Dermatitis. 2003 Jan;48(1): 17–25.
652. Roder E et al. Mitt Geb Lebensmitt Hyg. 1981;74:4.
653. Culvenor C et al. Aust J Chem. 1976;29:229–30.
654. Mroczek T et al. J Chromatogr A. 2002 Mar 8;949(1–2): 249–62.
655. Ryu JH et al. J Nat Prod. 1999 Oct;62(10):1437–8.
656. Wang CD et al. Yao Xue Xue Bao. 1989;24(12):913–6.
657. Hwang SB et al. Eur J Pharmacol. 1987 Sep 11;141(2): 269–81.
658. Kokoska L et al. J Ethnopharmacol. 2002 Sep;82(1):51–3.
659. Fu JX. Zhong Xi Yi Jie He Za Zhi. 1989 Nov;9(11):658–9.
660. Sperl W et al. Eur J Pediatr. 1995 Feb;154(2):112–6.
661. Roulet M et al. J Pediatr. 1988 Mar;112(3):433–6.
662. Spang R. J Pediatr. 1988;115:1025.
663. Prakash AS et al. Mutat Res/Genetic Toxicol Environ Mutag. 1999 Jul;443(1–2):53–67.
664. Kraus C et al. Planta Med. 1985;51(2):89–91.

Berberidaceae

1. The Local Food-Nutraceuticals Consortium. Pharmacol Res. 2005 Oct;52(4):353–66.
2. Fatehi M et al. J Ethnopharmacol. 2005 Oct;31;102(1):46–52.
3. Pozniakovskii VM et al. Vopr Pitan. 2003;72(4):46–9.
4. Arayne MS et al. Pak J Pharm Sci. 2007 Jan;20(1):83–92.
5. Sturm S, Stuppner H. Electrophoresis. 1998 Nov;19(16–17): 3026–32.
6. Domagalina E, Smajkiewicz A. Acta Pol Pharm. 1971;28(1): 81–7.
7. Suau R et al. Phytochemistry. 1998 Dec;49(8):2545–9.
8. Vilinski J et al. Pharm Biol. 2003;41(8):351–7.
9. Kathleen A. Altern Med Rev. 2000;5(2):175–7.
10. Martindale, The Extra Pharmacopoeia 26th Ed. Pharmaceutical Press London March 1973 p. 325.
11. Ryzhikova MA et al. Eksp Klin Farmakol. 1999 Mar–Apr; 62(2):36–8.
12. Cernakova M, Kostalova D. Folia Microbiol (Praha). 2002; 47(4):375–8.
13. Tran QL et al. J Ethnopharmacol. 2003 Jun;86(2–3): 249–52.
14. Sriwilaijareon N et al. Parasitol Int. 2002 Mar;51(1):99–103.
15. Park KS et al. J Antimicrob Chemother. 1999 May;43(5): 667–74.
16. Amin AH et al. Can J Microbiol. 1969;15:1067–76.
17. Rackova L at al. Bioorg Med Chem. 2004 Sep 1;12(17): 4709–15.
18. Muller K et al. Planta Med. 1995 Feb;61(1):74–5.
19. Gudima SO et al. Mol Biol (Mosk). 1994 Nov–Dec;28(6): 1308–14.
20. Lin SS et al. Phytomedicine. 2005 May;12(5):351–8.
21. Fukuda K et al. J Ethnopharmacol. 1999 Aug;66(2): 227–33.
22. Cernakova M et al. BMC Complement Altern Med. 2002 Feb 19;2:2.
23. Ivanovska N, Philipov S. Int J Immunopharmacol. 1996 Oct;18(10):553–61.
24. Kong W et al. Nat Med. 2000 Dec;10(12):1344–51.
25. Sheng WD et al. East Afr Med J. 1997 May;74(5):283–4.
26. Xu R et al. Leuk Res. 2005 Jul 13;2006 Jan;30(1):17–23.
27. Zi ZN et al. Planta Med. 2002 Jul;68(7):596–600.
28. Wang GY et al. J Zhejiang Univ Sci B. 2007 Apr;8(4):248–55.
29. Ju HS et al. Biochem Pharmacol. 1990 Jun 1;39(11):1673–8.
30. Bezakova L et al. Pharmazie. 1996 Oct;51(10):758–61.
31. Marshall SJ et al. Antimicrob Agents Chemother. 1994 Jan;38(1):96–103.
32. Guo ZB, Fu JG. Zhongguo Zhong Xi Yi Jie He Za Zhi. 2005 Aug;25(8):765–8.
33. Teh BS et al. Int J Immunopharmacol. 1990;12(3):321–6.
34. Pilch DS et al. Biochemistry. 1997 Oct;36(41):12542–53.
35. McCutcheon AR et al. J Ethnopharmacol. 1994 Dec; 44(3):157–69.
36. Misik V et al. Planta Med. 1995 Aug;61(4):372–3.
37. Bezakova L et al. Pharmazie. 1996 Oct;51(10):758–61.
38. Misik V et al. Planta Med. 1995 Feb;61(4):372–3.
39. Sotnikova R et al. Methods Find Exp Clin Pharmcol. 1997 Nov;19(9):589–97.
40. Claus EP. Pharmacognosy 4th Ed. Henry Kimpton. London 1961 p. 334.
41. Slobodnikova L et al. Phytother Res. 2004 Aug;18(8):674–6.
42. Vollekova A et al. Phytother Res. 2003 Aug;17(7):834–7.
43. Vollekova A et al. Folia Microbiol (Praha). 2001;46(2): 107–11.
44. Hajnicka V et al. Planta Med. 2002 Mar;68(3):266–8.
45. Kostalova D et al. Fitoterapia. 2001 Nov;72(7):802–6.
46. Kostalova D et al. Ceska Slov Farm. 2001 Nov;50(6):286–9.
47. Gulliver WP, Donsky HJ. Am J Ther. 2005 Sep–Oct;12(5): 398–406.
48. Augustin M et al. Forsch Komplementarmed. 1999 Apr; 6 Suppl 2:19–21.
49. Woldemariam TZ et al. J Pharm Biomed Anal. 1997 Mar; 15(6):839–43.
50. Betz JM et al. Phytochem Anal. 1998;9(5):232–6.
51. Kennelly EJ et al. J Nat Prod. 1999 Oct;62(10):1385–9.
52. Flom MS et al. J Pharm Sci. 1967 Nov;56(11):1515–7.
53. Jhoo JW et al. J Agric Food Chem. 2001 Dec;49(12):5969–74.
54. Finkel RS, Zarlengo KM. N Eng J Med. 2004 Jul 15;351(3): 302–3.
55. Jones TK, Lawson BM. J Pediatr. 1998 Mar;132(3 pt 1): 550–2.
56. Gunn TR, Wright IM. NZ Med J. 1996 Oct 25;109(1032): 410–1.
57. Bergener P. Medical Herbalism. 12(1):12–14.
58. Rao RB, Hoffman RS. Vet Hum Toxicol. 2002 Aug;44(4): 221–2.
59. Scott CC, Chen KK. J Pharm Exp Ther. 1943;79:334.

Betulaceae

1. Demirci B et al. Evid Based Complement Alternat Med. 2004 Dec;1(3):301–3.
2. Carnat A et al. Ann Pharm Fr. 1996;54(5):231–5.
3. Keinanen M, Julkunen-Tiitto R. J Chromatog A. 1998 Jan 16;793(2):370–7.
4. Patocka J. J Applied Biomed. 2003;1:7–12.
5. Taipale HT et al. Phytochemistry. 1993 Oct;34(3):755–8.
6. Mukhtar HM et al. Pharmazie. 2003 Sep;58(9):671–3.

7. Rickling B, Glombitza KW. Planta Med. 1993 Feb;59(1): 76–9.
8. Salminen JP et al. Z Naturforsch (C). 2002 Mar–Apr; 57(3–4):248–56.
9. Shul'ts EE et al. Prikl Biokhim Mikrobiol. 2005 Jan–Feb; 41(1):107–12.
10. Ossipov V et al. J Chromatog A. 1996 Jan;15;721(1):59–68.
11. Laitinen J et al. J Chem Ecol. 2005 Oct;31(10):2243–62.
12. Smite E et al. Phytochemistry. 1995 Sep;40(1):341–3.
13. Smite E et al. Phytochemistry. 1993 Jan 20;32(2):365–9.
14. Laitinen ML et al. J Chem Ecol. 2005 Apr;31(4):697–717.
15. Palme AE et al. Mol Ecol. 2004 Jan;13(1):167–78.
16. Nosik NN et al. Vopr Virusol. 2005 Sep–Oct;50(5):29–32.
17. Yamashita K et al. Clin Chim Acta. 2002 Nov;325(1–2):91–6.
18. Szuster-Ciesielska A, Kandefer-Szerszen M. Pharmcol Rep. 2005 Sep–Oct;57(5):588–95.
19. Pavlova NI et al. Fitoterapia. 2003 Jul;74(5):489–92.
20. Zdzisinska B et al. Pol J Pharmacol. 2003 Mar–Apr; 55(2):235–8.
21. Hiroya K et al. Bioorg Med Chem. 2002 Oct;10(10):3229–36.
22. Miura N et al. Mol Pharmacol. 1999;56(6):1324–8.
23. Zhou J et al. J Biol Chem. 2005 Dec 23;280(51):42149–55.
24. Bringmann G et al. Planta Med. 1993 Jun;63(3):255–7.
25. Chowdhury AR et al. Med Sci Monit. 2002 Jul;8(7):254–60.
26. Fulda S et al. J Biol Chem. 1998 Dec 18;273(51):33942–8.
27. Wick W et al. J Pharmacol Exp Ther. 1999 Jun;289(3): 1306–12.
28. Fulda S, Debatin KM. Neoplasia. 2005 Feb;7(2):162–70.
29. Bernard P et al. Phytochemistry. 2001 Nov;58(6):865–74.
30. Cosmes PM et al. Allergol Immunopathol (Madr). 2005 May–Jun;33(3):145–50.
31. Varela S et al. J Investig Allergol Clin Immunol. 2003; 13(2):124–30.

Bignonaceae

1. Oswald EH. Br J Phytotherapy. 1994 Summer;3(3):112–7.
2. Steinert J et al. J Chromatog A. 1996 Feb 2;723(1):206–9.
3. Park BS et al. J Ethnopharmacol. 2006 Apr 21;105(1–2): 255–62.
4. Koyama J et al. Chem Pharm Bull (Tokyo). 2000 Jun;48(6): 873–5.
5. Steinhert J et al. J Chromatog A. 1995 Feb 24;693(2):281–7.
6. Park BS et al. J Agric Food Chem. 2003 Jan 1;51(1):295–300.
7. Awale S et al. Chem Pharm Bull (Tokyo). 2005 Jun;53(6): 710–3.
8. Warashina T et al. Phytochemistry. 2005 Mar;66(5):589–97.
9. Warashina T et al. Chem Pharm Bull (Tokyo). 2006 Jan;54(1):14–20.
10. Warashina T et al. Phytochemistry. 2004 Jul;65(13):2003–11.
11. Koyama J et al. Phytochemistry. 2000 Apr;53(8):869–72.
12. Nakano K et al. Phytochemistry. 1993 Jan 20;32(2):371–3.
13. Anesini C, Perez C. J Ethnopharmacol. 1993 Jun;39(2): 119–28.
14. Machado TB et al. Int J Antimicrob Agents. 2003 Mar;21(3): 279–84.
15. Park BS et al. J Agric Food. 2005 Feb 23;53(4):1152–7.
16. Portillo A et al. J Ethnopharmcol. 2001 Jun;76(1):93–8.
17. Glen VL et al. J Chromatogr B:Biomed Sci Appl. 1997 Apr 25;692(1):181–6.

18. Ueda S et al. Phytochemistry. 1994 May;36(2):323–5.
19. Pinto AV et al. Arzneimittelforschung. 1997 Jan;47(1):74–9.
20. Menna-Bareto RF et al. J Antimicrob Chemother. 2005 Dec;56(6):1034–41.
21. Pinto CN et al. Arzneimittelforschung. 2000 Dec;50(12): 1120–8.
22. Carvalho LH et al. Brazilian J Med Biol Res. 1988;21(3): 485–7.
23. Renou SG et al. Pharmazie. 2003 Oct;58(10):690–5.
24. Lee H et al. Pharmacol Res. 2005 Jun;51(6):553–60.
25. Choi YH et al. J Biochem Mol Biol. 2003 Mar 31;36(2):223–9.
26. Woo HJ, Choi YH. Int J Oncol. 2005 Apr;26(4):1017–23.
27. Simamura E et al. Can Detect Prevent. 2003;27(1):5–13.
28. Choi BT et al. Anticancer Drugs. 2003 Nov;14(10):845–50.
29. Manna SK et al. Biochem Pharmacol. 1999 Apr 1;57(7): 763–74.
30. Gupta D et al. Experim Hematol. 2002 Jul;30(7):711–20.
31. Muller K et al. J Nat Prod. 1999 Aug;62(8):1134–6.

Boraginaceae

1. Franz G. Planta Med. 1969 Aug;17(3):217–20.
2. Luthy J et al. Pharm Acta Helv. 1984;59(9–10):242–6.
3. Griffiths G et al. Phytochemistry 1996 Sep;43(2):381–6.
4. Tyystjarvi P. Phytochemistry. 1993 Jul 23;33(5):1029–32.
5. Gonzalez CA et al. Cancer Epidemiol Biomarkers Prev. 1993 Mar–Apr;2(2):157–8.
6. Bandoniene D et al. J Chromatogr Sci. 2005 Aug;43(7): 372–6.
7. Nahrstedt A et al. Phytochemistry. 1989 Jan;28(2):623–4.
8. Medrano A et al. J Food Compost Anal. 1992 Dec;5(4): 313–8.
9. Bandoniene C, Murkovic M. J Biochem Biophys Methods. 2002 Oct–Nov;53(1–3):45–9.
10. Kast RE. Int Immunopharm. 2001 Nov;1(12):2197–9.
11. Henz BM et al. Br J Dermatol. 1999;140:685–8.
12. Frei H et al. Chemico-Biol Interact. 1992 Jun;15;83(1):1–22.
13. Dr Duke's Phytochemical and Ethnobotanical Databases. http://www.ars-grin.gov/duke/.
14. Dennis R et al. Acta Pharm Hung. 1987 Nov;57(6):267–74.
15. Franz G. Planta Med. 1969 Aug;17(3):217–20.
16. Roder E. Pharmazie. 1995;50:83–98.
17. Brauchli J et al. Experientia. 1982 Feb;10(2–3):183–8.
18. Oberlies NH et al. Public Health Nutr. 2004 Oct;7(7):919–24.
19. Rode D. Trends Pharmacol Sci. 2002 Nov;23(11):497–99.
20. Kim NC et al. J Nat Prod. 2001 Feb;64(2):251–3.
21. Gracza L et al. Arch Pharm (Weinheim). 1985 Dec;318(12): 1090–5.
22. Wagner H et al. Arnzeimittelforschung. 1970 May;20(5): 705–13.
23. Mohammad FV et al. Phytochemistry. 1995 Sep;40(1):213–8.
24. Ahmad VU et al. Phytochemistry. 1993 Mar;32(4):1003–6.
25. Ahmad VU et al. J Nat Prod. 1993 Mar;56(3):329–34.
26. Martindale, The Extra Pharmacopoeia 26th Ed. The Pharmaceutical. Press London March 1973 p. 557.
27. Tunon H et al. J Ethnopharmcol. 1995 Oct;48(2):61–76.
28. van den Dungen et al. Clin Exp Immunol. 1991 Oct; 86(Suppl 1):3.
29. Olinescu A et al. Roum Arch Microbiol Immunol. 1993 Apr–Jun;52(2):73–80.

30. Predel HG et al. Phytomedicine. 2005 Nov;12(10):707–14.
31. Kucera M et al. Wien Med Wochenschr. 2004 Nov; 154(21–22):498–507.
32. Koll R et al. Phytomedicine. 2004 Sep;11(6):470–7.
33. Koll R, Klingenburg S. Fortschr Med Orig. 2002;120(1):1–9.
34. Kucera M et al. Adv Ther. 2000 Jul–Aug;17(4):204–10.
35. Grube B et al. Phytomedicine. 2007;14:2–10.
36. Gafar M et al. Rev Chir Oncol Radiol O R L Oftamol Stomatol Ser Stomatol. 1989 Apr–Jun;36(2):91–8.
37. Suciu G et al. Rev Chir Oncol Radiol O R L Oftamol Stomatol Ser Stomatol. 1988 Jul–Sep;35(3):191–4.
38. Stickel F, Seitz HK. Public Health Nutr. 2000 Dec;3(4A): 501–8.
39. Prakash S et al. Mutat Res. 1999 Jul 15;443(1–2):53–67.
40. Mattocks AR. Lancet. 1980 Nov 22;2(8204):1136–7.
41. Couet CE et al. Nat Toxins. 1996;4(4):163–7.
42. Schanenberg BT et al. Phytochem Anal. 2004 Jan–Feb;15(1): 36–9.
43. Culvenor CC et al. Chemico-Biol Interact. 1976;12(3–4): 299–324.
44. Ridker PM, McDermott WV. Lancet. 1989 Mar 25;333(8639): 657–8.
45. Betz JM et al. J Pharm Sci. 1994 May;83(5):649–53.
46. Behninger C et al. Planta Med. 1989 Dec;55(6):518–22.

Brassicaceae

1. Li X, Kushad MM. J Agric Food Chem. 2004 Nov 17;52(23): 6950–5.
2. Song L et al. Anal Biochem. 2005 Dec 15;347(2):234–43.
3. Yu EY et al. Biochem Biophy Acta. 2001 Aug 15;1527(3): 156–60.
4. Dr Duke's Phytochemical and Ethnobotanical Databases. http://www.ars-grin.gov/duke/.
5. Weil MJ et al. J Agric Food Chem. 2005 Mar 9;53(5):1440–4.
6. Conaway CC et al. Nutr Cancer. 2000;38(2):168–78.
7. Shapiro TA et al. Cancer Epidemiol Biomarkers Prev. 1998 Dec;7(12):1091–100.
8. Weil MJ et al. Nutr Cancer. 2004;48(2):207–13.
9. Zhu CY, Loft S. Food Chem Toxicol. 2001 Dec;39(12):1 191–7.
10. Keum YS et al. Drug News Perspect. 2005 Sep;18(7):445–51.
11. Stoewsand GS. Food Chem Toxicol. 1995 Jun;33(6):537–43.
12. Agabeili RA et al. Tsitol Genet. 2004 Mar–Apr;38(2):40–5.
13. Leoni O et al. Bioorg Med Chem. 1997 Sep;5(9):1799–806.
14. Smith TK et al. Carcinogenesis. 2004 Aug;25(8):1409–15.
15. Brabban AD, Edwards C. J Appl Bacteriol. 1995 Aug;79(2): 171–7.
16. Iurrison S. Farmatsiia. 1973 Sep–Oct;22(5):34–5.
17. El-Abyad MS et al. Microbios. 1990;62(250):47–57.
18. Iurrison S. Tartu Riiliku Ulikooli Toim. 1971;270:71–9.
19. Kuroda K, Takagi K. Nature. 1968 Nov 16;220(168):707–8.
20. Kuroda K, Akao M. Gann. 1981 Oct;72(5):777–82.
21. Kuroda K, Kaku T. Life Sci. 1969 Feb 1;8(3):151–5.
22. Miyazawa M et al. Yaku Zasshi. 1979;99(10):1041–3.
23. Aksoy A et al. Sci Total Environ. 1999 Feb 9;226(2–3): 177–86.
24. Kuroda K, Takagi K. Nature. 1968 Nov 16;220(5168):707–8.
25. Kuroda K et al. Cancer Res. 1976 Jun;36(6):1900–3.

Burseraceae

1. British Herbal Medicine Association. British Herbal Compendium vol. 1 Bournemouth 1992:163–5.
2. Hanus LO et al. Biomed Pap Med Fac Univ Palacky Olomouc Czech Repub. 2005 Jul;149(1):3–28.
3. Tian J, Shi S. Zhongguo Zhong Yao Za Zhi. 1996 Apr;21(4): 235–7.
4. Brieskorn CH, Noble P. Phytochemistry. 1983;22(5): 1207–1211.
5. Dolara P et al. Planta Med. 2000 May;66(4):356–8.
6. Brieskorn CH, Noble P. Phytochemistry. 1983;22(1):187–9.
7. Marongiu B et al. J Agric Food Chem. 2005 Oct 5;53(20): 7939–43.
8. Mincione E, Iavarone C. Chim Ind (Milan). 1972;54:525–7.
9. Martindale, The Extra Pharmacopoeia 26th Ed. Pharmaceutical Press London March 1973 p. 313–4.
10. Hassan AM et al. J Egypt Soc Parasitol. 2003 Dec;33(3): 999–1008.
11. Allam AF et al. J Egypt Soc Parasitol. 2001 Dec;31(3): 683–90.
12. Massoud AM et al. J Egypt Soc Parasitol. 2001 Aug;31(2): 517–290.
13. Massoud AM, Labib IM. J Egypt Soc Parasitol. 2000 Apr;30(1):101–15.
14. Massoud AM et al. J Egypt Soc Parasitol. 2005 Aug;35(2): 667–86.
15. Dolara P et al. Planta Med. 2000 May;66(4):356–8.
16. Massoud A et al. Am J Trop Med Hyg. 2001 Aug;65(2):96–9.
17. Soliman OE et al. J Egypt Soc Parasitol. 2004 Dec;34(3): 941–66.
18. Abo-Maydan AA et al. J Egypt Soc Parasitol. 2004 Dec; 34(3):807–18.
19. Hegab MH, Hassan RM. J Egypt Soc Parasitol. 2003 Aug; 33(2):561–70.
20. Al-Mathal EM, Fouad MA. J Egypt Soc Parasitol. 2004 Aug; 34(2):713–20.
21. Abo-Maydan AA et al. J Egypt Soc Parasitol. 2004 Aug; 34(2):423–46.
22. El Baz MA et al. J Egypt Soc Parasitol. 2003 Dec; 33(3):761–76.
23. Sheir Z et al. Am J Trop Med Hyg. 2001 Dec;65(6):700–4.
24. Massoud AM et al. J Egypt Soc Parasitol. 2007 Aug; 37(2):395–410.
25. Massoud AM et al. J Egypt Soc Parasitol. 2004 Apr; 34(1):315–32.
26. Barakat R et al. Am J Trop Med Hyg. 2005 Aug;73(2):365–7.
27. Botros S et al. Am J Trop Med Hyg. 2005 Feb;72(2):119–23.
28. Southgate VR et al. J Helminthol. 2005 Sep;79(3):181–5.
29. Tipton DA et al. Toxicol In Vitro. 2006 Mar;20(2):248–55.
30. Assimopoulou AN et al. Food Chem. 2005 Oct;92(4):721–7.
31. Moussaieff A et al. J Ethnopharmacol. 2005 Oct 3;101(1–3): 16–26.
32. Mielck W. Dent Dienst. 1970 Nov;22(11):21.
33. Pannuti CM et al. Pesqui Odontol Bras. 2003;17(4):314–8.
34. Al-Rowais NA. Saudi Med J. 2002 Nov;23(11):1327–31.
35. Tipton DA et al. Toxicol In Vitro. 2003 Jun;17(3):301–10.
36. Gallo R et al. Contact Dermatitis. 1999 Oct;41(4):230–1.
37. Al-Suwaidan SW et al. Contact Dermatitis. 1998 Sep; 39(3):137.
38. Al Faraj S. Ann Trop Med Parasitol. 2005 Mar;99(2):219–20.

Cannabaceae

1. Bohr G et al. J Nat Prod. 2005 Oct;68(10):1545–8.
2. Zhang X et al. J Am Soc Mass Spectrom. 2004 Feb; 15(2):180–7.
3. Yasukawa K et al. Oncology. 1995 Mar–Apr;52(2):156–8.
4. Hecht S et al. Phytochemistry. 2004 Apr;65(8):1057–60.
5. Hoek AC et al. Phyotchem Anal. 2001 Jan–Feb;12(1):53–7.
6. Wohlfart R et al. Arch Pharm Wein. 1983;316:132–7.
7. Hartley RD, Fawcett CH. Phytochemistry. 1969 Mar; 8(3):637–43.
8. Hartley RD, Fawcett CH. Phytochemistry. 1969 Sep; 8(9):1793–6.
9. Kishimoto T et al. J Agric Food Chem. 2005 Jun 15; 53(12):4701–7.
10. Hartley RD, Fawcett CH. Phytochemistry. 1968 Aug; 7(8):1395–1400.
11. Steinhaus M, Schieberle P. J Agric Food Chem. 2000 May; 48(5):1776–83.
12. Roberts MT et al. J Sep Sci. 2004 Apr;27(5–6):473–8.
13. Zhao F et al. J Nat Prod. 2005 Jan;68(1):43–9.
14. He GQ et al. J Zhejiang Univ Sci B. 2005 Oct;6(10):999–1004.
15. Stevens JF et al. Phytochemistry. 1997 Apr;44(8):1575–85.
16. Tabata N et al. Phytochemistry. 1997 Oct;46(4):683–7.
17. Chadwick LR et al. J Nat Prod. 2004 Dec;67(12):2024–32.
18. Chadwick LR et al. J Nat Prod. 2004 Dec;67(12):2024–32.
19. Tekel' J et al. J Agric Food Chem. 1999 Dec;47(12):5059–63.
20. Nikolic D et al. J Mass Spectrom. 2005 Mar;40(3):289–99.
21. Bhandari PR. J Chromatogr. 1964 Oct;16:130–5.
22. Jerkovic V et al. J Agric Food Chem. 2005 May 18;53(10): 4202–6.
23. Taylor AW et al. J Agric Food Chem. 2003 Jul 2;51(14): 4101–10.
24. Stevens JF et al. J Agric Food Chem. 2002 Jun 5;50(12): 3435–43.
25. Qu Y et al. Z Naturoforsch [C]. 2003 Sep–Oct;58(9–10): 640–2.
26. Oosterveld A et al. Carbohydr Polym. 2002 Sep 1;49(4): 407–13.
27. Hampton R et al. Phytochemistry. 2003 Dec;61(7):855–62.
28. Auerbach RH et al. J AOAC Int. 2000 May–Jun;83(3):621–6.
29. Danilova TV et al. Genetika. 2003 Nov;39(11):1484–9.
30. Jakse J et al. Genome. 2004 Oct;47(5):889–99.
31. Stevens JF. Phytochemistry. 2000 Apr;53(7):759–75.
32. Sisek P et al. Pflugers Arch. 2000;439(3 Suppl):R16–8.
33. De Keukeleire J et al. J Agric Food Chem. 2003 Jul 16;51(15): 4436–41.
34. Martindale, The Extra Pharmacopoeia 26th Ed. Pharmaceutical Press London March 1973 p. 327.
35. Gerhauser C. Eur J Cancer. 2005 Sep;41(13):1941–54.
36. Dixon-Shanies D, Shaikh N. Oncol Rep. 1999 Nov–Dec;6(6): 1383–7.
37. Pan L et al. Mol Nutr Food Res. 2005 Sep;49(9):837–43.
38. Miranda CL et al. Food Chem Toxicol. 1999 Apr;37(4): 271–85.
39. Gerhauser C et al. Mol Cancer Ther. 2002 Sep;1(11):959–69.
40. Delmulle L et al. Phytomedicine. 2006 Nov;13(9–10):732–4.
41. Miranda CL et al. Drug Metab Dispos. 2000 Nov;28(11): 1297–302.
42. Dietz BM et al. Chem Res Toxicol. 2005 Aug;18(8):1296–305.
43. Liu G et al. Anal Chem. 2005 Oct 1;77(19):6407–14.
44. Albini A et al. FASEB J. 2006 Mar;20(3):527–9.
45. Vanhoecke B et al. Int J Cancer. 2005 Dec 20;117(6):889–95.
46. Chen WJ, Lin JK. J Agric Food Chem. 2004 Jan 14;52(1): 55–64.
47. Monteiro R et al. J Steroid Biochem Mol Biol. 2007 Jun–Jul; 105(1–5):124–30.
48. Milligan SR et al. J Clin Endocrinol Metab. 1999 Jun;84(6): 2249–52.
49. Bolca S et al. Br J Nutr. 2007 Nov;98(5):950–9.
50. Liu J et al. J Agric Food Chem. 2001 May;49(5):2472–9.
51. Overk CR et al. J Agric Food Chem. 2005 Aug 10;53(16): 6246–53.
52. Effenberger K et al. J Steroid Biochem Mol Biol. 2005 Sep;96(5):387–99.
53. Milligan SR et al. J Clin Endocrinol Metab. 2000 Dec; 85(12):4912–5.
54. Milligan SR et al. Reprod. 2002 Feb;123(2):235–42.
55. Sun J. J Altern Complement Med. 2003 Jun;9(3):403–9.
56. Heyerick A et al. Maturitas. 2006 May 20;54(2):164–75.
57. Bohr G et al. J Nat Prod. 2005 Oct;68(10):1545–8.
58. Lemay M et al. Asia Pac J Clin Nutr. 2004;13(Suppl):S110.
59. Lukaczer D et al. Phytother Res. 2005 Oct;19(10):864–9.
60. Buckwold VE et al. Antiviral Res. 2004 Jan;61(1):57–62.
61. Wang Q et al. Antiviral Res. 2004 Dec;64(3):189–94.
62. Gerhauser C. Mol Nutr Food Res. 2005 Sep;49(9):827–31.
63. Langezaal CR et al. Pharm Weekbl Sci. 1992 Dec 11;14(6): 353–6.
64. Simpson WJ, Smith AR. J Appl Bacteriol. 1992 Apr;72(4): 327–34.
65. Frolich S et al. J Antimicrob Chemother. 2005 Jun;55(6): 883–7.
66. Morinaga N et al. J Biol Chem. 2005 Jun 17;280(24): 23303–9.
67. Abourashed EA et al. Phytomedicine. 2004 Nov;11(7–8): 633–8.
68. Zanoli P et al. J Ethnopharmacol. 2005 Oct 31;102(1):102–6.
69. Hansel R et al. Z Naturforsch [C]. 1980 Nov–Dec;35(11–12): 1096–7.
70. Cerny A, Schmid K. Fitoterapia. 1999 Jun 1;70(3):221–8.
71. Morin CM et al. Sleep. 2005 Nov 1;28(11):1465–71.
72. Schmitz M, Jackel M. Wien Med Wochenschr. 1998; 148(13):291–8.
73. Gerhard U et al. Schweiz Rundsch Med Prax. 1996 Apr 9;85(15):473–81.
74. Dimpfel W et al. Eur J Med Res. 2004 Sep 29;9(9):423–31.
75. Schellenberg R et al. Planta Med. 2004 Jul;70(7):594–7.
76. Stevens JF et al. Chem Res Toxicol. 2003 Oct;16(10):1277–86.
77. Stevens JF et al. J Agric Food Chem. 2002 Jun 5;50(12): 3435–43.
78. Stevens JF et al. J Agric Food Chem. 2000 Sep;48(9):3876–84.
79. Liegeois C et al. J Agric Food Chem. 2000 Apr;48(4): 1129–34.
80. Krivenko VV et al. Vrach Delo. 1989 Mar;(3):76–8.
81. Yajima H et al. J Biol Chem. 2004 Aug 6;279(32):33456–62.
82. Possemiers S et al. J Agric Food Chem. 2005 Aug 10;53(16): 6281–8.
83. Nikolic D et al. J Mass Spectrom. 2005 Mar;40(3):289–99.
84. Zierau O et al. J Steroid Biochem Mol Biol. 2004 Sep; 92(1–2):107–10.
85. Spiewak R, Dutkiewicz J. Ann Agric Environ Med. 2002; 9(2):249–52.
86. Estrada JL et al. Contact Dermatitis. 2002 Feb;46(2):127.
87. Spiewak R et al. Ann Agric Environ Med. 2001;8(1):51–6.

88. Skorska C et al. Ann Uiv Mariae Curie Sklodowska [Med]. 2003;58(1):459–65.

89. Gora A et al. Ann Agric Environ Med. 2004;11(1):129–38.

90. Pradalier A et al. Allerg Immunol (Paris). 2002 Nov;34(9): 330–2.

91. Cobin JA, Johnson NA. J AOAC Int. 1996 Mar–Apr; 79(2):503–7.

92. Williams CS et al. Food Addit Contam. 1994 Sep–Oct; 11(5):615–9.

93. Humfrey CD. Nat Toxins. 1998;6(2):51–9.

94. Henderson MC et al. Xenobiotica. 2000 Mar;30(3):235–31.

Caprifoliaceae

1. WHO Monographs on Selected Medicinal Plants—Vol 2. WHO Geneva 2004 p. 269–275.

2. Gray AM et al. J Nutr. 2000 Jan;130(1):15–20.

3. Lamaison JL et al. Ann Pharm Fr. 1991;49(5):258–62.

4. Pietta P et al. J Chromatogr. 1992 Feb 28;593(1–2):165–70.

5. Jorgensen U et al. J Agric Food Chem. 2000 Jun;48(6): 2376–83.

6. Dellagreca M et al. Nat Prod Res. 2003 Jun;17(3):177–81.

7. D'Abrosca B et al. Phytochemistry. 2001 Dec;58(7):1073–81.

8. Girbes T et al. Cell Mol Biol (Noisy-le-grand). 2003 Jun;49(4): 537–45.

9. Kolodynska M, Praczko J. Ann Univ Mariae Curie Sklodowska [Med]. 1996;21:207–11.

10. Dr Duke's Phytochemical and Ethnobotanical Databases. http://www.ars-grin.gov/duke/

11. Kaack K, Austed T. Plants Foods Hum Nutr. 1998;52(3): 187–98.

12. Wu X et al. J Agric Food Chem. 2004 Dec 29;52(26):7846–56.

13. Thole JM et al. J Med Food. 2006 Dec;9(4):498–504.

14. Jensen SR, Nielsen BJ. Acta Chem Scand. 1973;27:2661–2.

15. Mach L et al. Biochem J. 1996 May 1;315(Pt 3):1061.

16. Van Damme EJ et al. Plant J. 1997 Dec;12(6):1251–60.

17. Martindale, The Extra Pharmacopoeia 26th Ed. Pharmaceutical Press London March 1973.

18. Serkedjievea J et al. Phytother Res. 1990;4(3):97–100.

19. Zakay-Rones Z et al. J Altern Complement Med. 1995 Winter;1(4):361–9.

20. [No authors listed]. Alt Med Rev. 2005;10(1):51–5.

21. Barak V et al. Isr Med Assoc J. 2002 Nov;4(11 Suppl): 919–22.

22. Barak V et al. Eur Cytokine Netw. 2001 Apr–Jun;12(2): 290–6.

23. Uncini Manganelli RE et al. J Ethnopharmacol. 2005 Apr 26;98(3):323–7.

24. Zakay-Rones Z et al. J Int Med Res. 2004 Mar–Apr; 32(2):132–40.

25. Harokopakis E et al. J Periodontal. 2006 Feb;77(2):271–9.

26. Yesilada E et al. J Ethnopharmacol. 1997 Sep;58(1):59–73.

27. Nakajima JI et al. J Biomed Biotechnol. 2004;2004(5):241–7.

28. Guarrera PM. Fitoterapia. 2005 Jan;76(1):1–25.

29. Cao G, Prior RL. Clin Chem. 1999;45:574–6.

30. Mulleder U et al. J Biochem Biophys Methods. 2002; 53:61–6.

31. Frank T et al. Methods Find Exp Clin Pharmacol. 2007 Oct; 29(8):525–33.

32. Celechovska O et al. Ceska Slov Farm. 2004 Nov; 53(6):336–9.

33. Vandecasteele B et al. Sci Total Environ. 2002 Nov 1; 229(1–3):191–205.

34. Forster-Waldl E et al. Clin Exp Allergy. 2003 Dec;33(12): 1703–10.

35. Bock K et al. Phytochemistry. 1978;17(4):753–7.

36. Horhammer L et al. Z Naturforsch B. 1967 Jul;22(7):768–76.

37. Nicholson JA et al. Proc Soc Exp Biol Med. 1972 Jun; 140(2):457–61.

38. Jarboe C et al. Nature. 1966 Nov 19;212(5064):837.

39. Smolinski D et al. J Altern Complement Med. 2005;11(3): 483–9.

40. Jarboe CH et al. J Med Chem. 1967;10:488.

41. Jarboe CH et al. J Org Chem. 1969 Dec;34(12):4202–3.

42. Smith ID et al. Prostaglandins. 1975 Jul;10(1):41–57.

Caryophyllaceae

1. Budzianowski J et al. Pol J Pharmacol Pharm. 1991 Sep–Oct;43(5):395–401.

2. Dong Q et al. Zhongguo Zhong Yao Za Zhi. 2007 Jun; 32(11):1048–51.

3. Jovanovic M et al. Contact Dermatitis. 2003 Jan;48(1):17–25.

4. Pande A et al. Phytochemistry. 1995 Jun;39(3):709–11.

5. Jamieson GR, Reid EH. Phytochemistry. 1971 Jul;10(7): 1575–7.

6. Guil JL et al. Plant Food Hum Nutr. 1997;51(2):99–107.

7. Pieroni A et al. Phytother Res. 2002 Aug;16(5):467–73.

8. Jovanovic M et al. Med Pregl. 2005 Mar–Apr;58(3–4):123–6.

9. Jovanovic M et al. Contact Dermatitis. 2004 Sep;51(3): 101–10.

Clusiaceae

1. WHO Monographs on Selected Medicinal Plants—Vol 2. WHO Geneva 2004 p. 149–71.

2. Chandrasekera DH et al. J Pharm Pharmacol. 2005 Dec; 57(12):1645–52.

3. Pellati F et al. J Chromatogr A. 2005 Sep 23;1088(1–2): 205–17.

4. Tolonen A et al. Phytochem Anal. 2003 Sep–Oct;14(5):306–9.

5. Von Eggelkraut-Gottanka SG et al. Phytochem Anal. 2002 May–Jun;13(3):170–6.

6. Tolonen A et al. Rapid Commun Mass Spectrom. 2002; 16(5):396–402.

7. Girzu-Amblard M et al. Ann Pharm Fr. 2000 Oct;58(5): 341–5.

8. Baugh SF. J AOAC Int. 2005 Nov–Dec;88(6):1607–12.

9. Schempp CM et al. Planta Med. 2002 Feb;68(2):171–3.

10. Liu F et al. J Pharm Biomed Anal. 2005 Feb 23;37(2):303–12.

11. Benkiki N et al. Z Naturforsch [C]. 2003 Sep–Oct;58(9–10): 655–8.

12. Vajs V et al. Fitoterapia. 2003 Jul;74(5):439–44.

13. Shan MD et al. J Nat Prod. 2001 Jan;64(1):127–30.

14. Verotta L et al. J Nat Prod. 1999 May;62(5):770–2.

15. Zou Y et al. J Agric Food Chem. 2004 Aug 11;52(16):5032–9.

16. Urbanek M et al. J Chromatogr A. 2002 Jun 7;958(1–2): 261–71.

17. Schulte-Lobbert S et al. J Pharm Biomed Anal. 2003 Sep 15;33(1):53–60.

18. Butterweck V et al. Psychopharmacology (Berl). 2002 Jul;162(2):193–202.
19. Juergenliemk G et al. Planta Med. 2003 Nov;69(11):1013–7.
20. Tekel'ova D et al. Planta Med. 2000 Dec;66(8):778–80.
21. Schwob I et al. C R Biol. 2002 Jul;325(7):781–5.
22. Ploss O et al. Pharmazie. 2001 Jun;56(6):509–11.
23. Seger C et al. Eur J Pharm Sci. 2004 Mar;21(4):453–63.
24. Jurgenliemk G, Nahrstedt A. Planta Med. 2002 Jan; 68(1):88–91.
25. Shan MD et al. Nat Prod Res. 2004 Feb;18(1):15–9.
26. Wirz A et al. Phytochemistry. 2000 Dec;55(8):941–7.
27. Murch SJ, Saxena PK. Naturwissenschaften. 2002 Dec; 89(12):555–60.
28. Southwell IA, Bourke CA. Phytochemistry. 2001 Mar; 56(5):437–41.
29. Kazlauskas S, Bagdonaite E. Medicina (Kaunas). 2004; 40(10):975–81.
30. Zobayed SM et al. Plant Physiol Biochem. 2005 Oct–Nov; 43(10–11):977–84.
31. Gray DE et al. Planta Med. 2003 Nov;69(11):1024–30.
32. Conforti F et al. Nat Prod Res. 2005 Apr;19(3):295–303.
33. Yi XP et al. Guang Pu Xue Yu Guang Pu Fen Xi. 2004 Jul;24(7):890–2.
34. Gomez MR et al. J Pharm Biomed Anal. 2004 Feb 18;34(3):569–76.
35. Fergert JM et al. J Child Adolesc Psychopharmacol. 2006;16(1–2):197–206.
36. Schroeder C et al. Clin Pharmacol Ther. 2004 Nov; 76(5):480–9.
37. Hansen RS et al. Eur J Pharmacol. 2005 Sep 20;519(3): 199–207.
38. Zanoli P. CNS Drug Rev. 2004 Fall;10(3):203–18.
39. Neary JT, Bu Y. Brain Res. 1999 Jan 23;816(2):358–63.
40. Butterweck V et al. Psychopharmacology (Berl). 2002 Jul;162(2):193–202.
41. Schulte-Lobbert S et al. J Pharm Pharmacol. 2004 Jun; 56(6):813–8.
42. Hanrahan JR et al. Bioorg Med Chem Lett. 2003 Jul 21;13(14):2281–4.
43. Simmen U et al. Pharmacopsychiatry. 2001 Jul;34 Suppl 1: S137–42.
44. Jensen Ag et al. Life Sci. 2001 Feb 23;68(14):1593–605.
45. Winkler C et al. Biol Chem. 2004 Dec;385(12):1197–202.
46. Denke A et al. Arzneimittelforschung. 2000 May;50(5): 415–9.
47. Murck H et al. Neuropsychobiology. 2004;50(2):128–33.
48. Murck H. Wien Med Wochenschr. 2002;152(15–16):398–403.
49. Schule C et al. Neuropsychobiology. 2004;49(2):58–63.
50. Franklin M, Cowen PJ. Pharmacopsychiatry. 2001 Jul; 34 Suppl 1:S29–37.
51. Schule C et al. Pharmacopsychiatry. 2001 Jul;34 Suppl 1: S127–33.
52. Franklin M et al. Biol Psychiatry. 1999 Aug 15;46(4):581–4.
53. Franklin M et al. Pharmacopsychiatry. 2006 Jan;39(1):13–5.
54. Patel J et al. Am J Ther. 2004 Jul–Aug;11(4):262–77.
55. Fiebich BL et al. Pharmacopsychiatry. 2001 Jul;34 Suppl 1: S26–8.
56. Thiele B et al. J Geriatr Psychiatry Neurol. 1994 Oct;7 Suppl 1:S60–2.
57. Harrer G. Schweiz Rundsch Med Prax. 2000 Dec 14; 89(50):2123–9.
58. Nathan PJ. J Psychopharmacol. 2001 Mar;15(1):47–54.
59. Muller WE, Rossol R. J Geriatr Psychiatry Neurol. 1994 Oct;7 Suppl 1:S63–4.
60. Caccia S. Curr Drug Metab. 2005 Dec;6(6):531–43.
61. Laakmann G et al. Pharmacopsychiatry. 1998 Jun;31 Suppl 1: 54–9.
62. Reichling J et al. Forsch Komplementarmed Klass Naturheilkd. 2003 Apr;10 Suppl 1:28–32.
63. Schulz V. Phytomedicine. 2006 Feb;13(3):199–204.
64. Laakmann G et al. Pharmacopsychiatry. 1998 Jun;31 Suppl 1: 54–9.
65. Mueller BM. Adv Ther. 1998 Mar–Apr;15(2):109–16.
66. Sommer H, Harrer G. J Geriatr Psychiatry Neurol. 1994 Oct;7 Suppl 1:S9–11.
67. Rychlik R et al. Fortschr Med Orig. 2001 Nov 29;119(3–4): 119–28.
68. Randlov C et al. Phytomedicine. 2006 Mar;13(4):215–21.
69. Uebelhack R et al. Adv Ther. 2004 Jul–Aug;21(4):265–75.
70. Lecrubier Y et al. Am J Psychiatry. 2002 Aug;159(8):1361–6.
71. Bhopal JS. Can J Psychiatry. 2001 Jun;46(5):456–7.
72. Holsboer-Trachsler E, Vanoni C. Schweiz Rundsch Med Prax. 1999 Sep 9;88(37):1475–80.
73. Schmidt U, Sommer H. Fortschr Med. 1993 Jul 10;111(19): 339–42.
74. Linde K, Knuppel L. Phytomedicine. 2005 Jan;12(1–2): 148–57.
75. Roder C et al. Fortschr Neurol Psychiatr. 2004 Jun;72(6): 330–43.
76. Gaster B, Holroyd J. Arch Intern Med. 2000 Jan 24; 160(2):152–6.
77. Linde K et al. BMJ. 1996 Aug 3;313(7052):253–8.
78. Simeon J et al. J Child Adolesc Psychopharmacol. 2005 Apr; 15(2):293–301.
79. Hubner WD, Kirste T. Phytother Res. 2001 Jun;15(4):367–70.
80. Muller D et al. Phytomedicine. 2003;10 Suppl 4:25–30.
81. Poldinger W. Schweiz Rundsch Med Prax. 2000 Dec 21; 89(51–52):2183–9.
82. Findling RL et al. J Am Acad Child Adolesc Psychiatry. 2003 Aug;42(8):908–14.
83. Volz HP. MMW Fortschr Med. 2004 Aug 19;146(33–34): 27–8, 30.
84. Muller T et al. Psychosom Med. 2004 Jul–Aug;66(4):538–47.
85. Volz HP et al. Psychopharmacology (Berl). 2002 Nov; 164(3):294–300.
86. Kasper S, Dienel A. Psychopharmacology (Berl). 2002 Nov; 164(3):301–8.
87. Whiskey E et al. Int Clin Psychopharmacol. 2001 Sep; 16(5):239–52.
88. Kim HL et al. J Nerv Ment Dis. 1999 Sep;187(9):532–8.
89. Gastpar M et al. Pharmacopsychiatry. 2006 Mar;39(2): 66–75.
90. Van Gurp G et al. Can Fam Physician. 2002 May;48:905–12.
91. Brenner R et al. Clin Ther. 2000 Apr;22(4):411–9.
92. Harrer G et al. J Geriatr Psychiatry Neurol. 1994 Oct; 7 Suppl 1:S24–8.
93. Behnke K et al. Adv Ther. 2002 Jan–Feb;19(1):43–52.
94. Friede M et al. Pharmacopsychiatry. 2001 Jul;34 Suppl 1: S38–41.
95. Schrader E. Int Clin Psychopharmacol. 2000 Mar;15(2):61–8.
96. Harrer G et al. Arzneimittelforschung. 1999 Apr;49(4): 289–96.
97. Woelk H. BMJ. 2000 Sep 2;321(7260):536–9.
98. Philipp M et al. BMJ. 1999 Dec 11;319(7224):1534–8.

99. Vorbach EU et al. J Geriatr Psychiatry Neurol. 1994 Oct; 7 Suppl 1:S19–23.

100. Hubner WD et al. J Geriatr Psychiatry Neurol. 1994 Oct; 7 Suppl 1:S12–4.

101. Hansgen KD et al. J Geriatr Psychiatry Neurol. 1994 Oct; 7 Suppl 1:S15–8.

102. Linde K et al. Br J Psychiatry. 2005 Feb;186:99–107.

103. Fava M et al. J Clin Psychopharmacol. 2005 Oct;25(5): 441–7.

104. Farabaugh A et al. Int Clin Psychopharmacol. 2005 Mar; 20(2):87–91.

105. Bjerkenstedt L et al. Eur Arch Psychiatry Clin Neurosci. 2005 Feb;255(1):40–7.

106. Murck H et al. Int J Neuropsychopharmacol. 2005 Jun;8(2):215–21.

107. Szegedi A et al. BMJ. 2005 Mar 5;330(7490):503.

108. Wheatley D. Pharmacopsychiatry. 1997 Sep;30 Suppl 2: 77–80.

109. Vorbach EU et al. Pharmacopsychiatry. 1997 Sep;30 Suppl 2:81–5.

110. Kobak KA et al. J Clin Psychopharmacol. 2005 Feb; 25(1):51–8.

111. Gelenberg AJ et al. J Clin Psychiatry. 2004 Aug; 65(8):1114–9.

112. Hypericum Depression Trial Study Group. JAMA. 2002 Apr 10;287(14):1807–14.

113. Shelton RC et al. JAMA. 2001 Apr 18;285(15):1978–86.

114. Linde K, Mulrow CD. Cochrane Database Syst Rev. 2000;(2):CD000448.

115. Werneke U et al. J Clin Psychiatry. 2004 May;65(5):611–7.

116. Williams JW Jr et al. Ann Intern Med. 2000 May 2;132(9): 743–56.

117. Wolsko PM et al. Am J Med. 2005 Oct;118(1):1087–93.

118. Linde K et al. Cochrane Database Syst Rev. 2005 Apr 18;(2):CD000448.

119. Vitiello B et al. J Clin Psychopharmacol. 2005 Jun; 25(3):243–9.

120. Kieser M, Szegedi A. Pharmacopsychiatry. 2005 Sep;38(5):194–200.

121. Czekalla J et al. Pharmacopsychiatry. 1997 Sep;30 Suppl 2:86–8.

122. Schellenberg R et al. Pharmacopsychiatry. 1998 Jun;31 Suppl 1:44–53.

123. Uebelhack R et al. Obstet Gynecol. 2006 Feb;107(2 Pt 1): 247–55.

124. Grube B et al. Adv Ther. 1999 Jul–Aug;16(4):177–86.

125. Stevinson C, Ernst E. BJOG. 2000 Jul;107(7):870–6.

126. Huang KL, Tsai SJ. Int J Psychiatry Med. 2003;33(3): 295–7.

127. Hicks SM et al. J Altern Complement Med. 2004 Dec;10(6):925–32.

128. Taylor LH, Kobak KA. J Clin Psychiatry. 2000 Aug; 61(8):575–8.

129. Kobak KA et al. Int Clin Psychopharmacol. 2005 Nov;20(6):299–304.

130. Murck H et al. Biol Psychiatry. 2006 Mar 1;59(5):440–5.

131. Martinez B et al. J Geriatr Psychiatry Neurol. 1994 Oct; 7 Suppl 1:S29–33.

132. Holsboer-Trachsler E. Schweiz Rundsch Med Prax. 2000 Dec 21;89(51–52):2178–82.

133. Sharpley AL et al. Psychopharmacology (Berl). 1998 Oct;139(3):286–7.

134. Krylov AA, Ibatov AN. Lik Sprava. 1993 Feb–Mar; (2–3):146–8.

135. Sarrell EM et al. Arch Pediatr Adolesc Med. 2001 Jul; 155(7):796–9.

136. Siepmann M et al. Br J Clin Pharmacol. 2002 Sep; 54(3):277–82.

137. Johnson D et al. J Geriatr Psychiatry Neurol. 1994 Oct;7 Suppl 1:S44–6.

138. Dimpfel W et al. Eur J Med Res. 1999 Aug 25;4(8):303–12.

139. Sindrup SH et al. Pain. 2001 Apr;91(3):361–5.

140. Barnes J et al. Planta Med. 2006 Mar;72(4):378–82.

141. Elllis KA et al. Behav Pharmacol. 2001 Jun;12(3):173–82.

142. Stavropoulos NE et al. J Photochem Photobiol B. 2006 Jul;3;84(1):64–9.

143. Skalkos D et al. Planta Med. 2005 Nov;71(11):1030–5.

144. Martarelli D et al. Cancer Lett. 2004 Jul 8;210(1):27–33.

145. Kapsokalyvas D et al. J Photochem Photobiol B. 2005 Sep 1; 80(3):208–16.

146. Roscetti G et al. Phytother Res. 2004 Jan;18(1):66–72.

147. Hostanska K et al. Pharmazie. 2002 May;57(5):323–31.

148. Vukovic-Gacic B, Simic D. Basic Life Sci. 1993;61:269–77.

149. Schempp CM et al. Oncogene. 2002 Feb 14;21(8):1242–50.

150. Dona M et al. Cancer Res. 2004 Sep 1;64(17):6225–32.

151. Quiney C et al. Leukaemia. 2006 Mar;20(3):491–7.

152. Matinez-Poveda B et al. Int J Cancer. 2005 Dec 10;117(5): 775–80.

153. Couldwell WT et al. Neurosurgery. 1994;35:705–10.

154. Schwarz D et al. Cancer Res. 2003 Nov 15;63(22):8062–8.

155. Chaudhary A, Willett KL. Toxicology. 2006 Jan 16;217(2–3): 194–205.

156. Hostanska K et al. J Pharm Pharmacol. 2003 Jul;55(7): 973–80.

157. Hostanska K et al. Eur J Pharm Biopharm. 2003 Jul;56(1): 121–32.

158. Kliewer SA. J Nutr. 2003 Jul;133(7 Suppl):2444–75.

159. Kliewer SA, Willson TM. J Lipid Res. 2002 Mar;43(3): 359–64.

160. Exarchou V et al. J Chromatogr A. 2006 Apr 21;1112(1–2): 293–302.

161. Herold A et al. Roum Arch Microbiol Immunol. 2003 Jul–Dec;62(3–4):217–27.

162. Conforti F et al. Nat Prod Res. 2005 Apr;19(3):295–303.

163. Hunt EJ et al. Life Sci. 2001 Jun 1;69(2):181–90.

164. Heilmann J et al. Planta Med. 2003 Mar;69(3):202–6.

165. Zou Y et al. J Agric Food Chem. 2004 Aug 1;52(16):5032–9.

166. Trommer H, Neubert RH. J Pharm Pharm Sci. 2005 Sep 15;8(3):494–506.

167. Albert D et al. Biochem Pharmacol. 2002 Dec 15;64(12): 1767–75.

168. Gobbi M et al. Planta Med. 2004 Jul;70(7):680–2.

169. de Prati AC et al. Curr Med Chem. 2005;12(16):1819–28.

170. Tedeschi E et al. J Pharmacol Exp Ther. 2003 Oct;307(1): 254–61.

171. Schempp CM et al. Br J Dermatol. 2000 May;142(5): 979–84.

172. Zhou C et al. J Clin Immunol. 2004 Nov;24(6):623–36.

173. Schempp CM et al. Phytomedicine. 2003;10 Suppl 4:31–7.

174. Darbinian-Sarkissian N et al. Gene Ther. 2006 Feb;13(4): 288–95.

175. Taher MM et al. IUBMB Life. 2002 Dec;54(6):357–64.

176. Avato P et al. Phytother Res. 2004 Mar;18(3):230–2.

177. Molochko VA et al. Vestn Dermatol Venerol. 1990;(8):54–6.

178. Reichling J et al. Pharmacopsychiatry. 2001 Jul;34 Suppl 1: S116–8.
179. Kolesnikova AG. Zh Mikrobiol Epidemiol Immunobiol. 1986 Mar;(3):75–8.
180. Barbagallo C, Chisari G. Fitoterapia. 1987;58(3):175–7.
181. Jacobson JM et al. Antimicrob Agents Chemother. 2001 Feb;45(2):517–24.
182. Gulick RM et al. Ann Intern Med. 1999 Mar 16;130(6): 510–4.
183. James JS. AIDS Treatment News. 1989 Feb;24:74.
184. Skalkos D et al. J Photochem Photobiol B. 2006 Feb 1; 82(2):146–51.
185. Kopleman SH et al. AAPS Pharm Sci. 2001;3(4):E26.
186. Sloley BD et al. Acta Pharmacol Sin. 2000 Dec;21(12): 1145–52.
187. Baillie N. Modern Phytotherapist. 1997;3(2):24–26.
188. Poutaraoud A et al. Phytochem Anal. 2001 Nov–Dec;12(6):355–62.
189. Ang CY et al. J Agric Food Chem. 2004 Oct 6;52(20): 6156–64.
190. Pellati F et al. J Chromatogr A. 2005 Sep 23;1088(1–2): 205–17.
191. Draves AH, Walker SE. Can J Clin Pharmacol. 2003 Fall; 10(3):114–8.
192. Bergonzi MC et al. Drug Dev Ind Pharm. 2001 Jul; 27(6):491–7.
193. Shah AK et al. Drug Dev Ind Pharm. 2005 Oct; 31(9):907–16.
194. De Jager LS et al. JAOAC Intl. 2004 Sep–Oct;87(5):1042–8.
195. Agrosi M et al. Phytomedicine. 2000 Dec;7(6):455–62.
196. Maisenbacher P, Kovar KA. Planta Med. 1992 Aug;58(4): 351–4.
197. Schulz HU et al. Arzneimittelforschung. 2005;55(10): 561–8.
198. Riedel KD et al. J Chromatogr B Analyt Technol Biomed Life Sci. 2004 Dec 25;813(1–2):27–33.
199. Staffeldt B et al. J Geriatr Psychiatry Neurol. 1994 Oct; 7 Suppl 1:S47–53.
200. Biber A et al. Pharmacopsychiatry. 1998 Jun;31 Suppl 1: 36–43.
201. Schempp CM et al. Photoderm Photoimmunol Photomed. 2000 Jun;16(3):125–8.
202. Gastpar M et al. Pharmacopsychiatry. 2005 Mar;38(2): 78–86.
203. Trautmann-Sponsel RD, Dienel A. J Affect Disord. 2004 Oct 15;82(2):303–7.
204. Bilia AR et al. Life Sci. 2002 May 17;70(26):3077–96.
205. Lenoir S et al. Phytomedicine. 1999 Jul;6(3):141–6.
206. Siepmann M et al. J Clin Psychopharmacol. 2004 Feb; 24(1):79–82.
207. Timoshanko A et al. Behav Pharmacol. 2001 Dec; 12(8):635–40.
208. Schulz V. Phytomedicine. 2001 Mar;8(2):152–60.
209. Ernst E et al. Eur J Clin Pharmacol. 1998 Oct;54(8):589–94.
210. Woelk H et al. J Geriatr Psychiatry Neurol. 1994 Oct;7 Suppl 1:S34–8.
211. Rodriguez-Landa JF, Contreras CM. Phytomedicine. 2003 Nov;10(8):688–99.
212. No authors listed. Int J Toxicol. 2001;20 Suppl 2:31–9.
213. Schempp CM et al. Phytother Res. 2003 Feb;17(2):141–6.
214. Brockmoller J et al. Pharmacopsychiatry. 1997 Sep; 30 Suppl 2:94–101.
215. Bernd A et al. Photochem Photobiol. 1999 Feb;69(2): 218–21.
216. Schempp CM et al. Hautarzt. 2002 May;53(5):316–21.
217. Beattie PE et al. Br J Dermatol. 2005 Dec;153(6):1187–91.
218. Taroni P et al. Photochem Photobiol. 2005 May–Jun; 81(3):524–8.
219. He YY et al. Photochem Photobiol. 2004 Nov–Dec;80(3): 444–9.
220. Capasso R et al. J Urol. 2005 Jun;173(6):2194–7.
221. Fahmi M et al. World J Biol Psychiatry. 2002 Jan;3(1): 58–9.
222. Guzelcan Y et al. Ned Tijdschr Geneeskd. 2001 Oct 6;145(40):1943–5.
223. Barbenel DLM et al. J Psychopharmacol. 2000 Mar;14(1): 84–6.
224. Nierenberg AA et al. Biol Psychiatry. 1999 Dec 15;46(12): 1707–8.
225. Stevinson C, Ernst E. Int J Clin Pharmacol Ther. 2004 Sep; 42(9):473–80.
226. Spinella M, Eaton LA. Brain Inj. 2002 Apr;16(4):359–67.
227. Demiroglu YZ et al. Acta Medica (Hradec Kralove). 2005; 48(2):91–4.
228. Nanayakkara PW et al. Ned Tijcschr Geneeskd. 2005 Jun 11;149(24):1347–9.
229. Andelic S. Vojnosasnit Pregl. 2003 May–Jun;60(3):361–4.
230. Cotterill JA. J Cosmet Laser Ther. 2001 Sep;3(3):159–60.
231. Golsch S et al. Hautarzt. 1997 Apr;48(4):248–52.
232. Lantz MS et al. J Geriatr Psychiatry Neurol. 1999 Spring; 12(1):7–10.
233. Ferko N, Levine MA. Pharmacotherapy. 2001 Dec;21(12): 1574–8.
234. Borges LV et al. Phytother Res. 2005 Oct;19(10):885–7.
235. Traynor NJ et al. Toxicol Lett. 2005 Sep 15;158(3):220–4.
236. Okpanyi SN et al. Arzneimittelforschung. 1990 Aug; 40(8):851–5.
237. Tschudin S, Lapaire O. Ther Umsch. 2005 Jan;62(1):17–22.
238. Lee A et al. J Clin Psychiatry. 2003 Aug;64(8):966–8.
239. Klier CM et al. Pharmacopsychiatry. 2002 Jan;35(1):29–30.
240. Weber CC et al. Pharmacopsychiatry. 2004 Nov;37(6): 292–8.
241. Wenk M et al. Br J Clin Pharmacol. 2004 Apr;57(4):495–9.
242. Mueller SC et al. Eur J Clin Pharmacol. 2006 Jan;62(1): 29–36.
243. Gurley BJ et al. Drugs Aging. 2005;22(6):525–39.
244. Wang Z et al. Clin Pharmacol Ther. 2001 Oct;70(4):317–26.
245. Karyekar CS et al. J Postgrad Med. 2002 Apr–Jun;48(2): 97–100.
246. Komoroski BJ et al. Drug Metab Dispos. 2004 May;32(5): 512–8.
247. Wang LS et al. J Clin Pharmacol. 2004 Jun;44(6):577–81.
248. Obach RS. J Pharmacol Exp Ther. 2000 Jul;294(1):88–95.
249. Krusekopf S, Roots I. Pharmacogenet Genomics. 2005 Nov; 15(11):817–29.
250. Perloff MD et al. Pharm Res. 2003 Aug;20(8):1177–83.
251. Zhou S et al. Drug Metab Rev. 2004 Feb;36(1):57–104.
252. Madabushi R et al. Eur J Pharmacol. 2006 Mar;62(3): 225–33.
253. Pal D, Mitra AK. Life Sci. 2006 Mar 27;78(18):2131–45.
254. Groning R et al. Eur J Pharm Biopharm. 2003 Sep;56(2): 231–6.
255. Dasgupta A et al. J Clin Lab Anal. 2006;20(2):62–7.

256. Komoroski BJ et al. Clin Cancer Res. 2005 Oct 1;11(19 Pt 1): 6972–9.
257. Wada A et al. Drug Metab Pharmcokinet. 2002;17(5): 467–74.
258. Peebles KA et al. Biochem Pharmacol. 2001 Oct 15; 62(8):1059–70.
259. Mills E et al. Ther Drug Monit. 2005 Oct;27(5):549–57.
260. Busti AJ et al. Pharmacotherapy. 2004 Dec;24(12):1732–47.
261. Zhou S et al. Drug Metab Drug Interact. 2004;20(3): 143–58.
262. Wolbold R et al. Hepatology. 2003 Oct;38(4):978–88.
263. Venkataramanan R et al. Life Sci. 2006 Mar 27;78(18): 2105–15.
264. Donovan JL et al. Phytother Res. 2005 Oct;19(10):901–6.
265. Mills E et al. BMJ. 2004 Jul 3;329(7456):27–30.
266. Arold G et al. Planta Med. 2005 Apr;71(4):331–7.
267. Burstein AH et al. Clin Pharmacol Ther. 2000 Dec; 68(6):605–12.
268. Rengelshausen J et al. Clin Pharmacol Ther. 2005 Jul;78(1):25–33.
269. Smith P et al. Pharmacotherapy. 2004 Nov;24(11):1508–14.
270. Frye RF et al. Clin Pharmacol Ther. 2004 Oct;76(4):323–9.
271. Mathijssen RH et al. J Natl Cancer Inst. 2002;Aug 21; 94(16):1247–9.
272. Mueller SC et al. Clin Pharmacol Ther. 2004 Jun;75(6): 546–57.
273. Johne A et al. Clin Pharmacol Ther. 1999 Oct;66(4):338–45.
274. Jiang X et al. Br J Clin Pharmacol. 2004 May;57(5):592–9.
275. Izzo AA et al. Int J Cardiol. 2005 Jan;98(1):1–14.
276. Sugimoto K et al. Clin Pharmacol Ther. 2001 Dec;70(6): 518–24.
277. Tannergren C et al. Clin Pharmacol Ther. 2004 Apr;75(4): 298–309.
278. Wang LS et al. Clin Pharmacol Ther. 2004 Mar;75(3): 191–7.
279. Hu Z et al. Drugs. 2005;65(9):1239–82.
280. Zhou S et al. J Psychopharmacol. 2004 Jun;18(2):262–76.
281. Murphy PA et al. Contraception. 2005 Jun;71(6):402–8.
282. Hall SD et al. Clin Pharmacol Ther. 2003 Dec;74(6):525–35.
283. Pfrunder A et al. Br J Clin Pharmacol. 2003 Dec;56(6): 683–90.
284. Schwarz UI et al. Br J Clin Pharmacol. 2003 Jan;55(1): 112–3.
285. Bauer S et al. Br J Clin Pharmacol. 2003 Feb;55(2):203–11.
286. Turton-Weeks SM et al. Prog Transplant. 2001 Jun;11(2): 116–20.
287. Beer AM, Ostermann T. Med Klin (Munich). 2001 Aug 15;96(8):480–3.
288. Karliova M et al. J Hepatol. 2000 Nov;33(5):853–5.
289. Mai I et al. Clin Pharmacol Ther. 2004 Oct;76(4):330–40.
290. Hebert MF et al. J Clin Pharmacol. 2004 Jan;44(1):89–94.
291. Mai I et al. Nephrol Dial Transplant. 2003 Apr;18(4): 819–22.
292. Johne A et al. J Clin Psycopharmacol. 2002 Feb;22(1): 46–54.
293. Kawaguchi A et al. Br J Clin Pharmacol. 2004 Oct;58(4): 403–10.
294. Eich-Hochli D et al. Pharmacopsychiatry. 2003 Jan;36(1): 35–7.
295. Markowitz JS et al. JAMA. 2003 Sep 17;290(11):1500–4.
296. Markowitz JS et al. Life Sci. 2000 Jan;21:66(9):PL133–9.
297. Morimoto T et al. J Clin Pharmacol. 2004 Jan;44(1): 95–101.
298. Dresser GK et al. Clin Pharmacol Ther. 2003 Jan;73(1): 41–50.
299. Wang Z et al. Clin Pharmacol Ther. 2002 Jun;71(6): 414–20.

Cupressaceae

1. Dr Duke's Phytochemical and Ethnobotanical Databases. http://www.ars-grin.gov/duke/.
2. Pepeljnjak S et al. Acta Pharm. 2005 Dec;55(4):417–22.
3. Cosentino S et al. J Food Prot. 2003 Jul;66(7):1288–91.
4. Barjaktarovic B et al. J Agric Food Chem. 2005 Apr 6; 53(7):2630–6.
5. Martin AM et al. Phytochem Anal. 2006 Jan–Feb;17(1):32–5.
6. Angioni A et al. J Agric Food Chem. 2003 May 7;51(10): 3073–8.
7. Chatzopoulou P et al. Planta Med. 2002 Sep;68(9):827–31.
8. Pashalina S et al. Pharm Acta Helv. 1995 Sep;70(3):247–53.
9. Martindale, The Extra Pharmacopoeia 26th Ed. Pharmaceutical Press London March 1973 p. 1242.
10. Gavini E et al. Pharm Dev Technol. 2005;10(4):479–87.
11. Mahady GB et al. Phytother Res. 2005 Nov;19(11):988–91.
12. Jimenez-Arellanes A et al. Phytother Res. 2003 Sep;17(8): 903–8.
13. Filipowicz N et al. Phytother Res. 2003 Mar;17(3):227–31.
14. Van der Weijden GA et al. J Clin Periodontol. 1998 May; 25(5):399–403.
15. Schneider I et al. Planta Med. 2004 May;70(5):471–4.
16. Tunon H et al. J Ethnopharmacol. 1995 Oct;48(2):61–76.
17. Na HJ et al. Clin Chim Acta. 2001 Dec;314(1–2):215–20.
18. Hart PH et al. Inflamm Res. 2000 Nov;49(11):619–26.
19. Schilcher H, Leuschner F. Arzneimittelforshung. 1997 Jul; 47(7):855–8.
20. Argentino A et al. Ann Ital Med Int. 2000 Apr–Jun;15(2): 139–43.
21. Larson DW. Exp Gerontol. 2001 Apr;36(4–6):651–73.
22. Naser B et al. Evid Based Complement Altern Med. 2005 Mar;2(1):69–87.
23. Chang LC et al. J Nat Prod. 2000 Sep;63(9):1235–8.
24. Kawai S et al. Phytochemistry. 1999 May;51(2):243–7.
25. Claus EP. Pharmacognosy 4th Ed. Henry Kimpton. London 1961 p. 228.
26. Offergeld R et al. Leukaemia. 1992;6 Suppl 3:189S–191S.
27. Arima Y et al. J Antimicrob Chemother. 2003 Jan;51(1): 113–22.
28. Budihas SR et al. Nucleic Acids Res. 2005 Mar 1;33(4): 1249–56.
29. Naser B et al. Phytomedicine. 2005 Nov;12(10):715–22.
30. Hauke W et al. Chemotherapy. 2002;48:259–66.
31. Khan T et al. JEADV. 1998 Sep;11(2):S150.

Dioscoreaceae

1. No authors listed. Int J Toxicol. 2004;23 Suppl 2:49–54.
2. Dr Duke's Phytochemical and Ethnobotanical Databases. http://www.ars-grin.gov/duke/.

3. Sautour M et al. Biochem Sys Ecol. 2006 Jan;34(1):60–3.
4. Applezweig N. Chem Week. 1969 May 17;104:57–72.
5. Laveaga GS. Stud Hist Philos Biol Biomed Sci. 2005 Dec; 36(4):743–60.
6. Rosser A. Nurs Times. 1985 May 1–7;81(18):47.
7. Rosenberg Z et al. Clin Chim Acta. 2001 Oct;312(1–2):213–9.
8. Zava DT et al. Proc Soc Exp Biol Med. 1998 Mar;217(3): 369–78.
9. Komesaroff PA et al. Climacteric. 2001 Jun;4(2):144–50.
10. Araghiniknam M et al. Life Sci. 1996;59(11):PL147–57.
11. Wang LJ et al. Zhongguo Zhong Yao Za Zhi. 2002 Oct; 27(10):777–9.
12. Corbiere C et al. Cell Res. 2004 Jun;14(3):188–96.
13. Hou R et al. Acta Pharmacol Sin. 2004 Aug;25(8):1077–82.
14. Liagre B et al. Int J Mol Med. 2005 Dec;16(6):1095–101.
15. Liu MJ et al. Cancer Chemother Pharmacol. 2005 Jan; 55(1):79–90.
16. Leger DY et al. Int J Oncol. 2004 Sep;25(3):555–62.
17. Liu MJ et al. Biol Pharm Bull. 2004 Jul;27(7):1059–65.
18. Li J et al. Anal Sci. 2005 May;21(5):561–4.
19. Raju J et al. Cancer Epidemiol Biomarkers Prev. 2004 Aug;13(8):1392–8.
20. Moalic S et al. FEBS Lett. 2001 Oct 12;506(3):225–30.
21. Shishodia S, Aggarwal BB. Oncogene. 2006 Mar 9;25(10): 1463–73.
22. Beneytout JL et al. Biochem Biophys Res Commun. 1995 Feb 6;207(1):398–404.
23. Wang YJ et al. Planta Med. 2006 Apr;72(5):430–6.
24. Turchan-Cholewo J et al. Neurobiol Dis. 2006 Jul; 23(1):109–19.
25. Turchan J et al. Neurology. 2003 Jan 28;60(2):307–14.
26. Ondeykal JG et al. Mol Divers. 2005;9(1–3):123–9.
27. Nappez C et al. Cancer Lett. 1995 Sep 4;96(1):133–40.
28. Liagre B et al. Arthritis Res Ther. 2004 Jun;6(4):R373–83.
29. Cayen MN et al. Atherosclerosis. 1979 May;33(1):71–87.

Droseraceae

1. Vinkenborg J et al. Pharm Weekbl. 1969 Jan 17;104(3):45–9.
2. Kamarainen T et al. Phytochemistry. 2003 Jun;63(3):309–14.
3. Budzianowski J. Phytochemistry. 1996 Jul;42(4):1145–7.
4. Budzianowski J. Phytochemistry. 1997 Jan;44(1):75–7.
5. Krenn L et al. Arzneimittelforschung. 2004 54(7):402–5.
6. Martindale, The Extra Pharmacopoeia 26th Ed. Pharmaceutical Press London March 1973 p. 2012.
7. Paper DH et al. Phytother Res. 2005 Apr;19(4):323–6.
8. Ferreira DT et al. Mem Inst Oswaldo Cruz. 2004 Nov; 99(7):753–5.
9. Didry N et al. J Ethnopharmacol. 1998 Feb;60(1):91–6.
10. Wang TC, Huang TL. J Chromatogr A. 2005 Nov 11; 1094(1–2):99–104.
11. Didry N et al. Pharmazie. 1994 Sep;49(9):681–3.
12. Mossa JS et al. Phytother Res. 2004 Nov;18(11):934–7.
13. Ding Y et al. J Pharm Pharmacol. 2005 Jan;57(1):111–6.
14. Shen Z et al. Planta Med. 2003 Jul;69(7):605–9.
15. Gebre-Mariam T et al. J Ethnopharmacol. 2006 Mar 8; 104(1–2):182–7.
16. Hsu YL et al. J Pharmacol Ther Exp. 2006 Aug;318(2): 484–94.
17. Nguyen AT et al. Fitoterapia. 2004 Jul;75(5):500–4.

18. De Paiva SR et al. Mem Inst Oswaldo Cruz. 2003 Oct;98(7): 959–61.
19. Croft S et al. Ann Trop Med Parasitol. 1985;79(6):651.
20. Murali PM et al. Respir Med. 2006 Jan;100(1):39–45.

Ephedraceae

1. Martindale, The Extra Pharmacopoeia 26th Ed. Pharmaceutical Press London. March 1973 p. 12.
2. WHO Monographs on Selected Medicinal Plants—Vol 1. WHO Geneva 1999.

Equisetaceae

1. Dos Santos JG et al. Fitoterapia. 2005 Sep;76(6):508–13.
2. Dr Duke's Phytochemical and Ethnobotanical Databases. http://www.ars-grin.gov/duke/.
3. Pietta P et al. J Chromatogr A. 1991 Aug;553(16):223–31.
4. Veit M et al. Phytochemistry. 1990;29(8):2555–60.
5. Veit M et al. Phytochemistry. 1995 Mar;38(4):881–91.
6. D'Agostino M et al. Boll Soc Ital Biol Sper. 1984 Dec 30; 60(12):22415.
7. Holzhuter G et al. Anal Bioanal Chem. 2003 Jun;376(4): 512–7.
8. Peggs A, Bowen H. Phytochemistry. 1984;23(8):1788–9.
9. Radulovic N et al. Phytother Res. 2006 Jan;20(1):85–8.
10. Oh H et al. J Ethnopharmacol. 2004 Dec;95(2–3):421–4.
11. Sakurai N et al. Yakugaku Zasshi. 2003 Jul;123(7):593–8.
12. Veit M et al. Phytochemistry. 1992 Oct;31(10):3483–5.
13. Veit M et al. Phytochemistry. 1991 Jan;30(2):527–9.
14. Phillipson JD, Melville C. J Pharm Pharmacol. 1960 Aug; 12:506–8.
15. Antoniuk VO, Dubits'kyi OL. Ukr Biokhim Zh. 2002 May–Jun;74(3):109–12.
16. Nagai T et al. Food Chemistry. 2005 Jul;91(3):389–94.
17. Martindale, The Extra Pharmacopoeia 26th Ed. Pharmaceutical Press London March 1973 p. 2013.
18. Mantle D et al. J Ethnopharmacol. 2000 Sep;72(1–2):47–51.
19. Myagnar BE, Aniya Y. Phytomedicine. 2000 Jun;7(3):221–9.
20. Mekhfi H et al. J Ethnopharmacol. 2004 Oct;94(2–3):317–22.
21. Torra i Bou JE et al. Rev Enferm. 2003 Jan;26(1):54–61.
22. Graefe EU, Veit M. Phytomedicine. 1999 Oct;6(4):239–46.
23. Kolettis TM et al. Europace. 2005 May;7(3):225–6.
24. Sudan BJ. Contact Dermatitis. 1985 Sep;13(3):201–2.

Ericaceae

1. Parejo I et al. Phytochem Anal. 2001 Jun;21(3):232–4.
2. Shimizu M et al. Antimicrob Agents Chemother. 2001 Nov;45(11):3198–201.
3. Blake O et al. Br J Phytother. 1994 Summer;3(3):124–7.
4. Dombrowicz E et al. Pharmazie. 1991 Sep;46(9):680–1.
5. Jahodar L et al. Pharmazie. 1978 Aug;33(8):536–7.
6. Karikas GA et al. Planta Med. 1987;53:307–8.
7. Amarowicz R et al. Food Chemistry. 2004 Mar;84(4):551–62.
8. Martindale, The Extra Pharmacopoeia 26th Ed. Pharmaceutical Press London March 1973.

9. Kruszewski H et al. Acta Pol Pharm. 2004 Dec;61 Suppl: 18–21.

10. Ritch-Krc EM et al. J Ethnopharmacol. 1996 Jun;52(2):85–94.

11. Annuk H et al. FEMS Microbiol Lett. 1999 Mar 1;172(1): 41–5.

12. Jahodar L et al. Cesk Farm. 1985 Jun;34(5):174–8.

13. NgT B et al. Gen Pharmacol. 1996 Oct;27(7):1237–40.

14. Kedzia B et al. Med Dosw Mikrobiol. 1975;27(3):305–14.

15. WHO Monographs on Selected Medicinal Plants—Vol 2. WHO Geneva 2004 p. 342–51.

16. Larsson B et al. Curr Ther Res Clin Exp. 1993;53(4):441–3.

17. Bousova I et al. J Pharm Biomed Anal. 2005 Apr 29; 37(5):957–62.

18. Barsoom BN et al. Spectrochim Acta Part A. 2006 Jul;64(4):844–52.

19. Matsuo K et al. Yakugaku Zasshi. 1997 Dec;117(12):1028–32.

20. Matsuda H et al. Yakugaku Zasshi. 1992 Apr;112(4):276–82.

21. Schindler G et al. J Clin Pharmacol. 2002 Aug;42(8):920–7.

22. Muller L, Kasper P. Mutat Res. 1996 Aug;360(3):291–2.

23. Siegers C et al. Phytomedicine. 2003;10 Suppl 4:56–60.

24. Turi M et al. APMIS. 1997 Dec;105(12):1028–32.

25. Glockl I et al. J Chromatogr B Biomed Sci Appl. 2001 Sep 25;761(2):261–6.

26. Quintus J et al. Planta Med. 2005 Feb;71(2):147–52.

27. Wang L, Del Priore LV. Am J Ophthalmol. 2004 Jun; 137(6):1135–7.

28. Towers GHN et al. Phytochemistry. 1966 Jul;5(4):677–81.

29. Ribnicky DM et al. J Neutraceut Funct Med Foods. 2003;4(12):39–52.

30. Le Grand F et al. J Agric Food Chem. 2005 Jun 29;53(13): 5125–9.

31. Jones N et al. J Ethnopharmacol. 2000 Nov;73(1–2):191–8.

32. Chan T. Postgrad Med J. 1996 Feb;72(844):109–12.

33. Baxter AJ et al. Amer J Emerg Med. 2003 Sep;21(5):448–9.

34. Botma M et al. Int J Pediatr Otorhinolaryngol. 2001 May 11;58(3):229–32.

35. Bell AJ, Duggin G. Emerg Med (Fremantle). 2002 Jun;14(2): 188–90.

36. Cuba R. Int J Aromather. 2000 Jan;19(1–2):37–49.

37. http//www.cfsan.fda.gov/~dms/ds-ill.html.

38. Corder EH, Buckley CE. J Clin Epidemiol. 1995 Oct;48(10): 1269–75.

39. Oiso N et al. Contact Dermatitis. 2004 Jul;51(1):34–5.

40. Wright AL, Minford A. Pediatr Dermatol. 1999 Nov–Dec;16(6):463–4.

41. Zhu DX et al. J Invest Allergol Clin Immunol. 1997 May–Jun;7(3):160–8.

42. deAzevedo Pribitkin E. Sem Integr Med. 2005 Mar;3(1): 17–23.

43. Nakajima JI et al. J Biomed Biotechnol. 2004;2004(5):241–7.

44. Ichiyanagi T et al. Chem Pharm Bull (Tokyo). 2004 May;52(5):628–30.

45. Zhang Z et al. J Agric Food Chem. 2004 Feb 25;52(4):688–91.

46. Ichiyanagi T et al. Chem Pharm Bull (Tokyo). 2004 Feb;52(2):226–9.

47. Nyman NA, Kumpulainen JT. J Agric Food Chem. 2001 Sep; 49(9):4183–7.

48. Du Q et al. J Chromatogr A. 2004 Aug 6;1045(1–2):59–63.

49. Dugo P et al. J Agric Food Chem. 2001 Aug;49(8):3987–92.

50. Faria A et al. J Agric Food Chem. 2005 Aug 24;53(17): 6896–902.

51. Maatta-Riihinen KR et al. J Agric Food Chem. 2005 Nov 2;53(22):8485–91.

52. Witzell J et al. Biochem Sys Ecol. 2003 Feb;31(2):115–27.

53. Hakkinen SH, Riitta Torronen A. Food Res Int. 2000 Jul; 33(6):517–24.

54. Jaakola LA et al. Planta. 2004 Mar;218(5):721–8.

55. Jaakola LA et al. Planta Physiol. 2002 Oct;130(2):729–39.

56. Ehala S et al. J Agric Food Chem. 2005 Aug 10;53(16): 6484–90.

57. Rimando AM et al. J Agric Food Chem. 2004 Jul 28;52(15): 4713–9.

58. Lyons MM et al. J Agric Food Chem. 2003 Sep 24;51(20): 5867–70.

59. Slosse P, Hootele C. Tetrahedron. 1981;37(24):4287–94.

60. Cunio L. Aust J Med Herbalism. 1993;5(4):81–5.

61. Fraisse D et al. Ann Pharm Fr. 1996;54(6):280–3.

62. Jensen HD et al. J Agric Food Chem. 2002 Nov 6;50(23): 6871–4.

63. Kallio H et al. J Agric Food Chem. 2006 Jan 25;54(2):457–62.

64. Krasnov MS et al. Radiats Biol Radioecol. 2003 May–Jun;43(3):269–72.

65. Madhavi J et al. Plant Sci. 1998 Jan 15;131(1):95–103.

66. DeSmet PAGM et al. (Eds) Adverse Effects of Herbal Drugs II. New York: Springer-Verlag. 1993;307–14.

67. Reimann C et al. Sci Total Environ. 2001 Oct 20;278(1–3): 87–112.

68. Gallaher RN et al. J Food Comp Anal. 2006 Aug;19(Suppl 1): S53–7.

69. Cao G et al. Am J Clin Nutr. 2001 May;73(5):920–6.

70. Mazza G et al. J Agric Food Chem. 2002 Dec 18;50(26): 7731–7.

71. Viljanen K et al. J Agric Food Chem. 2004 Dec 1;52(24): 7419–24.

72. Ryzhikov MA, Ryzhikova VO. Vopr Pitan. 2006;75(2):22–6.

73. Roy S et al. Free Radic Res. 2002 Sep;36(9):1023–31.

74. Galvano F et al. J Nutr Biochem. 2004 Jan;15(1):2–11.

75. Laplaud PM et al. Fundam Clin Pharmacol. 1997; 11(1):35–40.

76. Erlund I et al. Eur J Clin Nutr. 2003 Jan;57(1):37–42.

77. Zhao C et al. J Agric Food Chem. 2004 Oct 6;52(20): 6122–8.

78. Katsube N et al. J Agric Food Chem. 2003 Jan 1;51(1): 68–75.

79. Wedge DE et al. J Med Food. 2001;4(1):49–51.

80. Bagchi D et al. Biochem (Mosc). 2004 Jan;69(1):75–80.

81. Bomser J et al. Planta Med. 1996 Jun;62(3):212–6.

82. Cooke D et al. Eur J Can. 2005 Sep;41(13):1931–40.

83. Alfieri R, Sole P. C R Seances Soc Biol Fil. 1966;160(8): 1590–3.

84. Urso G. Ann Ottamol Clin Ocul. 1967 Sep;93(9):930–8.

85. Zavarise G. Ann Ottalmol Clin Ocul. 1968 Feb;94(2): 209–13.

86. Jayle GE et al. Ann Ocul (Paris). 1965 Jun;198(6):556–62.

87. Neumann L. Klin Monatsbl Augenheilkd. 1973 Jul; 163(1):96–103.

88. Cluzel C et al. Biochem Pharmacol. 1970 Jul;19(7): 2295–302.

89. Cluzel C et al. C R Seances Soc Biol Fil. 1969;163(1): 147–50.

90. Sparrow JR et al. J Biol Chem. 2003 May 16;278(2): 18207–13.

91. Jang YP et al. Photochem Photobiol. 2005 May–Jun; 81(3):529–36.
92. Canter PH, Ernst E. Surv Ophthalmol. 2004 Jan–Feb; 49(1):38–50.
93. Muth ER et al. Altern Med Rev. 2000 Apr;5(2):164–73.
94. Scharrer A, Ober M. Klin Monatsbl Augenheilkd. 1981 May;178(5):386–9.
95. Bravetti G. Ann Ottalmol Clin Ocul. 1989;115:109.
96. Casseli L. Arch Med Int. 1985;37:29–35.
97. Boniface R, Robert AM. Klin Monatsbl Augenheilkd. 1996;209(6):368–72.
98. Chatterjee A et al. Mol Cell Biochem. 2004 Oct; 265(1–2):19–26.
99. Puupponen-Pimia R et al. Biofactors. 2005;23(4):243–51.
100. Kokoska L et al. J Ethnopharmacol. 2002 Sep;82(1):51–3.
101. Fokina GI et al. Vopr Virusol. 1991 Jan–Feb;36(1):18–21.
102. Trouillas P et al. Food Chem. 2003 Mar;3(2):149–59.
103. Uno H et al. J Ethnopharmacol. 1995 Oct;48(2):61–76.
104. Wang H et al. J Nat Prod. 1999;62(2):294–6.
105. Pulliero G et al. Fitoterapia. 1989;60:69–75.
106. Ghiringhelli C et al. Minerva Cardioangiol. 1978 Apr; 26(4):255–76.
107. Alcocer A et al. Prensa Med Mex. 1972 Sep–Oct;37(9): 390–3.
108. Coget J, Merlen JF. Phlebologie. 1968 Apr–Jun;21(2):221–8.
109. Neumann L. Munch Med Wochenschr. 1973 May 18; 115(2):952–4.
110. Sevin R, Cuendet JF. Ophthalmologica. 1966;152(2): 109–17.
111. Barzaghi N et al. Ital J Gastroenterol. 1991 Jun;23(5): 249–52.
112. Rahm D. Aesthetic Surg J. 2004 Jul–Aug;24(4):385–90A.
113. Palmer ME. Thromb Res. 2005;117(1–2):33–8.
114. Fuchikami H et al. Drug Metab Dispos. 2006 Apr;34(4): 577–82.

Euphorbiaceae

1. Dr Duke's Phytochemical and Ethnobotanical Databases. http://www.ars-grin.gov/duke/.
2. Gupta DR, Garg SK. Bull Chem Soc Jpn. 1966 Nov;39(11): 2532–4.
3. Galvez J et al. Planta Med. 1993 Aug;59(4):333–6.
4. Chen L. Zhongguo Zhong Yao Za Zhi. 1991 Jan;16(1):38–9.
5. Mors WB et al. Phytochemistry. 2000 Nov;55(6):627–42.
6. Yoshida T et al. Chem Pharm Bull. 1988;36:2940–9.
7. Wallace PA et al. Food Chemistry. 1998 Mar 31;61(3):287–91.
8. Wang YC, Huang TL. FEMS Immunol Med Microbiol. 2005 Feb 1;43(2):395–300.
9. Wiart C et al. Fitoterapia. 2004 Jan;75(1):68–73.
10. Zirihi GN et al. J Ethnopharmacol. 2005 Apr 26;98(3):281–5.
11. Cano JH. J Ethnopharmacol. 2004 Feb;90(2–3):293–316.
12. Martindale, The Extra Pharmacopoeia 26th Ed. Pharmaceutical Press London March 1973 p. 709.
13. Adamu HM et al. J Ethnopharmacol. 2005 May 13;99(1):1–4.
14. Sudhakar M et al. Fitoterapia. 2006 Jul;77(5):378–80.
15. Hamill FA et al. J Ethnopharmacol. 2003 Jan;84(1):57–78.
16. Vijaya K et al. J Ethnopharmacol. 1995 Dec 1;49(2):115–8.
17. Vijaya K, Ananthan S. J Altern Complement Med. 1997 Spring;3(1):13–20.
18. Somchit MN et al. J Trop Med Plants. 2001;2(2):179–82.
19. Tona L et al. J Ethnopharmacol. 2004 Jul;93(1):27–32.
20. Tona L et al. J Ethnopharmacol. 1999 Dec 15;68(1–3): 193–203.
21. Moundipa PF et al. Afr J Tradit Cam. 2005;2(2):113–121.
22. Tona L et al. Phytomedicine. 2000 Mar;7(1):31–8.
23. Tona L et al. Phytomedicine. 1999 Mar;6(1):59–66.
24. Duez P et al. J Ethnopharmacol. 1991 Sep;34(2–3):235–46.
25. Martin M et al. Med Trop (Mars). 1964 May–Jun;24:250–61.
26. Singh AK et al. J Ethnopharmacol. 2003 Jan;81(1):31–41.
27. Johnson PB et al. J Ethnopharmacol. 1999 Apr;65(1):63–9.
28. Tabuti JRS et al. J Ethnopharmacol. 2003 Sep;88(1):19–44.
29. Noumi E, Dibakto TW. Fitoterapia. 2000 Aug;71(4):406–12.
30. Lanhers MC et al. J Ethnopharmacol. 1990 May;29(2): 189–98.

Fabaceae

1. Martindale, The Extra Pharmacopoeia 26th Ed. Pharmaceutical Press London March 1973.
2. Plugge PC. Fres J Anal Chem. 1897 Dec;36(1):408–9.
3. Wack M et al. Planta Med. 2005 Sep;71(9):814–8.
4. Wagner H et al. Arzneimittelforschung. 1984;34(6):659–61.
5. Egert D, Beuscher N. Planta Med. 1992 Apr;58(2):163–5.
6. Wagner H et al. Arzneimittelforschung. 1985;35(7):1069–75.
7. Naser B et al. Phytomedicine. 2005 Nov 15;12(10):715–22.
8. Wustenberg P et al. Adv Ther. 1999 Jan–Feb;16(1):51–70.
9. Kohler G et al. Wien Med Wochenschr. 2002;152(15–16): 393–7.
10. Wagner H, Jurcic K. Arzneimittelforschung. 1991 Oct; 41(10):1072–6.
11. WHO Monographs on Selected Medicinal Plants—Vol 1. WHO Geneva 1999 p. 241–58.
12. Shah SA et al. J Pharm Pharmacol. 2000 Apr;52(4):445–9.
13. Sun Y et al. Se Pu. 2004 Jan;22(1):38–50.
14. Bala S et al. Phytochem Anal. 2001 Jul–Aug;12(4):277–80.
15. Sun SW, Su HT. J Pharm Biomed. 2002 Jul 31;29(5):881–94.
16. Habib AA, El-Sebakhy NA. J Nat Prod. 1980 Jul–Aug; 43(4):452–8.
17. Lemli J, Cuveele J. Pharm Acta Helv. 1967 Jan;42(1):37–40.
18. Nakajima K et al. J Pharm Pharmacol. 1985 Oct;37(10): 703–6.
19. Terreaux C et al. Planta Med. 2002 Apr;68(4):349–54.
20. Franz G. Pharmacology. 1993 Oct;47 Suppl 1:2–6.
21. Muller BM et al. Planta Med. 1989 Dec;55(6):536–9.
22. Chaubey M, Kapoor VP. Carbohydr Res. 2001 Jun 15; 332(4):439–44.
23. Goppel M, Franz G. Planta Med. 2004 May;70(5):432–6.
24. Basgel S, Erdemoglu SB. Sci Total Environ. 2006 Apr 15; 359(1–3):82–9.
25. Langmead L, Rampton DS. Aliment Pharmacol Ther. 2001 Sep;15(9):1239–52.
26. Pahor M et al. Aging (Milano). 1995 Apr;7(2):128–35.
27. Heaton K, Cripps HA. Dig Dis Sci. 1993 Jun;38(6):1004–8.
28. Ahmed S et al. Pak J Pharm Sci. 1989 Jul;2(2):37–45.
29. Lemli J. Bull Acad Natl Med. 1995 Nov;179(8):1605–1.
30. Dobbs HE et al. Farmaco [Sci]. 1975 Feb;30(2):147–58.
31. De Witte P, Lemli L. Hepatogastroenterolgy. 1990 Dec; 37(6):601–5.
32. Staumont G et al. Pharmacology. 1988;36 Suppl 1:49–56.

33. Buhmann S et al. Invest Radiol. 2005 Nov;40(11):689–94.
34. Sogni P et al. Gastroenterol Clin Biol. 1992;16(1):21–4.
35. Rogers HJ et al. Br J Clin Pharmacol. 1978 Dec;6(6):493–7.
36. Buhmann S et al. Rofo. 2005 Jan;177(1):35–40.
37. Patanwala AE et al. Pharmacotherapy. 2006 Jul;26(7):896–902.
38. Thorpe DM. Curr Pain Headache Rep. 2001 Jun;5(3):237–40.
39. Ramesh PR et al. J Pain Symptom Manage. 1998 Oct;16(4):240–4.
40. Agra Y et al. J Pain Symptom Manage. 1998 Jan;15(1):1–7.
41. Radaelli F et al. Am J Gastroenterol. 2005 Dec;100(12):2674–80.
42. Borowitz SM et al. Pediatrics. 2005 Apr;115(4):873–7.
43. Sondheimer JM, Gervaise EP. J Pediatr Gastroenterol Nutr. 1982;1(2):223–6.
44. Prather CM. Curr Gastroenterol Rep. 2004 Oct;6(5):402–4.
45. Shelton MG. S Afr Med J. 1980 Jan 19;57(3):78–80.
46. Wang M et al. Zhongguo Zhong Xi Yi Jie He Za Zhi. 1998 Sep;18(9):540–2.
47. Corman ML. Dis Colon Rectum. 1979 Apr;22(3):149–51.
48. Maddi VI. J Am Geriatr Soc. 1979 Oct;27(10):464–8.
49. Kinnunen O et al. Pharmacology. 1993 Oct;47 Suppl 1:253–5.
50. Passmore AP et al. Pharmacology. 1993 Oct;47 Suppl 1:249–52.
51. Maddi VI. J Am Geriatr Soc. 1979 Oct;27(10):464–8.
52. Ewe K et al. Pharmacology. 1993 Oct;47 Suppl 1:242–8.
53. Kinnunen O, Salokannel J. Acta Med Scand. 1987;222(5):477–9.
54. Connolly P et al. Curr Med Res Opin. 1974–1975;2(10):620–5.
55. Bossi S et al. Acta Biomed Ateneo Parmense. 1986;57(5–6):179–86.
56. Marlett JA et al. Am J Gastroenterol. 1987 Apr;82(4):333–7.
57. Lin LT et al. Phytother Res. 2002 Aug;16(5):440–4.
58. al-Dakan AA et al. Pharmacol Toxicol. 1995 Oct;77(4):288–92.
59. Sydiskis RJ et al. Antimicrob Agents Chemother. 1991 Dec;35(12):2463–6.
60. Cuellar MJ et al. Fitoterapia. 2001 Mar;72(3):221–9.
61. Lewis SJ et al. Br J Cancer. 1997;76(3):395–400.
62. Lewis S et al. Eur J Clin Nutr. 1996 Aug;50(8):565–8.
63. Van Doorne H et al. Pharm Weekbl Sci. 1988 Oct 14;10(5):217–20.
64. Beyer J et al. Ther Drug Monit. 2005 Apr;27(2):151–7.
65. Krumbiegel G, Schulz HU. Pharmacology. 1993 Oct;47 Suppl 1:120–4.
66. Pers M, Pers B. J Int Med Res. 1983;11(1):51–3.
67. Obisesan AA, Osinaike I. Niger Med J. 1978 Nov;8(6):563–70.
68. Gould SR, Williams CB. Gastrointest Endosc. 1982 Feb;28(1):6–8.
69. Miltenburger HG, Mengs U. Pharmacology. 1993 Oct;47 Suppl 1:178–86.
70. Sandnes D et al. Pharmacol Toxicol. 1992 Sep;71(3 Pt 1):165–72.
71. Brusick D, Mengs U. Environ Mol Mutagen. 1997;29(1):1–9.
72. Hagemann TM. J Hum Lact. 1998 Sep;14(3):259–62.
73. Faber P, Strenge-Hesse A. Geburtshilfe Frauenheilkd. 1989 Nov;49(11):958–62.
74. Faber P, Strenge-Hesse A. Pharmacology. 1988;36 Suppl 1:212–20.
75. Sykes NP. J Pain Symptom Manage. 1996 Jun;11(6):363–9.
76. Fenandez Seara J et al. Rev Esp Enferm Dig. 1995 Nov;87(11):785–91.
77. Perkin JM. Curr Med Res Opin. 1977;4(8):540–3.
78. Marcus SN, Heaton KW. Gut. 1986 May;27(5):550–8.
79. Vanderperren B et al. Ann Pharmacother. 2005 Jul–Aug;39(7–8):1353–7.
80. Seybold U et al. Ann Intern Med. 2004 Oct 19;141(8):650–1.
81. Sonmez A et al. Acta Gastroenterol Belg. 2005 Jul–Sep;68(3):385–7.
82. Levine D et al. Lancet. 1981 Apr 25;1(8226):919–20.
83. Malmquist J et al. Postgrad Med J. 1980 Dec;56(662):862–4.
84. Armstrong RD et al. Br Med J (Clin Res Ed). 1981 Jun 6;282(6279):1836.
85. Spiller HA et al. Ann Pharmacother. 2003 May;37(5):636–9.
86. Raimondi F et al. J Pediatr Gastroenterol Nutr. 2002 May;34(5):529–34.
87. Gorkom BA et al. Digestion. 2000;61(2):113–20.
88. Benavides SH et al. Gastrointestin Endosc. 1997 Aug;46(2):131–8.
89. Xing JH, Soffer EE. Dis Colon Rectum. 2001 Aug;44(8):1201–9.
90. Ahmed S, Gunaratnam NT. N Engl J Med. 2003 Oct 2;349(14):1349.
91. Fireman Z et al. Cancer Lett. 1989 Apr;45(1):59–64.
92. van Gorkom BA et al. Aliment Phamacol Ther. 1999;13:443–52.
93. Bronder E et al. Soz Praventivmed. 1999;44(3):117–25.
94. Joo JS et al. J Clin Gastroenterol. 1998 Jun;26(4):283–6.
95. Lewis SJ et al. Eur J Gastroenterol Hepatol. 1998 Jan;10(1):33–9.
96. Murakoshi I et al. Phytochemistry. 1986 Jan;25(2):521–4.
97. Saito K et al. Phytochemistry. 1994 May;36(2):309–11.
98. Kurihara T, Kekuchi M. J Pharm Soc Japan. 1980;100:1054–7.
99. Harborne JB. Phytochemistry. 1969 Aug;8(8):1449–565.
100. Tocher RD, Tocher CS. Phytochemistry. 1972 May;11(5):1661–7.
101. Malin-Berdel J et al. Cytometry. 1984 Mar;5(2):204–9.
102. Sundararajan R et al. BMC Complement Altern Med. 2006 Mar 16;6:8.
103. Reuter G. Phytochemistry. 1962 Apr;1(2):63–5.
104. Schreiber K et al. Arch Pharm. 1962 Apr;295/67:271–5.
105. Piers C et al. Electron J Nat Subst. 2006;1:6–11 http://ejns.univ-lyon1.fr/fichiers/233.pdf.
106. Champavier Y et al. Chem Pharm Bull (Tokyo). 2000 Feb;48(2):281–2.
107. Grover JK et al. J Ethnopharmacol. 2002 Jun;81(1):81–100.
108. Lemus I et al. Phytother Res. 1999 Mar;13(2):91–4.
109. Vuksan V, Sievenpiper JL. Nutr Metab Cardiovasc Dis. 2005 Jun;15(3):149–60.
110. Pundarikakshudu K et al. J Ethnopharmacol. 2001 Sep;77(1):111–2.
111. Atanasov AT, Tchorbanov B. J Med Food. 2002 Winter;5(4):229–34.
112. Atanasov AT, Spasov V. J Ethnopharmacol. 2000 Mar;69(3):235–40.
113. Saloniemi H et al. Proc Soc Exp Biol Med. 1995 Jan;208(1):13–7.

114. Keeler RF et al. J Environ Pathol Toxicol Oncol. 1992 Mar–Apr;11(2):11–7.

115. Witters L. J Clin Invest. 2001 Oct 15;108(8):1105–7.

116. Parturier G. Rev Med Chir Mal Foie. 1951 Dec;26(12):5–8.

117. Heiss H. Wien Med Wochenschr. 1968 Jun 15;118(24):546–8.

118. WHO Monograph on Selected Medicinal Plants—Vol 1. WHO Geneva 1999 p. 183–94.

119. Sabbioni C et al. Phytochem Anal. 2006 Jan–Feb;17(1):25–31.

120. Hayashi H et al. Biol Pharm Bull. 1998 Sep;21(9):987–9.

121. Andrisano V et al. J Pharm Biomed Anal. 1995 Apr;13(4–5):597–605.

122. Elgamal MH et al. Z Naturoforsch [C]. 1990 Sep–Oct;45(9–10):937–41.

123. Elgamal MH, El-Tawil BA. Planta Med. 1975 Mar;27(2):159–63.

124. Li JR et al. J Asian Nat Prod Res. 2005 Aug;7(4):677–80.

125. Kinoshita T et al. Chem Pharm Bull (Tokyo). 2005 Jul;53(7):847–9.

126. Rauchensteiner F et al. J Pharm Biomed Anal. 2005 Jul 15;38(4):594–600.

127. Statti GA et al. Fitoterapia. 2004 Jun;75(3–4):371–4.

128. Vaya J et al. Free Radic Biol Med. 1997;23(2):302–13.

129. Kitagawa I et al. Chem Pharm Bull (Tokyo). 1994 May;42(5):1056–62.

130. Hatano T et al. Yakugaku Zasshi. 1991 Jun;111(6):311–21.

131. Okada K et al. Chem Pharm Bull (Tokyo). 1989 Sep;73(9):2528–30.

132. Takada K et al. Chem Pharm Bull (Tokyo). 1992 Sep;40(9):2487–90.

133. Kiss T et al. Acta Pharm Hung. 1998 Sep;68(5):263–8.

134. Shimizu N et al. Chem Pharm Bull (Tokyo). 1991 Aug;39(8):2082–6.

135. Mitscher LA et al. J Nat Prod. 1980 Mar–Apr;43(2):259–69.

136. Demizu S et al. Chem Pharm Bull (Tokyo). 1988 Sep;36(9):3474–9.

137. Zayed SM et al. Zentralbl Veterinarmed A. 1964 Jul;11(5):476–82.

138. Hatano T et al. Chem Pharm Bull (Tokyo). 1989 Nov;37(11):3005–9.

139. Raggi MA et al. Boll Chim Farm. 1995 Dec;134(11):634–8.

140. Rafi MM et al. J Agric Food Chem. 2002 Feb 13;50(4):677–84.

141. Hayashi H et al. Chem Pharm Bull (Tokyo). 2003 Nov;51(11):1338–40.

142. Wang ZY, Nixon DW. Nutr Cancer. 2001;39(1):1–11.

143. Mizutani K et al. Biosci Biotechnol Biochem. 1994 Mar;58(3):554–5.

144. Palermo M et al. Clin Endocrinol (Oxf). 1996 Nov;45(5):605–11.

145. Calo LA et al. J Clin Endocrinol Metab. 2004 Apr;89(4):1973–6.

146. Kato H et al. J Clin Endocrinol Metab. 1995 Jun;80(6):1929–33.

147. Ploeger B et al. Drug Metab Rev. 2001 May;33(2):125–47.

148. Armanini D et al. J Endocrinol Invest. 1989 May;12(5):303–6.

149. Armanini D et al. Clin Endocrinol (Oxf). 1983 Nov;19(5):609–12.

150. Bader T et al. Horm Metab Res. 2002 Nov–Dec;34(11–12):752–7.

151. Armanini D et al. J Endocrinol Invest. 2003 Jul;26(7):646–50.

152. Somjen D et al. J Steroid Biochem Mol Biol. 2004 Aug;91(4–5):241–6.

153. Somjen D et al. J Steroid Biochem Mol Biol. 2004 Jul;91(3):147–55.

154. Stewart PM et al. Lancet. 1987 Oct 10;2(8563):821–4.

155. Sigurjonsdottir HA et al. J Hum Hypertens. 2001 Aug;15(8):549–52.

156. Sigurjonsdottir HA et al. Blood Press. 2006;15(3):169–72.

157. Epstein MT et al. Br Med J. 1977 Feb 19;1(6059):488–90.

158. Epstein MT et al. J Clin Endocrinol Metab. 1978 Aug;47(2):397–400.

159. Forslund T et al. J Intern Med. 1989 Feb;225(2):95–9.

160. Dawson L et al. Ned Tijdschr Geneeskd. 1998 Aug;8:142(32):1826–9.

161. Murakami T, Uchikawa T. Life Sci. 1993;53(5):PL63–8.

162. Josephs RA et al. Lancet. 2001 Nov 10;358(9293):1613–4.

163. Aramanini D et al. Steroids. 2004 Oct–Nov;69(11–12):763–6.

164. Mattarello MJ et al. Steroids. 2006 May;71(5):403–8.

165. Armanini D et al. Exp Clin Endocrinol Diabetes. 2003 Sep;111(6):341–3.

166. Armanini D et al. N Engl J Med. 1999;341(15):1158.

167. Sigurjonsdottir HA et al. Horm Res. 2006 Feb;65(2):106–10.

168. Le Moli R et al. Neth J Med. 1999 Aug;55(2):71–5.

169. Kapadia GJ et al. Pharmacol Res. 2002 Mar;45(3):213–20.

170. Hsiang CY et al. Life Sci. 2002 Feb 22;70(14):1643–56.

171. Watanabe M et al. Biol Pharm Bull. 2002 Oct;25(10):1388–90.

172. Makino T et al. Basic Clin Pharmacol Toxicol. 2006 Apr;98(4):401–5.

173. Rafi MM et al. J Agric Food Chem. 2002 Feb 13;50(4):677–84.

174. Jung JI et al. J Nutr Biochem. 2006 Oct;17(10):689–96.

175. Frazier MC et al. Proteomics. 2004 Sep;4(9):2814–21.

176. Kanazawa M et al. Eur Urol. 2003 May;43(5):580–6.

177. Fu Y et al. Biochem Biophys Res Commun. 2004 Sep 10;322(1):263–70.

178. Jackson KM et al. Cancer Lett. 2002 Apr 25;178(2):161–5.

179. Rafi MM et al. Anticancer Res. 2000 Jul–Aug;20(4):2653–8.

180. Singletary K, MacDonald C. Cancer Lett. 2000 Jul 3;155(1):47–54.

181. Hsu YL et al. Planta Med. 2005 Feb;71(2):130–4.

182. Ma J et al. Planta Med. 2001 Nov;67(8):754–7.

183. Pan MH et al. J Agric Food Chem. 2003 Jul;51(14):3977–84.

184. Ii T et al. Cancer Lett. 2004 Apr 15;207(1):27–35.

185. Oerter Klein K et al. J Clin Endocrinol Metab. 2003 Sep;88(9):4077–9.

186. Zava DT et al. Proc Soc Exp Biol Med. 1998 Mar;217(3):369–78.

187. Tamir S et al. J Steroid Biochem Mol Biol. 2001 Sep;78(3):291–8.

188. Maggiolini M et al. J Steroid Biochem Mol Biol. 2002 Nov;82(4–5):315–22.

189. Tamir S et al. Cancer Res. 2000 Oct 15;60(20):5704–9.

190. Amato P et al. Menopause. 2002 Mar–Apr;9(2):145–50.

191. Liu J et al. J Agric Food Chem. 2001 May;49(5):2472–9.

192. Zani F et al. Planta Med. 1993 Dec;59(6):502–7.

193. Kuo S et al. Mutat Res. 1992 Jun;282:93–8.

194. Shankel DM, Clarke CH. Basic Life Sci. 1990;52:457–60.

195. Tanaka M et al. J Pharmacobiodyn. 1987 Dec;10(12):685–8.
196. Ikken Y et al. J Agric Food Chem. 1999 Aug;47(8):3257–64.
197. Sheela ML et al. Int Immunopharmacol. 2006 Mar;6(3): 494–8.
198. Hundertmark S et al. J Endocrinol. 1997 Oct;155(1): 171–80.
199. Wagner H, Jurcic K. Phytomedicine. 2002 Jul;9(5):390–7.
200. Barfod L et al. Int Immunopharmacol. 2002 Mar;2(4): 545–55.
201. Shinada M et al. Proc Soc Exp Biol Med. 1986 Feb;181(2): 205–10.
202. de la Taille A et al. J Altern Complement Med. 2000 Oct;6(5):449–51.
203. Brush J et al. Phytother Res. 2006 Aug;20(8):687–95.
204. Haggag EG et al. J Herb Pharmacother. 2003;3(4):41–54.
205. Amaryan G et al. Phytomedicine. 2003 May;10(4):271–85.
206. Kim DC et al. Mol Pharmacol. 2006 Aug;70(2):493–500.
207. Christensen E et al. Am J Gastroenterol. 1978 Mar; 69(3 Pt 1):272–82.
208. Kolarski V et al. Vutr Boles. 1987;26(3):56–9.
209. Brailski KH et al. Vutr Boles. 1983;22(1):12–18.
210. Mittelstaedt A, Schwick M. Fortschr Med. 1976 Feb 19; 94(16):343–6.
211. Larkworthy W, Holgate PF. Practitioner. 1975 Dec; 215(1290):787–92.
212. Brailski KH et al. Vutr Boles. 1975;14(4):101–6.
213. Shiratori K et al. Pancreas. 1986;1(6):483–7.
214. Takeuchi T et al. J Clin Gastroenterol. 1991;13 Suppl 1: S83–7.
215. Baas EU et al. Z Gastroenterol. 1976 Apr;14(2):273–6.
216. Rees WD et al. Scand J Gastroenterol. 1979;14(5):605–7.
217. Kassir ZA. Ir Med J. 1985;78(6):153–6.
218. Crotteau CA et al. J Fam Pract. 2006 Jul;55(7):634–6.
219. Madisch A et al. Digestion. 2004;69(1):45–52.
220. Madisch A et al. Z Gastroenterol. 2001 Jul;39(7):511–7.
221. De Bartolo et al. Biomaterials. 2005 Nov;26(33):6625–34.
222. Wu YT et al. Phytother Res. 2006 Aug;20(8):640–5.
223. Chan HT et al. Toxicology. 2003 Jun 30;188(2–3):211–7.
224. Jeuken A et al. J Agric Food Chem. 2003 Aug 27;51(18): 5478–87.
225. Sokol RJ et al. J Pediatr Gastroenterol Nutr. 2006 Jul; 43 Suppl 1:S4–9.
226. Arase Y et al. Cancer. 1997;79:1494–1500.
227. van Rossum et al. J Gastroenterol Hepatol. 1999; 14:1093–99.
228. Archakov AI et al. Vopr Med Khim. 2002 Mar–Apr; 48(2):139–53.
229. Eisenberg J. Fortschr Med. 1992 Jul 30;110(21):395–8.
230. Abe Y et al. Nippon Rinsho. 1994 Jul;52(7):1817–22.
231. Acharya SK et al. Indian J Med Res. 1993 Apr;98:69–74.
232. Coon JT, Ernst E. J Hepatol. 2004 Mar;40(3):491–500.
233. Da Nagao Y et al. J Gastroenterol. 1996 Oct;31(5):691–5.
234. Krausse R et al. J Antimicrob Chemother. 2004 Jul;54(1): 243–6.
235. O'Mahony R et al. World J Gastroenterol. 2005 Dec 21; 11(47):7499–507.
236. Fukai T et al. Life Sci. 2002 Aug 9;71(12):1449–63.
237. Hwang JK et al. Fitoterapia. 2004 Sep;75(6):596–8.
238. Nam C et al. Skin Pharmacol Appl Skin Physiol. 2003 Mar–Apr;16(2):84–90.
239. Hatano T et al. Phytochemistry. 2005 Sep;66(17):2047–55.
240. Fukai T et al. Fitoterapia. 2002 Oct;73(6):536–9.
241. Hatano T et al. Chem Pharm Bull (Tokyo). 2000 Sep;48(9): 1286–92.
242. Motsei ML et al. J Ethnopharmacol. 2003 Jun;86(2–3): 235–41.
243. Lin JC. Antiviral Res. 2003 Jun;59(1):41–7.
244. Pompei R et al. Nature. 1979 Oct 25;281(5733):689–90.
245. Cinatl J et al. Lancet. 2003 Jun 14;361(9374):2045–6.
246. Sasaki H et al. Pathobiology. 2002–2003;70(4):229–36.
247. De Clerq E. Med Res Rev. 2000 Sep;20(5):323–49.
248. Curreli F et al. J Clin Invest. 2005 Mar;115(3):642–52.
249. Sato H et al. Antiviral Res. 1996 May;30(2–3):171–7.
250. Takahara T et al. J Hepatol. 1994 Oct;21(4):601–9.
251. Badam L. J Commun Dis. 1997 Jun;29(2):91–9.
252. Friis-Moller A et al. Planta Med. 2002 May;68(5):416–9.
253. Chen M et al. Antimicrob Agents Chemother. 1993 Dec;37(12):2550–6.
254. Segal R et al. J Pharm Sci. 1985 Jan;74(1):79–81.
255. Edgar WM. J Dent Res. 1978 Jan;57(1):59–64.
256. Soderling E et al. Clin Oral Investig. 2006 Jun;10(2): 108–13.
257. Goultschin J et al. J Clin Periodontol. 1991 Mar;18(3): 210–2.
258. Steinberg D et al. Isr J Dent Sci. 1989 Oct;2(3):153–7.
259. Herold A et al. Roum Arch Microbiol Immunol. 2003 Jul–Dec;62(3–4):217–27.
260. Naik GH et al. Phytochemistry. 2003 May;63(1):97–104.
261. Okada K et al. Chem Pharm Bull (Tokyo). 1989 Sep;37(9): 2528–30.
262. Haraguchi H et al. J Pharm Pharmacol. 2000 Feb;52(2): 219–23.
263. Belinsky PA et al. Free Radic Biol Med. 1998 Jun;24(9): 1419–29.
264. Belinsky PA et al. Atherosclerosis. 1998 Mar;137(1):49–61.
265. Vaya J et al. Free Radic Biol Med. 1997;23(2):302–13.
266. Fiore C et al. Biochim Biophys Acta. 2004 Oct;1658(3): 195–201.
267. Fuhrman B et al. Am J Clin Nutr. 1997 Aug;66(2):267–75.
268. Fuhrman B et al. Nutrition. 2002 Mar;18(3):268–73.
269. Herold A et al. Roum Arch Microbiol Immunol. 2003 Jan–Jun;62(1–2):117–29.
270. Sajid TM et al. Pak J Pharm Sci. 1991 Jul;4(2):145–52.
271. Tokiwa T et al. Biol Pharm Bull. 2004 Oct;27(10):1691–3.
272. Tawata M et al. Eur J Pharmacol. 1992 Feb 25;212(1): 87–92.
273. Kang O et al. Int J Mol Med. 2005 Jun;15(6):981–5.
274. Kawakami F et al. J Biochem (Tokyo). 2003 Feb;133(2): 231–7.
275. Fujisawa Y et al. Microbiol Immunol. 2000;44(9):799–804.
276. Kroes BH et al. Immunology. 1997 Jan;90(1):115–20.
277. Taniguchi C et al. Planta Med. 2000 Oct;66(7):607–11.
278. Di Mambro VM, Fonseca MJ. J Pharm Biomed Anal. 2005 Feb 23;37(2):287–95.
279. Rossi T et al. In Vivo. 2005 Jan–Feb;19(1):319–22.
280. Nerya O et al. J Agric Food Chem. 2003 Feb 26;51(5): 1201–7.
281. Khanom F et al. Biosci Biotechnol Biochem. 2000 Sep;64(9):1967–9.
282. Halder RM, Richards GM. Skin Therapy Lett. 2004 Jun–Jul;9(6):1–3.
283. Morteza-Semnani K et al. J Cosmet Sci. 2003 Nov–Dec; 54(6):551–8.
284. Armanini D et al. Steroids. 2005 Jul;70(8):538–42.

285. Saeedi M et al. J Dermatolog Treat. 2003 Sep;14(3):153–7.
286. Das SK et al. J Assoc Physicians India. 1989 Oct;37(10):647.
287. Hatano T et al. Yakugaku Zasshi. 1991 Jun;111(6):311–21.
288. Ofir R et al. J Mol Neurosci. 2003 Apr;20(2):135–40.
289. Imagawa M et al. Jpn Heart J. 1982 Mar;23(2):201–9.
290. Datla R et al. Indian J Physiol Pharmacol. 1981 Jan–Mar; 25(1):59–63.
291. van Gelderen CE et al. Hum Exp Toxicol. 2000 Aug; 19(8):434–9.
292. Cantelli-Forti G et al. Environ Health Perspect. 1994 Nov;102 Suppl 9:65–8.
293. Isbrucker RA, Burdock GA. Regul Toxicol Pharmacol. 2006 Dec;46(3):167–92.
294. Ploeger B et al. Pharm Res. 2000 Dec;17(12):1516–25.
295. Krahenbuhl S et al. J Clin Endocrinol Metab. 1994 Mar;78(3):581–5.
296. Terasawa K et al. J Pharmacobiodyn. 1986 Jan;9(1):95–100.
297. Kerstens MN et al. J Intern Med. 1999 Dec;246(6):539–47.
298. Asano T et al. J Ethnopharmacol. 2003 Dec;89(2–3):285–9.
299. Sigurjonsdottir HA et al. J Hum Hypertens. 2003 Feb;17(2):125–31.
300. Ferrari P et al. Hypertension. 2001 Dec 1;38(6):1330–6.
301. Palermo M et al. Arq Bras Endocrinol Metabol. 2004 Oct;48(5):687–96.
302. Khanna A, Kurtzman NA. J Nephrol. 2006 Mar–Apr; 19 Suppl 9:S86–96.
303. Nobata S et al. Hinyokika Kiyo. 2001 Sep;47(9):633–5.
304. Brouwers AJ, van der Meulen J. Ned Tijdschr Geneeskd. 2001 Apr 14;145(15):744–7.
305. Woywodt A et al. Postgrad Med J. 2000 Jul;76(897):426–8.
306. Doeker BM, Andler W. Horm Res. 1999;52(5):253–5.
307. Seelen MA et al. Ned Tijdschr Geneeskd. 1996 Dec 28; 140(52):2632–5.
308. Heikens J et al. Neth J Med. 1995 Nov;47(5):230–4.
309. Negro A et al. Ann Ital Med Int. 2000 Oct–Dec;15(4): 296–300.
310. Shintani S et al. Eur Neurol. 1992;32(1):44–51.
311. Janse A et al. Neth J Med. 2005 Apr;63(4):149–50.
312. Cheng CJ et al. Support Care Cancer. 2004 Nov; 12(11):810–2.
313. Ishiguchi T et al. Intern Med. 2004 Jan;43(1):59–62.
314. Yoshida S, Takayama Y. Clin Neurol Neurosurg. 2003 Sep;105(4):286–7.
315. Armanini D et al. J Endocrinol Invest. 1996 Oct;19(9): 624–9.
316. Kageyama K et al. Endocr J. 1997 Aug;44(4):631–2.
317. de Klerk GJ et al. BMJ. 1997 Mar 8;314(7082):731–2.
318. Bernardi M et al. Life Sci. 1994;55(11):863–72.
319. Firenzuoli F, Gori L. Recenti Prog Med. 2002 Sep;93(9):482–3.
320. van den Bosch AE et al. Neth J Med. 2005 Apr;63(4):146–8.
321. Sardi A et al. Ann Ital Med Int. 2002 Apr–Jun;17(2):126–9.
322. Elinav E, Chajek-Shaul T. Mayo Clin Proc. 2003 Jun;78(6): 767–8.
323. Lin SH et al. Am J Sci. 2003 Mar;325(3):153–6.
324. Hussain RM. Postgrad Med J. 2003 Feb;79(928):115–6.
325. Cumming AM et al. Postgrad Med J. 1980 Jul;56(657): 526–9.
326. Russo S et al. Am J Nephrol. 2000 Mar–Apr;20(2):145–8.
327. van der Zwan A. Clin Neurol Neurosurg. 1993 Mar;95(1): 35–7.
328. Fraunfelder FW. Am J Ophthalmol. 2004 Oct;138(4): 639–47.
329. Dobbins KR, Saul RF. J Neuroophthalmol. 2000 Mar; 20(1):38–41.
330. Bocker D, Breithardt G. Z Kardiol. 1991 Jun;80(6):389–91.
331. Eriksson JW et al. J Intern Med. 1999 Mar;245(3):307–10.
332. Cuzzolin L et al. Eur J Clin Pharmacol. 2006 Jan; 62(1):37–42.
333. Maser E et al. Chem Biol Interact. 2003 Feb 1;143–144: 435–48.
334. Strandberg TE et al. Am J Epidemiol. 2001 Jun 1;153(11): 1085–8.
335. Strandberg TE et al. Am J Epidemiol. 2002 Nov 1; 156(9):803–5.
336. Zhou S et al. Life Sci. 2004 Jan 9;74(8):935–68.
337. Tsukamoto S et al. Biol Pharm Bull. 2005 Oct;28(10):2000–2.
338. Budzinski JW et al. Phytomedicine. 2000 Jul;7(4):273–82.
339. Kent UM et al. Drug Metab Dispos. 2002 Jun;30(6):709–15.
340. Folkersen L et al. Ugeskr Laeger. 1996 Dec 16;158(51): 7420–1.
341. Harada T et al. Cardiology. 2002;98(4):218.
342. Santeusanio F et al. Minerva Med. 1982 Sep 15;73(35): 2279–86.
343. Polyakov NE et al. J Phys Chem B. 2005 Dec 29;109(51): 24526–30.
344. Marhro E et al. J Chromaogr A. 2006 Sep 1;1125(2):147–51.
345. Milauskas G et al. Food Chemistry. 2004 Apr;85(2):231–7.
346. Hirakawa T et al. Chem Pharm Bull (Tokyo). 2000 Feb;48(2): 286–7.
347. Gilania AH, Atta-ur-Rahman. J Ethnopharmacol. 2005 Apr;100(1–2):43–9.
348. Benson ME et al. Am J Vet Res. 1981 Nov;42(11):2014–5.
349. Trouillas P et al. Food Chemistry. 2003 Mar;80(3):399–407.
350. Minghetti P et al. Eur J Pharm Sci. 2000 Apr;10(2):111–7.
351. Consoli A. Minerva Cardioangiol. 2003 Aug;51(4):411–6.
352. Cataldi A et al. Minerva Cardioangiol. 2001 Apr;49(2): 159–63.
353. Vettorello G et al. Minerva Cardioangiol. 1996 Sep;44(9): 447–55.
354. Pastura G et al. Clin Ter. 1999 Nov–Dec;150(6):403–8.
355. Kinney BM. Aesthet Surg J. 1999 Sep;19(5):429–30.
356. Lis-Balchin M. Phytother Res. 1999 Nov;13(7):627–9.
357. Leporatti ML, Ivancheva S. J Ethnopharmacol. 2003 Aug; 87(2–3):123–142.
358. Felter SP et al. Food Chem Toxicol. 2006 Apr;44(4):462–75.
359. de Azevedo Pribitkin E. Sem Integr Med. 2005 Mar;3(1):17–23.
360. Marder VJ. Thromb Res. 2005;117(1–2):7–13.
361. Heck AM et al. Am J Health Syst Pharm. 2000 Jul 1; 57(13):1221–7.
362. Moriyama M et al. Tetrahedron Lett. 1990;31(46):6667–8.
363. Tahara S et al. Phytochemistry. 1993 Aug 3;34(1):303–15.
364. Labbiento L et al. Phytochemistry. 1986 May 22; 25(6):1505–6.
365. Schwarza SP et al. Tetrahedron. 1964;20(5):1317–30.
366. Redaellia C, Santaniellob E. Phytochemistry. 1984;23(12): 2976–7.
367. Falshawa CP et al. Tetrahedron. 1966;22(Suppl 7):333–48.
368. Moriyama M et al. Phytochemistry. 1993 Sep 9;34(2):545–52.
369. Pietta P, Zio C. J Chromatogr A. 1983;260:497–501.

370. Tahara S, Ibrahim RK. Phytochemistry. 1995 Mar; 38(5):1073–94.
371. Caceres A et al. J Ethnopharmacol. 1991 Mar;31(3):263–76.
372. Molina-Jimenez MF et al. Toxicol Appl Phamacol. 2005 Dec 15;209(3):214–25.
373. Sherer TB et al. J Neurosci. 2002 Aug 15;22(16):7006–15.
374. Dr Duke's Phytochemical and Ethnobotanical Databases. Agric Res Serv. Apr 2004. www.ars-grin.gov/duke.
375. Tsao R et al. J Agric Food Chem. 2006 Aug 9;54(16): 5797–5805.
376. Booth NL et al. J Altern Complement Med. 2006 Mar; 12(2):133–9.
377. Wu Q et al. J Chromatogr A. 2003 Oct 24;1016(2):195–209.
378. Han EH et al. Arch Pharm Res. 2006 Jul;29(7):570–6.
379. Peng YY, Ye JN. Fitoterapia. 2006 Feb 22;54(4):1277–82.
380. Lin LZ et al. J Agric Food Chem. 2000 Feb;48(2):354–65.
381. Sivakumaran S et al. J Agric Food Chem. 2004 Mar 24; 52(6):1581–5.
382. Booth NL et al. J Agric Food Chem. 2006 Feb 22;54(4): 1277–82.
383. Swinny EE, Ryan KG. J Agric Food Chem. 2005 Oct 19; 53(21):8273–8.
384. Sivesind E, Seguin P. J Agric Food Chem. 2005 Aug 10; 53(16):6397–402.
385. Boue SM et al. J Agric Food Chem. 2003 Apr;51(8):2193–9.
386. Overk CR et al. J Agric Food Chem. 2005 Aug 10;53(16): 6246–53.
387. Beck V et al. J Steroid Biochem Mol Biol. 2005 Apr;94(5): 499–518.
388. Beck V et al. J Steroid Biochem Mol Biol. 2003 Feb;84(2–3): 259–68.
389. Liu J et al. J Agric Food Chem. 2001 May;49(5):2472–9.
390. Lukaczer D et al. Altern Ther Health Med. 2005 Sep–Oct;11(5):60–5.
391. Atkinson C et al. Am J Clin Nutr. 2004 Feb;79(2):326–33.
392. Clifton-Bligh PB et al. Menopause. 2001 Jul–Aug;8(4): 259–65.
393. Howes JB et al. Diabetes Obes Metab. 2003 Sep;5(5): 325–32.
394. Atkinson C et al. Breast Cancer Res. 2004;6(3):R170–9.
395. Tice JA et al. JAMA. 2003 Jul 9;290(2):207–14.
396. Howes JB et al. Climacteric. 2004 Mar;7(1):70–7.
397. Simoncini T et al. Menopause. 2005 Jan–Feb;12(1):69–77.
398. Garcia-Martinez MC et al. Acta Obstet Gynecol Scand. 2003 Aug;82(8):705–10.
399. Hidalgo LA et al. Gynecol Endocrinol. 2005 Nov;21(5): 257–64.
400. Campbell MJ et al. Eur J Clin Nutr. 2004 Jan;58(1):173–9.
401. Blakesmith SJ et al. Br J Nutr. 2003 Apr;89(4):467–74.
402. Atkinson C et al. J Nutr. 2004 Jul;134(7):1759–64.
403. Nelson HD et al. JAMA. 2006 May 3;295(17):2057–71.
404. Carroll DG. Am Fam Physician. 2006 Feb 1;73(3):457–64.
405. Barentsen R. J Br Menopause Soc. 2004 Mar;10 Suppl 1:4–7.
406. Huntley AL, Ernst E. Menopause. 2003 Sep–Oct;10(5): 465–76.
407. Low Dog T. Am J Med. 2005 Dec 19;118(12 Suppl 2): 98–108.
408. Booth NL et al. Menopause. 2006 Mar–Apr;13(2):251–64.
409. Teede HJ et al. Arterioscler Thromb Vasc Biol. 2003 Jun 1; 23(6):1066–71.
410. Nestel P et al. Eur J Clin Nutr. 2004 Mar;58(3):403–8.

411. Jarred RA et al. Cancer Epidemiol Biomarkers Prev. 2002 Dec;11(12):1689–96.
412. Wende K et al. Planta Med. 2004 Oct;70(10):1003–5.
413. Roberts DW et al. J Agric Food Chem. 2004 Oct 20;52(21): 6623–32.
414. Lam AN et al. Nutr Cancer. 2004;49(1):89–93.
415. Chan HY et al. Br J Nutr. 2003 Jul;90(1):87–92.
416. Stephens FO. Med J Aust. 1997 Aug 4;167(3):138–40.
417. Georgetti SR et al. AAPS PharmSci. 2003;5(2):E20.
418. Kroyer GTH. Innov Food Sci Emerg Tech. 2004 Mar;5(1): 101–5.
419. Howes J et al. J Altern Complement Med. 2002 Apr;8(2): 135–42.
420. Heinonen SM et al. J Agric Food Chem. 2004 Nov 3;52(22): 6802–9.
421. Johnson BM et al. Chem Res Toxicol. 2001 Nov;14(11): 1546–51.
422. Piersen CE et al. Curr Med Chem. 2004 Jun;11(11): 1361–74.
423. Bodinet C, Freudenstein J. Menopause. 2004 May–Jun; 11(3):281–9.
424. Budzinski JW et al. Phytomedicine. 2000 Jul;7(4):273–82.
425. Taylor WG et al. J Agric Food Chem. 2002 Oct 9;50(21): 5994–7.
426. Yang WX et al. Zhongguo Zhong Yao Za Zhi. 2005 Sep; 30(18):1428–30.
427. Hibasami H et al. Int J Mol Med. 2003 Jan;11(1):23–6.
428. Yoshikawa M et al. Chem Pharm Bull (Tokyo). 1997 Jan; 45(1):81–7.
429. Murakami T et al. Chem Pharm Bull (Tokyo). 2000 Jul;48(7):994–1000.
430. Shang M et al. Zhongguo Zhong Yao Za Zhi. 1998 Oct; 23(10):614–6.
431. Awadalla MZ et al. Z Ernahrungswiss. 1980 Dec;19(4): 244–7.
432. Fowden L et al. Phytochemistry. 1973 Jul;12(7):1707–11.
433. Shang M et al. Zhong Yao Cai. 1998 Apr;21(4):188–90.
434. Shang MY et al. Zhongguo Zhong Yao Za Zhi. 2002 Apr;27(4):277–9.
435. Singh J et al. Plant Foods Hum Nutr. 1994 Jul;46(1):77–84.
436. Srinivasan K. Int J Food Sci Nutr. 2005 Sep;56(6):399–414.
437. Rababah TM et al. J Agric Food Chem. 2004 Aug 11;52(16): 5183–6.
438. Rosser A. Nurs Times. 1985 May 1–7;81(18):47.
439. Bajpai M et al. Int J Food Sci Nutr. 2005 Nov;56(7):473–81.
440. Madar Z. Int J Obes. 1987;11 Suppl 1:57–65.
441. Vijayakumar MV et al. Br J Pharmacol. 2005 Sep;146(1): 41–8.
442. Sauvaire Y et al. Diabetes. 1998 Feb;47(2):206–10.
443. Bhardwaj PK et al. J Assoc Physicians India. 1994 Jan; 42(1):33–5.
444. Kochhar A, Nagi M. J Med Food. 2005 Dec;8(4):545–9.
445. Madar Z et al. Eur J Clin Nutr. 1988 Jan;42(1):51–4.
446. Sharma RD et al. Nutr Res. 1996 Aug;16(8):1331–9.
447. Sharma RD. Nutr Res. 1986 Dec;12(6):1353–64.
448. Sharma RD, Raghuram TC. Nutr Res. 1990 Jul;10(7): 731–9.
449. Gupta A et al. J Assoc Physicians India. 2001 Nov;49: 1057–61.
450. Sharma RD et al. Eur J Clin Nutr. 1990 Apr;44(4):301–6.
451. Basch E et al. Altern Med Rev. 2003 Feb;8(1):20–7.
452. Grover JK et al. J Ethnopharmacol. 2002 Jun;81(1):81–100.

453. Saxena A, Vikram NK. J Altern Complement Med. 2004 Apr;10(2):223–5.
454. Ruby BC et al. Amino Acids. 2005 Feb;28(1):71–6.
455. Sowmya P, Rajyalakshmi P. Plant Foods Hum Nutr. 1999; 53(4):359–65.
456. Thompson Coon JS, Ernst E. J Fam Pract. 2003 Jun;52(6): 468–78.
457. Bordia A et al. Prostaglandins Leukot Essent Fatty Acids. 1997 May;56(5):379–84.
458. Damanik R et al. Asia Pac J Clin Nutr. 2006;15(2):267–74.
459. Betzold CM. J Midwifery Womens Health. 2004 Mar–Apr; 49(2):151–4.
460. Kaviarasan S et al. Alcohol Alcohol. 2006 May–Jun;41(3): 267–73.
461. Jung K et al. Spectrochim Acta A Mol Biomol Spectrosc. 2006 Mar 13;63(4):846–50.
462. Kaviarasan S et al. Plant Foods Hum Nutr. 2004 Fall;59(4): 143–7.
463. Langmead L et al. Aliment Pharmacol Ther. 2002 Feb; 16(2):197–205.
464. Yetim H et al. Meat Sci. 2006 Oct;74(2):354–8.
465. Shishodia S, Aggarwal BB. Oncogene. 2006 Mar 9;25(10): 1463–73.
466. Raju J et al. Cancer Epidemiol Biomarkers Prev. 2004 Aug;13(8):1392–8.
467. El-Basheir ZM, Fouad MA. J Egypt Soc Parasitol. 2002 Dec;32(3):725–36.
468. Flammang AM et al. Food Chem Toxicol. 2004 Nov; 42(11):1769–75.
469. Patil SP et al. Ann Allergy Asthma Immunol. 1997 Mar;78(3):297–300.
470. Adish AA et al. Public Health Nutr. 1999 Sep;2(3):243–5.
471. Sewell AC et al. N Engl J Med. 1999 Sep 2:341(10):769.
472. Yalcin SS et al. Pediatr Int. 1999 Feb;41(1):108–9.
473. Korman SH et al. J Paediatr Child Health. 2001 Aug; 37(4):403–4.
474. Lambert JP, Cormier J. Pharmacotherapy. 2001 Apr;21(4): 509–12.
475. Abebe W. J Clin Pharm Ther. 2002 Dec;27(6):391–401.
476. Heck AM et al. Am J Health Syst Pharm. 2000 Jul 1;57(13): 1221–7.

Fagaceae

1. Martindale, The Extra Pharmacopoeia 26th Ed. Pharmaceutical Press London March 1973 p. 266.
2. Kuliev ZA et al. Chem Nat Comp. 1997 Nov;33(6):642–52.
3. Vovk I et al. J Chromatogr A. 2003 Apr 4;991(2):267–74.
4. Vrkococa P et al. Biochem Syst Ecol. 2000 Dec 1;28(10): 933–47.
5. Dr Duke's Phytochemical and Ethnobotanical Databases. http://www.ars-grin.gov/duke/.
6. Coart E et al. Theor Appl Genet. 2002 Aug;105(2–3):431–9.
7. Masaki H et al. Biol Pharm Bull. 1995 Jan;18(1):162–6.
8. Molochko VA et al. Vestn Dermatol Venerol. 1990;(8):54–6.
9. Andrensek S et al. Int J Food Microbiol. 2004 Apr 15;92(2): 181–7.
10. Jeuken A et al. J Agric Food Chem. 2003 Aug 27;51(18): 5478–87.

11. Goun EA et al. J Ethnopharmacol. 2002 Aug;81(3):337–42.
12. Grimme H, Augustin M. Forsch Komplementarmed. 1999 Apr;6 Suppl 2:5–8.
13. Eshchar J, Friedman G. Am J Dig Dis. 1974 Sep;19(9):825–9.
14. Halkes S et al. Burns. 2002 Aug;28(5):449–53.
15. Cai K et al. Biochem Pharmacol. 2006 May 28;71(11): 1570–80.
16. Chung KT et al. Trends Food Sci Technol. 1998 Apr;9(4): 168–75.

Fumariaceae

1. Sturm S et al. J Chromatogr A. 2006 Apr 21;1112(1–2): 331–8.
2. Seger C et al. Magn Reson Chem. 2004 Oct;42(10):882–6.
3. Mardirossian ZH et al. Phytochemistry. 1983;22(3):759–61.
4. Torck M et al. Ann Pharm Fr. 1971 Dec;29(12):591–6.
5. Hentshcel C et al. Fortschr Med. 1995 Jul 10;113(19):291–2.
6. Leporatti ML et al. J Ethnopharmacol. 2003 Aug;87(2–3): 123–42.
7. Brinkhaus B et al. Scand J Gastroenterol. 2005 Aug;40(8): 936–43.

Gentianaceae

1. Dr Duke's Phytochemical and Ethnobotanical Databases. http://www.ars-grin.gov/duke/.
2. Bricout J. Phytochemistry. 1974 Dec;13(12):2819–23.
3. Kakuda R et al. Chem Pharm Bull (Tokyo). 2003 Jul;51(7): 885–7.
4. Carnat A et al. J Sci Food Agric. 2005 Mar;85(4):598–602.
5. Hayashi T, Yamagishi T. Phytochemistry. 1998;27(11): 3696–9.
6. Carpenter I et al. Phytochemistry. 1969 Oct;8(10):2013–26.
7. Evan IR et al. Acta Crystallogr Sect E Struct Rep Online. 2004 Sep;60(9):1557–9.
8. Atkinson JE et al. Tetrahedron. 1969;25(7):1507–11.
9. Pettei MJ, Hostettmann K. J Chromatogr A. 1978 Jul; 154:106.
10. Toriumi Y et al. Chem Pharm Bull (Tokyo). 2003 Jan; 51(1):89–91.
11. Martindale, The Extra Pharmacopoeia 26th Ed. Pharmaceutical Press London March 1973 p. 326.
12. Blanca G et al. Biol Conserv. 1998 Sep;85(3):269–85.
13. Glatzel H, Hackenberg K. Planta Med. 1967;15(3):223–32.
14. Mahady GB et al. Phytother Res. 2005 Nov;19(11):988–91.
15. Sluis van der WG et al. J Chromatogr A. 1983 Jan;259:522–6.
16. Suzuki O et al. Biochem Pharm. 1978;27(16):2075–8.
17. Menkovic N et al. Pharm Pharmacol Lett. 1999;9(2):74–5.
18. Morimoto I et al. Mutat Res. 1983 Feb;116(2):103–117.
19. Matsushima T et al. Mutat Res. 1985 Jun–Jul;150(1–2):141–6.
20. Zagler B et al. Wien Klin Wochenschr. 2005 Feb;117(3): 106–8.
21. Festa M et al. Minerva Anestesiol. 1996 May;62(5):195–6.
22. Garnier R et al. Ann Med Interne (Paris). 1985;136(2):125–8.

Geraniaceae

1. Dr Duke's Phytochemical and Ethnobotanical Databases. http://www.ars-grin.gov/duke/.
2. Claus EP. Pharmcognosy 4th Ed. Henry Kimpton. London 1961.

Ginkgoaceae

1. Ding S et al. Rapid Commun Mass Spectrom. 2006;20(18): 2753–60.
2. WHO Monographs on Selected Medicinal Plants—Vol 1. WHO Geneva 1999 p. 154–67.
3. Dubber MJ, Kanfer I. J Chromatogr A. 2006 Jul 28; 1122(1–2):266–74.
4. Reuter HD. Br J Phytotherapy. 1995–6 Summer;4(1):3–20.
5. Aguilar-Sanchez R et al. J Pharm Biomed Anal. 2005 Jun 15; 38(2):239–49.
6. Tang Y et al. Phytochemistry. 2001 Dec;58(8):1251–6.
7. Gray DE et al. Phytochem Anal. 2006 Jan–Feb;17(1):56–62.
8. Chi JD et al. Yao Xue Xue Bao. 1997 Aug;32(8):625–8.
9. Wang H et al. Zhongguo Zhong Yao Za Zhi. 2000 Jul; 25(7):408–10.
10. Fan Y et al. Zhongguo Zhong Yao Za Zhi. 1998 May; 23(5):267–9, 319.
11. Zhang Y et al. Zhongguo Zhong Yao Za Zhi. 2002 Apr; 27(4):254–7, 320.
12. Wang Y et al. Yao Xue Xue Bao. 2001 Aug;36(8):606–8.
13. Balz JP et al. Planta Med. 1999 Oct;65(7):620–6.
14. Ellnain-Wojtaszek M. Acta Pol Pharm. 1997 May–Jun;54(3): 229–32.
15. Zheng W, Wang SY. J Agric Food Chem. 2001;49(11): 5165–70.
16. Choi YH et al. Phytochem Anal. 2004 Sep–Oct;15(5):325–30.
17. Yang LQ et al. Yao Xue Xue Bao. 2002 Jul;37(7):555–8.
18. Chen GH et al. Hunan Yi Ke Da Xue Xue Bao. 2001 Aug 28;64(4):335–6.
19. Beek TA. J Chromatogr A. 2002 Aug 16;967(1):21–55.
20. Stefanovits-Banyai E et al. Life Sci. 2006 Feb 2;78(10): 1049–56.
21. Bilia AR. Fitoterapia. 2002 Jun;73(3):276–9.
22. Scholtyssek H et al. Chem Biol Interact. 1997 Oct 24;106(3): 183–90.
23. Huang P et al. Wie Sheng Yan Jiu. 2004 Jul;33(4):453–4.
24. Pietta P et al. J Pharm Biomed Anal. 2000 Aug 1;23(1): 223–6.
25. Lugasi A et al. Phytother Res. 1999 Mar;13(2):160–2.
26. Ellnain-Wojtaszek M et al. Fitoterapia. 2003 Feb;74(1–2):1–6.
27. Kose K, Dogan P. J Int Med Res. 1995 Jan–Feb;23(1):9–18.
28. Bedir E et al. J Agric Food Chem. 2002 May 22;50(11): 3150–5.
29. Pincemail J et al. Experientia. 1989 Aug 15;45(8):708–12.
30. Rimbach G et al. Biofactors. 2001;15(1):39–52.
31. Voss P et al. Free Radic Res. 2006 Jul;40(7):673–83.
32. Huang P et al. Zhong Yao Cai. 2004 Sep;27(9):654–6.
33. Yan LJ et al. Biochem Biophys Res Commun. 1995 Jul 17; 212(2):360–6.
34. Maitra I et al. Biochem Pharmacol. 1995 May 26;49(11): 1649–55.
35. Ergun U et al. Cell Biol Int. 2005 Aug;29(8):717–20.
36. Zhu QX et al. Skin Pharmacol Physiol. 2005 Jul–Aug;18(4): 160–9.
37. Kim SJ. J Dermatol. 2001 Apr;28(4):193–9.
38. Akiba S et al. Biochem Mol Biol Int. 1998 Dec;46(6):1243–8.
39. Barth SA et al. Biochem Pharmacol. 1991 May 15;41(10): 1521–6.
40. Di Mambro VM, Fonseca MJ. J Pharm Biomed Anal. 2005 Feb 23;37(2):287–95.
41. Sarikcioglu SB et al. Phytother Res. 2004 Oct;18(10): 837–40.
42. Kudolo GB et al. Diabetes Res Clin Pract. 2005 Apr;68(1): 29–38.
43. Kose K et al. Jpn J Pharmacol. 1997 Nov;75(3):253–8.
44. Kudolo GB et al. J Herb Pharmcother. 2003;3(4):1–15.
45. Balashova TS, Kubatiev AA. Ter Arkh. 1998;70(12):49–54.
46. Pietschmann A et al. Z Gesamte Inn Med. 1992 Nov;47(11): 518–22.
47. Mantle D et al. J Altern Complement Med. 2003 Oct;9(5): 625–9.
48. Noda Y et al. Biochem Mol Biol Int. 1997 Jun;42(1):35–44.
49. Maclennan KM et al. Prog Neurobiol. 2002 Jun;67(3): 235–57.
50. Stromgaard K et al. J Med Chem. 2002 Aug 29;45(18): 4038–46.
51. Nunez D et al. Eur J Pharmacol. 1986 Apr 16;123(2): 197–205.
52. Pincemail J et al. Experientia. 1987 Feb 15;43(2):181–4.
53. Kurihara K et al. J Allergy Clin Immunol. 1989 Jan;83(1): 83–90.
54. Simon MF et al. Thromb Res. 1987 Feb 15;43(2):181–4.
55. Lenoir M et al. Biochem Pharmacol. 2002 Apr 1;63(7): 1241–9.
56. Dutta-Roy AK et al. Platelets. 1999 Oct;10(5):298–305.
57. Grino JM. Ann Intern Med. 1994 Sep 1;121(5):345–7.
58. Wang XX et al. Yao Xue Xue Bao. 2004 Aug;39(8):656–60.
59. Chen J et al. J Cardiovasc Pharmacol. 2004 Mar;43(3): 347–52.
60. Chen JW et al. Arterioscler Thromb Vasc Biol. 2003 Sep 1;23(9): 1559–66.
61. Yang PY et al. Yao Xue Xue Bao. 2002 Feb;37(2):86–9.
62. Mao YJ et al. Yao Xue Xue Bao. 2006 Jan;41(1):36–40.
63. Arnould T et al. J Cardiovasc Pharmacol. 1998 Mar;31(3): 456–63.
64. Janssens D et al. Biochem Pharmacol. 1995;50(7):991–9.
65. Janssens D et al. Br J Pharmacol. 2000 Aug;130(7):1513–24.
66. Dell'Agli M et al. Planta Med. 2006 Apr;72(5):468–70.
67. Bochu W et al. Colloids Surf B Biointerfaces. 2005 Jul 10; 43(3–4):194–7.
68. Li Z et al. Clin Exp Pharmacol Physiol. 2001 May–Jun; 28(5–6):441–5.
69. Cheung F et al. Biochem Pharmacol. 1999 Nov 15;58(10): 1665–73.
70. Cheung F et al. Biochem Pharmacol. 2001 Feb 15;61(4): 503–10.
71. Woo CW et al. Mol Cell Biochem. 2003 Jan;243(1–2):37–47.
72. Zhu GY et al. Zhongguo Zhong Xi Yi Jie He Za Zhi. 2004 Dec;24(12):1069–72.
73. Heiss WD. Bull Schweiz Akad Med Wiss. 1980 Apr;36(1–3): 183–207.
74. Mehlsen J et al. Clin Physiol Funct Imaging. 2002 Nov;22(6):375–8.

75. Jung F et al. Arzneimittelforschung. 1990 May;40(5):589–93.
76. Santos RF et al. Pharmacopsychiatry. 2003 Jul; 36(4):127–33.
77. Witte S et al. Fortschr Med. 1992 May 10;110(13):247–50.
78. Schaffler K, Reeh PW. Arzneimittelforschung. 1985;35(8): 1283–6.
79. Kudolo GB. J Clin Pharmacol. 2000 Jun;40(6):647–54.
80. Boelsma E et al. Planta Med. 2004 Nov;70(11):1052–7.
81. Kudolo GB et al. Thromb Res. 2002 Nov 1;108(2–3): 151–60.
82. Liadov KV et al. Angiol Sosud Khir. 2005;11(4):91–8.
83. Pokrovskii AV et al. Angiol Sosud Khir. 2005;11(3):47–52.
84. Palade R et al. Chirurgia (Bucur). 1997 Jul–Aug;92(4): 249–55.
85. Sumboonnanonda K, Lertsithichai P. J Med Assoc Thai. 2004 Feb;87(2):137–42.
86. Hep A et al. Vnitr Lek. 2000 May;46(5):282–5.
87. Chen K et al. Zhongguo Zhong Xi Yi Jie He Za Zhi. 1996 Jan;16(1):24–6.
88. Li DZ et al. Chin J Integr Med. 2005 Dec;11(4):260–3.
89. Dziak LA, Golik VA. Lik Sprava. 1998 Aug;(6):125–7.
90. Deng YK et al. Zhongguo Zhong Xi Yi Jie He Za Zhi. 2006 Apr;26(4):316–8.
91. Huang SY et al. Clin Nutr. 2004 Aug;23(4):615–21.
92. Schweizer J, Hautmann C. Arzneimittelforschung. 1999 Nov;49(11):900–4.
93. Peters H et al. Vasa. 1998 May;27(2):106–10.
94. Blume J et al. Vasa. 1996;25(3):265–74.
95. Mouren X et al. Angiology. 1994 Jun;45(6):413–7.
96. Thomson GJ et al. Int Angiol. 1990 Apr–Jun;9(2):75–8.
97. Li AL et al. Zhongguo Yao Li Xue Bao. 1998 Sep;19(5): 417–21.
98. Drabaek H et al. Ugeskr Laeger. 1996 Jul 1;158(27): 3928–31.
99. Bauer U. Presse Med. 1986 Sep 25;15(31):1546–9.
100. Muir AH et al. Vasc Med. 2002;7(4):265–7.
101. Pepe C et al. Minerva Cardioangiol. 1999 Jun;47(6): 223–30.
102. Lagrue G, Behar A. J Mal Vasc. 1989;14(3):231–5.
103. Lagrue G et al. Presse Med. 1986 Sep 25;15(31):1550–3.
104. Rostoker G et al. Nephron. 2000 Jul;85(3):194–200.
105. Koltringer P et al. Fortschr Med. 1993 Apr 10;111(10): 170–2.
106. Koltringer P et al. Wien Klin Wochenschr. 1989 Mar 17; 101(6):198–200.
107. Ivaniv OP. Lik Sprava. 1998 Dec;(8):13–8.
108. Kupnovyts'ka MIu et al. Lik Sprava. 1997 Sep–Oct;(5): 142–5.
109. Eckmann F. Fortschr Med. 1990 Oct 10;108(29):557–60.
110. Gerhardt G et al. Fortschr Med. 1990 Jun 30;108(19):384–8.
111. Limanova OA et al. Eksp Klin Farmakol. 2002 Nov–Dec; 65(6):28–31.
112. Raabe A et al. Klin Monatsbl Augenheilkd. 1991 Dec;199(6): 432–8.
113. Merte HJ, Merkle W. Klin Monatsbl Augenheilkd. 1980 Nov;177(5):577–83.
114. Hopfenmuller W. Arzneimittelforschung. 1994 Sep;44(9): 1005–13.
115. Kleijnen J, Knipschild P. Br J Clin Pharmacol. 1992 Oct; 34(4):352–8.
116. Liu J. Explore (NY). 2006 May;2(3):262–3.
117. Zeng X et al. Cochrane Database Syst Rev. 2005 Oct;19(4): CD003691.
118. Roncin JP et al. Aviat Space Environ Med. 1996 May;67(5): 445–52.
119. Chow T et al. Arch Intern Med. 2005 Feb 14;165(3): 296–301.
120. Gertsch JH et al. BMJ. 2004 Apr 3;328(7443):797.
121. Gertsch JH et al. High Alt Med Biol. 2002 Spring;3(1): 29–37.
122. Jowers C et al. High Alt Med Biol. 2004 Winter;5(4):445–9.
123. Ramassamy C et al. Free Radic Biol Med. 1999 Sep;27(5–6): 544–53.
124. Smith JV, Luo Y. J Alzheimers Dis. 2003 Aug;5(4):287–300.
125. Kumar V. Phytother Res. 2006 Dec;20(12):1023–35.
126. Ramassamy C. Eur J Pharmacol. 2006 Sep 1;545(1):51–64.
127. Nitti M et al. Free Radic Biol Med. 2005 Apr 1;38(7): 846–56.
128. Zhuang H et al. Cell Mol Biol (Noisy-le-grand). 2002 Sep; 48(6):647–53.
129. Siddique MS et al. Acta Neurochir Suppl. 2000;76:87–90.
130. Gsell W et al. J Neural Transm Suppl. 1995;45:271–9.
131. Yao ZX et al. J Nutr Biochem. 2004 Dec;15(12):749–56.
132. Chromy BA et al. Biochemistry. 2003 Nov 11;42(44): 12749–60.
133. Bate C et al. J Neuroinflammation. 2004 May 11;1(1):4.
134. Lee JH et al. Planta Med. 2004 Dec;70(12):1228–30.
135. Huang SH et al. Eur J Pharmacol. 2004 Jun 28;494(2–3): 131–8.
136. Huang S et al. Eur J Pharmacol. 2003 Mar 7;464(1):1–8.
137. Ivic L et al. J Biol Chem. 2003 Dec 5;278(49):49279–85.
138. Fowler JS et al. Methods. 2002 Jul;27(3):263–77.
139. Fowler JS et al. Life Sci. 2000 Jan 21;66(9):PL141–6.
140. Kanowski S, Hoerr R. Phamacospsychiatry. 2003 Nov; 36(6):297–303.
141. Le Bars et al. Dement Geriatr Cogn Discord. 2000 Jul–Aug; 11(4):230–7.
142. Maurer K et al. J Psychiatr Res. 1997 Nov–Dec;31(6): 645–55.
143. Le Bars PL et al. JAMA. 1997 Oct 22–29;278(16):1327–32.
144. Kanowski S et al. Pharmacopsychiatry. 1996 Mar;29(2): 47–56.
145. Mazza M et al. Eur J Neurol. 2006 Sep;13(9):981–5.
146. Le Bars PL et al. Neuropsychobiology. 2002;45(1):19–26.
147. Wettstein A. Phytomedicine. 2000 Jan;6(6):393–401.
148. Itil TM et al. Psychopharmacol Bull. 1998;34(3):391–7.
149. Schreiter Gasser U, Gasser T. Fortschr Med Orig. 2001 Nov 29;119(3–4):135–8.
150. Schulz V. Phytomedicine. 2003;10 Suppl 4:74–9.
151. Itil TM et al. Am J Ther. 1996 Jan;3(1):63–73.
152. Kennedy DO et al. Pharmacol Biochem Behav. 2003 Jun; 75(3):701–9.
153. Heinen-Kammerer T et al. MMW Fortschr Med. 2005 Oct 6;147 Suppl 3:127–33.
154. Haan J, Horr R. Wien Med Wochenschr. 2004 Nov; 154(21–22):511–4.
155. Le Bars PL. Pharmacopsychiatry. 2003 Jun;36 Suppl 1: S50–61.
156. Hoerr R. Pharmacopsychiatry. 2003 Jun;36 Suppl 1: S56–61.
157. Blasko I et al. Neurobiol Aging. 2005 Aug–Sep;26(8): 1135–43.

158. Andrieu S et al. J Gerontol A Biol Sci Med Sci. 2003 Apr; 58(4):372–7.
159. DeKosky ST et al. Contemp Clin Trials. 2006 Jun;27(3): 238–53.
160. Schneider LS et al. Curr Alzheimer Res. 2005 Dec;2(5): 541–51.
161. van Dongen MC et al. J Am Geriatr Soc. 2000 Oct;48(10): 1183–94.
162. van Dongen M et al. J Clin Epidemiol. 2003 Apr;56(4): 367–76.
163. Bidzan L et al. Psychiatr Pol. 2005 May–Jun;39(3):559–66.
164. Semlitsch HV et al. Pharmacopsychiatry. 1995 Jul;28(4): 134–42.
165. Birks J et al. Cochrane Database Syst Rev. 2002;(4): CD003120.
166. Ihl R. MMW Fortschr Med. 2002 May 6;Suppl 2:24–6, 28–9.
167. Oken BS et al. Arch Neurol. 1998 Nov;55(11):1409–15.
168. Loew D. Wien Med Wochenschr. 2002;152(15–6):418–22.
169. Stoppe G et al. Pharmacopsychiatry. 1996 Jul;29(4):150–5.
170. Atmaca M et al. Psychiatry Clin Neurosci. 2005 Dec; 59(6):652–6.
171. Zhang XY et al. J Clin Psychiatry. 2001 Nov;62(11):878–83.
172. Zhou D et al. Chin Med J (Engl). 1999 Dec;112(12):1093–6.
173. Luo HC et al. Zhongguo Zhong Xi Yi Jie He Za Zhi. 1997 Mar;17(3):139–42.
174. Zhang XY et al. Psychpharmacolgy (Berl). 2006 Sep;188(1): 12–7.
175. Woelk H et al. J Psychiatry Res. 2007 Sep;41(6):472–8.
176. Johnson SK et al. Explore (NY). 2006 Jan;2(1):19–24.
177. Choung YH et al. J Laryngol Otol. 2006 Apr;120(4):343–52.
178. Cockle SM et al. Hum Psychopharmacol. 2000 Jun;15(4): 227–35.
179. Kennedy DO et al. Physiol Behav. 2002 Apr 15;75(5): 739–51.
180. Trick L et al. Phytother Res. 2004 Jul;18(7):531–7.
181. Cieza A et al. Fortschr Med Orig. 2003;121(1):5–10.
182. Cieza A et al. Arch Med Res. 2003 Sep–Oct;34(5):373–81.
183. Solomon PR et al. JAMA. 2002 Aug 21;288(7):835–40.
184. Hemmeter U et al. Pharmacopsychiatry. 2001 Mar;34(2): 50–9.
185. Holsboer-Trachsler E. Schweiz Rundsch Med Prax. 2000 Dec 21;89(51–52):2178–82.
186. Wang XM et al. Zhongguo Zhong Xi Yi Jie He Za Zhi. 2004 May;24(5):392–5.
187. Hartley DE et al. Pharmacol Biochem Behav. 2003 Jun; 75(3):711–20.
188. Burns NR et al. Hum Psychopharmacol. 2006 Jan;21(1): 27–37.
189. Subhan Z, Hindmarch I. Int J Clin Pharmacol Res. 1984;4(2): 89–93.
190. Kennedy DO et al. Nutr Neurosci. 2001;4(5):399–412.
191. Moulton PL et al. Physiol Behav. 2001 Jul;73(4):659–65.
192. Page JW et al. J Gerontol A Biol Sci Med Sci. 2005 Oct; 60(10):1246–51.
193. Karazhaeva MI et al. Vestn Oftalmol. 2004 Jul–Aug;120(4): 14–8.
194. Bernardczyk-Meller J et al. Klin Oczna. 2004;106(4–5): 569–71.
195. Lanthony P, Cosson JP. J Fr Ophthalmol. 1988;11(10): 671–4.

196. Chung HS et al. J Ocul Pharmacol Ther. 1999 Jun;15(3): 233–40.
197. Quaranta L et al. Ophthalmology. 2003 Feb;110(2):359–62.
198. Fies P, Dienel A. Wien Med Woshcenschr. 2002;152(15–16): 423–6.
199. Lebuisson DA et al. Presse Med. 1985 Sep 25;15(31): 1556–8.
200. Pal'chun VT et al. Vestn Otorinolaringol. 2005;(5):7–10.
201. Morgenstern C, Biermann E. Int J Clin Pharmacol Ther. 2002 May;40(5):188–97.
202. Meyer B. Presse Med. 1985 Sep 25;15(31):1562–4.
203. Meyer B. Ann Otolaryngol Chir Cervicofac. 1986;103(3): 185–8.
204. Holstein N. Fortschr Med Orig. 2001 Jan 11;118(4):157–64.
205. Drew S, Davies E. BMJ. 2001 Jan 13;322(7278):73.
206. Holgers KM et al. Audiology. Mar–Apr;33(2):85–92.
207. Smith PF et al. J Ethnopharmacol. 2005 Aug 22;100(1–2): 95–9.
208. Rejali D et al. Clin Otolaryngol Allied Sci. 2004 Jun;29(3): 226–31.
209. Hilton M, Stuart E. Cochrane Database Syst Rev. 2004;(2): CD003852.
210. Issing W et al. J Altern Complement Med. 2005 Feb;11(1): 155–60.
211. Parfenov VA. Ter Arkh. 2005;77(1):56–9.
212. Hamann KF. HNO. 2007 Apr;55(4):258–63.
213. Cesarani A et al. Adv Ther. 1998 Sep–Oct;15(5):291–304.
214. Haguenauer JP et al. Presse Med. 1985 Sep 25;15(31): 1569–72.
215. Claussen CF. Presse Med. 1985 Sep 25;15(31):1565–8.
216. Smith PF, Darlington CL. J Vestib Res. 1994 May–Jun; 4(3):169–79.
217. Hahn A, Stolbova K. Int Tinnitus J. 2000;6(1):54–5.
218. Orendorz-Fraczkowska K et al. Otolaryngol Pol. 2002; 56(1):83–8.
219. Burschka MA et al. Eur Arch Otorhinolaryngol. 2001 Jul; 258(5):213–9.
220. Dubreuil C. Presse Med. 1986 Sep 25;15(31):1559–61.
221. Reisser CH, Weidauer H. Acta Otolaryngol. 2001 Jul; 121(5):579–84.
222. Hoffman F et al. Layrngorhinootologie. 1994 Mar;73(3): 149–52.
223. Mix JA, Crews WD. Hum Psychopharmacol. 2002 Aug; 17(6):267–77.
224. Polich J, Gloria R. Hum Psychopharmacol. 2001 Jul;16(5): 409–16.
225. Elsabagh S et al. Psychopharmacology (Berl). 2005 May; 179(2):437–46.
226. Scholey AB, Kennedy DO. Hum Psychopharmacol. 2002 Jan;17(1):35–44.
227. Kennedy DO et al. Psychopharmacology (Berl). 2000 Sep; 151(4):416–23.
228. Rigney Y et al. Phytother Res. 1999 Aug;13(5):408–15.
229. Hindmarch I. Presse Med. 1986 Sep 25;15(31):1592–4.
230. Stough C et al. Int J Neuropsychopharmacol. 2001 Jun;4(2): 131–4.
231. Mix JA, Crews WD. J Altern Complement Med. 2000 Jun; 6(3):219–29.
232. Singh B et al. Altern Ther Health Med. 2004 Jul–Aug; 10(4):52–6.
233. Nathan PJ et al. Hum Psychopharmacol. 2002 Jan;17(1): 45–9.

234. Nathan PJ et al. Hum Psychopharmacol. 2004 Mar;19(2): 91–6.
235. Persson J et al. Psychopharmcology (Berl). 2004 Apr; 172(4):430–4.
236. Warot D et al. Therapie. 1991 Jan–Feb;46(1):33–6.
237. Allain H et al. Clin Ther. 1993 May–Jun;15(3):549–58.
238. Rai GS et al. Curr Med Res Opin. 1991;12(6):350–5.
239. Taillandier J et al. Press Med. 1986 Sep 25;15(31):1583–7.
240. Voelp A, Klasser M. Arzneimittelforschung. 1985;35(9): 1459–65.
241. Grassel E. Fortschr Med. 1992 Feb 20;110(5):73–6.
242. Hofferberth B. Arzneimittelforschung. 1989 Aug;39(8): 918–22.
243. Elsabagh S et al. J Psychopharmacol. 2005 Mar;19(2): 173–81.
244. Neznamov GC et al. Eksp Klin Farmakol. 2002 Jan–Feb; 65(1):19–23.
245. Wesnes KA et al. Psychopharmacol Bull. 1997;33(4): 677–83.
246. Krasnov VN, Vet'tishev DI. Zh Nevro Psikhiatr Im S S Korsakova. 1999;9(7):37–40.
247. Koltringer P et al. Acta Med Austriaca. 1989;16(2):35–7.
248. Lyon MR et al. J Psychiatry Neurosci. 2001 May;26(3): 221–8.
249. Shprakh VV et al. Zh Nevrol Psikhiatr Im S S Korsakova. 2000;100(3):33–5.
250. Oh SM, Chung KH. J Steroid Biochem Mol Biol. 2006 Aug; 100(4–5):167–76.
251. Oh SM, Chung KH. Life Sci. 2004 Jan 30;74(11):1325–35.
252. Pretner E et al. Anticancer Res. 2006 Jan–Feb;26(1A):9–22.
253. Chao JC, Chu CC. World J Gastroenterol. 2004 Jan;10(1): 37–41.
254. Li W et al. Cell Mol Biol (Noisy-le-grand). 2002 Sep;48(6): 655–62.
255. Papadopoulos V et al. Anticancer Res. 2000 Sep–Oct; 20(5A):2835–47.
256. Kim KS et al. Oral Oncol. 2005 Apr;41(4):383–9.
257. DeFeudis FV et al. Fundam Clin Pharmacol. 2003 Aug; 17(4):405–17.
258. Moon YJ et al. Toxicol In Vitro. 2006 Mar;20(2):187–210.
259. Chang TK et al. Toxicol Appl Pharmacol. 2006 May 15; 213(1):18–26.
260. Emerit I et al. Free Radic Biol Med. 1995 Jun;18(6):985–91.
261. Emerit I et al. Radiat Res. 1995 Nov;144(2):198–205.
262. Hauns B et al. Phytother Res. 2001 Feb;15(1):34–8.
263. Hauns B et al. Arzneimittelforschung. 1999 Dec;49(12): 1030–4.
264. Tian WX et al. Life Sci. 2004 Mar 26;74(19):2389–99.
265. Paick JS, Lee JH. J Urol. 1996 Nov;156(5):1876–80.
266. Ito TY et al. J Sex Marital Ther. 2006 Oct–Dec;32(5):369–78.
267. Ito TY et al. J Sex Marital Ther. 2001 Oct–Dec;27(5):541–9.
268. Waynberg J, Brewer S. Adv Ther. 2000 Sep–Oct;17(5): 255–62.
269. Markowitz JS et al. Pharmacotherapy. 2005 Oct;25(10): 1337–40.
270. Wheatley D. Hum Psychopharmacol. 2004 Dec;19(8): 545–8.
271. Kang BJ et al. Hum Psychopharmacol. 2002 Aug;17(6): 279–84.
272. Ellison JM, DeLuca P. J Clin Psychiatry. 1998 Apr;59(4): 199–200.
273. Cohen AJ, Bartlik B. J Sex Marital Ther. 1998 Apr–Jun; 24(2):139–43.
274. Tamborini A, Taurelle R. Rev Fr Gynecol Obstet. 1993 Jul–Sep;88(7–9):447–57.
275. Jezova D et al. J Physiol Pharmacol. 2002 Sep;53(3): 337–48.
276. Zhu HW et al. Zhongguo Zhong Xi Yi Jie He Za Zhi. 2005 Oct;25(10):889–91.
277. Lu J, He H. Chin J Integr Med. 2005 Sep;11(3):226–8.
278. Kudolo GB. J Clin Pharmacol. 2001 Jun;41(6):600–11.
279. Kudolo GB et al. Clin Nutr. 2006 Feb;25(1):123–34.
280. Boonkaew T, Camper ND. Phytomedicine. 2005 Apr; 12(4):318–23.
281. Osawa K et al. Bull Tokyo Dent Coll. 1991 Feb;32(1):1–7.
282. Lee HS, Kim MJ. J Agric Food Chem. 2002 Mar 27;50(7): 1840–4.
283. Mazzanti G et al. J Ethnopharmacol. 2000 Jul;71(1–2):83–8.
284. Atzori C et al. Antimicrob Agents Chemother. 1993 Jul; 37(7):1492–6.
285. Huang X et al. FEBS Lett. 2000 Jul 28;478(1–2):123–6.
286. Kim SJ et al. Skin Pharmacol. 1997;10(4):200–5.
287. Kudolo GB et al. J Herb Pharmacother. 2004;4(4):13–26.
288. Cheng SM et al. Biochem Pharmacol. 2003 Aug 15;66(4): 679–89.
289. He M et al. Zhongguo Zhong Xi Yi Jie He Za Zhi. 2005 Mar;25(3):222–4.
290. Li MH et al. Zhongguo Zhong Xi Yi Jie He Za Zhi. 2001 Nov;21(11):819–21.
291. Li MH et al. Zhongguo Zhong Xi Yi Jie He Za Zhi. 1997 Apr;17(4):216–8.
292. Parsad D et al. Clin Exp Dermatol. 2003 May;28(3):285–7.
293. Li W et al. Zhongguo Zhong Xi Yi Jie He Za Zhi. 1995 Oct;15(10):593–5.
294. Lister RE. J Int Med Res. 2002 Mar–Apr;30(2):195–9.
295. Hibatallah J et al. J Pharm Pharmacol. 1999 Dec;51(12): 1435–40.
296. Ihl R. Pharmacopsychiatry. 2003 Jun;36 Suppl 1:S38–43.
297. Wolsko PM et al. Am J Med. 2005 Oct;118(10):1087–93.
298. Kressmann S et al. J Pharm Pharmacol. 2002 May;54(5): 661–9.
299. Dubber MJ et al. J Pharm Biomed Anal. 2005 Apr 1;37(4): 723–31.
300. Ganzera M et al. Chem Pharm Bull (Tokyo). 2001 Sep;49(9): 1170–3.
301. Li XF et al. Analyst. 2002 May;127(5):641–6.
302. Liu C et al. Analyst. 2005 Mar;130(3):325–9.
303. Kressmann S et al. J Pharm Pharmacol. 2002 Nov;54(11): 1507–14.
304. Elosta S et al. J Sep Sci. 2006 May;29(8):1174–9.
305. Wang Y et al. J Pharm Pharmacol. 2005 Jun;57(6):751–8.
306. Wang FM et al. Eur J Drug Metab Pharmokinet. 2003 Jul–Sep;28(3):173–7.
307. Fourtillan JB et al. Therapie. 1995 Mar–Apr;50(2):137–44.
308. Drago F et al. J Ocul Pharmacol Ther. 2002 Apr;18(2): 197–202.
309. Mauri P et al. Rapid Commun Mass Spectrom. 2001; 15(12):929–34.
310. Fuzzati N et al. Fitoterapia. 2003 Apr;74(3):247–56.
311. Ndjoko K et al. J Chromtogr B Biomed Sci Appl. 2000 Jul 21;744(20):249–55.
312. Lawrence GA, Scott PM. J AOAC Int. 2005 Jan–Feb;88(1): 26–9.

313. Petty HR et al. Chem Res Toxicol. 2001 Sep;14(9):1254–8.
314. Le Bars PL, Kastelan J. Public Health Nutr. 2000 Dec; 3(4A):495–9.
315. Pennisi RS. Med J Aust. 2006 Jun 5;184(11):583–4.
316. Yuste M et al. Actas Dermosifiliogr. 2005 Nov;96(9): 589–92.
317. Cianfrocca C et al. Ital Heart J. 2002 Nov;3(11):689–91.
318. MacVie OP, Harney BA. Br J Ophthalmol. 2005 Oct;89(10): 1378–9.
319. Schneider C et al. J Fr Ophtalmol. 2002 Sep;25(7):731–2.
320. Benjamin J et al. Postgrad Med J. 2001 Feb;77(904):112–3.
321. Bebbington A et al. J Arthroplasty. 2005 Jan;20(1):125–6.
322. Destro MW et al. Br J Plast Surg. 2005 Jan;58(1):100–1.
323. Fong KC, Kinnear PE. Postgrad Med J. 2003 Sep;79(935): 531–2.
324. Hauser D et al. Transpl Int. 2002 Jul;15(7):377–9.
325. Fessenden JM et al. Am Surg. 2001 Jan;67(1):33–5.
326. Yagmur E et al. Am J Hematol. 2005 Aug;79(4):343–4.
327. Miller LG, Freeman B. J Herb Pharmacother. 2002;2(2): 57–63.
328. Kupiec T, Raj V. J Anal Toxicol. 2005 Oct;29(7):755–8.
329. Granger AS. Age Aging. 2001 Nov;30(6):523–5.
330. Hecker H et al. Toxicology. 2002 Aug 15;177(2–3):167–77.
331. Hasegawa S et al. Pediatr Neurol. 2006 Oct;35(4):275–6.
332. Harms SL et al. Epilepsia. 2006 Feb;47(2):323–9.
333. Kohler S et al. Blood Coagul Fibrinolysis. 2004 Jun;15(4): 303–9.
334. Halil M et al. Blood Coagul Fibrinolysis. 2005 Jul;16(5): 349–53.
335. Bal Dit Sollier C et al. Clin Lab Haematol. 2003 Aug;25(4): 251–3.
336. Koch E. Phytomedicine. 2005 Jan;12(1–2):10–16.
337. Gaus W et al. Methods Inf Med. 2005;44(5):697–703.
338. Bent S et al. J Gen Intern Med. 2005 Jul;20(7):657–61.
339. Mossabeb R et al. Wien Klin Wochenschr. 2001 Aug 16; 113(15–16):580–7.
340. Fuchikami H et al. Drug Metab Dispos. 2006 Apr;34(4): 577–82.
341. Moltke LL et al. J Pharm Pharmacol. 2004 Aug;56(8): 1039–44.
342. Gaudineau C et al. Biochem Biophys Res Commun. 2004 Jun 11;318(4):1072–8.
343. Zou L et al. Life Sci. 2002 Aug 16;71(13):1579–89.
344. Yale SH, Glurich K. J Altern Complement Med. 2005 Jun; 11(3):433–9.
345. He N, Edeki T. Am J Ther. 2004 May–Jun;11(3):206–12.
346. Mohutsky MA et al. Am J Ther. 2006 Jan–Feb;13(1):24–31.
347. Chatterjee SS et al. J Pharm Pharmacol. 2005 May;57(5): 641–50.
348. Jiang X et al. Br J Clin Pharmacol. 2005 Apr;59(4):425–32.
349. Gurley BJ et al. Drugs Aging. 2005;22(6):525–39.
350. Dergal JM et al. Drugs Aging. 2002;19(11):879–86.
351. Aruna D, Naidu MU. Br J Clin Pharmacol. 2007 Mar;63(3): 333–8.
352. Wolf HR. Drugs RD. 2006;7(3):163–72.
353. Lu WJ et al. J Clin Pharmacol. 2006 Jun;46(6):628–34.
354. Greenblatt DJ et al. J Clin Pharmacol. 2006 Feb;46(2): 214–21.
355. Engelsen J et al. Ugeskr Laeger. 2003 Apr 28;165(18): 1868–71.
356. Kudolo GB et al. Clin Nutr. 2006 Aug;25(4):606–16.
357. Yasui-Furukori N et al. J Clin Pharmacol. 2004 May;44(5): 538–42.
358. Mauro VF et al. Am J Ther. 2003 Jul–Aug;10(4):247–51.
359. Duche JC et al. Int J Clin Pharmacol Res. 1989;9(3):165–8.
360. Yin OQ et al. Pharmacogenetics. 2004 Dec;14(12):841–50.
361. Yoshioka M et al. Biol Pharm Bull. 2004 Dec;27(12): 2006–9.
362. Meisel C et al. Atherosclerosis. 2003 Apr;167(2):367.
363. Galluzzi S et al. J Neurol Neurosurg Psychiatry. 2000 May; 68(5):679–80.
364. Delgoda R, Westlake AC. Toxicol Rev. 2004;23(4):239–49.
365. Glintborg B et al. Eur J Clin Pharmacol. 2005 Oct;61(9): 675–81.

Hammelidaceae

1. WHO Monographs on Selected Medicinal Plants—Vol 2. WHO Geneva 2004 p. 124–36.
2. Wang H et al. J Pharm Biomed Anal. 2003 Nov 24;33(4): 539–44.
3. Dauer A et al. Planta Med. 2003 Jan;69(1):89–91.
4. Deters A et al. Phytochemistry. 2001 Nov;58(6):949–58.
5. Iauk L et al. Phytother Res. 2003 Jun;17(6):599–604.
6. Brantner A, Greinl E. J Ethnopharmacol. 1994;44(1):35–40.
7. Gloor M et al. Forsch Komplementarmed Klass Naturheilkd. 2002 Jun;9(3):153–9.
8. Dauer A et al. Planta Med. 1998 May;64(4):324–7.
9. Dauer A et al. Phytochemistry. 2003 May;63(2):199–207.
10. Periera da Silva A et al. Phytother Res. 2000 Dec;14(8): 612–6.
11. Choi HR et al. Phytother Res. 2002 Jun;16(4):364–7.
12. Masaki H et al. Biol Pharm Bull. 1995 Jan;18(1):162–6.
13. Masaki H et al. Free Rad Res Comm. 1993;19(5):333–40.
14. Erdelmeier CA et al. Planta Med. 1996 Jun;62(3):241–5.
15. Habtemariam S. Toxicon. 2002 Jan;40(1):83–8.
16. Hartisch C et al. Planta Med. 1997 Apr;63(2):106–10.
17. Hughes-Formella BJ et al. Skin Pharmacol Appl Skin Physiol. 2002 Mar–Apr;15(2):125–32.
18. Hughes-Formella BJ et al. Dermatology. 1998;196(3):316–22.
19. Korting HC et al. Eur J Clin Pharmacol. 1993;44(4):315–8.
20. Swoboda M, Meurer J. Z Phytother. 1991;12:114–7.
21. Korting HC et al. Eur J Clin Pharmacol. 1995;48(6):461–5.
22. Martindale, The Extra Pharmacopoeia 26th Ed. Pharmaceutical Press London March 1973 p. 265.
23. Granlund H. Contact Dermatitis. 1994 Sep;31(3):195.

Hippocastanaceae

1. WHO Monographs on Selected Medicinal Plants—Vol 2. WHO Geneva 2004 p. 127–48.
2. Sirtori CR. Pharmacol Res. 2001 Sep;44(3):183–93.
3. Yoshikawa M et al. Yakugaku Zasshi. 1999 Jan;119(1):81–7.
4. Yoshikawa M et al. Chem Pharm Bull (Tokyo). 1998 Nov; 46(11):1764–9.
5. Konoshima T, Lee KH. J Nat Prod. 1986 Jul–Aug;49(4): 650–6.
6. Stankovic SK et al. Phytochemistry. 1985;24(1):119–21.
7. Stankovic SK et al. Phytochemistry. 1984;23(11):2677–9.
8. Antoniuk VO. Ukr Biokhim Zh. 1992 Sep–Oct;64(5):47–52.

9. Martindale, The Extra Pharmacopoeia 26th Ed. Pharmaceutical Press London March 1973 p. 1781.
10. Facino RM et al. Arch Pharm (Weinheim). 1995 Oct;328(10):
    720–4.
11. Brunner F et al. Br J Clin Pharmacol. 2001 Mar;51(3):219–24.
12. Belcaro G et al. Angiology. 2004 May–Jun;55(Suppl 1):
    S15–18.
13. Ruffini I et al. Angiology. 2004 May–Jun;55(Suppl 1):
    S19–21.
14. Cesarone MR et al. Angiology. 2004 May–Jun;55(Suppl 1):
    S23–25.
15. Ricci A et al. Angiology. 2004 May–Jun;55(Suppl 1):S11–14.
16. Incandela L et al. Angiology. 2001 Dec;52(Suppl 3):S69–72.
17. De Sanctis MT et al. Angiology. 2001 Dec;52(Suppl 3):
    S49–55.
18. Cesarone MR et al. Angiology. 2001 Dec;52(Suppl 3):S43–8.
19. Incandela L et al. Angiology. 2001 Dec;52(Suppl 3):S35–41.
20. De Sanctis MT et al. Angiology. 2001 Dec;52(Suppl 3):
    S29–34.
21. Incandela L et al. Angiology. 2001 Dec;52(Suppl 3):S23–27.
22. Neumann-Mangoldt P. Fortschr Med. 1979 Dec;197(45):
    2117–9.
23. Bisler H et al. Dtsch Med Wochenschr. 1986 Aug 29;111(35):
    1321–9.
24. Bogdanets LI et al. Angiol Sosud Khir. 2005;11(3):55–9.
25. Dickson S et al. J Herb Pharmacother. 2004;4(2):19–23.
26. Greeske K, Pohlmann BK. Fortschr Med. 1996 May 30;114(15):
    196–200.
27. Rehn D et al. Arzneimittelforschung. 1996 May;46(5):483–7.
28. Diehm C et al. Vasa. 1992;21(2):188–92.
29. Koch R. Phytother Res. 2002 Mar;16 Suppl 1:S1–5.
30. Diehm C et al. Lancet. 1996 Feb 3;347(8997):292–4.
31. Ottillinger B, Greeske K. BMC Cardiovasc Disord.
    2001;1:5.
32. Leach MJ et al. Ostomy Wound Mange. 2006 Apr;52(4):
    68–70, 72–4, 76–8.
33. Suter A et al. Adv Ther. 2006 Jan–Feb;23(1):179–90.
34. Pittler MH, Ernst E. Cochrane Database Syst Rev. 2006 Jan 25;
    (1):CD003230.
35. Pittler MH, Ernst E. Cochrane Database Syst Rev. 2004;(2):
    CD003230.
36. Siebert U et al. Int Angiol. 2002 Dec;21(4):305–15.
37. Tiffany N et al. J Herb Pharmacother. 2002;2(1):71–85.
38. Endl J, Auinger W. Wien Klin Wochenschr. 1977 Apr 29;
    89(9):304–7.
39. Cazzola D. Clin Ter. 1975 Sep 30;74(6):559–78.
40. Miyasaka A, Imoto T. Proc Jap Sympos Taste Smell. 1988;
    22:269–72.
41. Wu CY et al. Proc Natl Acad Sci USA. 2004 Jul 6;101(27):
    10012–7.
42. Fujimura T et al. J Cosmet Sci. 2006 Sep–Oct;57(5):369–76.
43. Schrader E et al. Pharmazie. 1995 Sep;50(9):623–7.
44. Loew D et al. Methods Find Exp Clin Pharmacol. 2000 Sep;
    22(7):537–42.
45. Bassler D et al. Adv Ther. 2003 Sep–Oct;20(5):295–304.
46. Takegoshi K et al. Gastroenterol Jpn. 1986 Feb;21(1):62–5.
47. Comaish JS, Kersey PJ. Contact Dermatitis. 1980 Jan;6(2):
    150–1.
48. Walli F et al. Schweiz Med Wochenschr. 1981 Sep 19;111(38):
    1398–405.
49. Schuff-Werner P, Berg PA. Klin Wochenschr. 1980 Sep 15;
    58(18):935–41.
50. Hellberg K et al. Thoraxchir Vask Chir. 1975 Aug;23(4):
    396–9.
51. Grases F et al. Clin Ther. 2004 Dec;26(12):2045–55.

Iridaceae

1. Dr Duke's Phytochemical and Ethnobotanical Databases.
   http://www.ars-grin.gov/duke/.
2. Claus EP. Pharmacognosy 4th Ed. Henry Kimpton. London
   1961.
3. Winston D, Dattner AM. Clin Dermatol. 1999 Jan 2;17(1):
   53–6.
4. Amenta A et al. Fitoterapia. 2000 Aug 1;71(Suppl 1):S13–20.

Juglandaceae

1. Dr Duke's Phytochemical and Ethnobotanical Databases.
   http://www.ars-grin.gov/duke/.
2. Claus EP. Pharmacognosy 4th Ed. Henry Kimpton. London
   1961.
3. Omar S et al. J Ethnopharmacol. 2000 Nov;73(1–2):161–70.
4. Ficker CE et al. Mycoses. 2003 Feb;46(1–2):29–37.
5. Inbaraj JJ, Chignell CF. Chem Res Toxicol. 2004 Jan;17(1):
   55–62.
6. Paulsen MT, Ljungman M. Toxicol Appl Pharmacol. 2005
   Nov 15;209(1):1–9.
7. Kamei H et al. Am Cancer Biother Radiopharm. 1998 Jun;
   13(3):185–8.
8. Cenas N et al. J Biol Chem. 2006 Mar 3;281(9):5593–603.
9. Segura-Aguilar J et al. Leuk Res. 1992 Jun–Jul;16(6–7):
   631–7.
10. Varga Z et al. Biochem Biophys Res Commun. 1996 Jan 26;
    218(3):828–32.
11. Neamatallah A et al. Lett Appl Microbiol. 2005;41(1):94–6.
12. Didry N et al. Pharmazie. 1994 Sep;49(9):681–3.
13. Cai L et al. J Agric Food Chem. 2000 Mar;48(3):909–14.
14. Clark AM et al. Phytother Res. 1990 Feb;4(1):11–14.
15. Park BS et al. J Ethnopharmacol. 2006 Apr 21;105(1–2):
    255–62.
16. Min BS et al. Phytother Res. 2002 Mar;16 Suppl 1:S57–62.
17. Akerman SE, Muller S. J Biol Chem. 2005 Jan 7;280(1):
    564–70.
18. Montoya J et al. Biochem Biophys Res Commun. 2004 Dec 24;
    325(4):1517–23.
19. Bhargarva UC et al. J Pharm Sci. 1968 Oct;57(10):1728–32.
20. Gupta SR et al. Phytochemistry. 1972 Aug;11(8):2634–6.
21. Choi HR et al. Phytother Res. 2002 Jun;16(4):364–7.
22. Han DH et al. Anticancer Res. 2006 Sep–Oct;26(5A):3601–6.
23. Amaral RM et al. Food Chemistry. 2004 Dec;88(3):373–9.
24. Babula P et al. J Chromatogr B Analyt Technol Biomed Life
    Sci. 2006 Sep 14;842(1):28–35.
25. Muetzel S, Becker K. Animal Feed Sci Technol. 2006 Jan 6;
    125(1–2):139–49.
26. Buttery RG et al. J Agric Food Chem. 2000 Jul;48(7):
    2858–61.
27. Qadan F et al. Am J Chin Med. 2005;33(2):197–204.
28. Nariman F et al. Helicobacter. 2004 Apr;9(2):146–51.
29. Ali-Shtayeh MS, Abu Ghdeib SI. Mycoses. 1999;42(11–12):
    665–72.

30. Alkhawajah AM. J Chin Med. 1997;25(2):175–80.
31. Ashri N, Gazi M. Oral Surg Oral Med Oral Pathol. 1990 Oct;70(4):445–9.
32. Kaur K et al. J Environ Pathol Toxicol Oncol. 2003;22(1): 59–67.
33. Arora S et al. Teratog Carcinog Mutagen. 2003;Suppl 1: 295–300.
34. Cortes B et al. J Am Coll Cardiol. 2006 Oct 17;48(8):1666–71.
35. Marangoni F et al. Nutr Metab Cardiovasc Dis. 2007 Jul;17(6): 457–61.
36. Chauhan N et al. Curr Alzheimer Res. 2004 Aug;1(3):183–8.
37. Saad B et al. Evid Based Complement Alternat Med. 2006 Mar;3(1):93–8.
38. Arora S et al. J Environ Pathol Toxicol Oncol. 2005;24(3): 193–200.
39. Tikkanen L et al. Mutat Res. 1983 Oct;124(1):25–34.
40. Neri I et al. Contact Dermatitis. 2006 Jul;55(1):62–3.
41. Bonamonte D et al. Contact Dermatitis. 2001 Feb;44(2):102.

Lamiaceae

1. Dr Duke's Phytochemical and Ethnobotanical Databases. http://www.ars-grin.gov/duke/.
2. Seidel V et al. Ann Pharm Fr. 1998;56(1):31–5.
3. Bruno M et al. Phytochemistry. 1986 Jan 22;25(2):538–9.
4. Bertrand M et al. Biochem Syst Ecol. 2000 Dec 1;28(10): 1031–3.
5. Seidel V et al. Phytother Res. 2000 Mar;14(2):93–8.
6. Seidel V et al. Phytochemistry. 1997 Feb;44(4):691–3.
7. Didry N et al. J Ethnopharmacol. 1999 Nov 1;67(2):197–202.
8. Citoglu GS et al. J Ethnopharmacol. 2004 Jun;92(2–3): 275–80.
9. Daels-Rakotoarison DA et al. Arzneimittelforschung. 2000 Jan;50(1):16–23.
10. Tomas-Barberan FA et al. Phytochemistry. 1988;27(8): 2631–45.
11. Zieba J. Pol J Pharmacol Pharm. 1973 Nov–Dec;25(6):593–7.
12. Liu J. J Ethnopharmacol. 1995;49(2–1):57–68.
13. Lawrence BM et al. Phytochemistry. 1972 Aug;11(8): 2636–38.
14. Komprda T et al. Arch Tierernahr. 1999;52(1):95–105.
15. Grayer RJ et al. Phytochemistry. 2003 Sep;64(2):519–28.
16. Kuhn H et al. Eur J Biochem. 1989 Dec 8;186(1–2):155–62.
17. Kumarasamy Y et al. Tetrahedron. 2003 Aug 18;59(34): 6403–7.
18. Wang W et al. Plant Physiol. 2003 Jul;132(3):1322–34.
19. Widen B, Widen M. Hereditas. 2000;132(3):229–41.
20. Blanco E et al. J Ethnopharmacol. 1999 May;65(2):113–24.
21. Kumarasamy Y et al. Fitoterapia. 2002 Dec;73(7–8):721–3.
22. Tokuda H et al. Cancer Lett. 1986 Dec;33(3):279–85.
23. Henry DY et al. Eur J Biochem. 1987 Dec 30;170(1–2): 389–94.
24. Tognolini M et al. Life Sci. 2006 Feb 23;78(13):1419–32.
25. Bate-Smith EC, Westall RC. Biochim Biophys Acta. 1950;4: 427–40.
26. Janicsak G et al. Biochem Syst Ecol. 2006 May;34(5):392–6.
27. Zgorka G, Glowniak K. J Pharm Biomed Anal. 2001 Aug; 26(1):79–87.
28. Matsuura H et al. Phytochemistry. 2004 Jan;65(1):91–7.
29. Grayer RJ et al. Phytochemistry. 2003 Sep;64(2):519–28.

30. Gollapudi S et al. Biochem Biophys Res Comm. 1995 May 5; 210(1):145–51.
31. Varga E et al. Acta Pharm Hung. 1998 May;68(3):183–8.
32. Newton SM et al. J Ethnopharmacol. 2002 Feb;79(1):57–67.
33. Bedoya LM et al. Phytother Res. 2002 Sep;16(6):550–4.
34. Kries W et al. Antiviral Res. 1990 Dec;14(6):323–37.
35. Marino M et al. Int J Food Microbiol. 2001 Aug 5;67(3): 187–95.
36. Ghfir B et al. Mycopathologia. 1997 Jul;138(1):7–12.
37. Miyazaki H et al. J Nutr Sci Vitaminol (Tokyo). 2003 Oct;49(5): 346–9.
38. Millet Y et al. Rev Electroencephalogr Neurophysiol Clin. 1979 Jan–Mar;9(1):12–18.
39. Burkhard PR et al. J Neurol. 1999 Aug;246(8):667–70.
40. Millet Y et al. Clin Toxicol. 1981 Dec;18(12):1485–98.
41. Buzianowski J, Skrzypczak L. Phytochemistry. 1995 Mar; 38(4):997–1001.
42. Glennie CW, Harborne JB. Phytochemistry. 1971 Jun;10(6): 1325–9.
43. Paduch R et al. J Ethnopharmacol. 2007 Mar 1;110(1):69–75.
44. Pedersen JA. Biochem Syst Ecol. 2000 Mar;28(3):229–53.
45. Alipieva KI et al. Biochem Syst Ecol. 2007 Jan;35(1):17–22.
46. Alipieva KI et al. Biochem Syst Ecol. 2006 Jan;34(1):88–91.
47. Damtoft S. Phytochemistry. 1992 Jan;31(1):175–8.
48. Savchenko T et al. Biochem Syst Ecol. 2001 Oct;29(9): 891–900.
49. Damtoft S, Jensen SR. Phytochemistry. 1995 Jul;39(4):923–4.
50. Sarker SD et al. Phytochemistry. 1997 Aug;45(7):1431–3.
51. Matkowski A, Piotrowska M. Fitoterapia. 2006 Jul;77(5): 346–53.
52. Chudnicka A, Matysik G. J Ethnopharmacol. 2005 Jun 3; 99(2):281–6.
53. Tunon H et al. J Ethnopharmacol. 1995 Oct;48(2):61–76.
54. Trouillas P et al. Food Chemistry. 2003 Mar;80(3):399–407.
55. Kokoska L et al. J Ethnopharmacol. 2002 Sep;82(1):51–3.
56. Bartram T. Encyclopedia of Herbal Medicine. 1st Edition, 1995 Grace Publishers, Stour Rd, Christchurch.
57. Fakhari AR et al. J Chromatogr A. 2005 Dec 9;1098(1–2): 14–18.
58. Daferera DJ et al. J Agric Food Chem. 2002 Sep 25;50(2): 5503–7.
59. Upson TM et al. Biochem Syst Ecol. 2000 Dec 1;28(10): 991–1007.
60. Nitzsche A et al. J Agric Food Chem. 2004 May 19;52(10): 2915–23.
61. Rota C et al. J Food Prot. 2004 Jun;67(6):1252–6.
62. Schwiertz A et al. Int J Aromather. 2006;16(3–4):169–74.
63. Mahady GB et al. Phytother Res. 2005 Nov;19(11):988–91.
64. Sterer N, Rubinstein Y. Quintessence Int. 2006 Sep;37(8): 653–8.
65. Takarada K et al. Oral Microbiol Immunol. 2004 Feb;19(1): 61–4.
66. Cavanagh HM, Wilkinson JM. Phytother Res. 2002 Jun;16(4): 301–8.
67. D'Auria FD et al. Med Mycol. 2005 Aug;43(5):391–6.
68. Shin S. Arch Pharm Res. 2003 May;26(5):389–93.
69. Inouye S et al. Mycoses. 2000;43(1–2):17–23.
70. Moon T et al. Parasitol Res. 2006 Nov;99(6):722–8.
71. Giordani R et al. Phytother Res. 2004 Dec;18(12):990–5.
72. Daferera DJ et al. J Agric Food Chem. 2000 Jun;48(6): 2576–81.
73. Ferreira A et al. J Ethnopharmacol. 2006 Nov 3;108(1):31–7.

74. Hohmann J et al. Planta Med. 1999 Aug;65(6):576–8.
75. Lee KG, Shibamoto T. J Agric Food Chem. 2002 Aug 14; 50(17):4947–52.
76. Adsersen A et al. J Ethnopharmacol. 2006 Apr 6;104(3): 418–22.
77. Wiseman DA et al. J Pharm Exp Ther. 2007 Mar;320(3): 1163–70.
78. Clark SS. Oncology. 2006;70(1):13–18.
79. Da Fonseca CO et al. Surg Neurol. 2006;65 Suppl 1:S1: 2–1:8.
80. Da Fonseca CO et al. Surg Neurol. 2006 Dec;66(6):611–5.
81. Lewith GT et al. J Altern Complement Med. 2005 Aug; 11(4):631–7.
82. Goel N et al. Chronobiol Int. 2005;22(5):889–904.
83. Nagai M et al. Neurosci Lett. 2000 Aug 11;289(3):227–9.
84. Sanders C et al. J Int Neurosci. 2002 Nov;112(11):1305–20.
85. Morris N. Complement Ther Med. 2002 Dec;10(4):223–8.
86. Vernet-Maury E et al. J Auton Nerv Syst. 1999 Feb 15; 75(2–3):176–83.
87. Moss M et al. Int J Neurosci. 2003 Jan;113(1):15–38.
88. Akhondzadeh S et al. Prog Neuropsychopharmacol Biol Psychiatry. 2003 Feb;27(1):123–7.
89. Dimpfel W et al. Eur J Med Res. 2004 Sep 29;9(9):423–31.
90. Motomura N et al. Percept Mot Skills. 2001 Dec;93(3): 713–8.
91. Lee SY. Taehan Kanho Hakhoe Chi. 2005 Apr;35(2): 303–12.
92. Holmes C et al. Int J Geriatr Psychiatry. 2002 Apr;17(4): 305–8.
93. Saeki Y. Complement Ther Med. 2000 Mar;8(1):2–7.
94. Cornwell S, Dale A. Mod Midwife. 1995 Mar;5(3):31–3.
95. Dale A, Cornwell S. J Adv Nurs. 1994 Jan;19(1):89–96.
96. Hay IC et al. Arch Dermatol. 1998 Nov;134(11):1349–52.
97. Sysoev NP. Stomatologiia (Mosk). 1991 Jan–Feb;70(1): 12–13.
98. Hajhashemi V et al. J Ethnopharmacol. 2003 Nov;89(1): 67–71.
99. Heuberger E et al. Neuropsychopharmacology. 2004 Oct; 29(10):1925–32.
100. Evandri MG et al. Food Chem Toxicol. 2005 Sep;43(9): 1381–7.
101. Prashar A et al. Cell Prolif. 2004 Jun;37(3):221–9.
102. Coulson IH, Khan AS. Contact Dermatitis. 1999 Aug; 41(2):111.
103. Sugiura M et al. Contact Dermatitis. 2000 Sep;43(3): 157–60.
104. Benito M et al. Ann Allergy Asthma Immunol. 1996 May; 76(5):416–8.
105. Duskova J, Dusek J. Ceska Slov Farm. 2004 Jan;53(1): 39–41.
106. Tomas-Barberan FA et al. Biochem Syst Ecol. 1993 Jun;21(4): 531–2.
107. Papanova GY et al. Phytochemistry. 1998 Mar;47(6): 1149–51.
108. Malakov P et al. Phytochemistry. 1985;24(10):2341–3.
109. Tschesche R et al. Phytochemistry. 1980;19:2783.
110. Pedersen JA. Biochem Syst Ecol. 2000 Mar;28(3):229–53.
111. Milkowska-Leyck K et al. J Ethnopharmacol. 2002 Apr; 80(1):85–90.
112. Lawrence BM et al. Phytochemistry. 1972 Aug;11(8): 2636–8.

113. Geller SE, Studee L. Maturitas. 2006 Nov;55(Suppl 1): S3–S13.
114. Mantle D et al. J Ethnopharmacol. 2000 Sep;72(1–2):47–51.
115. Matkowski A, Piotrowska M. Fitoterapia. 2006 Jul;77(5): 346–53.
116. Chen CX, Kwan CY. Life Sci. 2001 Jan;68(8):953–60.
117. Kong YC et al. Am J Chin Med (Gard City NY). 1976 Winter;4(4):373–82.
118. Wang Z et al. J Asian Nat Prod Res. 2004 Dec;6(4):281–7.
119. Zou QZ et al. Am J Clin Med. 1989;17(1–2):65–70.
120. Lamaison JL et al. Ann Pharm Fr. 1990;48(2):103–8.
121. Auf'mkolk M et al. Endocrinology. 1985 May;116(5): 1677–86.
122. Wagner H et al. Arzneimittelforschung. 1970 May;20(5): 705–13.
123. Gumbinger HG et al. Planta Med. 1992 Feb;58(1):49–50.
124. Hussein AA et al. Tetrahedron. 1999 Jun 4;55(23):7375–88.
125. Hussein AA, Rodriguez B. J Nat Prod. 2000 Mar;63(3): 419–21.
126. Jeremi D et al. Tetrahedron. 1985;41(2):357–64.
127. Nahrstedt A et al. Planta Med. 1990 Aug;56(4):395–8.
128. Gumbinger HC et al. Contraception. 1981 Jun;23(6):661–6.
129. Rompel A et al. FEBS Lett. 1999 Feb 19;445(1):103–10.
130. Auf'mkolk M et al. Endocrinology. 1984 Aug;115(2): 527–34.
131. Auf'mkolk M et al. Endocrinology. 1985 May;116(5): 1687–93.
132. Kong LD et al. J Ethnopharmacol. 2000 Nov;73(1–2): 199–207.
133. Lamaison JL et al. Ann Pharm Fr. 1991;66(7):185–8.
134. Gibbons S et al. Phytochemistry. 2003 Jan;62(1):83–7.
135. Vonhoff C et al. Life Sci. 2006 Feb 2;78(10):1063–70.
136. El Bardai S et al. Br J Pharmacol. 2003 Dec;140(7):1211–6.
137. Tomas-Barberan FA et al. Phytochemistry. 1992 Sep;31(9): 3097–102.
138. Saleh MM, Glombitza KW. Planta Med. 1989;55:105.
139. Sahpaz S et al. Nat Prod Lett. 2002 Jun;16(3):195–9.
140. Saphaz S et al. J Ethnopharmacol. 2002 Mar;79(3):389–92.
141. Martindale, The Extra Pharmacopoeia 26th Ed. Pharmaceutical Press London March 1973.
142. Matkowski A, Piotrowska M. Fitoterapia. 2006 Jul;77(5): 346–53.
143. VanderJagt TJ et al. Life Sci. 2002 Jan 18;70(9):1035–40.
144. Berrougui H et al. Life Sci. 2006 Dec 14;80(2):105–12.
145. Martin-Nizard F et al. J Pharm Pharmacol. 2004 Dec; 56(12):1607–11.
146. Al-Bakri AG, Afifi FU. J Microbiol Methods. 2007 Jan; 68(1):19–25.
147. Newall CA et al. Herbal Medicines. The Pharmaceutical Press London 1996.
148. Herrera-Arellano A et al. Phytomedicine. 2004 Nov; 11(7–8):561–6.
149. Eddouks M et al. J Ethnopharmacol. 2002 Oct;82(2–3): 97–103.
150. WHO Monographs on Selected Medicinal Plants—Vol 2. WHO Geneva 2004 p. 180–7.
151. Nhu-Trang TT et al. Anal Bioanal Chem. 2006 Dec;386(7–8): 2141–52.
152. de Sousa AC et al. J Pharm Pharmacol. 2004 May;56(5): 677–81.
153. Mrlianova M et al. Planta Med. 2002 Feb;68(2):178–80.

154. Patora J et al. Acta Pol Pharm. 2003 Sep–Oct;60(5): 395–400.
155. Carnat AP et al. Pharm Acta Helv. 1998 Jan;72(5):301–5.
156. Karasova G et al. J Sep Sci. 2005 Dec;28(18):2468–76.
157. Ziakova A et al. J Chromatogr A. 2003 Jan 3;983(1–2): 271–5.
158. Lamaison JL et al. Ann Pharm Fr. 1990;48(2):103–8.
159. Janicsak G et al. Biochem Syst Ecol. 2006 May;34(5):392–6.
160. Herodez S et al. Food Chem. 2003 Feb;80(2):275–82.
161. Patora J, Klimek B. Acta Pol Pharm. 2002 Mar–Apr;59(2): 139–43.
162. Heitz A et al. Fitoterapia. 2000 Apr;71(2):201–2.
163. Apak R et al. Int J Food Sci Nutr. 2006 Aug–Sep;57(5): 292–304.
164. Germann I et al. Phytomedicine. 2006;13 Suppl 1:45–50.
165. Ferreira A et al. J Ethnopharmacol. 2006 Nov 3;108(1): 31–7.
166. Ivanova D et al. J Ethnopharmacol. 2005 Jan 4;96(1–2): 145–50.
167. Blomhoff R. Tidsskr Nor Laegeforen. 2004 Jun 17;124(12): 1643–5.
168. Dragland S et al. J Nutr. 2003 May;133(5):1286–90.
169. Hohmann J et al. Planta Med. 1999 Aug;65(6):576–8.
170. Trommer H, Neubert RH. J Pharm Pharm Sci. 2005 Sep 15; 8(3):494–506.
171. Mimica-Dukic N et al. J Agric Food Chem. 2004 May 5; 52(9):2485–9.
172. Petersen M, Simmonds MSJ. Phytochemistry. 2003 Jan; 62(2):121–5.
173. Wake G et al. J Ethnopharmacol. 2000 Feb;69(2):105–14.
174. Dos Santos-Neto LL et al. Evid Based Complement Alternat Med. 2006 Dec;3(4):441–5.
175. Akhondzadeh S et al. J Neurol Neurosurg Psychiatry. 2003 Jul;74(7):863–6.
176. Ballard CG et al. J Clin Psychiatry. 2002 Jul;63(7):553–8.
177. Kennedy DO et al. Psychosom Med. 2004 Jul–Aug;66(4): 607–13.
178. Kennedy DO et al. Neuropsychopharmacology. 2003 Oct; 28(10):1871–81.
179. Kennedy DO et al. Pharmacol Biochem Behav. 2002 Jul; 72(4):953–64.
180. Muller SF, Klement S. Phytomedicine. 2006 Jun;13(6): 383–7.
181. Cerny A, Schmid K. Fitoterapia. 1999 Jun;70(3):221–8.
182. Kennedy DO et al. Phytother Res. 2006 Feb;20(2):96–102.
183. Dimpfel W et al. Eur J Med Res. 2004 Sep 29;9(9):423–31.
184. Yamasaki K et al. Biol Pharm Bull. 1998 Aug;21(8):829–33.
185. Nolkemper S et al. Planta Med. 2006 Dec;75(15):1378–82.
186. Dimitrova Z et al. Acta Microbiol Bulg. 1993;29:65–72.
187. Allahverdiyev A et al. Phytomedicine. 2004 Nov;11(7–8): 657–61.
188. Iauk L et al. Phytother Res. 2003 Jun;17(6):599–604.
189. Larrondo JV et al. Microbios. 1995;82(332):171–2.
190. Mahady G et al. Phytother Res. 2005 Nov;19(11):988–91.
191. Mikus J et al. Planta Med. 2000 May;66(4):366–8.
192. Friedman M et al. J Agric Food Chem. 2004 Sep 22;52(19): 6042–8.
193. Koytchev R et al. Phytomedicine. 1999 Oct;6(4):225–30.
194. Wolbling RH, Leonhardt K. Phytomedicine. 1994;1:25–31.
195. Kwon YI et al. Asia Pac J Clin Nutr. 2006;15(1):107–18.
196. Santini F et al. J Endocrinol Invest. 2003 Oct;26(10):950–5.
197. Vejdani R et al. Dig Dis Sci. 2006 Aug;51(8):1501–7.
198. Madisch A et al. Digestion. 2004;69(1):45–52.
199. Madisch A et al. Z Gastroenterol. 2001 Jul;39(7):511–7.
200. Chakurski I et al. Vutr Boles. 1981;20(6):51–4.
201. Savino F et al. Phytother Res. 2005 Apr;19(4):335–40.
202. de Sousa AC et al. J Pharm Pharmacol. 2004 May;56(5): 677–81.
203. Dudai N et al. Planta Med. 2005 May;71(5):484–8.
204. Galasinski W et al. Acta Pol Pharm. 1996 Sep–Oct;53(5): 311–8.
205. Chlabicz J, Galasinski W. J Pharm Pharmacol. 1986 Nov; 38(11):791–4.
206. Peake PW et al. Int J Immunopharmacol. 1991;13(7): 853–7.
207. Ramos Ruiz A et al. J Ethnopharmacol. 1996 Jul 5;52(3): 123–7.
208. Duband F et al. Ann Pharm Fr. 1992;50(3):146–55.
209. Monograph on Selected Medicinal Plants—Vol 2. WHO Geneva p. 188–98.
210. Marin C, Schippa C. J Agric Food Chem. 2006 Jun 28; 54(13):4814–9.
211. Rohloff J et al. J Agric Food Chem. 2005 May 18;53(10): 4143–8.
212. Gershenzon J et al. Plant Physiol. 2000 Jan;122(1):205–14.
213. Rohloff J. J Agric Food Chem. 1999 Sep;47(9):3782–6.
214. Kjonaas R, Croteau R. Arch Biochem Biophys. 1983 Jan; 220(1):79–89.
215. Gasic O et al. Biochem Syst Ecol. 1987 May;15(3):335–40.
216. Burbott AJ, Loomis WD. Plant Physiol. 1967 Jan;42(1): 20–8.
217. Areias FM et al. Food Chem. 2001 May;73(3):307–11.
218. Voirin B et al. Phytochemistry. 1999 Apr 10;50(7):1189–93.
219. Jullien F et al. Phytochemisty. 1984;23(12):2972–3.
220. de Almeida-Muradian LB et al. Boll Chim Farm. 1998 Jul–Aug;137(7):290–4.
221. Lozak A et al. Sci Total Environ. 2002 Apr 22;289(1–3): 33–40.
222. Gallaher RN et al. J Food Comp Anal. 2006 Aug;19 (Suppl 1): S53–7.
223. Mahady GB et al. Phytother Res. 2005 Nov;19(11):988–91.
224. Shkurupii VA et al. Probl Tuberk. 2002;(4):36–9.
225. Betoni JE et al. Mem Inst Oswaldo Cruz. 2006 Jun;101(4): 387–90.
226. Vidal F et al. Exp Parasitol. 2007 Jan;115(1):25–31.
227. Tassou C et al. Food Res Int. 2000 Apr;33(3–4):273–80.
228. Schelz Z et al. Fitoterapia. 2006 Jun;77(4):279–85.
229. Burt S. Int J Food Microbiol. 2004 Aug 1;94(3):223–53.
230. Tassou CC et al. J Appl Bacteriol. 1995 Jun;78(6):593–600.
231. Inouye S et al. J Infect Chemother. 2001 Dec;7(4):251–4.
232. Shapiro S et al. Oral Microbiol Immunol. 1994 Aug;9(4): 202–8.
233. Yadegarinia D et al. Phytochemistry. 2006 Jun;67(12): 1249–55.
234. Tampieri MP et al. Mycopathologia. 2005 Apr;159(3): 339–45.
235. Duarte MC et al. J Ethnopharmacol. 2005 Feb 28;97(2): 305–11.
236. Mimica-Dukic N et al. Planta Med. 2003 May;69(5):413–9.
237. Imai H et al. Microbios. 2001;106 Suppl 1:31–9.
238. Pattnaik S et al. Microbios. 1996;86(349):237–46.
239. Pattnaik S et al. Microbios. 1995;84(340):195–9.
240. el-Naghy MA et al. Zentralbl Mikrobiol. 1992;147(3–4): 214–20.

241. Schuhmacher A et al. Phytomedicine. 2003;10(6–7):504–10.
242. Veal L. Complement Ther Nurs Midwifery. 1996 Aug;2(4): 97–101.
243. Sroka Z et al. Z Naturoforsch [C]. 2005 Nov–Dec;60(11–12): 826–32.
244. Kaliora AC, Andrikopoulos NK. Phytother Res. 2005 Dec; 19(12):1077–9.
245. Atoui AK et al. Food Chem. 2005 Jan;89(1):27–36.
246. Blomhoff R. Tidsskr Nor Laegeforen. 2004 Jun 17;124(12): 1643–5.
247. Dragland S et al. J Nutr. 2003 May;133(5):1286–90.
248. Germann I et al. Phytomedicine. 2006;13 Suppl 1:45–50.
249. Schempp H et al. Phytomedicine. 2006;13 Suppl 1:36–44.
250. Grigoleit HG, Grigoleit P. Phytomedicine. 2005 Aug;12(8): 612–6.
251. Melzer J et al. Aliment Pharmacol Ther. 2004 Dec;20(11–12): 1279–87.
252. Madisch A et al. Digestion. 2004;69(1):45–52.
253. Madisch A et al. Z Gastroenterol. 2001 Jul;39(7):511–7.
254. Yamamoto N et al. J Gastroenterol Hepatol. 2006 Sep; 21(9):1394–8.
255. Mizuno S et al. J Gastroenterol Hepatol. 2006 Aug;21(8): 1297–301.
256. Hiki N et al. Gastrointest Endosc. 2003 Apr;57(4):475–82.
257. Asao T et al. Clin Radiol. 2003 Apr;58(4):301–5.
258. Asao T et al. Gastrointest Endosc. 2001 Feb;53(2):172–7.
259. Sparks MJ et al. Br J Radiol. 1995 Aug;68(812):841–3.
260. Grigoleit HG, Grigoleit P. Phytomedicine. 2005 Aug;12(8): 607–11.
261. Micklefield G et al. Phytother Res. 2003 Feb;17(2):135–40.
262. Pimentel M et al. J Clin Gastroenterol. 2001 Jul;33(1): 27–31.
263. Kline RM et al. J Pediatr. 2001 Jan;138(1):125–8.
264. Liu JH et al. J Gastroenterol. 1997 Dec;32(6):765–8.
265. Freise J, Kohler S. Pharmazie. 1999 Mar;54(3):210–5.
266. Grigoleit HG, Grigoleit P. Phytomedicine. 2005 Aug;12(8): 601–6.
267. Thompson Coon J, Ernst E. Aliment Pharmacol Ther. 2002 Oct;16(10):1689–99.
268. May B et al. Aliment Pharmacol Ther. 2000 Dec;14(12): 1671–7.
269. Madisch A et al. Arzneimittelforschung. 1999 Nov;49(11): 925–32.
270. May B et al. Arzneimittelforschung. 1996 Dec;46(12): 1149–53.
271. Goerg KJ, Spilker T. Aliment Pharmacol Ther. 2003 Feb; 17(3):445–51.
272. Tate S. J Adv Nurs. 1997 Sep;26(3):543–9.
273. Lee VM, Linden RW. Exp Physiol. 1992 Jan;77(1):221–4.
274. Logan AC, Beaulne TM. Altern Med Rev. 2002 Oct;7(5): 410–7.
275. Shkurupii VA et al. Probl Tuberk Bolezn Legk. 2006;(9): 43–5.
276. Mahieu F et al. J Biol Chem. 2007 Feb;282:3325–36.
277. Koo HN et al. J Mol Neurosci. 2001 Dec;17(3):391–6.
278. Norrish MI, Dwyer KL. Int J Psychophysiol. 2005 Mar;55(3):291–8.
279. Barker S et al. Percept Mot Skills. 2003 Dec;97(3 Pt 1): 1007–10.
280. Sullivan TE et al. J Clin Exp Neuropsychol. 1998 Apr; 20(2):227–36.

281. Gobel H et al. Nervenarzt. 1996 Aug;67(8):672–81.
282. Davies SJ et al. Clin J Pain. 2002 May–Jun;18(3):200–2.
283. Kumar A et al. Biofactors. 2004;22(1–4):87–91.
284. Satsu H et al. Biofactors. 2004;21(1–4):137–9.
285. Nielsen JB. Basic Clin Pharmacol Toxicol. 2006 Jun;98(6): 575–81.
286. Nair B. Int J Toxicol. 2001;20 Suppl 3:61–73.
287. Mascher H et al. Wien Med Wochcenschr. 2002;152(15–16): 432–6.
288. Kaffenberger RM, Doyle MJ. J Chromatogr. 1990 Apr 27; 527(1):59–66.
289. Romero-Jimenez M et al. Mutat Res. 2005 Aug 1;585(1–2): 147–55.
290. Lazutka JR et al. Food Chem Toxicol. 2001 May;39(5): 485–92.
291. Hurrell RF et al. Br J Nutr. 1999 Apr;81(4):289–95.
292. Morton CA et al. Contact Dermatitis. 1995 May;32(5): 281–4.
293. Rogers SN, Pahor AL. Dent Update. 1995 Jan–Feb;22(1): 36–7.
294. Foti C et al. Contact Dermatitis. 2003 Dec;49(6):312–3.
295. Sainio EL, Kanerva L. Contact Dermatitis. 1995 Aug;33(2): 100–5.
296. Wilkinson SM, Beck MH. Contact Dermatitis. 1994 Jan; 30(1):42–3.
297. Hausen BM. Dtsch Med Wochenschr. 1984 Feb 24;109(8): 300–2.
298. Dooms-Goossens A et al. Contact Dermatitis. 1977 Dec; 3(6):304–8.
299. Andersen KE. Contact Dermatitis. 1978 Aug;4(4):195–8.
300. Sadlo S et al. Rocz Panstw Zakl Hig. 2006;57(3):211–6.
301. Unger M, Frank A. Rapid Commun Mass Spectrom. 2004; 18(19):2273–81.
302. Dresser GK et al. Clin Pharmacol Ther. 2002;72(3):247–55.
303. Regnier LFE et al. Phytochemistry. 1967;6:1281–9.
304. Baranauskiene R et al. J Agric Food Chem. 2003 Jun 18; 51(13):3840–8.
305. Xie S et al. Phytochemistry. 1988;27(2):469–72.
306. Murai F et al. Chem Pharm Bull (Tokyo). 1984 Jul;32(7): 2809–14.
307. Proestos C et al. Food Chem. 2006 Apr;95(4):664–71.
308. Klimek B, Modnicki D. Acta Pol Pharm. 2005 May–Jun; 62(3):231–5.
309. Claus EP. Pharmacognosy. 4th Ed. Henry Kimpton. London 1961.
310. Nostro A et al. Int J Antimicrob Agents. 2001 Dec;18(6): 583–5.
311. Zhu J et al. J Am Mosq Control Assoc. 2006 Sep;22(3): 515–22.
312. Pavela R. Fitoterapia. 2005 Dec;76(7–8):691–6.
313. Chauhan KR et al. J Med Entomol. 2005 Jul;42(4):643–6.
314. Osterhoudt KC et al. Vet Hum Toxicol. 1997 Dec;39(6): 373–5.
315. Angioni A et al. J Agric Food Chem. 2004 Jun 2;52(11): 3530–5.
316. Ramirez P et al. J Pharm Biomed Anal. 2006 Aug 28;41(5): 1606–13.
317. Flamini G et al. J Agric Food Chem. 2002 Jun 5;50(12): 3512–7.
318. Richheimer SL et al. JAOCS. 1996 Apr;73(4):507–14.
319. Mahmoud AA et al. Phytochemistry. 2005 Jul;66(14): 1685–90.

320. Cantrell CL et al. J Nat Prod. 2005 Jan;68(1):98–100.
321. Hidalgo PJ et al. J Agric Food Chem. 1998 Jul;46(7):2624–7.
322. Wellwood CR, Cole RA. J Agric Food Chem. 2004 Oct 6; 52(20):6101–7.
323. Peng Y et al. J Pharm Biomed Anal. 2005 Sep 15;39(3–4): 431–7.
324. del Bano MJ et al. J Agric Food Chem. 2004 Aug 11;52(16): 4987–92.
325. Ibanez E et al. J Agric Food Chem. 2003 Jan 15;51(2):375–82.
326. Okamura N et al. Phytochemistry. 1994 Nov;37(5):1463–6.
327. Swain AR et al. J Am Diet Assoc. 1985 Aug;85(8):950–60.
328. Abe F et al. Biol Pharm Bull. 2002 Nov;25(11):1485–7.
329. Munne-Bosch S, Alegre L. Planta. 2000 May;210(6):925–31.
330. Torre J et al. J Chromatogr A. 2001 Jun 15;919(2):305–11.
331. Tahraoui A et al. J Ethnopharmacol. 2007 Mar 1;110(1): 105–17.
332. Almela L et al. J Chromatogr A. 2006 Jul 7;1120(1–2):221–9.
333. Moreno S et al. Free Radic Res. 2006 Feb;40(2):223–31.
334. Choi HR et al. Phytother Res. 2002 Jun;16(4):364–7.
335. Masuda T et al. J Agric Food Chem. 2002 Oct 9;50(21): 5863–9.
336. Kaliora AC, Andrikopoulos NK. Phytother Res. 2005 Dec; 19(12):1077–9.
337. Zeng HH et al. Acta Pharmacol Sin. 2001 Dec;22(12):1094–8.
338. Valenzuela A et al. Int J Food Sci Nutr. 2004 Mar;55(2): 155–62.
339. del Bano JM et al. J Agric Food Chem. 2003 Jul 16;51(15): 4247–53.
340. Santoyo S et al. J Food Prot. 2005 Apr;68(4):790–5.
341. Prabuseenivasan S et al. BMC Complement Altern Med. 2006 Nov 30;6:39.
342. Yano Y et al. Int J Food Microbiol. 2006 Aug 15;111(1):6–11.
343. Mahady GB et al. Phytother Res. 2005 Nov;19(11):988–91.
344. Lopez P et al. J Agric Food Chem. 2005 Aug 24; 53(17):6939–46.
345. Del Campo J et al. J Food Prot. 2000 Oct;63(10):1359–68.
346. Oluwatuyi M et al. Phytochemistry. 2004 Dec;65(24): 3249–54.
347. Shin S. Arch Pharm Res. 2003 May;26(5):389–93.
348. Giodani R et al. Phytother Res. 2004 Dec;18(12):990–5.
349. Aruoma OI et al. Food Chem Toxicol. 1996 May;34(5): 449–56.
350. Paris A et al. J Nat Prod. 1993 Aug;56(8):1426–30.
351. Gutierrez ME et al. Life Sci. 2003 Apr 11;72(21):2337–60.
352. Perez-Fons L et al. Arch Biochem Biophys. 2006 Sep 15; 453(2):224–36.
353. Kim SJ et al. Neuroreport 2006 Nov;17(16):1729–33.
354. Slamenova D et al. Cancer Lett. 2002 Mar 28;177(2):145–53.
355. del Bano MJ et al. J Agric Food Chem. 2006 Mar 22;54(6): 2064–8.
356. Offord EA et al. Cancer Lett. 1997 Mar 19;114(1–2):275–81.
357. Offord EA et al. Carcinogenesis. 1995 Sep;16(9):2057–62.
358. Saito Y et al. Biosci Biotechnol Biochem. 2004 Apr;68(4): 781–6.
359. Offord EA et al. Free Radic Biol Med. 2002 Jun 15;32(12): 1293–303.
360. Calabrese V et al. Int J Tissue React. 2001;23(2):51–8.
361. Vitaglione P et al. Crit Rev Food Sci Nutr. 2004;44(7–8): 575–86.
362. Kaziulin AN et al. Vopr Pitan. 2006;75(2):40–4.
363. Adsersen A et al. J Ethnopharmacol. 2006 Apr 6;104(3): 418–22.
364. Kosaka K, Yokoi T. Biol Pharm Bull. 2003 Nov;26(11):1620–2.
365. Moss M et al. Int J Neurosci. 2003 Jan;113(1):15–38.
366. Sanders C et al. Int J Neurosci. 2002 Nov;112(11):1305–20.
367. Diego MA et al. Int J Neurosci. 1998 Dec;96(3–4):217–24.
368. Plouzek CA et al. Eur J Cancer. 1999 Oct;35(10):1541–5.
369. Rau O et al. Planta Med. 2006 Aug;72(10):881–7.
370. Visanji JM et al. Cancer Lett. 2006 Jun 8;237(1):130–6.
371. Steiner M et al. Nutr Cancer. 2001;41(1–2):135–44.
372. Dorrie J et al. Cancer Lett. 2001 Sep 10;170(1):33–9.
373. al-Sereiti MR et al. Indian J Exp Biol. 1999 Feb;37(2):124–30.
374. Waliwitiya R et al. J Econ Entomol. 2005 Oct;98(5):1560–5.
375. Choi WS et al. J Am Mosq Control Assoc. 2002 Dec;18(4): 348–51.
376. Browning AM et al. J Pharm Pharmacol. 2005 Aug;57(8): 1037–42.
377. Nicolaides AN. Angiology. 2003 Jul–Aug;54 Suppl 1:S33–44.
378. Pecking AP et al. Angiology. 1997 Jan;48(1):93–8.
379. Amiel M, Barbe R. Ann Cardiol Angeiol (Paris). 1998 Mar; 47(3):185–8.
380. Korthuis RG, Gute DC. Adv Exp Med Biol. 2002;505: 181–90.
381. Filis KA et al. Int Angiol. 1999 Dec;18(4):327–30.
382. Manuel y Keenoy B et al. Diabetes Nutr Metab. 1999 Aug; 12(4):256–63.
383. Valensi PE et al. Diabet Med. 1996 Oct;13(10):882–8.
384. Lukaczer D et al. Phytother Res. 2005 Oct;19(10):864–9.
385. Fuchs SM et al. Skin Pharmacol Physiol. 2005 Jul–Aug; 18(4):195–200.
386. Hay IC et al. Arch Dermatol. 1998 Nov;134(11):1349–52.
387. Minnunni M et al. Mutat Res. 1992 Oct;269(2):193–200.
388. Samman S et al. Am J Clin Nutr. 2001 Mar;73(3):607–12.
389. Martinez-Gonzalez MC et al. Contact Dermatitis. 2007 Jan; 56(1):49–50.
390. Inui S, Katayama I. J Dermatol. 2005 Aug;32(8):667–9.
391. Serra E et al. Contact Dermatitis. 2005 Sep;53(3):179–80.
392. Gonzalez-Mahave I et al. Contact Dermatitis. 2006 Apr; 54(4):210–2.
393. Armisen M et al. Contact Dermatitis. 2003 Jan;48(1):52–3.
394. Laitinen LA et al. Pharm Res. 2004 Oct;21(10):1904–16.
395. Daferera DJ et al. J Agric Food Chem. 2002 Sep 25;50(20): 5503–7.
396. Richter J, Schellenberg I. Anal Bioanal Chem. 2007 Mar; 387(6):2207–17.
397. Velickovic DT et al. Ultrason Sonochem. 2006 Feb;13(2): 150–6.
398. Perry NB et al. J Agric Food Chem. 1999 May;47(5): 2048–54.
399. Funk C et al. Arch Biochem Biophys. 1992 Apr;294(1): 306–13.
400. Baskan S et al. Food Chem. 2007;101(4):1748–52.
401. Brieskorn CH, Fuchs A. Chem Ber. 1962;95:3034–41.
402. Bandoniene D et al. J Chromatogr Sci. 2005 Aug;43(7): 372–6.
403. Ben Hameda A et al. J Sep Sci. 2006 May;29(8):1188–92.
404. Zgorka G, Glowniak K. J Pharm Biomed Anal. 2001 Aug; 26(1):79–87.
405. Lu Y, Foo LY. Tetrahedron Lett. 2001 Nov 12;42(46): 8223–5.

406. Lu Y, Foo LY. Phytochemistry. 2002 Jan;59(2):117–40.
407. Lu Y, Foo LY. Phytochemistry. 2000 Oct;55(3):263–7.
408. Miura K et al. Phytochemistry. 2001 Dec;58(8):1171–5.
409. Capek P et al. Int J Biol Macromol. 2003 Nov;33(1–3):113–9.
410. Grassi P et al. Phytochem Anal. 2004 May–Jun;15(3): 198–203.
411. Santos-Gomes PC, Fernandes-Ferreira M. J Agric Food Chem. 2001 Jun;49(6):2908–16.
412. Basgel S, Erdemoglu SB. Sci Total Environ. 2006 Apr 15; 359(1–3):82–9.
413. Otoom SA et al. J Herb Pharmacother. 2006;6(2):31–41.
414. Bors W et al. Biol Res. 2004;37(2):301–11.
415. Matsingou TC et al. J Agric Food Chem. 2003 Nov 5;51(23): 6696–701.
416. Miura K et al. J Agric Food Chem. 2002 Mar 27;50(7): 1845–51.
417. Lu Y, Foo LY. Food Chem. 2001 Nov;75(2):197–202.
418. Zheng W, Wang SY. J Agric Food Chem. 2001 Nov;49(11): 5165–70.
419. Hohmann J et al. Planta Med. 1999 May;51(5):527–34.
420. Apak S et al. Int J Food Sci Nutr. 2006 Aug–Sep;57(5–6): 292–304.
421. Feres M et al. J Int Acad Periodontol. 2005 Jul;7(3):90–6.
422. Osawa K et al. Bull Tokyo Dent Coll. 1991 Feb;32(1):1–7.
423. Longaray Delamere AP et al. Food Chem. 2007;100(2): 603–8.
424. Pereira RS et al. Rev Saude Publica. 2004 Apr;38(2):326–8.
425. Pavlenko LV et al. Antibiot Khimioter. 1989 Aug;34(8):582–5.
426. Tada M et al. Phytochemistry. 1994 Jan;35(2):53941.
427. Capek P, Hribalova V. Phytochemistry. 2004 Jul;65(13): 1983–92.
428. Hubbert M et al. Eur J Med Res. 2006 Jan 31;11(1):20–6.
429. Saller R et al. Forsch Komplementarmed Klass Naturheilkd. 2001 Dec;8(6):373–82.
430. Kennedy DO et al. Neuropsychopharmacology. 2006 Apr; 31(4):845–52.
431. Savelev SU et al. Phytother Res. 2004;18(4):315–24.
432. Ferreira A et al. J Ethnopharmacol. 2006 Nov 3;108(1): 31–7.
433. Kavvadias D et al. Planta Med. 2003 Feb;69(2):113–7.
434. Akhondzadeh S et al. J Clin Pharm Ther. 2003 Feb;28(1): 53–9.
435. Vukovic-Gacic B et al. Food Chem Toxicol. 2006 Oct;44(10): 1730–8.
436. Simic D et al. Mutat Res. 1998 Jun 18;402(1–2):51–7.
437. Petersen M, Simmonds MS. Phytochemistry. 2003 Jan;62(2): 121–5.
438. De Leo V et al. Minerva Ginecol. 1998 May;50(5):207–11.
439. Shubina LP et al. Vrach Delo. 1990 May;(5):66–7.
440. Hellum BH et al. Basic Clin Pharmacol Toxicol. 2007 Jan; 100(1):23–30.
441. Bergeron C et al. J Agric Food Chem. 2005 Apr 20;53(8): 3076–80.
442. Yagmhai MS. Flav Frag J. 1988;3:27–31.
443. Bruno M et al. Phytochemistry. 1998 Jun;48(4):687–91.
444. Murch SJ et al. The Lancet. 1997 Nov 29;350(9091):1598–9.
445. Awad R et al. Phytomedicine. 2003 Nov;10(8):640–9.
446. Gafner S et al. J Nat Prod. 2003 Apr;66(4):535–7.
447. Gabrielska J et al. J Naturforsch [C]. 1997 Nov–Dec; 52(11–12):817–23.
448. Ma Z et al. Blood. 2005 Apr 15;105(8):3312–8.
449. Ding YZ et al. Biochem Biophys Res Commun. 1999 Dec 20;266(2):392–399.
450. Lyu SY et al. Arch Pharm Res. 2005 Nov;28(11):1293–301.
451. Zhang GH et al. Biochem Biophys Res Commun. 2005 Sep 2;334(3):812–6.
452. Huang Y et al. Curr Drug Targets Cardiovasc Haematol Disord. 2005 Apr;5(2):177–84.
453. Wolfson P, Hoffmann DL. Altern Ther Health Med. 2003 Mar–Apr;9(2):74–8.
454. MacGregor FB et al. BMJ. 1989 Nov 4;299(6708):1156–7.
455. Gafner S et al. J AOAC Int. 2003 May–Jun;86(3):453–60.
456. Kouzi SA et al. Chem Res Toxicol. 1994 Nov;7(6):850–6.
457. Haznaagy-Radnai E et al. Fitoterapia. 2006 Dec;77(7–8): 521–4.
458. Meremeti A et al. Biochem Sys Ecol. 2004 Feb;32(2):139–51.
459. Miyase T et al. Phytochemistry. 1996 Sep;43(2):475–9.
460. Vundac VB et al. Biochem Sys Ecol. 2006 Dec;34(12): 875–81.
461. Radnai E et al. ISHS Acta Horticulturae 597 International Conference on Medicinal and Aromatic Plants (Part II).
462. Matkowski A, Piotrowska M. Fitoterapia. 2006 Jul;77(5): 346–53.
463. Matkowski A, Wolniak D. BMC Plant Biol. 2005;5(Suppl 1):S23.
464. Jordan MJ et al. Indust Crops Prod. 2006 Nov;24(3): 253–63.
465. Echeverrigaray S et al. J Agric Food Chem. 2001 Sep;49(9): 4220–3.
466. Thompson JD et al. J Chem Ecol. 2003 Apr;29(4):859–80.
467. Guillen MD, Manzanos MJ. Food Chem. 1998 Nov;63(3): 373–83.
468. Diaz-Maroto MC et al. J Agric Food Chem. 2005 Jun 29; 53(13):5385–9.
469. Hudaib M et al. J Pharm Biomed Anal. 2002 Jul 20;29(4): 691–700.
470. Raal A et al. Medicina (Kaunas). 2004;40(8):795–800.
471. Proestos C et al. J Agric Food Chem. 2005 Feb 23;53(4): 1190–5.
472. Morimitsu Y et al. Biosci Biotechnol Biochem. 1995 Nov; 59(11):2018–21.
473. Chun H et al. Biol Pharm Bull. 2001 Aug;24(8):941–6.
474. Wang M et al. J Agric Food Chem. 1999 May;47(5):1911–4.
475. Agbor GA et al. J Agric Food Chem. 2005 Aug 24;53(17): 6819–24.
476. Dapkevicius A et al. J Nat Prod. 2002 Jun;65(6):892–6.
477. Nakatani N. Biofactors. 2000;13(1–4):141–6.
478. Haraguchi H et al. Planta Med. 1996 Jun;62(3):217–21.
479. Lee KG, Shibamoto T. J Agric Food Chem. 2002 Aug 14; 50(17):4947–52.
480. Zheng W, Wang SY. J Agric Food Chem. 2001 Nov;49(11): 5165–70.
481. Braga PC et al. Pharmacology. 2006;76(2):61–8.
482. Braga PC et al. Pharmacology. 2006;77(3):130–6.
483. Yano Y et al. Int J Food Microbiol. 2006 Aug 15;111(1): 6–11.
484. Fan M, Chen J. Wei Sheng Wu Xue Bao. 2001 Aug;41(4): 499–504.
485. Essawi T, Srour M. J Ethnopharmacol. 2000 Jun;70(3): 343–9.
486. Lall N, Meyer JJ. J Ethnopharmacol. 1999 Sep;66(3):347–54.
487. Tabak M et al. J Appl Bacteriol. 1996 Jun;80(6):667–72.

488. Ghazaleh BM. Jpn J Infect Dis. 2000 Jun;53(3):111–5.
489. Fujita M et al. Microbiol Immunol. 2005;49(4):391–6.
490. Kohlert C et al. J Clin Pharmacol. 2002 Jul;42(7):731–7.
491. Marino M et al. J Food Prot. 1999 Sep;62(9):1017–23.
492. Penalver P et al. APMIS. 2005 Jan;113(1):1–6.
493. Nguefack J et al. Lett Appl Microbiol. 2004;39(5):395–400.
494. Pina-Vaz C et al. J Eur Acad Dermatol Venereol. 2004 Jan; 18(1):73–8.
495. Bozin B et al. J Agric Food Chem. 2006 Mar 8;54(5):1822–8.
496. Dusan F et al. Toxicol In Vitro. 2006 Dec;20(8):1435–45.
497. Rasooli I et al. Int J Infect Dis. 2006 May;10(3):236–41.
498. Schelz Z et al. Fitoterapia. 2006 Jun;77(4):279–85.
499. Burt SA, Reinders RD. Lett Appl Microbiol. 2003;36(3): 162–7.
500. Inouye S et al. J Infect Chemother. 2001 Dec;7(4):251–4.
501. Inouye S et al. J Antimicrob Chemother. 2001 May;47(5): 565–73.
502. Inouye S et al. Mycoses. 2000;43(1–2):17–23.
503. Agnihotri S, Vaidya AD. Indian J Exp Biol. 1996 Jul;34(7): 712–5.
504. Juven BJ et al. J Appl Bacteriol. 1994 Jun;76(6):626–31.
505. Smith-Palmer A et al. J Med Microbiol. 2002 Jul;51(7): 567–74.
506. Hersch-Martinez P et al. Fitoterapia. 2005 Jul;76(5):453–7.
507. Inouye S et al. Mycoses. 2001 May;44(3–4):99–107.
508. Soliman KM, Badeaa RI. Food Chem Toxicol. 2002 Nov; 40(11):1669–75.
509. Bonjar GH. Fitoterapia. 2004 Jan;75(1):74–6.
510. Giordani R et al. Phytother Res. 2004 Dec;18(12):990–5.
511. Santoro GF et al. Parasitol Res. 2007 Mar;100(4):783–90.
512. Mikus J et al. Planta Med. 2000 May;66(4):366–8.
513. Fuselli SR et al. Rev Argent Microbiol. 2006 Apr–Jun;38(2): 89–92.
514. Park BS et al. J Am Mosq Control Assoc. 2005 Mar;21(1): 80–3.
515. Kluth D et al. Free Radic Biol Med. 2007 Feb 1;42(3): 315–25.
516. Aydin S et al. J Agric Food Chem. 2005 Feb 23;53(4): 1299–305.
517. Aydin S et al. Mutat Res. 2005 Mar 7;581(1–2):43–53.
518. Zava DT et al. Proc Soc Exp Biol Med. 1998 Mar;217(3): 369–78.
519. Jukic M et al. Phytother Res. 2007 Mar;21(3):259–61.
520. Jager AK et al. J Ethnopharmacol. 2006 Apr;21;105(1–2): 294–300.
521. Priestley CM et al. Br J Pharmacol. 2003 Dec;140(8):1363–72.
522. Sterer N, Rubinstein Y. Quintessence Int. 2006 Sep;37(8): 653–8.
523. Okazaki K et al. Phytother Res. 2002 Jun;16(4):398–9.
524. Kemmerich B et al. Arzneimittelforschung. 2006;56(9): 652–60.
525. Buechi S et al. Forsch Komplementarmed Klass Naturheilkd. 2005 Dec;12(6):328–32.
526. Gruenwald J et al. Arzneimittelforschung. 2005;55(11): 669–76.
527. Hagedorn M. Z Hautkr. 1989 Sep 15;64(9):810, 813–4.
528. Manou I et al. J Appl Microbiol. 1998 Mar;217(3):369–78.
529. Zani F et al. Planta Med. 1991 Jun;57(3):237–41.
530. Golec M et al. Ann Agric Environ Med. 2005;12(1):5–10.
531. Mackiewcz B et al. Ann Agric Environ Med. 1999;6(2): 167–70.
532. Lemiere C et al. Allergy. 1996 Dec;51(9):647–9.
533. Spiewak R et al. Contact Dermatitis. 2001 Apr;44(4):235–9.
534. Armisen M et al. Contact Dermatitis. 2003 Jan;48(1):52–3.
535. Foster BC et al. Phytomedicine. 2003 May;10(4):334–42.

Lauraceae

1. Jayatilaka A et al. Anal Chim Acta. 1995 Feb;302(2–3):147–62.
2. Wijseskera RO. CRC Crit Rev Food Sci Nutr. 1978;10(1):1–30.
3. Channe Gowda D, Sarathy C. Carbohydr Res. 1987 Sep 1; 166(2):263–9.
4. Martindale, The Extra Pharmacopoeia 26th Ed. Pharmaceutical Press London March 1973 p. 1237.
5. Mancini-Filho J et al. Boll Chim Farm. 1998 Dec;137(11):443–7.
6. Chericoni S et al. J Agric Food Chem. 2005 Jun 15;53(12):4762–5.
7. Hersch-Martinez P et al. Fitoterapia. 2005 Jul;76(5):453–7.
8. Prabuseenivasan S et al. BMC Complement Altern Med. 2006 Nov 30;6:39–46.
9. Raybaudi-Massilia RM et al. J Food Prot. 2006 Jul;69(7): 1579–86.
10. Lopez P et al. J Agric Food Chem. 2005 Aug 24;53(17): 6939–46.
11. Inouye S et al. Int J Aromather. 2003;13(1):33–41.
12. Tabak M et al. J Appl Bacteriol. 1996;80(6):667–72.
13. Raharivelomanana PJ et al. Arch Inst Pasteur Madagascar. 1989;56(1):261–71.
14. Smith-Palmer A et al. J Med Microbiol. 2002 Jul;51(7):567–74.
15. Pawar VC, Thaker VS. Mycoses. 2006 Jul;49(4):316–23.
16. Tampieri MP et al. Mycopathologia. 2005 Apr;159(3):339–45.
17. Simic A et al. Phytother Res. 2004 Sep;18(9):713–7.
18. Soliman KM, Badeaa RI. Food Chem Toxicol. 2002 Nov;40(11): 1669–75.
19. Singh HB et al. Allergy. 1995 Dec;50(12):995–9.
20. Lima EO et al. Mycoses. 1993 Sep–Oct;36(9–10):333–6.
21. Quale JM et al. Am J Chin Med. 1996;24(2):103–9.
22. Yang YC et al. Int J Parasitol. 2005 Dec;35(14):1595–600.
23. Raj RK. Indian J Physiol Pharmacol. 1975 Jan–Mar;19(1): unknown.
24. Rosti L, Gastaldi G. Pediatrics. 2005 Oct;116(4):1057.
25. Ka H et al. Cancer Lett. 2003 Jul 10;196(2):143–52.
26. Huss U et al. J Nat Prod. 2002 Nov;65(11):1517–21.
27. Hamdan II, Afifi FU. J Ethnopharmacol. 2004 Jul;93(1): 117–21.
28. Verspohl EJ et al. Phytother Res. 2005 Mar;19(3):203–6.
29. Ungsurungsie M et al. Food Chem Toxicol. 1984 Feb;22(2): 109–12.
30. Sparks T. West J Med. 1985 Jun;142(6):835.
31. Endo H, Rees TD. Compend Contin Educ Dent. 2006 Jul; 27(7):403–9.
32. Hoskyn J, Guin JD. Contact Dermatitis. 2005 Mar;52(3):160–1.
33. Cohen DM, Bhattacharyya I. J Am Dent Assoc. 2000 Jul; 131(7):929–34.
34. Nadiminti H et al. Contact Dermatitis. 2005 Jan;52(1):46–7.
35. Garcia-Abujeta JL et al. Contact Dermatitis. 2005 Apr; 52(4):234.
36. Kanerva L et al. Contact Dermatitis. 1996 Sep;35(3):157–62.
37. Nixon R. Australas J. Dermatol. 1995 Feb;36(1):41.
38. Goh CL, Ng SK. Derm Beruf Umwelt. 1988 Nov–Dec; 36(6):186–7.
39. White A et al. Inflamm Bowel Dis. 2006 Jun;12(6):508–14.
40. Westra WH et al. Head Neck. 1998 Aug;20(5):430–3.

Liliaceae

1. Claus EP. Pharmacognosy 4th Ed. Henry Kimpton. London 1961.
2. Dr Duke's Phytochemical and Ethnobotanical Databases. http://www.ars-grin.gov/duke/.
3. Felter HW, Lloyd JU. 1898. King's American Dispensatory, 18th ed., reprinted by Eclectic Medical Publications, Portland, OR.
4. Ichikawa M et al. J Agric Food Chem. 2006 Jun 28;54(13): 4849–54.
5. Amagase H. J Nutr. 2006 Mar;136(3Suppl):716S–25S.
6. Zheng P et al. Se Pu. 2006 Jul;24(4):351–3.
7. Miean KH, Mohamed S. J Agric Food Chem. 2001 Jun; 49(6):3106–12.
8. Mochizuki E et al. J AOAC Int. 2004 Sep–Oct;87(5):1063–9.
9. Arnault I, Auger J. J Chromatogr A. 2006 Apr 21;1112(1–2): 23–30.
10. Gorinstein S et al. J Agric Food Chem. 2005 Apr 6;53(7): 2726–32.
11. Dumont E et al. Anal Bioanal Chem. 2006 Mar;384(5): 1196–206.
12. Horn-Ross PL et al. Cancer Causes Control. 2000 Apr;11(4): 289–98.
13. Baumgartner S et al. Carbohydr Res. 2000 Sep 8;328(2):177–83.
14. Wang HX, Ng TB. Life Sci. 2001 Dec 7;70(3):357–65.
15. Xia L, Ng TB. Peptides. 2005 Feb;26(2):177–83.
16. Lee J, Harnly JM. J Agric Food Chem. 2005 Nov 16;53(23): 9100–4.
17. Ichikawa M et al. J Agric Food Chem. 2006 Mar 8;54(5): 1535–40.
18. Hughes J et al. Plant Foods Hum Nutr. 2006 Jun;61(2):81–5.
19. Ryback ME et al. J Agric Food Chem. 2004 Feb 25;52(4): 682–7.
20. Arnault I et al. J Pharm Biomed Anal. 2005 Apr 29;37(5): 963–70.
21. WHO Monographs on Selected Medicinal Plants—Vol 1. WHO Geneva 1999 p. 16–32.
22. Lonsdale D. Med Sci Monit. 2004 Sep;10(9):RA199–203.
23. Shukla Y, Kalra N. Cancer Lett. 2007 Mar 18;247(2):167–81.
24. Dumont E et al. Anal Bioanal Chem. 2006 Aug;385(7):1304–23.
25. Fox TE et al. Int J Vitam Nutr Res. 2005 May;75(3):179–86.
26. Lavilla I et al. J Agric Food Chem. 1999 Dec;47(12):5072–7.
27. Wang XP, Xiang SL. Guang Pu Xue Yu Guang Pu Fen Xi. 2006 Oct;26(10):1907–11.
28. Kroes BH. J Nutr. 2006 Mar;136(3S):732S–35S.
29. Freeman F, Kodera Y. J Agric Food Chem. 1995 Sep;43(9): 2332–8.
30. Lawson LD, Gardner CD. J Agric Food Chem. 2005 Aug 10; 53(16):6254–61.
31. Kim HK et al. J Med Food. 2005 Winter;8(4):476–81.
32. Lawson LD, Wang ZJ. J Agric Food Chem. 2005 Mar 23;53(6): 1974–83.
33. Amagase H et al. J Nutr. 2001 Mar;131(3S):955S–62S.
34. Ariga T, Seki T. Biofactors. 2006 26(2):93–103.
35. Lawson LD et al. Planta Med. 2001 Feb;67(1):13–8.
36. Lawson LD, Wang ZJ. J Agric Food Chem. 2001 May;49(5): 2592–9.
37. Spigelski D, Jones PJ. Nutr Rev. 2001 Jul;59(7):236–41.
38. Zhang XH et al. J Nutr. 2001 May;131(5):1471–8.
39. Chung LY. J Med Food. 2006 Summer;9(2):205–13.
40. Okada Y et al. Redox Rep. 2005;10(2):96–102.
41. Yin MC et al. J Agric Food Chem. 2002 Oct 9;50(21):6143–7.
42. Siegers CP et al. Phytomedicine. 1999 Mar;6(1):13–6.
43. Stajner D et al. Phytother Res. 2006 Jul;20(7):581–4.
44. Pedraza-Chaverri J et al. Food Chem Toxicol. 2007 Apr; 45(4):622–7.
45. Pedraza-Chaverri J et al. Nutr J. 2004 Sep 1;3:10.
46. Leelarungrayub N et al. Nutrition. 2006 Mar;22(3):266–74.
47. Harris JC et al. Appl Microbiol Biotechnol. 2001 Oct;57(3): 282–6.
48. Iwalokun BA et al. J Med Food. 2004 Fall;7(3):327–33.
49. Lee YL et al. Nutrition. 2003 Nov–Dec;19(11–12):994–6.
50. Unal R et al. J Food Prot. 2001 Feb;64(2):189–94.
51. Jonkers D et al. Antimicrob Agents Chemother. 1999 Dec; 43(12):3045.
52. Cutler RR, Wilson P. Br J Biomed Sci. 2004;61(2):71–4.
53. Gomaa NF, Hashish MH. J Egypt Public Health Assoc. 2003; 78(5–6):361–72.
54. Ruddock PS et al. Phytother Res. 2005 Apr;19(4):327–34.
55. Dikasso D et al. Ethiop Med J. 2002 Jul;40(3):241–9.
56. Canizares P et al. Biotechnol Prog. 2004 Jan–Feb;20(1):32–7.
57. Mahady GB et al. Am J Gastroenterol. 2001 Dec;96(12):3454–5.
58. O'Gara EA et al. Appl Environ Microbiol. 2000 May;66(5): 2269–73.
59. Sasaki J, Kita J. J Nutr Sci Vitaminol (Tokyo). 2003 Aug;49(4): 297–9.
60. Ankri S, Mirelman D. Microbes Infect. 1999 Feb;1(2):125–9.
61. Bakri IM, Douglas CW. Arch Oral Biol. 2005 Jul;50(7):645–51.
62. Groppo FC et al. Int Dent J. 2002 Dec;52(6):433–7.
63. Tsao SM, Yin MC. J Med Microbiol. 2001 Jul;50(7):646–9.
64. Sivam GP. J Nutr. 2001 Mar;131(3s):1106S–8S.
65. Betoni JE et al. Mem Inst Oswaldo Cruz. 2006 Jun;101(4): 387–90.
66. Ward P et al. J Food Prot. 2002 Mar;65(3):528–33.
67. Ross ZM et al. Appl Environ Microbiol. 2001 Jan;67(1): 475–80.
68. Sasaki J et al. J Nutr Sci Vitaminol (Tokyo). 1999 Dec;45(6): 785–90.
69. Ledezma E, Apitz-Castro R. Rev Iberoam Micol. 2006 Jun; 23(2):75–80.
70. Thamburan S et al. Phytother Res. 2006 Oct;20(1):844–50.
71. Shuford JA et al. Antimicrob Agents Chemother. 2005 Jan; 49(1):473.
72. Lemar KM et al. J Eukaryot Microbiol. 2003;50 Suppl:685–6.
73. Davis SR et al. J Antimicrob Chemother. 2003 Mar;51(3):593–7.
74. Shadkchan Y et al. J Antimicrob Chemother. 2004 May;53(5): 832–6.
75. Shams-Ghahfarokhi M et al. Fitoterapia. 2006 Jun;77(4):321–3.
76. Avato P et al. Phytomedicine. 2000 Jun;7(3):239–43.
77. Visbal G et al. Curr Drug Targets Infect Disord. 2005 Sep;5(3): 211–26.
78. Lemar KM et al. Microbiology. 2005 Oct;151(Pt 10):3257–65.
79. Ogita A et al. Planta Med. 2006 Oct;72(13):1247–50.
80. Pyun MS, Shin S. Phytomedicine. 2006 Jun;13(6):394–400.
81. Lemar KM et al. J Appl Microbiol. 2002;93(3):398–405.
82. Zhen H et al. Antiviral Res. 2006 Oct;72(1):68–74.
83. Shu SN et al. Zhongguo Zhong Yao Za Zhi. 2003 Oct;28(10): 967–70.
84. Fang F et al. J Tongji Med Univ. 1999;19(4):271–4.
85. Luo R et al. Zhonghua Shi Yan He Lin Chuang Bing Du Xue Za Zhi. Jun;15(2):135–8.
86. No authors listed. Treatment Update. 1998 May;10(3):1–2.
87. Harris JC et al. Microbiology. 2000 Dec;146 Pt 12:3119–27.

88. Anthony JP et al. Trends Parasitol. 2005 Oct;21(10):462–8.
89. Ledzema E et al. Parasitol Res. 2002 Aug;88(8):748–53.
90. Coppi A et al. Antimicrob Agents Chemother. 2006 May; 50(5):1731–7.
91. Sabitha P et al. Trop Doct. 2005 Apr;35(2):99–100.
92. Sarrell EM et al. Pediatrics. 2003 May;111(5 Pt 1):e574–9.
93. Sarrell EM et al. Arch Pediatr Adolesc Med. 2001 Jul; 155(7):796–9.
94. Ledezma E et al. J Am Acad Dermatol. 2000 Nov;43(5 Pt 1): 829–32.
95. Ledezma E et al. Arzneimittelforschung. 1999 Jun;49(6): 544–7.
96. Xie XL et al. Zhong Nan Da Xue Xue Bao Yi Xue Ban. 2004 Jun;29(3):330–1.
97. Dehghani F et al. Int J Dermatol. 2005 Jul;44(7):612–5.
98. You WC et al. Int J Epidemiol. 1998 Dec;27(6):941–4.
99. Salih BA, Abasiyanik FM. Saudi Med J. 2003 Aug; 24(8):842–5.
100. McNulty CA et al. Helicobacter. 2001 Sep;6(3):249–53.
101. Josling P. Adv Ther. 2001 Jul–Aug;18(4):189–93.
102. Andrianova IV et al. Ter Arkh. 2003;75(3):53–6.
103. Davis SR. Mycoses. 2005 Mar;48(2):95–100.
104. Knowles LM, Milner JA. J Nutr. 2001 Mar;131(3S):1061S–6S.
105. Song K, Milner JA. J Nutr. 2001 Mar;131(3S):1054S–7S.
106. Pinto JT et al. J Nutr. 2006 Mar;136(3S):835S–41S.
107. Milner JA et al. J Nutr. 2006 Mar;136(3S):827S–31S.
108. Xiao D et al. Cancer Res. 2003 Oct 15;63(20):6825–37.
109. Hosono T et al. J Biol Chem. 2005 Dec 16;280(50):41487–93.
110. Xiao D, Singh SV. Carcinogenesis. 2006 Mar;27(3):533–40.
111. Xiao D et al. Mol Cancer Ther. 2005 Sep;4(9):1388–98.
112. Li M et al. Carcinogenesis. 2002 Apr;23(4):573–9.
113. Zhang YW et al. Arch Pharm Res. 2006 Dec;29(12):1125–31.
114. Karmakar S et al. Apoptosis. 2007 Apr;12(4):671–84.
115. Xiao D et al. Oncogene. 2005 Sep 15;24(41):6256–69.
116. Gunadharini DN et al. Cell Biochem Funct. 2006 Sep–Oct; 24(5):407–12.
117. Arunkumar A et al. Biol Pharm Bull. 2005 Apr;28(4):740–3.
118. Arunkumar A et al. Cancer Lett. 2007 Jun 18;251(1):59–67.
119. Arunkumar A et al. Mol Cell Biochem. 2006 Aug;288(1–2): 107–13.
120. Xiao XL et al. Ai Zheng. 2006 Oct;25(10):1247–51.
121. Ling H et al. Cell Mol Biol Lett. 2006;11(3):408–23.
122. Ha MW et al. World J Gastroenterol. 2005 Sep 21;11(35): 5433–7.
123. Park SY et al. Cancer Lett. 2005 Jun 16;224(1):123–32.
124. Wu XJ et al. Mutat Res. 2005 Nov 11;579(1–2):115–24.
125. Hong YS et al. Exp Mol Med. 2000 Sep 30;32(3):127–34.
126. Hirsch K et al. Nutr Cancer. 2000;38(2):245–54.
127. Lund T et al. Br J Cancer. 2005 May 9;92(9):1773–81.
128. Chang HS et al. Cancer Lett. 2005 Jun 1;223(1):47–55.
129. Hassan HT. Leuk Res. 2004 Jul;28(7):667–71.
130. Xu B et al. Fundam Clin Pharmacol. 2004 Apr;18(2):171–80.
131. Kwon KB et al. Biochem Pharmacol. 2002 Jan 1;63(1):41–7.
132. Dirsch VM et al. Leukaemia. 2002 Jan;16(1):74–83.
133. Wu CC et al. Food Chem Toxicol. 2004 Dec;42(12):1937–47.
134. De Martino A et al. J Nutr Biochem. 2006 Nov;17(11):742–9.
135. Wen J et al. Biochem Pharmacol. 2004 Jul 15;68(2):323–31.
136. Jakubikova J, Sedlak J. Neoplasma. 2006;53(3):191–9.
137. Su CC et al. In Vivo. 2006 Jan–Feb;20(1):85–90.
138. Chung JG et al. Food Chem Toxicol. 2004 Feb;42(2):195–202.
139. Yu FS et al. Food Chem Toxicol. 2005 Jul;43(7):1029–36.
140. Lu HF et al. Food Chem Toxicol. 2004 Oct;42(10):1543–52.
141. Chung JG. Drug Chem Toxicol. 1999 May;22(2):343–58.
142. Nakagawa H et al. Carcinogenesis. 2001 Jun;22(6):891–7.
143. Pinto JT, Rivlin RS. J Nutr. 2001 Mar;131(3S):1058S–60S.
144. Tsai CW et al. J Agric Food Chem. 2007 Feb 7;55(3):1019–26.
145. Chen C et al. Free Radic Biol Med. 2004 Nov 15;37(10): 1578–90.
146. Sabayan B et al. Med Hypotheses. 2007;68(3):512–4.
147. Yadav S et al. Bull Environ Contam Toxicol. 2006 Oct; 77(4):477–83.
148. Bhattacharya K et al. Toxicol Lett. 2004 Nov 28;153(3): 327–32.
149. Lohani M et al. Toxicol Lett. 2003 Jun 5;143(1):45–50.
150. Belloir C et al. Food Chem Toxicol. 2006 Jun;44(6):827–34.
151. Yu FL et al. Cancer Detect Prev. 2003;27(5):370–9.
152. Siddique YH, Afzal M. J Environ Biol. 2005 Jul;26(3):547–50.
153. Siddique YH, Afzal M. Indian J Exp Biol. 2004 Apr;42(4): 437–8.
154. L'vova GN, Zasukhina GD. Genetika. 2002 Mar;38(3): 306–9.
155. Vasil'eva IM, Zasukhina GD. Genetika. 2002 Mar;38(3): 422–5.
156. Son EW et al. Int Immunopharmacol. 2006 Dec 5;6(12): 1788–95.
157. Seki T et al. Cancer Lett. 2000 Nov 10;160(1):29–35.
158. Chu Q et al. Carcinogenesis. 2006 Nov;27(11):2180–9.
159. Mousa AS, Mousa SA. Nutr Cancer. 2005;53(1):104–10.
160. Xiao D et al. Nutr Cancer. 2006;55(1):94–107.
161. Ahmed N et al. Anticancer Res. 2001 Sep–Oct;21(5):3519–23.
162. Galeone C et al. Am J Clin Nutr. 2006 Nov;84(5):1027–32.
163. Fleischauer AT, Arab L. J Nutr. 2001 Mar;131(3S):1032S–40S.
164. Challier B et al. Eur J Epidemiol. 1998 Dec;14(8):737–47.
165. Schulz M et al. Cancer Epidemiol Biomarkers Prev. 2005 Nov;14(11 Pt 1):2531–5.
166. Fleischauer AT et al. Am J Clin Nutr. 2000 Oct;72(4): 1047–52.
167. Takezaki T et al. Jpn J Cancer Res. 2001 Nov;92(11):1157–65.
168. Gonzalez CA et al. Int J Cancer. 2006 May 15;118(10): 2559–66.
169. Setiawan VW et al. Asian Pac J Cancer Prev. 2005 Jul–Sep; 6(3):387–95.
170. Zickute J et al. Medicina (Kaunas). 2005;41(9):733–40.
171. Hsing AW et al. J Natl Cancer Inst. 2002 Nov 6;94(21): 1648–51.
172. Chung MJ et al. Cancer Lett. 2002 Aug 8;182(1):1–10.
173. Tilli CMLJ et al. Arch Dermatol Res. 2003 Jul 1;295(3):117–23.
174. Cavagnaro PF et al. J Agric Food Chem. 2007 Feb 21;55(4): 1280–8.
175. Fukao H et al. Biosci Biotechnol Biochem. 2007 Jan;71(1): 84–90.
176. Pierre S et al. Platelets. 2005 Dec;16(8):469–73.
177. Bordia A. Atherosclerosis. 1978 Aug;30(4):355–60.
178. Briggs WH et al. J Agric Food Chem. 2000 Nov;48(11): 5731–5.
179. Ali M et al. Prostaglandins Leukot Essent Fatty Acids. 1999 Jan;60(1):43–7.
180. Lawson LD et al. Thromb Res. 1992 Jan 15;65(2):141–56.
181. Suboh SM et al. Phytother Res. 2004 Apr;18(4):280–4.
182. Zhang JL et al. Zhongguo Zhong Xi Yi Jie He Za Zhi. 2002 Jun;22(6):423–5.
183. Rassoul F et al. Phytomedicine. 2006 Mar;13(4):230–5.
184. Siegel G et al. Phytomedicine. 2004 Jan;11(1):24–35.
185. Ho SE et al. Phytomedicine. 2001 Jan;8(1):39–46.

186. Ou CC et al. Lipids. 2003 Mar;38(3):219–24.
187. Huang CN et al. J Agric Food Chem. 2004 Jun 2;52(11): 3674–8.
188. Rahman K, Lowe GM. J Nutr. 2006 Mar;136(3S):736S–40S.
189. Mathew BC et al. Kathmandu Univ Med J (KUMJ). 2004 Apr–Jun;2(2):100–2.
190. Xu S, Simon Cho BH. J Nutr Biochem. 1999 Nov;10(11): 654–9.
191. Gupta N, Porter TD. J Nutr. 2001 Jun 13;131(16):1662–7.
192. Lin MC et al. J Nutr. 2002 Jun;132(6):1165–8.
193. Orekhov AN, Tertov VV. Lipids. 1997 Oct;32(10):1055–60.
194. Makris A et al. Placenta. 2005 Nov;26(10):828–34.
195. Garcia Gomez LJ, Sanchez-Muniz FJ. Arch Latinoam Nutr. 2000 Sep;50(3):219–29.
196. Banerjee SK, Maulik SK. Nutr J. 2002 Nov;19;1:4.
197. Stevinson C et al. Ann Intern Med. 2000 Sep 19;133(6): 420–9.
198. van Doorn MB et al. Am J Clin Nutr. 2006 Dec;84(6):1324–9.
199. Mahmoodi M et al. Pak J Pharm Sci. 2006 Oct;19(4):295–8.
200. Dhawan V, Jain S. Mol Cell Biochem. 2005 Jul;275(1–2): 85–94.
201. Qidwai W et al. J Pak Med Assoc. 2000 Jun;50(6):204–7.
202. Capraz M et al. Int J Cardiol. 2007 Sep 14;121(1):130–1.
203. Koscielny J et al. Atherosclerosis. 1999 May;144(1):237–49.
204. Siegel G, Klussendorf D. Atherosclerosis. 2000 Jun;150(2): 437–8.
205. Breithaupt-Grogler K et al. Circulation. 1997 Oct 21;96(8): 2649–55.
206. Kiesewetter H et al. Int J Clin Pharmacol Ther Toxicol. 1991 Apr;29(4):151–5.
207. Manoharan A et al. Am J Hematol. 2006 Sep;81(9):676–83.
208. Anim-Nyame N et al. J Nutr Biochem. 2004 Jan;15(1):30–6.
209. Wohlrab J et al. Arzneimittelforschung. 2000 Jul;50(7): 606–12.
210. Jepson RG et al. Cochrane Database Syst Rev. 2000;(2): CD000095.
211. Sobenin IA et al. Klin Med (Mosk). 2005;83(4):52–5.
212. Verma SK et al. Indian J Physiol Pharmacol. 2005 Jan;49(1): 115–8.
213. Najafi Sani M et al. World J Gastroenterol. 2006 Apr 21; 12(15):2427–31.
214. Akyuz F et al. Eur J Intern Med. 2005 Apr;16(2):126–8.
215. Abrams GA, Fallon MB. J Clin Gastroenterol. 1998 Oct; 27(3):232–5.
216. Rapp A et al. Forsch Komplementarmed. 2006 Jun;13(3): 141–6.
217. Meher S, Duley L. Cochrane Database Syst Rev. 2006 Jul 19;3:CD006065.
218. Ziaei S et al. Eur J Obstet Gynecol Reprod Biol. 2001 Dec 1; 99(2):201–6.
219. Cho SJ et al. Nutrition. 2006 Nov–Dec;22(11–12):1177–84.
220. Lamm DL, Riggs DR. Urol Clin North Am. 2000 Feb;27(1): 157–62.
221. Spelman K et al. Altern Med Rev. 2006 Jun;11(2):128–50.
222. Keiss HP et al. J Nutr. 2003 Jul;133(7):2171–5.
223. Hodge G et al. Cytometry. 2002 Aug 1;48(4):209–15.
224. Salman H et al. Int J Immunopharmacol. 1999 Sep;21(9): 589–97.
225. Hassan ZM et al. Int Immunopharmacol. 2003 Oct;3(10–11): 1483–9.
226. Lang A et al. Clin Nutr. 2004 Oct;23(5):1199–208.
227. Romano EL et al. Immunopharmacol Immunotoxicol. 1997 Feb;19(1):15–36.
228. Sela U et al. Immunology. 2004 Apr;111(4):391–9.
229. Elango EM et al. J Appl Genet. 2004;45(4):469–71.
230. Nijhawan S et al. Trop Gastroenterol. 2000 Oct–Dec; 21(4):177–9.
231. Chakrabarti K et al. Asian J Androl. 2003 Jun;5(2):131–5.
232. Jarial MS. J Med Entomol. 2001 May;38(3):446–50.
233. Berspalov VG et al. Vopr Onkol. 2004;50(1):81–5.
234. Denisov LM et al. Ter Arkh. 1999;71(8):55–8.
235. Jabbari A et al. Lipids Health Dis. 2005 May 19;4:11.
236. Valerio L, Maroli M. Ann Ist Super Sanita. 2005;41(2):253–6.
237. Rajan RV et al. Med Vet Entomol. 2005 Mar;19(1):84–9.
238. Staba EJ et al. J Nutr. 2001 Mar;131(3S):1118S–9S.
239. Miron T et al. Biochim Biophys Acta. 2000 Jan 15;1463(1): 20–30.
240. Rosen RT et al. J Nutr. 2001 Mar;131(3S):968S–71S.
241. Tamaki T, Sonoki S. J Nutr Sci Vitaminol (Tokyo). 1999 Apr; 45(2):213–22.
242. Teyssier C et al. Drug Metab Dispos. 1999 Jul;27(7):835–41.
243. Suarez F et al. Am J Physiol. 1999 Feb;276(2 Pt 1):G425–30.
244. Verhagen H et al. Br J Nutr. 2001 Aug;86 Suppl 1:S111–4.
245. Mennella JA, Beauchamp GK. Pediatr Res. 1993 Dec; 34(6):805–8.
246. Guyonnet D et al. Mutat Res. 2001 Aug 22;495(1–2):135–45.
247. Ackermann RT et al. Arch Intern Med. 2001 Mar 26;161(6): 813–24.
248. Friedman T et al. Int J Dermatol. 2006 Oct;45(10):1161–3.
249. Baruchin AM et al. Burns. 2001 Nov;27(7):781–2.
250. Kao SH et al. J Allergy Clin Immunol. 2003;50 Suppl:685–6.
251. Moneret-Vautrin DA et al. Allerg Immunol (Paris). 2002 Apr;34(4):135–40.
252. Pires G et al. Allergy. 2002 Oct;57(10):957–8.
253. Hughes TM et al. Contact Dermatitis. 2002 Jul;47(1):48.
254. Lerbaek A et al. Contact Dermatitis. 2004 Aug;51(2):79–83.
255. Jappe U et al. Am J Contact Dermat. 1999 Mar;10(1):37–9.
256. Fernandez-Vozmediano JM et al. Contact Dermatitis. 2000 Feb;42(2):108–9.
257. Alvarez MS et al. Am J Contact Dermatol. 2003 Sep;14(3): 161–5.
258. Jimenez-Timon A et al. Allergol Immunopathol (Madr). 2002 Sep–Oct;30(5):295–9.
259. Perez-Pimiento AJ et al. Allergy. 1999 Jun;54(6):626–9.
260. Ruocco V et al. Dermatology. 1996;192(4):373–4.
261. Carden SM et al. Clin Experiment Ophthalmol. 2002 Aug; 30(4):303–4.
262. Patel J et al. Am J Ther. 2004 Jul–Aug;11(4):262–77.
263. Sparreboom A et al. J Clin Oncol. 2004 Jun 15;22(12): 2489–503.
264. Fujita K, Kamataki T. Drug Metab Dispos. 2001 Jul;29(7): 983–9.
265. Foster BC et al. J Pharm Pharm Sci. 2001 May–Aug;4(2): 176–84.
266. Demeule M et al. Biochem Biophys Res Commun. 2004 Nov 12;324(2):937–45.
267. Maldonado PD et al. Phytother Res. 2005 Mar;19(3):252–4.
268. Cox MC et al. Clin Cancer Res. 2006 Aug;2(15):4636–40.
269. Piscitelli SC et al. Clin Infect Dis. 2002 Jan 15;34(2):234–8.
270. Gallicano K et al. Br J Clin Pharmacol. 2003 Feb;55(2): 199–202.
271. Hu Z et al. Drugs. 2005;65(9):1239–82.
272. Pathak A et al. Therapie. 2003 Jul–Aug;58(4):380–1.

273. Markowitz JS et al. Clin Pharmacol Ther. 2003 Aug;74(2): 170–7.
274. Gurley BJ et al. Drugs Aging. 2005;22(6):525–39.
275. Loizou GD, Cocker J. Hum Exp Toxicol. 2001 Jul;20(7): 321–7.
276. Wilkinson GR. Adv Drug Deliv Rev. 1997 Sep 15;27(2–3): 129–59.
277. Boudreau MD, Beland FA. J Environ Sci Health C Environ Carcinog Ecotoxicol Rev. 2006 Apr;24(1):103–54.
278. Choi S, Chung M-H. Sem Integr Med. 2003 Mar;1(1):53–62.
279. Okamura N et al. Phytochemistry. 1997 Aug;45(7):1519–22.
280. Huang D et al. Se Pu. 2006 Jan;24(1):42–5.
281. Yang Y et al. Biomed Chromatogr. 2004 Mar;18(2):112–6.
282. ElSohly MA et al. Int Immunopharmacol. 2004 Dec 20; 4(14):1739–44.
283. Kuzuya H et al. J Chromatogr B Biomed Sci Appl. 2001 Mar 5;752(1):91–7.
284. Pan X et al. Se Pu. 2005 Jan;23(1):96–9.
285. Lee KY et al. Free Radic Biol Med. 2000 Jan 15;28(2):261–5.
286. Park MK et al. Planta Med. 1996 Aug;62(4):363–5.
287. Yagi A, Takeo S. Yakugaku Zasshi. 2003 Jul;123(7):517–32.
288. Zhang XF et al. Bioorg Med Chem Lett. 2006 Feb 15; 16(4):949–53.
289. Saccu D et al. J Agric Food Chem. 2001 Oct;49(10):4526–30.
290. Im SA et al. Int Immunopharmacol. 2005 Feb;5(2):271–9.
291. WHO Monographs on Selected Medicinal Plants—Vol 1 WHO Geneva 1999 p. 33–58.
292. Ni Y et al. Int Immunopharmacol. 2004 Dec 20;4(14):1745–55.
293. Eberendu AR et al. J AOAC Int. 2005 May–Jun;88(3):684–91.
294. Tai-Nin Chow J et al. Carbohydr Res. 2005 May 2;340(6): 1131–42.
295. Pugh N et al. J Agric Food Chem. 2001 Feb;49(2):1030–4.
296. Turner CE et al. Int Immunopharmacol. 2004 Dec 20;4(14): 1727–37.
297. Esua MF, Rauwald JW. Carbohydr Res. 2006 Feb 27;341(3): 355–64.
298. Kostalova D et al. Ceska Slov Farm. 2004 Sep;53(5):248–51.
299. Akev N, Can A. Phytother Res. 1999 Sep;13(6):489–93.
300. Tanaka M et al. Biol Pharm Bull. 2006 Jul;29(7):1418–22.
301. Moon EJ et al. Angiogenesis. 1999;3(2):117–23.
302. Afzal M et al. Planta Med. 1991 Feb;57(1):38–40.
303. Lee KH et al. J Pharm Pharmacol. 2000 May;52(5):593–8.
304. Esteban A et al. Planta Med. 2000 Dec;66(8):724–7.
305. Fujita K et al. Biochem Pharmacol. 1979 Apr;28(7):1261–2.
306. Sabeh F et al. Enzyme Protein. 1996;49(4):212–21.
307. Rajasekaran S et al. Biol Trace Elem Res. 2005 Winter; 108(1–3):195–95.
308. Hou D et al. Wei Sheng Yan Jiu. 2004 Nov;33(6):747–9.
309. Eshun K, He Q. Crit Rev Food Sci Nutr. 2004;44(2):91–6.
310. Shindo T et al. Shokuhin Eiseigaku Zasshi. 2002 Jun;43(3): 122–6.
311. Chang XL et al. J Food Eng. 2006 Jul;75(2):245–51.
312. Bozzi A et al. Food Chem. 2007;103(1):22–30.
313. Turner CE et al. Int Immunopharmacol. 2004 Dec 20;4(14): 1727–37.
314. Kim KH et al. Arch Pharm Res. 1998 Oct;21(5):514–20.
315. Womble D, Helderman JH. Int J Immunopharmacol. 1988; 10(8):967–74.
316. Chen XD et al. Zhongguo Wei Zhong Bing Ji Jiu Yi Xue. 2005 May;17(5):296–8.
317. 't Hart LA et al. Int J Immunopharmacol. 1990;12(4):427–34.
318. Avila H et al. Toxicon. 1997 Sep;35(9):1423–30.
319. Dutta A et al. Glycoconj J. 2007 Jan;24(1):81–6.
320. Tian B et al. Zhongguo Zhong Yao Za Zhi. 2003 Nov; 28(11):1034–7.
321. Sydiskis RJ et al. Antimicrob Agents Chemother. 1991 Dec; 35(12):2463–6.
322. Barrantes E, Guinea M. Life Sci. 2003 Jan 3;72(7):843–50.
323. Ferro VA et al. Antimicrob Agents Chemother. 2003 Mar; 47(3):1137–9.
324. Rojas L et al. Rev Cubana Med Trop. 1995;47(3):181–4.
325. Iljazovic E et al. Eur J Surg Oncol. 2006 Nov;Suppl 1:S73.
326. Xiao B et al. Oral Oncol. 2007 Oct;43(9):905–10.
327. Guo J et al. Cancer Biol Ther. 2007 Jan 29;6(1).
328. Lin JG et al. J Urol. 2006 Jan;175(1):343–7.
329. Kuo PL et al. Life Sci. 2002 Sep 6;71(16):1879–92.
330. Pecere T et al. Cancer Res. 2000 Jun 1;60(11):2800–4.
331. Lee KH et al. J Pharm Pharmacol. 2000 Aug;52(8):1037–41.
332. Esmat AY et al. Cancer Biol Ther. 2005 Jan;4(1):108–12.
333. Cardenas C, Quesada AR. Cell Mol Life Sci. 2006 Dec; 63(24):3083–9.
334. Mueller SO, Stopper H. Biochim Biophys Acta. 1999 Aug 5; 1428(2–3):406–14.
335. Yoo EJ, Lee BM. J Toxicol Environ Health A. 2005 Nov 12; 68(21):1841–60.
336. Lissoni P et al. Nat Immun. 1998;16(1):27–33.
337. Abdullah KM et al. J Altern Complement Med. 2003 Oct; 9(5):711–8.
338. Chen XD et al. Zhonghua Shao Shang Za Zhi. 2005 Dec; 21(6):430–3.
339. Choi SW et al. Br J Dermatol. 2001 Oct;145(4):535–45.
340. Yagi A et al. Planta Med. 1997 Feb;63(1):18–21.
341. Lee KY et al. Biochem Mol Biol Int. 1997 Feb;41(2):285–92.
342. Wang ZW et al. Ai Zheng. 2005 Apr;24(4):438–42.
343. Wang ZW et al. J Radiat Res (Tokyo). 2004 Sep;45(3):447–54.
344. Vath Pe et al. Photochem Photobiol. 2002 Apr;75(4):346–52.
345. Xia Q et al. Toxicol Lett. 2007 Jan 30;168(2):165–75.
346. Strickland FM et al. Cutis. 2004 Nov;74(5 Suppl):24–8.
347. Puentes Sanchez J et al. Rev Enferm. 2006 Oct;29(10): 25–30.
348. Dal'Belo SE et al. Skin Res Technol. 2006 Nov;12(4):241–6.
349. West DP, Zhu YF. Am J Infect Control. 2003 Feb;31(1):40–2.
350. Hayes SM. Gen Dent. 1999 May–Jun;47(3):268–72.
351. Akhtar MA, Hatwar SK. J Clin Epidemiol. 1996 Jan; 49(Suppl 1):S24.
352. Visuthikosol V et al. J Med Assoc Thai. 1995 Aug;78(8): 403–9.
353. Syed TA et al. Trop Med Int Health. 1996 Aug;1(4):505–9.
354. Paulsen E et al. J Eur Acad Dermatol Venereol. 2005 May; 19(3):326–31.
355. Poor MR et al. J Oral Maxillofac Surg. 2002 Apr;60(4): 374–9.
356. Garnick JJ et al. Oral Surg Oral Med Oral Pathol Oral Radiol Endod. 1998 Nov;86(5):550–6.
357. Thomas DR et al. Adv Wound Care. 1998 Oct;11(6):273–6.
358. Puvabanditsin P, Vongtongsri R. J Med Assoc Thai. 2005 Sep;88(Suppl 4):S173–6.
359. Schmidt JM, Greenspoon JS. Obstet Gynecol. 1991 Jul; 78(1):115–7.
360. Olsen D et al. Oncol Nurs Forum. 2001 Apr;28(3):543–7.
361. O'Brien A et al. Radiother Oncol. 2005 Sep;76(Suppl 1): S40–S41.
362. Williams M et al. Int J Rad Oncol Biol Phy. 1996 Sep 1; 36(2):345–9.

363. Heggie S et al. Cancer Nurs. 2002 Dec;25(6):442–51.
364. Su CK et al. Int J Rad Oncol Biol Phy. 2004 Sep 1;60(1):171–7.
365. Maddocks-Jennings W et al. Complement Ther Clin Pract. 2005 Nov;11(4):224–31.
366. Richardson J et al. Clin Oncol (R Coll Radiol). 2005 Sep;17(6):478–84.
367. Yagi A et al. Planta Med. 2003 Mar;69(3):269–71.
368. Bezakova L et al. Ceska Slov Farm. 2005 Jan;54(1):43–6.
369. Khattak S et al. Nat Prod Res. 2005 Sep;19(6):567–71.
370. Langmead L et al. Aliment Pharmacol Ther. 2004 Mar 1;19(5):521–7.
371. Hu Y et al. J Agric Food Chem. 2003 Dec 17;51(26):7788–91.
372. Davis K et al. Int J Clin Pract. 2006 Sep;60(9):1080–6.
373. Langmead L et al. Aliment Pharmacol Ther. 2004 Apr 1;19(7):739–47.
374. Fahim MS, Wang M. Contraception. 1996 Apr;53(4):231–6.
375. Grover JK et al. J Ethnopharmacol. 2002 Jun;81(1):81–100.
376. Vinson JA et al. Phytomedicine. 2005 Nov;12(10):760–5.
377. Kirdpon S et al. J Med Assoc Thai. 2006 Aug;89(8):1199–205.
378. Kirdpon S et al. J Med Assoc Thai. 2006 Aug;89 Suppl 2:S9–14.
379. Ghannam N et al. Horm Res. 1986;24(4):288–94.
380. Chalaprawat M. J Clin Epidemiol. 1997 Jan;50(Suppl 1):S3.
381. Vogler BK, Ernst E. Br J Gen Pract. 1999 Oct;49(447):823–8.
382. Reynolds T, Dweck AG. J Ethnopharmacol. 1999 Dec 15;68(1–3):3–37.
383. Martindale, The Extra Pharmacopoeia 26th Ed. Pharmaceutical Press London March 1973.
384. Canigueral S, Roser V. Br J Phytotherapy. 1993 Winter;3(2):67–75.
385. Reider N et al. Contact Dermatitis. 2005 Dec;53(6):332–4.
386. Morrow DM et al. Arch Dermatol. 1980 Sep;116(9):1064–5.
387. Dominguez-Soto L. Int J Dermatol. 1992 May;31(5):372.
388. Hunter D, Frumkin A. Cutis. 1991 Mar;47(3):193–6.
389. Kim EJ et al. Nephrology. 2007 Feb;12(1):109.
390. Evangelos C et al. Eur J Intern Med. 2005 Feb;16(1):59–60.
391. Rabe C et al. World J Gastroenterol. 2005 Jan 14;11(2):303–4.
392. Kanat O et al. Eur J Intern Med. 2006 Dec;17(8):589.
393. Pigatto PD, Guzzi G. Arch Med Res. 2005 Sep–Oct;36(5):608.
394. Paes-Leme AA et al. J Ethnopharmacol. 2005 Nov 14;102(2):197–210.
395. Lee A et al. Ann Pharmacother. 2004 Oct;38(10):1651–4.
396. Schenk B et al. Planta Med. 1980 Sep;40(1):1–11.
397. Loffelhardt W et al. Phytochemistry. 1979;18(8):1289–91.
398. Hipsz M et al. Acta Pol Pharm. 1975;32(6):695–701.
399. Kubelka W. Planta Med. 1971;Suppl 4:153–9.
400. Mahato SB et al. Phytochemistry. 1982 Jun 2;21(5):959–78.
401. Kopp B, Loffelhardt W. Z Naturforsch [C]. 1980 Jan–Feb;35(1–2):41–4.
402. Malinowski J, Strzelecka H. Acta Pol Pharm. 1976;33(6):767–76.
403. Liu H. Se Pu. 1999 Jul;17(4):410–2.
404. Bohm BA. Arch Biochem Biophys. 1966 Jul;115(1):181–6.
405. Jager AK et al. J Ethnopharmacol. 2006 Apr 21;105(1–2):294–300.
406. Lamminpaa A, Kinos M. Hum Exp Toxicol. 1996 Mar;15(3):245–9.
407. Eriksson NE et al. Allergy. 1987 Jul;42(5):374–81.
408. Fraunfelder FW. Amer J Ophthalmol. 2004 Oct;138(4):639–47.
409. Gaillard Y, Pepin G. J Chromatogr B Biomed Sci Appl. 1999 Oct 15;733(1–2):181–229.
410. Satour M et al. Planta Med. 2006 Jun;72(7):667–70.
411. Satour M et al. J Nat Prod. 2005 Oct;68(10):1489–93.
412. Yuan JZ et al. Zhongguo Zhong Yao Za Zhi. 2004 Sep;29(9):867–70.
413. Du Q et al. J Chromatogr A. 2005 Jun 3;1077(1):98–101.
414. Guo J et al. Clin Chem. 2007 Mar;53(3):465–71.
415. Chen T et al. Planta Med. 1999 Feb;65(1):56–9.
416. Yi Y et al. Yao Xue Xue Bao. 1998 Nov;33(11):873–5.
417. Chu KT, Ng TB. Biochem Biophys Res Commun. 2006 Feb 3;340(1):118–24.
418. Ooi LS et al. J Agric Food Chem. 2004 Oct 6;52(20):6091–5.
419. Caceres A et al. J Ethnopharmacol. 1991 Mar;31(3):263–76.
420. Thabrew MI et al. Life Sci. 2005 Aug 5;77(12):1319–30.
421. Iddamaldeniya SS et al. J Carcinog. 2003 Oct 18;2(1):6.
422. Jiang J, Xu Q. J Ethnopharmacol. 2003 Mar;85(1):53–9.
423. Chen Z. Zhong Xi Yi Jie He Za Zhi. 1990 Feb;10(2):71–4, 67.
424. Rollier R. Int J Lepr. 1959 Oct–Dec;27:328–40.
425. Paris R et al. Ann Pharm Fr. 1952 May;10(5):328–35.
426. Thurmon FM. New Engl J Med. 1942;227(4):128–33.
427. Marker RE et al. J Am Chem Soc. 1943 Apr;65(4):739.
428. Iizuka M et al. Chem Pharm Bull (Tokyo). 2001 Mar;49(3):282–6.
429. Krenn L et al. Fitoterapia. 2000 Apr;71(2):126–9.
430. Kopp B et al. Phytochemistry. 1996 May;42(2):513–22.
431. Fernandez M et al. Phytochemistry 1972 Apr;11(4):1534.
432. Fernandez M et al. Phytochemistry 1975 Feb;14(2):586.
433. Aliotta G et al. J Nephrol. 2004 Mar–Apr;17(2):342–7.
434. Stauch M et al. Klin Wochenschr. 1977 Jul 15;55(14):705–6.
435. Tuncok Y et al. J Toxicol Clin Toxicol. 1995;33(1):83–6.

Linaceae

1. Dybing C, Zimmerman DC. Plant Physiol. 1966 Nov;41(9):1465–70.
2. Sorensen BM et al. Lipids. 2005 Oct;40(10):1043–9.
3. Bacala R, Barthet V. J AOAC Int. 2007 Jan–Feb;90(1):153–61.
4. Frehner M et al. Plant Physiol. 1990 Sep;94(1):28–34.
5. Warrand J et al. Biomacromolecules. 2005 Jul–Aug;6(4):1871–6.
6. Warrand J et al. Int J Biol Macromol. 2005 Apr;35(3–4):121–5.
7. Warrand J et al. J Agric Food Chem. 2005 Mar 9;53(5):1449–52.
8. Muir AD. J AOAC Int. 2006 Jul–Aug;89(4):1147–57.
9. Coran SA et al. J Chromatogr A. 2004 Aug 6;1045(1–2):217–22.
10. Liggins J et al. Anal Biochem. 2000 Dec 1;287(1):102–9.
11. Meagher LP et al. J Agric Food Chem. 1999 Aug;47(8):3173–80.
12. Degenhardt A et al. J Chromatogr A. 2002 Jan 18;943(2):299–302.
13. Kamal-Eldin A et al. Phytochemistry. 2001 Oct;58(4):587–90.
14. Kraushofer T, Sontag G. J Chromatogr B Analyt Technol Biomed Life Sci. 2002 Sep 25;777(1–2):61–6.
15. Sicilia T et al. J Agric Food Chem. 2003 Feb 26;51(5):1181–8.

16. Bloedon LT, Szapary PO. Nutr Rev. 2004 Jan;62(1):18–27.
17. Eliasson C et al. J Chromatogr A. 2003 Sep 19;1012(2):151–9.
18. Stefanowicz P. Acta Biochim Pol. 2001;48(4):1125–9.
19. Luyengi L et al. J Nat Prod. 1993 Nov;56(11):2012–5.
20. Martindale, The Extra Pharmacopoeia 26th Ed. Pharmaceutical Press London March 1973 p. 1084.
21. Brooks JD, Thompson LU. J Steroid Biochem Mol Biol. 2005 Apr;94(5):461–7.
22. Paschos GK et al. Angiology. 2005 Jan–Feb;56(1):49–60.
23. Rallidis LS et al. Atherosclerosis. 2004 May;174(1):127–32.
24. Harper CR et al. J Nutr. 2006 Jan;136(1):83–7.
25. Cao J et al. Clin Chem. 2006 Dec;52(12):2265–72.
26. Freese R, Mutanen M. Am J Clin Nutr. 1997 Sep;66(3):591–8.
27. Harper CR et al. J Nutr. 2006 Nov;136(11):2844–8.
28. Goh YK et al. Diabetologia. 1997 Jan;40(1):45–52.
29. McManus RM et al. Diabetes Care. 1996 May;19(5):463–7.
30. St-Onge MP et al. J Nutr. 2003 Jun;133(6):1815–20.
31. Lucas EA et al. J Clin Endocrinol Metab. 2002 Apr;87(4):1527–32.
32. Ridges L et al. Asia Pac J Clin Nutr. 2001;10(3):204–11.
33. Mandasescu S et al. Rev Med Chir Soc Med Nat Iasi. 2005 Jul–Sep;109(3):502–6.
34. Jenkins DJ et al. Am J Clin Nutr. 1999 Mar;69(3):395–402.
35. Tohgi N. Diabetes Care. 2004 Oct;27(10):2563–4.
36. Hallund J et al. J Nutr. 2006 Jan;136(1):112–6.
37. Dodin S et al. J Clin Endocrinol Metab. 2005 Mar;90(3):1390–7.
38. Hallund J et al. J Nutr. 2006 Sep;136(9):2314–8.
39. Stuglin C, Prasad K. J Cardiovasc Pharmacol Ther. 2005 Mar;10(1):23–7.
40. Tarpila S et al. Eur J Clin Nutr. 2002 Feb;56(2):157–65.
41. Nesbitt PD, Thompson LU. Nutr Cancer. 1997;29(3):222–7.
42. Knust U et al. Food Chem Toxicol. 2006 Jul;44(7):1038–49.
43. Arjmandi BH. J Am Coll Nutr. 2001 Oct;20(5 Suppl):398S–402S.
44. Danbara N et al. Anticancer Res. 2005 May–Jun;25(3B):2269–76.
45. Waldschlager J et al. Anticancer Res. 2005 May–Jun;25(3A):1817–22.
46. Lewis JE et al. Menopause. 2006 Jul–Aug;13(4):631–42.
47. Brooks JD et al. Am J Clin Nutr. 2004 Feb;79(2):318–25.
48. Lemay A et al. Obstet Gynecol. 2002 Sep;100(3):495–504.
49. Spence JD et al. J Am Coll Nutr. 2003 Dec;22(6):494–501.
50. Hutchins AM et al. Nutr Cancer. 2001;39(1):58–65.
51. Haggans CJ et al. Nutr Cancer. 1999;33(2):188–95.
52. Thompson LU et al. Clin Cancer Res. 2005 May 15;11(10):3828–35.
53. Demark-Wahnefried W et al. Urology. 2001 Jul;58(1):47–52.
54. Demark-Wahnefried W et al. Urology. 2004 May;63(5):900–4.
55. Dalais F et al. Urology. 2004 Sep;64(3):510–5.
56. Dahl WJ et al. J Med Food. 2005 Winter;8(4):508–11.
57. Ruchala P et al. Biopolymers. 2003 Dec;70(4):497–511.
58. Bell A et al. Acta Pol Pharm. 2000 Nov;57 Suppl:134–6.
59. Picur B et al. J Pept Sci. 2006 Sep;12(9):569–74.
60. Hosseinian FS et al. Org Biomol Chem. 2007 Feb 21;5(4):644–54.
61. Ford JD et al. J Nat Prod. 2001 Nov;64(11):1388–97.
62. Kitts DD et al. Mol Cell Biochem. 1999 Dec;202(1–2):91–100.
63. Prozorovskaia NN et al. Vopr Pitan. 2003;72(2):13–8.
64. Ipatova OM et al. Biomed Khim. 2004 Jan–Feb;50(1):25–43.

65. Rossetti RG et al. J Leukoc Biol. 1997 Oct;62(4):438–43.
66. Joshi K et al. Prostaglandins Leukot Essent Fatty Acids. 2006 Jan;74(1):17–21.
67. Johannson G et al. Gerodontology. 2001 Dec;18(2):87–94.
68. Ranich T et al. J Ren Nutr. 2001 Oct;11(4):183–93.
69. Clark WF et al. J Am Coll Nutr. 2001 Apr;20(2 Suppl):143–8.
70. Velasquez MT, Bhathena SJ. Am J Kidney Dis. 2001 May;37(5):1056–68.
71. Kuijsten A et al. J Nutr. 2005 Dec;135(12):2812–6.
72. Hyvarinen HK et al. J Agric Food Chem. 2006 Jan 11;54(1):48–53.
73. Frische EJ et al. J Am Coll Nutr. 2003 Dec;22(6):550–4.
74. Cunnane SC et al. Br J Nutr. 1993 Mar;69(2):443–53.
75. Lampe JW et al. J AOAC Int. 2006 Jul–Aug;89(4):1174–81.
76. Woodside JV et al. J Nutr Biochem. 2006 Mar;17(3):211–5.
77. Hutchins AM et al. Cancer Epidemiol Biomarkers Prev. 2000 Oct;9(10):1113–8.
78. Jacobs E et al. J Steroid Biochem Mol Biol. 1999 Mar;68(5–6):211–8.
79. Knust U et al. Food Chem Toxicol. 2006 Jul;44(7):1057–64.
80. Nesbitt PD et al. Am J Clin Nutr. 1999 Mar;69(3):549–55.
81. Wanasundara PK, Shahidi F. Adv Exp Med Biol. 1998;434:307–25.
82. Knudsen VK et al. BJOG. 2006 May;113(5):536–43.
83. Rojas-Molina M et al. Environ Mol Mutagen. 2005;45(1):90–5.
84. Leon F et al. Allergol Immunopathol (Madr). 2003 Jan–Feb;31(1):47–9.
85. Lezaun A et al. Allergy. 1998 Jan;53(1)105–6.
86. Gruver DI. Plast Reconstr Surg. 2003 Sep;112(3):934.

Lobeliaceae

1. Kang B, Chang S. Tetrahedron. 2004 Aug 16;60(34):7353–9.
2. Subarnas A et al. J Pharm Pharmacol. 1993 Jun;45(6):545–50.
3. Felpin FX, Lebreton J. J Org Chem. 2002 Dec 27;67(26):9192–9.
4. Martindale, The Extra Pharmacopoeia 26th Ed. Pharmaceutical Press London March 1973.
5. Raj H et al. Resp Physiol Neurobiol. 2005 Jan;145(1):79–90.
6. Felpin FX, Lebreton J. Tetrahedron. 2004 Nov 1;60(45):10127–53.
7. Dwoskin LP, Crooks PA. Biochem Pharmacol. 2002 Jan 15;63(2):89–98.
8. Gaillard Y, Pepin G. J Chromatogr B:Biomed Sci Appl. 1999 Oct 15;733(1–2):191–229.

Loganiaceae

1. Martindale, The Extra Pharmacopoeia 26th Ed. Pharmaceutical Press London March 1973.
2. Lina L-Z et al. Phytochemistry. 1991 Jan 2;30(2):679–83.
3. Kogure N et al. Tetrahedron Lett. 2005 Aug 29;46(35):5857–61.
4. Claus EP. Pharmacognosy 4th Ed. Henry Kimpton. London 1961 p. 351.

Loranthaceae

1. Martindale, The Extra Pharmacopoeia 26th Ed. Pharmaceutical Press London March 1973 p. 803.
2. Stein GM et al. Anticancer Res. 1999 Mar–Apr;19(2A): 1037–42.
3. Schaller G et al. Planta Med. 1998 Oct;64(7):677–8.
4. Urech K et al. Arzneimittelforschung. 2006 Jun;56(6A): 428–34.
5. Franz H et al. Biochem J. 1981 May 1;195(2):481–4.
6. Jager S et al. Planta Med. 2007 Feb;73(2):157–62.
7. Urech K et al. J Pharm Pharmacol. 2005 Jan;57(1):101–9.
8. Orhan DD et al. Z Naturforsch [C]. 2006 Jan–Feb;61(1–2): 26–30.
9. Wagner H et al. Planta Med. 1986 Apr;52(2):102–4.
10. Khwaja TA et al. Oncology. 1986;43 Suppl 1:42–50.
11. Reviatskaia AP. Farm Zh. 1965;20(6):27–30.
12. Luczkiewicz M et al. Acta Pol Pharm. 2001 Sep–Oct;58(5): 373–9.
13. Deliorman D et al. Fitoterapia. 2001 Feb;72(2):101–5.
14. Stein GM et al. Anticancer Res. 1999 Sep–Oct;19(5B):3907–14.
15. Elluru S et al. Arzneimittelforschung. 2006 Jun;56(6A):461–6.
16. Urech K et al. Anticancer Res. 2006 Jul–Aug;26(4B):3049–55.
17. Lavastre V et al. Leuk Res. 2005 Dec;29(12):1443–53.
18. Mueller EA, Anderer FA. Cancer Immunol Immunother. 1990;32(4):221–7.
19. Mueller EA et al. Immunopharmacology. 1980 Jan–Feb; 17(1):11–18.
20. Tabiasco J et al. Eur J Biochem. 2002 May;269(10):2591–600.
21. Eggenschwiler J et al. Arzneimittelforschung. 2006 Jun; 56(6A):483–96.
22. Zuzak TJ et al. Anticancer Res. 2006 Sep–Oct;26(5A): 3485–92.
23. Kovacs E. Phytother Res. 2002 Mar;16(2):143–7.
24. Bussing A et al. Cancer Lett. 1995 Aug 1;94(2):199–205.
25. Burger AM et al. Anticancer Res. 2003 Sep–Oct;23(5A): 3801–6.
26. Styczynski J, Wysocki M. Pediatr Blood Cancer. 2006 Jan; 46(1):94–8.
27. Lavastre V et al. Clin Exp Immunol. 2004 Aug;137(2):272–8.
28. Lyu SY et al. Arch Pharm Res. 2004 Jan;27(1):118–26.
29. Grossarth-Maticek R, Ziegler R. Eur J Med Res. 2006 Nov 30;11(11):485–95.
30. Maldacker J. Arzneimittelforschung. 2006 Jun;56(6A):461–6.
31. Mengs U et al. Anticancer Res. 2002 May–Jun;22(3): 1399–407.
32. Bar-Sela G et al. Harefuah. 2006 Jan;145(1):42–6, 77.
33. Mansky PJ. Semin Oncol. 2002 Dec;29(6):589–94.
34. Stauder H, Kreuser ED. Onkologie. 2002 Aug;25(4):374–80.
35. Frank U et al. Eur J Clin Microbiol Infect Dis. 2003 Aug; 22(8):501–3.
36. Stein GM et al. Anticancer Res. 1999 Mar–Apr;19(2A): 1037–42.
37. Schmidt KH. Planta Med. 1989 Oct;55(5):455–7.
38. Coeugniet EG, Elek E. Onkologie. 1987 Jun;10(3 Suppl): 27–33.
39. Kovacs E. J Altern Complement Med. 2004 Apr;10(2):241–6.
40. Stein GM et al. Anticancer Res. 2002 Jan–Feb;22(1A):267–74.
41. Onay-Ucar E et al. Fitoterapia. 2006 Dec;77(7–8):556–60.
42. Tenorio FA et al. Fitoterapia. 2005 Mar;76(2):204–9.
43. Sener B et al. Gazi Uni Eczac Fac Derg. 1996;13(2):143–6.
44. Onal S et al. Prep Biochem Biotechnol. 2005;35(1):29–36.
45. Karagoz A et al. Phytother Res. 2003 May;17(5):560–2.
46. Basaran AA et al. Teratog Carcinog Mutagen. 1996;16(2): 125–38.
47. Bussing A et al. Arzneimittelforschung. 1995 Jan;45(1):81–3.

Malvaceae

1. Nosal'ova G et al. J Carbohydr Chem. 1993;12(4–5):589–96.
2. Gudej J. Planta Med. 1991 Jun;57(3):284–5.
3. Tomas-Barberan FA et al. Biochem Syst Ecol. 1993 Jun;21(4): 487–97.
4. Capek P et al. Carbohydr Res. 1987 Jul;164:443–52.
5. Kardosova A, Machova E. Fitoterapia. 2006 Jul;77(5): 367–73.
6. Martindale, The Extra Pharmacopoeia 26th Ed. Pharmaceutical Press London March 1973 p. 1074.
7. Iauk L et al. Phytother Res. 2003 Jun;17(6):599–604.
8. Kobayashi A et al. Biol Pharm Biol. 2002 Feb;25(2):229–34.
9. Ebringerova A et al. Int J Biol Macromol. 2002 Mar;30(1): 1–6.
10. Buechi S et al. Forsch Komplementarmed Klass Naturheilkd. 2005 Dec;12(6):328–32.
11. Puodziuniene G et al. Medicina (Kaunas). 2005;41(6):500–5.
12. Rouhi H, Ganji F. Pakistan J Nutr. 2007;6(3):256–8.

Menyanthaceae

1. Janeczko Z et al. Phytochemistry. 1990 Jan;29(12):3885–7.
2. Junior P. Planta Med. 1989 Feb;55(1):83–7.
3. Damtoft S et al. Phytochemistry. 1997 Jun;45(4):743–50.
4. Krebs GK, Matern J. Arch Pharm Ber Dtsch Pharm Ges. 1958 Apr;291/63(4):163–5.
5. Swiatek L et al. Planta Med. 1986 Dec;52(6):530.
6. Kuduk-Jaworska J et al. Z Naturoforsch [C]. 2004 Jul–Aug; 59(7–8):485–93.
7. Martindale, The Extra Pharmacopoeia 26th Ed. Pharmaceutical Press London March 1973 p. 327.
8. Tuno H et al. J Ethnopharmacol. 1995 Oct;48(2):61–76.

Monimiaceae

1. Vogel H et al. Planta Med. 1999 Feb;65(1):90–1.
2. Vila R et al. Planta Med. 1999 Mar;65(2):178–9.
3. Hughes DW et al. J Pharm Sci. 1968 Sep;57(9):1619–20.
4. Hughes DW et al. J Pharm Sci. 1968 Jun;57(6):1023–5.
5. O'Brien P et al. Chem Biol Interact. 2006 Jan;159(1):1–17.
6. Krug H, Borkowski B. Pharmazie. 1965 Nov;20(11):692–8.
7. Leitao GG et al. J Ethnopharmacol. 1999 May;65(2):87–102.
8. Schmeda-Hirschmann G et al. Free Radic Res. 2003 Apr; 37(4):447–52.
9. Martindale, The Extra Pharmacopoeia 26th Ed. Pharmaceutical Press London March 1973 p. 639.
10. Speisky H et al. Phytother Res. 2006 Jun;20(6):462–7.
11. Speisky H, Cassels BK. Pharmacol Res. 1994 Jan–Feb;29(1): 1–12.

12. Jimenez I et al. Phytother Res. 2000 Aug;14(5):339–43.
13. Silva E et al. Photochem Photobiol. 2002 Jun;75(6):585–90.
14. Rancan F et al. J Photochem Photobiol B. 2002 Nov;68(2–3): 133–9.
15. Kringstein P, Cederbaum AI. Free Radic Biol Med. 1995 Mar; 18(3):559–63.
16. Morello A et al. Comp Biochem Physiol C. 1994 Mar; 107(3pt3):367–71.
17. Gonzalez-Cabello R et al. J Invest Allerg Clin Immunol. 1994; 4(3):139–45.
18. Johnson MA, Croteau R. Arch Biochem Biophys. 1984 Nov 15; 235(1):254–66.
19. Gotteland M et al. Rev Med Chil. 1995 Aug;123(8):955–60.
20. Tavares DC, Takahashi CS. Mutat Res. 1994 May;321(3): 139–45.
21. Moreno PR et al. Mutat Res. 1991 Jun;260(2):145–52.
22. Pizarro F et al. Arch Latinoam Nutr. 1994 Dec;44(4):277–80.
23. Monzon S et al. Allergy. 2004 Sep;59(9):1019–20.
24. Agarwal SC et al. Int J Cardiol. 2006 Jan 13;106(2):260–1.
25. Piscaglia F et al. Scand J Gastroenterol. 2005 Feb;40(2): 236–9.
26. Lambert JP, Cormier J. Pharmacother. 2001 Apr;21(4): 509–12.

Myricaceae

1. Martindale, The Extra Pharmacopoeia 26th Ed. Pharmaceutical Press London March 1973 p. 263.
2. Paul BD et al. J Pharm Sci. 1974 Jun;63(6):958–9.
3. Chistokhodova N et al. J Ethnopharmacol. 2002 Jul;81(2): 277–80.
4. Yokomizo A, Moriwaki M. Biosci Biotechnol Biochem. 2005 Sep;69(9):1774–6.

Nymphaceae

1. Lavid N et al. Planta. 2001 Feb;212(3):323–31.
2. Bertol E et al. J R Soc Med. 2004 Feb;97(2):84–5.
3. Collins BS et al. Bioresour Technol. 2005 May;96(8):937–48.
4. Vajpayee P et al. Chemosphere. 2000 Oct;41(7):1075–82.
5. Khan N, Sultana S. Mol Cell Biochem. 2005 Mar;27(1–2): 1–11.
6. Khan N, Sultana S. J Enzyme Inhib Med Chem. 2005 Jun; 20(3):275–83.

Oleaceae

1. Boyer L et al. Phytochem Anal. 2005 Sep–Oct;16(5):375–9.
2. Gulcin I et al. Afr J Biotechnol. 2007 Feb 19;6(4):410–18.
3. Paiva-Martins F, Gordon MH. J Agric Food Chem. 2001 Sep; 49(9):4214–9.
4. Karioti A et al. Biosci Biotechnol Biochem. 2006 Aug;70(8): 1898–903.
5. Briante R et al. J Agric Food Chem. 2002 Aug 14;50(17): 4934–40.
6. Meirinhos J et al. Nat Prod Res. 2005 Feb;19(2):189–95.

7. Ranalli A et al. J Agric Food Chem. 2006 Jan 25;54(2): 434–40.
8. Paiva-Martins F et al. J Agric Food Chem. 2007 May 16;55(10): 4139–43.
9. Japon-Lujan R, Luque de Castro MD. J Chromatogr A. 2006 Dec 15;1136(2):185–91.
10. Japon-Lujan R et al. J Chromatogr A. 2006 Mar 3;1108(1): 76–82.
11. Pieroni A et al. Pharmazie. 1996 Oct;51(10):765–8.
12. Saija A, Uccella IN. Trends Food Sci Tech. 2000 Sep 10; 11(9–10):357–63.
13. Saimaru H et al. Chem Pharm Bull (Tokyo). 2007 May; 55(5):784–8.
14. Campeol E et al. J Agric Food Chem. 2003 Mar 26;51(7): 1994–9.
15. Flamini G et al. J Agric Food Chem. 2003 Feb 26;51(5): 1382–6.
16. Campeol E et al. Carbohydr Res. 2004 Nov 15;339(16): 2731–2.
17. Tabera J et al. J Agric Food Chem. 2004 Jul 28;52(15):4774–9.
18. Tuck KL, Hayball PJ. J Nutr Biochem. 2002 Nov; 13(11):636–44.
19. De la Puerta C et al. Food Chem. 2007 Jan;104(2):609–12.
20. Visioli F et al. J Agric Food Chem. 1999;47(8):3397–401.
21. Cervellati R et al. J Agric Food Chem. 2002 Dec 18;50(26): 7504–9.
22. Benavente-Garcia O et al. Food Chem. 2000 Mar;68(4): 457–62.
23. Wojcikowski K et al. J Altern Complement Med. 2007 Jan–Feb;13(1):103–9.
24. O'Brien NM et al. J Med Food. 2006 Summer;9(2):187–95.
25. Katsiki M et al. Rejuvenation Res. 2007 Jun;10(2):157–72.
26. Lee-Huang S et al. Biochem Biophy Res Commun. 2003 Aug 8;307(4):1029–37.
27. Bao J et al. FEBS Lett. 2007 Jun 12;581(14):2737–42.
28. Lee-Huang S et al. Biochem Biophy Res Commun. 2007 Mar 23;354(4):872–8.
29. Markin D et al. Mycoses. 2003 Apr;46(3–4):132–6.
30. Pereira AP et al. Molecules. 2007 May 26;12(5):1153–62.
31. Baycin D et al. J Agric Food Chem. 2007 Feb 21;55(4): 1227–36.
32. Bisignano G et al. J Pharm Pharmacol. 1999 Aug 1; 51(8):971–4.
33. Aziz NH et al. Microbios. 1998;93(374):43–54.
34. Furneri PM et al. Antimicrob Agents Chemother. 2004 Dec; 48(12):4892–4.
35. Micol V et al. Antiviral Res. 2005 Jun;66(2–3):129–36.
36. Abaza L et al. Biosci Biotechnol Biochem. 2007 May; 71(5):1306–12.
37. Singh I et al. Nutr Metab Cardiovasc Dis. 2008 Feb;18(2): 127–32.
38. Saija A et al. J Sci Food Agric. 1999 May 11;79(3):476–80.
39. Cherif S et al. J Pharm Belg. 1996 Mar–Apr;51(2):69–71.
40. Ziyyat A et al. J Ethnopharmacol. 1997 Sep;58(1):45–54.
41. Bartram T. Encyclopedia of Herbal Medicine 1st Ed. Grace Publishers Dorset. 1995.
42. Tsarbopoulos A et al. J Chromatogr B Anal Tech Biomed Life Sci. 2003 Feb;785(1):157–64.
43. Visoli F et al. FEBS Lett. 2000 Feb;468(2–3):159–60.
44. Martindale, The Extra Pharmacopoeia 26th Ed. Pharmaceutical Press London March 1973 p. 1260.

Papaveraceae

1. Then M et al. J Chromatogr A. 2000 Aug 11;889(1–2):69–74.
2. Saglam H, Arar G. Fitoterapia. 2003 Feb;74(1–2):127–9.
3. Fulde G, Wilchlt M. Dtsche Apoth Ztg. 1994;134(12):17–21.
4. Stuppner H, Ganzera M. J Chromatogr A. 1995 Nov; 717(1–2):271–7.
5. Walterova D et al. Planta Med. 1984 Apr;50(2):149–51.
6. Colombo ML, Bosisio E. Pharmacol Res. 1996 Feb;33(2): 127–34.
7. Tome F, Colombo ML. Phytochemistry. 1995 Sep;40(1):37–9.
8. Taborska E et al. Ceska Slov Farm. 1995 Apr;44(2):71–5.
9. Hahn R, Nahrstedt A. Planta Med. 1993 Feb;59(1):71–5.
10. Nawrot R et al. Phytochemistry. 2007 Jun;68(12):1612–22.
11. Nawrot R et al. Fitoterapia. 2007 Dec;78(7–8):496–501.
12. Bilka F et al. Ceska Slov Farm. 2007 Apr;56(2):90–4.
13. Fik E et al. Acta Biochim Pol. 2000;47(2):423–20.
14. Rogelj B et al. Phytochemistry. 1998 Nov;49(6):1645–9.
15. Fik E et al. Acta Microbiol Pol. 1997;46(3):325–7.
16. Cheng RB et al. Shanghai Kou Qiang Yi Xue. 2007 Feb;16(1): 68–72.
17. Cheng RB et al. Shanghai Kou Qiang Yi Xue. 2006 Jun; 15(3):318–20.
18. Tosun R et al. J Ethnopharmacol. 2004 Dec;95(2):273–5.
19. Gerencer M et al. Antiviral Res. 2006 Nov;72(2):153–6.
20. Matos OC et al. J Ethnopharmacol. 1999 Aug;66(2):151–8.
21. Parsons LG et al. J Clin Periodontol. 1987 Aug;14(7):381–5.
22. Laster LL, Lobene RR. J Can Dent Assoc. 1990;56(7 Suppl): 19–30.
23. Boulware RT, Southard GL. J Soc Cosmet Chem. 1985; 36:297–302.
24. Khmel'nitskaia NM et al. Vestn Otorinolaringol. 1998; (4):39–42.
25. Kemeny-Beke A. Cancer Lett. 2006 Jun 8;237(1):67–75.
26. Habermehl D et al. BMC Cancer. 2006 Jan;17;6:14.
27. Ding Z et al. Biochem Pharm. 2002 Apr;63(8):1415–21.
28. Gansauge F et al. Gastroenterology. 2001 Apr;120(5): A617–8.
29. Spiridonov NA et al. Phytother Res. 2005 May;19(5):428–32.
30. Vavreckova C et al. Planta Med. 1996 Dec;62(6):491–4.
31. Ernst E, Schmidt K. BMC Cancer. 2005 Jul 1;5(1):69.
32. Xian MS et al. Acta Med Okayama. 1989 Dec;43(6):345–51.
33. Kuznetsova LP et al. Tsitologiia. 2001;43(11):1046–50.
34. Cho KM et al. Biol Pharm Bull. 2006 Nov;29(11):2317–20.
35. Haberlein H et al. Planta Med. 1996 Jun;62(3):227–31.
36. Schempp H et al. Phytomedicine. 2006 Nov 24;13(Suppl 1): 36–44.
37. Vavreckova C et al. Planta Med. 1996 Oct;62(5):397–401.
38. Agarwal S et al. Oral Microbiol Immunol. 1991 Feb; 6(1):51–61.
39. Jeng JH et al. Atherosclerosis. 2007 Apr;191(2):250–8.
40. Mantle D et al. J Ethnopharm. 2000 Sep 1;72(1–2):47–51.
41. Kliachko LL et al. Vestn Otorinolaringol. 1994 Mar–Apr;(2): 31–3.
42. Niederau C, Gopfert E. Med Klin (Munich). 1999 Aug 15; 94(8):425–30.
43. Adler M et al. Toxicol Lett. 2006 Sep 20;164(Suppl 1): S210–11.
44. Benninger J et al. Gastroenterology. 1999 Nov;117(5):1234–7.
45. Greving I et al. Pharmacoepidemiol Drug Saf. 1998 Aug; 7(Suppl 1):S66–9.
46. Rifai K et al. Internist (Berl). 2006 Jul;47(7):749–51.
47. Stickel F et al. Scand J Gastroenterol. 2003 May;38(5):565–8.
48. Crijns AP et al. Ned Tijdschr Geneeskd. 2002 Jan 19;146(3): 124–8.
49. Pinto Garcia V et al. Sangre (Barc). 1990 Oct;35(5):401–3.
50. Etxenagusia MA et al. Contact Dermatitis. 2000 Jul;43(1):47.
51. Klvana M et al. Phytochem Anal. 2006 Jul;17(4):236–42.
52. Gafner S et al. J Nat Prod. 2006 Mar;69(3):432–5.
53. Paul LD, Maurer HH. J Chromatogr B Analyt Technol Biomed Life Sci. 2003 Jun 5;789(1):43–57.
54. Beck MA, Haberlein H. Phytochemistry. 1999 Jan;50(2): 329–32.
55. MacLeod BP, Facchini PJ. Methods Mol Biol. 2006;318: 357–68.
56. Mortesza-Semnani K et al. Fitoterapia. 2003 Jul;74(5):493–6.
57. Mahady GB et al. Phytother Res. 2003 Mar;17(3):217–21.
58. Chia YC et al. Planta Med. 2006 Oct;72(13):1238–41.
59. Satou T et al. Vet Parasitol. 2002 Mar 1;104(2):131–8.
60. Hanus M et al. Curr Med Res Opin. 2004 Jan;20(1):63–71.
61. Rolland A et al. Planta Med. 1991 Jun;57(3):212–6.
62. Suchomelova J et al. J Pharm Biomed Anal. 2007 May 9;44(1): 283–7.
63. Graf TN et al. J Agric Food Chem. 2007 Feb 21;55(4): 1205–11.
64. Salmore AK, Hunter MD. J Chem Ecol. 2001 Sep;27(9): 1729–47.
65. Bambagiotti-Alberti M et al. J Pharm Biomed Anal. 1991; 9(10–12):1083–7.
66. Claus EP. Pharmacognosy. 4th Ed. London Henry Kimpton London 1961.
67. Mahady GB et al. Phytother Res. 2003 Mar;17(3):217–21.
68. Newton SM et al. J Ethnopharmacol. 2002 Jan;79(1):57–67.
69. Eisenberg AD et al. Caries Res. 1991;25(3):185–90.
70. Southard GL. J Am Dent Assoc. 1984 Mar;108(3):338–41.
71. Tenenbaum H et al. J Periodontol. 1999 Mar;70(3):307–11.
72. Kopczyk RA et al. J Periodontol. 1991 Oct;62(10):617–22.
73. Harper DS et al. J Periodontol. 1990 Jun;61(6):359–63.
74. Harper DS et al. J Periodontol. 1990 Jun;61(6):352–8.
75. Miller NA et al. J Paradontol. 1990 Feb;9(1):37–43.
76. Hannah JJ et al. Am J Orthod Dentofacial Orthop. 1989 Sep; 96(3):199–207.
77. Parsons LG et al. J Clin Periodontol. 1987 Aug;14(7):381–5.
78. Wennstrom J, Lindhe J. J Clin Periodontol. 1985 Nov;12(10): 867–72.
79. Cullinan MP et al. Aust Dent J. 1997 Feb;42(1):47–51.
80. Mallatt ME et al. J Periodontol. 1989 Feb;60(2):91–5.
81. Mauriello SM, Bader JD. J Periodontol. 1988 Apr;59(4): 238–43.
82. Etemadzadeh H, Ainamo J. J Clin Periodontol. 1987 Mar; 14(3):176–80.
83. Allen CL et al. Gen Dent. 2001 Nov–Dec;49(6):608–14.
84. Eversole LR et al. Oral Surg Oral Med Oral Pathol Oral Radiol Endod. 2000 Apr;89(4):455–64.
85. Damm DD et al. Oral Surg Oral Med Oral Pathol Oral Radiol Endod. 1999 Jan;87(1):61–6.
86. Frankos VH et al. J Can Dent Assoc. 1990;56(7 Suppl): 41–7.
87. Munro IC et al. Regul Toxicol Pharmacol. 1999 Dec;30(3): 182–96.
88. Kuftinec MM et al. J Can Dent Assoc. 1990;56(7 Suppl): 31–3.
89. Laster LL, Lobene RR. J Can Dent Assoc. 1990;56(7 Suppl): 19–30.

90. Chang MC et al. Toxicol Appl Pharmacol. 2007 Jan 12; 218(2):143–51.
91. Adhami VM et al. Mol Cancer Ther. 2004 Aug;3(8):933–40.
92. Adhami VM et al. Clin Cancer Res. 2003 Aug 1;9(8): 3176–82.
93. Ding Z et al. Biochem Pharm. 2002 Apr 15;63(8):1415–21.
94. Hussain AR et al. Cancer Res. 2007 Apr 15;67(8):3888–97.
95. Chaturvedi M et al. J Biol Chem. 1997 Nov 28;272(48): 30129–34.
96. Ahmad N et al. Clin Cancer Res. 2000 Apr;6(4):1524–8.
97. Eun JP, Koh GY. Biochem Biophys Res Commun. 2004 Apr 30;317(2):618–24.
98. Jellinek N, Maloney ME. J Am Acad Dermatol. 2005 Sep; 53(3):486–94.
99. McDaniel S, Goldman GD. Arch Dermatol. 2002 Dec; 138(12):1593–6.
100. Elston DM. J Am Acad Dermatol. 2005 Sep;53(3):522–4.
101. Vrba JV et al. Chemico-Biol Inter. 2004 Jan;147(1):35–47.
102. Jeng JH et al. Atherosclerosis. 2007 Apr;19(2):250–8.
103. Vrba JV et al. Toxicol Lett. 2004 Jul;151(2):375–87.
104. Ulrichova J et al. Toxicol Lett. 2001 Nov;125(1):125–31.

Passifloraceae

1. Dhawan K et al. Fitoterapia. 2001 Dec;72(8):922–6.
2. Chimichi S et al. Nat Prod Lett. 1998;11(3):225–32.
3. Pereira CA et al. Phytochem Anal. 2004 Jul–Aug;15(4):241–8.
4. Rehwald A et al. Pharm Acta Helv. 1994 Dec;69(3):153–8.
5. Qimin L et al. J Chromatogr. 1991 Jan 2;562(1–2):435–46.
6. Dhawan K et al. J Ethnopharmacol. 2001 Dec;78(2–3):165–70.
7. Tsuchiya H et al. Phytochem Anal. 1999 Sep;10(5):247–53.
8. Aoyagi N et al. Chem Pharm Bull (Tokyo). 1974 May;22(5): 1008–13.
9. Spencer KC, Seigler DS. Planta Med. 1984;50:356–7.
10. Buchbauer G et al. Flav Frag J. 1992;7(6):329–32.
11. Dhawan K et al. J Med Food. 2001 Autumn;4(3):137–44.
12. Dhawan K et al. Fitoterapia. 2001 Aug;72(6):698–702.
13. Martindale, The Extra Pharmacopoeia 26th Ed. Pharmaceutical Press London March 1973 p. 2029.
14. Simmen U et al. J Recept Signal Transduct Res. 1999 Jan–Jul; 19(1–4):59–74.
15. Gramowski A et al. Eur J Neurosci. 2006 Jul;24(2):455–65.
16. Schellenberg V et al. Schizophren Res. 1993;9(2–3):249–50.
17. Bourin M et al. Fundam Clin Pharmacol. 1997;11(2):127–32.
18. Akhondzadeh S et al. J Clin Pharm Ther. 2001 Oct;26(5): 369–73.
19. Akhondzadeh S et al. J Clin Pharm Ther. 2001 Oct;26(5): 363–7.
20. Mori A et al. Clin Eval. 1993;21:383–440.
21. Miyasaka LS et al. Cochrane Database Syst Rev. 2007 Jan 24; (1):CD004518.
22. Mahady GB et al. Phytother Res. 2005 Nov;19(11):988–91.
23. Kapadia GJ et al. Pharmacol Res. 2002 Mar;45(3):213–20.
24. Ramos Ruiz A et al. J Ethnopharmacol. 1996 Jul 5;52(3):123–7.
25. Madle E et al. Mutat Res Gen Toxicol. 1981 Dec;90(4): 433–42.
26. Rehwald A et al. Phytochem Anal. 1995 Mar–Apr;6(2): 96–100.
27. Fisher AA et al. J Toxicol Clin Toxicol. 2000;38(1):63–6.
28. Solbakken AM et al. Tidsskr Nor Laegeforen. 1997 Mar 20; 117(8):1140–1.
29. Dattikio L, Suddaby B. Pediatr Nurs. 2002 Nov–Dec;28(6): 612–3.
30. Smith GW et al. Br J Rheumatol. 1993 Jan;32(1):87–8.
31. Dhawan K et al. J Ethnopharmacol. 2004 Sep;94(1):1–23.
32. Argento A et al. Ann Ital Med Int. 2000 Apr–Jun;15(2): 139–43.

Pedaliaceae

1. Schmidt AH. J Chromatogr A. 2005 May 6;1073(1–2):377–81.
2. Clarkson C et al. J Nat Prod. 2006;69(9):1280–8.
3. Qi J et al. Phytochemistry. 2006 Jul;67(13):1372–7.
4. Gunther M, Schmidt PC. J Pharm Biomed Anal. 2005 Apr 1; 37(4):817–21.
5. Munkombwe NM. Phytochemistry. 2003 Apr;62(8):1231–4.
6. Grant L et al. Phytother Res. 2007 Mar;21(3):199–209.
7. Boje K et al. Planta Med. 2003 Sep;69(9):820–5.
8. Stewart KM, Cole D. J Ethnopharmacol. 2005 Sep 14;100(3): 225–36.
9. Baghdikian B et al. Planta Med. 1997 Apr;63(2):171–6.
10. Schulze-Tanzil G et al. Arzneimittelforschung. 2004;54(4): 213–20.
11. Fiebich BL et al. Phytomedicine. 2001 Jan;8(1):28–30.
12. Loew D et al. Clin Pharmacol Ther. 2001 May;69(5):356–64.
13. Spelman K et al. Altern Med Rev. 2006 Jun;11(2):128–50.
14. Gunther M et al. Phytochem Anal. 2006 Jan–Feb;17(1):1–7.
15. Huang TH et al. J Ethnopharmacol. 2006 Mar 8;104(1–2): 149–55.
16. Chrubasik S et al. Phytomedicine. 2002 Apr;9(3):181–94.
17. Chrubasik S et al. Eur J Anaesthesiol. 1999 Feb;16(2):118–29.
18. Laudahn D, Walper A. Phytother Res. 2001 Nov;15(7): 621–4.
19. Chrubasik S et al. Phytomedicine. 2005 Jan;12(1–2):1–9.
20. Wegener T, Lupke NP. Phytother Res. 2003 Dec;17(10): 1165–72.
21. Chantre P et al. Phytomedicine. 2000 Jun;7(3):177–83.
22. Leblan D et al. Joint Bone Spine. 2000;67(5):462–7.
23. Gobel H et al. Schmerz. 2001 Feb;15(1):10–8.
24. Wegener T. Wien Med Wochenschr. 2002;152(15–16):389–92.
25. Grahame R, Robinson BV. Ann Rheum Dis. 1981 Dec; 40(6):632.
26. Moussard C et al. Prostaglandins Leukot Essent Fatty Acids. 1992 Aug;46(4):283–6.
27. Crubasik JE et al. Phytother Res. 2007 Jul;21(7):675–83.
28. Gagnier JJ et al. Spine. 2007 Jan 1;32(1):82–92.
29. Brien S et al. J Altern Complement Med. 2006 Dec;12(10): 981–93.
30. Ameye LG et al. Arthritis Res Ther. 2006;8(4):R127.
31. Weckesser S et al. Phytomedicine. 2007 Aug 6;14(7–8):508–16.
32. Clarkson C et al. Planta Med. 2003 Aug;69(8):720–4.
33. Betancor-Fernandez A et al. J Pharm Pharmacol. 2003 Jul; 55(7):981–6.
34. Langmead L et al. Aliment Pharmacol Ther. 2002 Feb;16(2): 197–205.
35. Chrubasik S. Orthopade. 2004 Jul;33(7):804–8.
36. Chrubasik S. Phytother Res. 2004 Feb;18(2):187–9.
37. Chrubasik S et al. Phytomedicine. 2003;10(6–7):613–23.
38. Baghdikian B et al. Planta Med. 1999 Mar;65(2):164–6.
39. Unger M, Frank A. Rapid Commun Mass Spectrom. 2004; 18(19):2273–81.
40. Shaw D et al. Drug Saf. 1997;17:342–56.

Phaeophyceae

1. Martindale, The Extra Pharmacopoeia 26th Ed. Pharmaceutical Press London March 1973 p. 263.
2. Koivikko R et al. Phytochem Anal. 2007 Jul;18(4):326–32.
3. Truus K et al. Anal Bioanal Chem. 2004 Jul;379(5–6):849–52.
4. Nishino T et al. Carbohydr Res. 1994 Mar 4;255:213–24.
5. Ferreiros CM, Criado MT. Rev Esp Fisiol. 1983 Mar;39(1): 51–9.
6. Duperon R et al. Phytochemistry. 1983;22(2):535–8.
7. Deal MS et al. Oecologia. 2003 Jun;136(1):107–14.
8. Pawlik-Skowronska B et al. Aquatic Toxicol. 2007 Jul 20; 80(3):190–9.
9. Amer HA et al. J Environ Monit. 1999 Feb;1(1):97–104.
10. Skibola CF et al. J Nutr. 2005 Feb;135(2):296–300.
11. Skibola SF et al. BMC Complement Altern Med. 2004 Aug 4;4:10.
12. Moro CO, Basile G. Fitoterapia. 2000 Aug;71 Suppl 1:S73–82.
13. Couper R, Couper J. The Lancet. 2000 Aug;356(9230):673–5.
14. Curro F, Amadeo A. Arch Med Interna. 1976;28:19–32.
15. Nagayama, K et al. J Antimicrob Chemother. 2002;50(6): 889–893.
16. Criado MT, Ferreiros CM. Rev Esp Fisiol. 1984 Jun;40(2): 227–30.
17. Criado MT, Ferreiros CM. Ann Microbiol (Paris). 1983 Mar–Apr;134A(2):149–54.
18. Ahn M-J et al. Biol Pharm Bull. 2004 Apr;27(4):544–547.
19. Beress A et al. J Nat Prod. 1993 Apr;56(4):478–88.
20. Baba M et al. Antimicrob Agents Chemother. 1988 Nov; 32(11):1742–5.
21. Shibata H et al. J Nutr Sci Vitaminol (Tokyo). 1999 Jun;45(3): 325–36.
22. Shibata H et al. Biofactors. 2000;11(4):235–45.
23. Angulo Y, Lomonte B. Biochem Pharmacol. 2003 Nov 15; 66(10):1993–2000.
24. O'Leary R et al. Biol Pharm Bull. 2004 Feb;27(2):266–70.
25. Fujimura T et al. Biol Pharm Bull. 2000 Oct;23(10):1180–4.
26. Cumashi A et al. Glycobiology. 2007 May;17(5):541–52.
27. Durig J et al. Thromb Res. 1997 Mar 15;85(6):479–91.
28. Patankar MS et al. J Biol Chem. 1993 Oct 15;268(29): 21770–6.
29. Hsu HY et al. J Biol Chem. 1998 Jan;273(2):1240–6.
30. Ruperez P et al. J Agric Food Chem. 2002 Feb 13;50(4): 840–5.
31. Kang HS et al. Arch Pharm Res. 2004 Feb;27(2):194–8.
32. Fujimura T et al. J Cosmet Sci. 2002 Jan–Feb;53(1):1–9.
33. Murphy V et al. Water Res. 2007 Feb;41(4):731–40.
34. Riekie GJ et al. Chemosphere. 2006 Oct;65(2):332–42.
35. Merrifield ME et al. Chem Res Toxicol. 2006 Mar;19(3): 365–75.
36. Merrifield ME et al. Biochem Biophys Res Commun. 2004 Nov 5;324(1):127–32.
37. Conz PA et al. Nephrol Dial Transplant. 1998 Feb;13(2):526–7.
38. Agarwal SC et al. Int J Cardiol. 2006 Jan 13;106(2):260–1.

Phytolaccaceae

1. Woo WS. Phytochemistry. 1974 Dec;13(12):2887–9.
2. Woo WS, Kang SS. Phytochemistry. 1976 Jan;15(8):1315–7.
3. Kang SS, Woo WS. Planta Med. 1987 Aug;53(4):338–40.
4. Jeong SI et al. Planta Med. 2004 Aug;70(8):736–9.

5. Sussner U et al. Planta Med. 2004 Oct;70(10):942–7.
6. Hayashida M et al. J Mol Biol. 2003 Nov 28;334(3):551–65.
7. Reisfeld RA et al. Proc Natl Acad Sci USA. 1967 Nov;58(5): 2020–7.
8. Fujii T et al. Acta Crystallogr D Biol Crystallogr. 2004 Apr; 60(Pt4):665–73.
9. Funyama S, Hikino H. J Nat Prod. 1979 Nov–Dec;42(6): 672–4.
10. Martindale, The Extra Pharmacopoeia 26th Ed. Pharmaceutical Press London March 1973 p. 2032.
11. Jeong SI et al. Phytomedicine. 2004 Feb;11(2–3):175–81.
12. Yang JS et al. Clin Vaccine Immunol. 2006 Mar;13(3):309–13.
13. Ichiki T et al. Int Immunol. 1992 Jul;4(7):747–54.
14. Waxdal MJ. Biochemistry. 1974 Aug 27;13(18):3671–7.
15. Cho SY et al. Arch Pharm Res. 2003 Dec;26(12):1102–8.
16. Rau E. Adv Ther. 2000 Jul–Aug;17(4):197–203.
17. Zhao Y et al. Zhongguo Zhong Yao Za Zhi. 1991 Aug;16(8): 467–9, 511.

Piperaceae

1. Ganzera M, Kahn IA. Chromatographia. 1999 Dec;50(11–12): 649–53.
2. He X et al. Planta Med. 1997;63:70–4.
3. Warburton E et al. Phytochem Anal. 2007 Mar;18(2):98–102.
4. Gautz LD et al. J Agric Food Chem. 2006 Aug 23;54(17): 6147–52.
5. Janeczko Z et al. Acta Pol Pharm. 2001 Nov–Dec;58(6):463–8.
6. Bilia AR et al. J Agric Food Chem. 2002 Aug 28;50(18): 5016–25.
7. Bilia AR et al. J Chromatogr B Analyt Technol Biomed Life Sci. 2004 Dec 5;812(1–2):203–14.
8. Meissner O, Haberlein H. J Chromatogr B Analyt Technol Biomed Life Sci. 2005 Nov 5;826(1–2):46–9.
9. Dharmaratne HR et al. Phytochemistry. 2002 Feb;59(4): 429–33.
10. Smith RM. Tetrahedron. 1979;35(3):437–9.
11. Dragull K et al. Phytochemistry. 2003 May;63(2):193–8.
12. Cheng D et al. Biomed Environ Mass Spectrom. 1998 Nov; 17(5):371–6.
13. Dinh LD et al. Planta Med. 2001 Jun;67(4):306–11.
14. Boonen G, Haberlein H. Planta Med. 1998 Aug;64(6):504–6.
15. Uebelhack R et al. Pharmacopsychiatry. 1998 Sep;31(5): 187–92.
16. Grunze H et al. Prog Neuropsychopharmacol Biol Psychiatry. 2001 Nov;25(8):1555–70.
17. Gleitz J et al. Eur J Pharmacol. 1996 Nov 7;315(1):89–97.
18. Cagnacci A et al. Maturitas. 2003 Feb 25;44(2):103–9.
19. De Leo V et al. Maturitas. 2001 Aug 25;39(2):185–8.
20. De Leo V et al. Minerva Ginecol. 2000 Jun;52(6):263–7.
21. Warnecke G. Fortschr Med. 1991 Feb 10;109(4):119–22.
22. Geller SE, Studee L. Menopause. 2007 May–Jun;14(3 Pt 1): 541–9.
23. Geier FP, Konstantinowicz T. Phytother Res. 2004 Apr;18(4): 297–300.
24. Scherer J. Adv Ther. 1998 Jul–Aug;15(4):261–9.
25. Volz HP, Kieser M. Pharmacopsychiatry. 1997 Jan;30(1):1–5.
26. Boerner RJ. Phytother Res. 2001 Nov;15(7):646–7.
27. Kinzler E et al. Arzneimittelforschung. 1991 Jun;41(6): 584–8.

28. Witte S et al. Phytother Res. 2005 Mar;19(3):183–8.
29. Pittler MH, Ernst E. Cochrane Database Syst Rev. 2003;(1): CD003383.
30. Malsch U, Kieser M. Psychopharmacology (Berl). 2001 Sep; 157(3):277–83.
31. Gastpar M, Klimm HD. Phytomedicine. 2003 Nov; 10(8):631–9.
32. Watkins LL et al. J Psychopharmacol. 2001 Dec;15(4):283–6.
33. Boerner RJ et al. Phytomedicine. 2003;10 Suppl 4:38–49.
34. Neuhaus W et al. Zentralbl Gynakol. 2000;122(11):561–5.
35. Pittler MH, Ernst E. J Clin Psychopharmacol. 2000 Feb; 20(1):84–9.
36. Ernst E. Phytomedicine. 2006 Feb;13(3):205–8.
37. Cairney S et al. Aust NZ J Psychiatry. 2002 Oct;36(5):657–62.
38. Pittler MH, Ernst E. Cochrane Database Syst Rev. 2002;(2): CD003383.
39. Pittler MH, Ernst E. Cochrane Database Syst Rev. 2001;(4): CD003383.
40. Connor KM et al. Int Clin Psychopharmacol. 2006 Sep;21(5): 249–53.
41. Abraham KC et al. J Altern Complement Med. 2004 Jun; 10(3):556–9.
42. Connor KM et al. Int Clin Psychopharmacol. 2002 Jul;17(4): 185–8.
43. Thompson R et al. Hum Psychopharmacol. 2004 Jun;19(4): 243–50.
44. Lehrl S. J Affect Disord. 2004 Feb;78(2):101–10.
45. Wheatley D. Hum Psychopharmacol. 2001 Jun;16(4):353–56.
46. Wheatley D. J Psychopharmacol. 2005 Jul;19(4):414–21.
47. Jacobs BP et al. Medicine (Baltimore). 2005 Jul;84(4):197–207.
48. Cropley M et al. Phytother Res. 2002 Feb;16(1):23–7.
49. Munte TF et al. Neuropsychobiology. 1993;27(1):46–53.
50. Bilia AR et al. Life Sci. 2002 Apr 19;70(22):2581–97.
51. Steiner GG. Pac Health Dialog. 2001 Sep;8(2):335–9.
52. Wu D et al. Phytomedicine. 2002 Jan;9(1):41–7.
53. Wu D et al. J Agric Food Chem. 2002 Feb 13;50(4):701–5.
54. Folmer F et al. Biochem Pharmacol. 2006 Apr 14;71(8): 1206–18.
55. Gleitz J et al. Planta Med. 1997 Feb;63(1):27–30.
56. Kapadia GJ et al. Pharmacol Res. 2002 Mar;45(3):213–20.
57. Zi X, Simoneau AR. Cancer Res. 2005 Apr 15;65(8):3479–86.
58. Locher CP et al. J Ethnopharmacol. 1995 Nov 17;49(1): 23–32.
59. Guerin JC, Reveillere HP. Ann Pharm Fr. 1984;42:553–9.
60. Steiner GG. Hawaii Med J. 2000 Nov;59(11):420–2.
61. Hu L et al. J AOAC Int. 2005 Jan–Feb;88(1):16–25.
62. Krochmal R et al. Evid Based Complement Altern Med. 2004 Dec;1(3):305–13.
63. Matthias A et al. J Clin Pharm Ther. 2007 Jun;32(3):233–9.
64. Prescott J et al. Drug Alcohol Rev. 1993;12(1):49–57.
65. Duffield AM et al. J Chromatogr. 1989 Jul;28;475:273–81.
66. Connor KM et al. CNS Spectr. 2001 Oct;6(10):848, 850–3.
67. Clough AR et al. Intern Med. 2003 Aug;33(8):336–40.
68. Norton SA, Ruze P. J Am Acad Dermatol. 1994 Jul;31(1): 89–97.
69. Ruze P. Lancet. 1990 Jun 16;335(8703):1442–5.
70. Clough AR et al. Eur J Clin Nutr. 2004 Jul;58(7):1090–3.
71. Clough AR et al. J Epidemiol Community Health. 2004 Feb; 58(2):140–1.
72. Clough AR et al. Epidemiol Infect. 2003 Aug;131(1):627–35.
73. Cairney S et al. Neuropsychopharmacology. 2003 Feb;28(2): 389–96.
74. Garner LF, Klinger JD. J Ethnopharmacol. 1985 Jul;13(3): 307–11.
75. Perez J, Holmes JF. J Emerg Med. 2005 Jan;28(1):49–51.
76. Cairney S et al. Hum Psychopharmacol. 2003 Oct;18(7): 525–33.
77. Leung N. Emerg Med Australas. 2004 Feb;16(1):94.
78. Sibon I et al. Rev Neurol (Paris). 2002 Dec;158(12 Pt 1): 1205–6.
79. Meseguer E et al. Mov Disord. 2002 Jan;17(1):195–6.
80. Schmidt P, Boehncke WH. Contact Dermatitis. 2000 Jun; 42(6):363–4.
81. Suss R, Lehmann P. Hautarzt. 1996 Jun;47(6):459–61.
82. Spillane PK et al. Med J Aust. 1997 Aug 4;167(3):172–3.
83. Jappe U et al. J Am Acad Dermatol. 1998 Jan;38(1):104–6.
84. Donadio V et al. Neurol Sci. 2000 Apr;21(2):124.
85. Jhoo JW et al. J Agric Food Chem. 2006 Apr 9;54(8):3157–62.
86. Zou L et al. Phytomedicine. 2004;11(4):285–94.
87. Nerurkar PV et al. Toxicol Sci. 2004 May;79(1):106–11.
88. Zou L et al. Planta Med. 2004 Apr;70(4):289–92.
89. Anke J et al. Phytomedicine. 2006 Feb;13(3):192–5.
90. Estes JD et al. Arch Surg. 2003 Aug;138(8):852–8.
91. Stickel F et al. J Hepatol. 2003 Jul;39(1):62–7.
92. Schulze J et al. Phytomedicine. 2003;10 Suppl 4:68–73.
93. Humbertson CL et al. J Toxicol Clin Toxicol. 2003;41(2): 109–13.
94. Gow PJ et al. Med J Aust. 2003 May 5;178(9):442–3.
95. Kraft M et al. Dtsch Med Wochenschr. 2001 Sep 7;126(36): 970–2.
96. Russmann S et al. Ann Intern Med. 2001 Jul 3;135(1):68–9.
97. Strahl S et al. Dtsch Med Wochenschr. 1998 Nov 20;123(47): 1410–4.
98. Musch E et al. Dtsch Med Wochenschr. 2006 May;26: 131(21):1214–7.
99. Rietjens IM et al. Mol Nutr Food Res. 2005 Feb;49(2): 131–58.
100. Teschke R et al. Phytomedicine. 2003;10(5):440–6.
101. Ernst E. Br J Clin Pharmacol. 2007 Oct;64(4):415–7.
102. Anke J, Ramzan I. Planta Med. 2004 Mar;70(3):193–6.
103. Thomsen M et al. Med J Aust. 2004 Feb 16;180(4):198–9.
104. Clouatre DL. Toxicol Lett. 2004 Apr 15;150(1):85–96.
105. Richardson WN, Henderson L. Br J Clin Pharmacol. 2007 Oct;64(4):418–20.
106. Loew D et al. Phytomedicine. 2003;10(6–7):610–2.
107. Cote CS et al. Biochem Biophys Res Commun. 2004 Sep 10; 322(1):147–52.
108. Johnson BM et al. Chem Res Toxicol. 2003 Jun;16(6):733–40.
109. Singh YN. J Ethnopharmacol. 2005 Aug 22;100(1–2):108–13.
110. Wanwirolmuk S et al. Eur J Clin Pharmacol. 1998;54:431–5.
111. Whitton PA et al. Phytochemistry. 2003 Oct;64(3):673–9.
112. Brown AC et al. Clin Toxicol (Phila). 2007 Jun–Aug;45(5): 549–56.
113. Clough AR et al. J Toxicol Clin Toxicol. 2003;41(6):821–9.
114. Russmann S et al. Eur J Gastroenterol Hepatol. 2003 Sep; 15(9):1033–6.
115. Clough A et al. Drug Alcohol Rev. 2000;19(3):319–23.
116. Stevinson C et al. Drug Saf. 2002;25(4):251–61.
117. Teschke R. Z Gastroenterol. 2003 May;41(5):395–404.
118. Mills SY, Steinhoff B. Phytomedicine. 2003 Mar;10(2–3): 261–2.
119. Denham A et al. J Altern Complement Med. 2002 Jun;8(3): 237–63.
120. Ernst E. NZ Med J. 2004 Nov 5;117(1205):U1143.

121. Singh YN, Singh NN. CNS Drugs. 2002;16(11):731–43.
122. Mathews JM et al. Drug Metab Dispos. 2005 Oct;33(10): 1555–63.
123. Yueh MF et al. Drug Metab Dispos. 2005 Jan;33(1):38–48.
124. Jeurissen SM et al. J Chromatogr A. 2007 Feb 2;1141(1): 81–9.
125. Unger M, Frank A. Rapid Commun Mass Spectrom. 2004; 18(19):2273–81.
126. Ma Y et al. Drug Metab Dispos. 2004 Nov;32(11):1317–24.
127. Mathews JM et al. Drug Metab Dispos. 2002 Nov; 30(11):1153–7.
128. Weiss J et al. Drug Metab Dispos. 2005 Nov;33(11):1580–3.
129. Anke J, Razman I. J Ethnopharmacol. 2004 Aug;93(2–3): 153–60.
130. Gurley BJ et al. Clin Pharmacol Ther. 2008 Jan;83(1):61–9.
131. Gurley BJ et al. Clin Pharmacol Ther. 2005 May;77(5): 415–26.
132. Gurley BJ et al. Drug Metab Dispos. 2007 Feb;35(2):240–5.
133. Russmann S et al. Clin Pharmacol Ther. 2005 May;77(5): 453–4.
134. Foo H, Lemon J. Drug Alcohol Rev. 1997 Jun;16(2):147–55.
135. Herberg KW. Blutalkohol. 1993 Mar;30(2):96–105.
136. Almeida J, Grimsley E. Ann Int Med. 1996;125:940–1.
137. Schelosky L et al. J Neurol Neurosurg Psychiatry. 1995 May; 58(5):639–40.

Plantaginaceae

1. Jurisic R et al. Z Naturforsch [C]. 2004 Jan–Feb;59(1–2): 27–31.
2. Suomi J et al. J Chromatogr A. 2002 Sep 13;970(1–2):287–96.
3. Harvey JA et al. J Chem Ecol. 2005 Feb;31(2):287–302.
4. Fuchs A, Bowers MD. J Chem Ecol. 2004 Sep;30(9):1723–41.
5. Marak HB et al. J Chem Ecol. 2002 Dec;28(12):2429–48.
6. Tamura Y, Nishibe S. J Agric Food Chem. 2002 Apr 24;50(9): 2514–8.
7. Hausmann M et al. Clin Exp Immunol. 2007 May;148(2): 373–81.
8. Murai M et al. Planta Med. 1995 Oct;61(5):479–80.
9. Fleer H, Verspohl EJ. Phytomedicine. 2007 Jun;14(6):409–15.
10. Brautigam M, Franz G. Planta Med. 1985 Aug;51(4):293–7.
11. Chudnicka A, Matysik GJ. J Ethnopharmacol. 2005 Jun; 99(2):281–6.
12. Galvez M et al. J Agric Food Chem. 2005 Mar 23;53(6): 1927–33.
13. Kardosova A, Machova E. Fitoterapia. 2006 Jul;77(5): 367–73.
14. Herold A et al. Roum Arch Microbiol Immunol. 2003 Jul–Dec; 62(3–4):217–27.
15. Herold A et al. Roum Arch Microbiol Immunol. 2003 Jan–Jun; 62(1–2):117–29.
16. Galvez M et al. J Ethnopharmacol. 2003 Oct;88(2–3):125–30.
17. Ho JN et al. Biosci Biotechnol Biochem. 2005 Nov;69(11): 2227–31.
18. Lee KW et al. Carcinogenesis. 2007 Sep;28(9):1928–36.
19. Lee KY et al. Biol Pharm Bull. 2006 Jan;29(1):71–4.
20. Kozan E et al. J Ethnopharmacol. 2006 Nov 24;108(2):211–6.
21. Ramos Ruiz A et al. J Ethnopharmacol. 1996 Jul 5;52(3): 123–7.
22. Taskova R et al. Phytochemistry. 1999 Dec;52(8):1443–5.

23. Ronsted N et al. Plant Syst Evol. 2003 Nov;242(1–4):63–82.
24. Samuelsen AB. J Ethnopharmacol. 2000 Jul;71(1–2):1–21.
25. Ringbom T et al. J Nat Prod. 1998 Oct;61(10):1212–5.
26. Bogacheva AM et al. Biochimie. 2001 Jun;83(6):481–6.
27. Ringbom T et al. J Nat Prod. 2001 Jun;64(6):745–9.
28. Chiang LC et al. Am J Chin Med. 2003;31(2):225–34.
29. Holetz FB et al. Mem Inst Oswaldo Cruz. 2002 Oct;97(7): 1027–31.
30. Chiang LC et al. Antiviral Res. 2002 Jul;55(1):53–62.
31. Velasco-Lezama R et al. J Ethnopharmacol. 2006 Jan 3;103(1): 36–42.
32. Ponce-Macotela M et al. Rev Invest Clin. 1994 Sep–Oct; 46(5):343–7.
33. Chiang LC et al. Planta Med. 2003 Jul;69(7):600–4.
34. Chiang LC et al. Am J Chin Med. 2003;31(1):37–46.
35. Matev M et al. Vutr Boles. 1982;21(2):133–7.
36. Basaran AA et al. Teratog Carcinog Mutagen. 1996;16(2): 125–38.
37. Pimenta VM, Nepomuceno JC. Environ Mol Mutagen. 2005; 45(1):56–61.
38. Slifman NR et al. N Eng J Med. 1998 Sep 17;339(12):806–11.
39. Dasgupta A et al. Ann Clin Biochem. 2006 May;43(3):223–5.
40. Fischer MH et al. Carbohydr Res. 2004 Aug 2;339(11): 2009–17.
41. Marlett JA, Fischer MH. Proc Nutr Soc. 2003 Feb;62(1): 207–9.
42. Kennedy JF. Carbohydr Res. 1979 Oct 75:265–74.
43. Nakamura Y et al. Nutr Cancer. 2005;51(2):218–25.
44. Li L et al. J Chromatogr A. 2005 Jan 21;1063(1–2):161–9.
45. Martindale, The Extra Pharmacopoeia 26th Ed. Pharmaceutical Press London March 1973.
46. Al-Khaldi SF et al. Curr Microbiol. 1999 Oct;39(4):231–1.
47. Ashraf W et al. Aliment Pharmacol Ther. 1995 Dec;9(6): 639–47.
48. Marteau P et al. Gut. 1994 Dec;35(12):1747–52.
49. Chaplin MF et al. Proc Nutr Soc. 2003 Feb;62(1):217–22.
50. Blackwood AD et al. J R Soc Health. 2000 Dec;120(4):242–7.
51. Marlett JA et al. Am J Clin Nutr. 2000 Sep;72(3):784–9.
52. Bianchi M et al. Dig Liver Dis. 2002 Sep;34 Suppl 2:S129–33.
53. Kanuchi O et al. Curr Pharm Des. 2003;9(4):333–46.
54. Ewe K et al. Pharmacology. 1993 Oct;47 Suppl 1:242–8.
55. Tomas-Ridocci M et al. Rev Esp Enferm Dig. 1992 Jul;82(1): 17–22.
56. Soifer LO et al. Acta Gastroenterol Latinoam. 1987;17(4): 317–23.
57. Washington N et al. Am J Clin Nutr. 1998 Feb;67(2):317–21.
58. Fernandez-Banares F. Best Prac Res Clin Gastroenterol. 2006; 20(3):575–87.
59. Voderholzer WA et al. Am J Gastroenterol. 1997 Jan;92(1): 95–8.
60. Bossi S et al. Acta Biomed Ateneo Parmense. 1986;57(5–6): 179–86.
61. Ramkumar D, Rao SS. Am J Gastroenterol. 2005 Apr;100(4): 936–71.
62. McRorie JW et al. Aliment Pharmacol Ther. 1998 May; 12(5):491–7.
63. Dettmar PW, Sykes J. Curr Med Res Opin. 1998;14(4): 227–33.
64. Passmore AP et al. Pharmacology. 1993 Oct;47 Suppl 1: 249–52.
65. Kinnunen O et al. Pharmacology. 1993 Oct;47 Suppl 1: 253–5.

66. Ashraf W et al. Mov Disord. 1997 Nov;12(6):946–51.
67. Qvitzau S et al. Scand J Gastroenterol. 1988 Dec;23(10): 1237–40.
68. Smalley JR et al. J Pediatr Gastroenterol Nutr. 1982;1(3): 361–3.
69. Murphy J et al. Can Oncol Nurs J. 2000 Summer;10(3): 96–100.
70. Cavaliere H et al. Int J Obes Relat Metab Disord. 2001 Jul; 25(7):1095–9.
71. Sherman DS, Fish DN. Clin Infect Dis. 2000 Jun;30(6): 908–14.
72. Bliss DZ et al. Nurs Res. 2001 Jul–Aug;50(4):203–13.
73. Kecmanovic D et al. Acta Chir Iugosl. 2005;52(1):115–6.
74. Perez-Miranda M et al. Hepatogastroenterology. 1996 Nov–Dec;43(12):1504–7.
75. Kecmanovic DM et al. Phytother Res. 2006 Aug;20(8):655–8.
76. Kecmanovic D et al. Acta Chir Iugosl. 2004;51(3):121–3.
77. Hallert C et al. Scand J Gastroenterol. 1991;26:747–50.
78. Fernandez-Banares F et al. Am J Gastroenterol. 1999 Feb; 94(2):427–33.
79. Fujimori S et al. J Gastroenterol Hepatol. 2007 Aug;22(8): 1199–204.
80. Misra SP et al. Q J Med. 1989 Oct;73(270):931–9.
81. Chapman ND et al. Br J Clin Pract. 1990 Nov;44(11):461–6.
82. Hotz J, Plein K. Med Klin (Munich). 1994 Dec 15;89(12): 645–51.
83. Bijkerk CJ et al. Aliment Pharmacol Ther. 2004 Feb 1; 19(3):245–51.
84. Frati-Munari AC et al. Arch Invest Med (Mex). 1989 Apr–Jun;20(2):147–52.
85. Sierra M et al. Eur J Clin Nutr. 2001 Apr;55(4):235–43.
86. Cherbut C et al. Br J Nutr. 1994 May;71(5):675–85.
87. Pastors JG et al. Am J Clin Nutr. 1991 Jun;53(6):1431–5.
88. Singh B. Int J Pharm. 2007 Apr 4;334(1–2):1–14.
89. Ziai SA et al. J Ethnopharmacol. 2005 Nov 14;102(2):202–7.
90. Rodriguez-Moran M et al. J Diabetes Complications. 1998 Sep–Oct;12(5):273–8.
91. Sierra M et al. Eur J Clin Nutr. 2002 Sep;56(9):830–42.
92. Anderson JW et al. Am J Clin Nutr. 1999 Oct;70(4):466–73.
93. Frati-Munari AC et al. Arch Med Res. 1998 Summer; 29(2):137–41.
94. Clark CA et al. Eur J Clin Nutr. 2006 Sep;60(9):1122–9.
95. Uribe M et al. Gastroenterology. 1985 Apr;88(4):901–7.
96. Enzi G et al. Pharmatherapeutica. 1980;2(7):421–8.
97. Turnbull WH, Thomas HG. Int J Obes Relat Metab Disord. 1995 May;19(5):338–42.
98. Bergmann JF et al. Gut. 1992 Aug;33(8):1042–3.
99. Rigaud D et al. Eur J Clin Nutr. 1998 Apr;52(4):239–45.
100. Moreno LA et al. J Physiol Biochem. 2003 Sep;59(3): 235–42.
101. Miettinen TA, Tarpila S. Clin Chim Acta. 1989 Aug 31; 183(3):253–62.
102. Ganji V, Kies CV. Eur J Clin Nutr. 1994 Aug;48(8):595–7.
103. Chaplin MF et al. J Steroid Biochem Mol Biol. 2000 Apr; 72(5):283–92.
104. Bell LP et al. Am J Clin Nutr. 1990;52(6):1020–26.
105. Brown L et al. Am J Clin Nutr. 1999 Jan;69(1):30–42.
106. Lerman Garber I et al. Arch Inst Cardiol Mex. 1990 Nov–Dec; 0(6):535–9.
107. Shrethsa S et al. J Nutr. 2007 May;137(5):1165–70.
108. Jenkins DJ et al. Am J Clin Nutr. 2002 May;75(5):834–9.
109. Anderson JW et al. Am J Clin Nutr. 2000 Jun;71(6):1433–8.
110. Anderson JW et al. Am J Clin Nutr. 2000 Feb;71(2):472–9.
111. MacMahon M, Carless J. J Cardiovasc Risk. 1998 Jun;5(3): 167–72.
112. Davidson MH et al. Am J Clin Nutr. 1998 Mar;67(3): 367–76.
113. Van Rosendaal GM et al. Nutr J. 2004 Sep 28;3:17.
114. Kris-Etherton PM et al. J Am Diet Soc. 1988 Nov;88(11): 1373–400.
115. Davidson MH et al. Am J Clin Nutr. 1996 Jan;63(1): 96–102.
116. Reid R et al. Can J Diet Pract Res. 2002 Winter;63(4): 169–75.
117. Jensen CD et al. Am J Cardiol. 1997 Jan 1;79(1):34–7.
118. Jenkins DJ et al. Am J Clin Nutr. 2005 Feb;81(2):380–7.
119. Moreyra AE et al. Arch Intern Med. 2005 May 23;165(10): 1161–6.
120. Maciejko JJ et al. Arch Fam Med. 1994 Nov;3(11):955–60.
121. Wolever TM et al. Am J Clin Nutr. 1994 May;59(5):1055–9.
122. Vega-Lopez S et al. J Nutr. 2003 Jan;133(1):67–70.
123. Vega-Lopez S et al. Metabolism. 2002 Apr;51(4):500–7.
124. Vega-Lopez S et al. Am J Clin Nutr. 2001 Oct;74(4):435–41.
125. Schectman G et al. Am J Cardiol. 1993 Apr;1;71(10): 759–65.
126. Sola R et al. Am J Clin Nutr. 2007 Apr;85(4):1157–63.
127. Kinnunen O, Salokannel J. J Int Med Res. 1989 Sep–Oct; 17(5):442–54.
128. Gelissen IC et al. Am J Clin Nutr. 1994 Feb;59(2):395–400.
129. Moran S et al. Rev Gastroenterol Mex. 1997 Oct–Dec; 62(4):266–72.
130. Sauter G et al. Digestion. 1995;56(6):523–7.
131. Juarranz M et al. Eur J Cancer Prev. 2002 Oct;11(5):465–72.
132. Pylkas AM et al. J Med Food. 2005 Mar;8(1):113–6.
133. Friedman E et al. Cancer Lett. 1988 Dec 1;43(1–2):121–4.
134. Nordgaard I et al. Scand J Gastroenterol. 1996 Oct;31(10): 1011–20.
135. Bonithon-Kopp C et al. Lancet. 2000 Oct 14;356(9238): 1300–6.
136. Deters AM et al. Planta Med. 2005 Jan;71(1):33–9.
137. Westerhof W et al. Drugs Exp Clin Res. 2001;27(5–6): 165–75.
138. Zaman V et al. Phytother Res. 2002 Feb;16(1):78–9.
139. Burke V et al. Hypertension. 2001 Oct;38(4):821–6.
140. Kumar A et al. Gut. 1987 Feb;28(2):150–5.
141. Wolever TM et al. J Am Coll Nutr. 1991 Aug;10(4):364–71.
142. Heaney RP, Weaver CM. J Am Geriatr Soc. 1995 Mar; 43(3):261–3.
143. Oliver SD. J R Soc Health. 2000 Jun;120(2):107–11.
144. Leng-Peschlow E. Digestion. 1989;44(4):200–10.
145. Gonlachanvit S et al. Gut. 2004 Nov;53(11):1577–82.
146. Levitt MD et al. Ann Intern Med. 1996 Feb 15;124(4): 422–4.
147. Pittler MH et al. Obes Rev. 2005 May;6(2):93–111.
148. Aleman AM et al. Med Clin (Barc). 2001 Jan 13;116(1):20–2.
149. Machado L et al. Allergy. 1979 Feb;34(1):51–5.
150. Arlian LG et al. J Allergy Clin Immunol. 1992 Apr;89(4): 866–76.
151. Freeman GL. Ann Allergy. 1994 Dec;73(6):490–2.
152. Suhonen R et al. Allergy. 1983 Jul;38(5):363–5.
153. Khalili B et al. Ann Allergy Asthma Immunol. 2003 Dec; 91(6):579–84.
154. Vaswani SK et al. Allergy. 1996 Apr;51(4):266–8.
155. Herrle F et al. Obes Surg. 2004 Aug;14(7):1022–4.

156. Salguero Molpeceres O et al. Gastroenterol Hepatol. 2003 Apr;26(4):248–50.
157. Sauerbruch T et al. Endoscopy. 1980 Mar;12(2):83–5.
158. Shulman LM et al. Neurology. 1999 Feb;52(3):670–1.
159. Hunsaker DM, Hunsaker JC. Am J Forensic Med Pathol. 2002 Jun;23(2):149–54.
160. Fed Regist. 2007 Mar 29;72(60):14669–74.
161. Agha FP et al. Am J Gastroenterol. 1984 Apr;79(4):319–21.
162. Perez-Piqueras J et al. Endoscopy. 1994 Oct;26(8):710.
163. Schneider RP. South Med J. 1989 Nov;82(11):1449–50.
164. Agha FP et al. Am J Gastroenterol. 1984 Apr;79(4):319–21.
165. Berman JI, Schultz MJ. J Am Geriatr Soc. 1980 May;28(5):224–6.
166. Fraquelli M et al. J Hepatol. 2000 Sep;33(3):505–8.
167. Fernandez N et al. Eur Neuropsychopharmacol. 2005 Oct;125(5):505–9.
168. Chiu AC, Sherman SI. Thyroid. 1998 Aug;8(8):667–71.
169. Nordstrom M et al. Drug Nutr Interact. 1987;5(2):67–9.
170. Perlman BB. Lancet. 1990;335(8686):416.
171. Roe DA et al. J Am Diet Assoc. 1988 Feb;88(2):211–3.

Poaceae

1. Chen CY et al. J Nutr. 2007 Jun;137(6):1375–82.
2. Mattila P et al. J Agric Food Chem. 2005 Oct 19;53(21):8290–5.
3. Matsukawa T et al. Z Naturforsch [C]. 2000 Jan–Feb; 55(1–2):30–6.
4. Guth H, Grosch W. Z Lebensm Unters Forsch. 1994 Sep; 199(3):195–7.
5. Tschesche R, Schmidt W. Z Naturforsch. 1966;21:896–897.
6. Comai S et al. Food Chem. 2007 Jan;100(4):1350–55.
7. Adeli K, Altosaar I. Plant Physiol. 1984 May;75(1):225–7.
8. Kurtz ES, Wallo W. J Drugs Dermatol. 2007 Feb;6(2):167–70.
9. Reyna-Villasmil N et al. Am J Ther. 2007 Mar–Apr;14(2):203–12.
10. Ajithkumar A et al. J Agric Food Chem. 2005 Apr 6;53(4):1205–9.
11. Fu YC et al. J Agric Food Chem. 2005 Apr 6;53(7):2392–8.
12. Banas A et al. J Exp Bot. 2007 Aug;58(10):2463–70.
13. Hamberg M et al. Lipids. 1998 Apr;33(4):355–63.
14. Hauksson JB et al. Chem Phys Lipids. 1995 Oct 22;78(1):97–102.
15. Beringer H. Plant Physiol. 1971 Oct;48(4):433–6.
16. Chronakis IS et al. Colloids Surf B Biointerfaces. 2004 Jun 1;35(3–4):175–84.
17. Vahvaselka M et al. J Agric Food Chem. 2004 Mar 24;52(6):1749–52.
18. Peterson DM. J Cereal Sci. 2001 Mar;33(2):115–129.
19. Schneider E. Z Phytother. 1985;6:165–167.
20. Wenzig E et al. J Nat Prod. 2005 Feb;68(2):289–92.
21. Biosnic S et al. Int J Tissue React. 2005;27(3):83–9.
22. Aries MF et al. Biol Pharm Bull. 2005 Apr;28(4):601–6.
23. Boisnic S et al. Int J Tissue React. 2003;25(2):41–6.
24. Grimalt R et al. Dermatology. 2006 Dec;214(1):61–7.
25. Vie K et al. Skin Pharmacol Appl Skin Physiol. 2002 Mar–Apr; 15(2):120–4.
26. Matheson JD et al. J Burn Care Rehabil. 2001 Jan–Feb;22(1):76–81.
27. Nie L et al. Atherosclerosis. 2006 Jun;186(2):260–6.
28. Liu L et al. Atherosclerosis. 2004 Jul;175(1):39–49.
29. Makelainen H et al. Eur J Clin Nutr. 2007 Jun;61(6):779–85.
30. Maki KC et al. Eur J Clin Nutr. 2007 Jun;61(6):786–95.
31. Anderson JW et al. Am J Clin Nutr. 1990;52(3):495–9.
32. Queenan KM et al. Nutr J. 2007 Mar;26;6:6.
33. Kerckhoffs DA et al. J Nutr. 2002 Sep;132(9):2494–505.
34. Sayar S et al. J Agric Food Chem. 2006 Jul 12;54(14):5142–8.
35. Lia A et al. Am J Clin Nutr. 1995 Dec;62(6):1245–51.
36. Andersson M et al. Am J Clin Nutr. 2002 Nov;76(5):1111–6.
37. Salzman E et al. J Nutr. 2001 May;131(5):1465–70.
38. Davy BM et al. J Nutr. 2002 Mar;132(3):394–8.
39. Jacobs DR Jr et al. Br J Nutr. 2002 Aug;88(2):111–6.
40. Perez-Jimenez J, Saura-Calixto F. J Agric Food Chem. 2005 Jun 15;53(12):5036–40.
41. Chen CY et al. J Nutr. 2004 Jun;134(6):1459–66.
42. Bratt K et al. J Agric Food Chem. 2003 Jan 29;51(3):594–600.
43. Zielinski H, Kozlowska H. J Agric Food Chem. 2000 Jun; 48(6):2008–16.
44. Emmons CL et al. J Agric Food Chem. 1999 Dec;47(12)4894–8.
45. Bryngelsson S et al. J Agric Food Chem. 2002 Mar 27;50(7):1890–6.
46. Jin JS et al. J Ethnopharmacol. 2003 May;86(1):15–20.
47. Schmidt K, Geckeler K. Int J Clin Pharmacol Biopharm. 1976 Oct;14(3):214–6.
48. Anand CL. Nature. 1971 Oct 15;233(5320):496.
49. Bye C et al. Nature. 1974 Dec 13;252(5484):580–1.
50. Garsed K, Scott BB. Scand J Gastroenterol. 2007 Feb;42(2):171–8.
51. Pazzaglia M et al. Contact Dermatitis. 2000 Jun;42(6):364.
52. Pigatto P et al. Am J Contact Dermat. 1997 Dec;8(4):207–9.
53. Stoop JMH et al. Trends Plant Sci. 1996 May;1(5):139–44.
54. Mudd JB et al. Plant Physiol. 1959 Mar;34(2):144–8.
55. Martindale, The Extra Pharmacopoeia 26th Ed. Pharmaceutical Press London March 1973.
56. Friebe A et al. Phytochemistry. 1995 Mar;38(5):1157–9.
57. Koetter U et al. Planta Med. 1994 Oct;60(5):488–9.
58. Glinwood R et al. J Chem Ecol. 2003 Feb;29(2):261–74.
59. Mueller SO et al. Food Chem Toxicol. 1999 May;37(5):481–91.
60. Warren SE, Blantz RC. Arch Intern Med. 1981 Mar;141(4):493–7.
61. Guo BZ et al. J Econ Entomol. 2004 Dec;97(6):2117–26.
62. Maksimovic Z et al. Bioresour Technol. 2005 May;96(8):873–7.
63. Snook ME et al. J Agric Food Chem. 1993;41(9):1481–5.
64. Zhang HE, Xu DP. Zhong Yao Cai. 2007 Feb;30(2):164–6.
65. Flath RA et al. J Agric Food Chem. 1978 Nov;26(6):1290–3.
66. Maksimovic Z et al. Pharmazie. 2004 Jul;59(7):524–7.
67. Farsi DA et al. Phytother Res. 2008 Jan;22(1):108–12.
68. Rau O et al. Pharmazie. 2006 Nov;61(11):952–6.
69. Maksimovic ZA, Kovacevic N. Fitoterapia. 2003 Feb;74(1–2):144–7.
70. Romero CD et al. J Ethnopharmacol. 2005 Jun;99(2):253–7.
71. Habtemariam S. Planta Med. 1998 May;64(4):314–8.
72. Du Nat D et al. J Ethnopharmacol. 1992 Jun;36(3):225–31.

Polygonaceae

1. Lin CC et al. J Sep Sci. 2006 Nov;29(17):2584–93.
2. Komatsu K et al. Chem Pharm Bull (Tokyo). 2006 Jul;54(11):1491–9.
3. Komatsu K et al. Chem Pharm Bull (Tokyo). 2006 Jul;54(7):941–7.

4. Verhaeren EH et al. Planta Med. 1982 May;45(5):15–9.
5. Su X et al. J Chromatogr A. 2007 Jun 22;1154(1–2):132–7.
6. Lu H et al. J Pharm Biomed Anal. 2007 Jan 4;43(1):352–7.
7. Koyama J et al. Chem Pharm Bull (Tokyo). 2005 May;53(5): 573–5.
8. Sun SW, Yeh PC. J Pharm Biomed Anal. 2005 Jan 4;36(5): 995–1001.
9. Ding M, Ni W. Se Pu. 2004 Nov;22(6):605–8.
10. Shi YQ et al. Anticancer Res. 2001 Jul–Aug;21(4A):2847–53.
11. Usui T et al. J Endocrinol. 2002 Nov;175(2):289–96.
12. Abe I et al. Eur J Biochem. 2001 Jun;268(11):3354–9.
13. Liu R et al. J Chromatogr A. 2004 Oct 15;1052(1–2):217–21.
14. Li M et al. Zhong Yao Cai. 2006 Apr;29(4):381–3.
15. Ye M et al. J Am Soc Mass Spectrom. 2007 Jan;18(1):82–91.
16. Martindale, The Extra Pharmacopoeia 26th Ed. Pharmaceutical Press London March 1973 p. 1633.
17. Wojcikowski K et al. J Atlern Complement Med. 2007 Jan–Feb;13(1):103–9.
18. Cai Y et al. J Agric Food Chem. 2004 Dec 29;52(26):7884–90.
19. Iizuka A et al. J Ethnopharmacol. 2004 Mar;91(1):89–94.
20. Matsuda H et al. Bioorg Med Chem. 2001 Jan;9(1):41–50.
21. Zou H et al. Yao Xue Xue Bao. 1997 Apr;32(4):310–3.
22. Lu GD et al. Carcinogenesis. 2007 Sep;28(9):1937–45.
23. Kuo PL et al. Planta Med. 2004 Jan;70(1):12–16.
24. Muto A et al. Mol Cancer Ther. 2007 Mar;6(3):987–94.
25. Chen YC et al. Biochem Pharmacol. 2002 Dec 15;64(12): 1713–24.
26. Lin S et al. Arch Biochem Biophys. 2003 Oct 15;418(2): 99–107.
27. Chen YC et al. Biochem Pharmacol. 2002 Dec 15;64(12): 1713–24.
28. Xiao B et al. Oral Oncol. 2007 Oct;43(9):905–10.
29. Guo J et al. Cancer Biol Ther. 2007 Jan;6(1):85–8.
30. Kang SC et al. Phytother Res. 2006 Nov;20(11):1017–9.
31. Zhou X et al. Bioorg Med Chem Lett. 2006 Feb;16(3):563–8.
32. Shoemaker M et al. Phytother Res. 2005 Jul;19(7):649–51.
33. Su YT et al. Biochem Pharmacol. 2005 Jul 15;70(2):229–41.
34. Lee HZ et al. Int J Cancer. 2005 Mar 1;113(6):971–6.
35. Yeh FT et al. Int J Cancer. 2003 Aug 10;106(1):26–33.
36. Lee HZ et al. Eur J Pharmacol. 2001 Nov 23;431(3):287–95.
37. Lee HZ. Br J Pharmacol. 2001 Sep;134(1):11–20.
38. Campbell MJ et al. Anticancer Res. 2002 Nov–Dec;22(6C): 3843–52.
39. Yim H et al. Planta Med. 1999 Feb;65(1):9–13.
40. Horikawa K et al. Mutagenesis. 1994 Nov;9(6):523–6.
41. Lee H, Tsai SJ. Food Chem Toxicol. 1991 Nov;29(11):765–70.
42. Sun M et al. Biosci Biotechnol Biochem. 2000 Jul;64(7):1373–8.
43. Huang Q et al. Cancer Res. 2006 Jun 1;66(11):5807–15.
44. Huang Q et al. Cell Mol Life Sci. 2005 May;62(10):1167–75.
45. Huang Q et al. Biochem Pharmacol. 2004 Jul 15;68(2):361–71.
46. Kwak HJ et al. Int J Cancer. 2006 Jun 1;118(11):2711–20.
47. Huang Q et al. Med Res Rev. 2007 Sep;27(5):609–30.
48. Leonard SS et al. J Ethnopharmacol. 2006 Jan 16;103(2):288–96.
49. Yu HM et al. Lung Cancer. 2008 Feb;59(2):219–26.
50. Cai J et al. Zhong Xi YI Jie He Xue Bao. 2005 May;3(3): 195–8.
51. Zick SM et al. J Althern Complement Med. 2006 Dec;12(10): 971–80.
52. Al-Sukhni W et al. Can J Urol. 2005 Oct;12(5):2841–2.
53. Tamayo C et al. Phytother Res. 2000 Feb;14(1):1–14.
54. Chen M. J Tradit Chin Med. 1995 Dec;15(4):252–5.
55. Xu F, Fu HM. Zhongguo Zhong Xi Yi Jie He Za Zhi. 1993 Nov;13(11):655–7, 643.
56. Liu YF et al. Am J Chin Med. 2007;35(4):583–95.
57. Wang Z, Song H. Zhongguo Zhong Xi Yi Jie He Za Zhi. 1999 Dec;19(12):725–7.
58. Zhang ZJ et al. Zhonghua Fu Chan ke Za Zhi. 1994 Aug; 29(8):463–4, 509.
59. Sydiskis RJ et al. Antimicrob Agents Chemother. 1991 Dec; 35(12):2463–6.
60. Ho TY et al. Antiviral Res. 2007 May;74(2):92–101.
61. Li Z et al. Chemotherapy. 2007;53(5):320–6.
62. Liu N et al. Zhong Yao Cai. 2004 Jun;27(6):419–21.
63. Kim TG et al. Phytother Res. 2001 Dec;15(8):718–20.
64. Zhang B et al. Zhong Yao Cai. 1998 Oct;21(10):524–6.
65. Barnard DL et al. Antiviral Res. 1992;17(1):63–77.
66. Hsiang CY et al. Am J Chin Med. 2001;29(3–4):459–67.
67. Wang Z et al. Zhongguo Zhong Yao Za Zhi. 1996 Jun;21(6): 364–6, 384.
68. Blaszczyk T et al. Phytother Res. 2000 May;14(3):210–2.
69. Wang S et al. Zhonghua Kou Qiang Yi Xue Za Zhi. 2001 Sep; 36(5):385–7.
70. Bae EA et al. Biol Pharm Bull. 1998 Sep;21(9):990–2.
71. Cyong J et al. J Ethnopharmacol. 1987 May;19(3):279–83.
72. Ubbink-Kok T et al. Antimicrob Agents Chemother. 1986; 30(1):147–51.
73. Yang ZC et al. Colloids Surf B Biointerfaces. 2005 Mar 25; 41(2–3):79–81.
74. Alves DS et al. Biochem Pharmacol. 2004 Aug 1;68(3): 549–61.
75. Chen DC et al. Zhongguo Wei Zhong Bing Ji Jiu Yi Xue. 2007 Mar;19(3):150–2.
76. Fang XL et al. Zhong Xi Yi Jie He Za Zhi. 2006 Feb;26(2): 128–30.
77. Chen D et al. Zhongguo Zhong Xi Yi Jie He Za Zhi. 2000 Jul;20(7):515–8.
78. Dong CM et al. Zhongguo Wei Zhong Bing Ji Jiu Yi Xue. 2003 Nov;15(11):666–8.
79. Saller R et al. Forsch Komplementared Klass Naturheilkd. 2001 Dec;8(6):373–82.
80. Peng A et al. Ann Acad Med Singapore. 2005 Jan;34(1):44–51.
81. Nakagawa T et al. Am J Chin Med. 2005;33(5):817–29.
82. Fu DC, Yu CY. Zhongguo Zhong Xi Yi Jie He Za Zhi. 2005 Aug;25(8):744–7.
83. Zhang JH et al. Chin Med J. 1990 Oct;103(10):778–93.
84. Li LS, Liu ZH. Zhong Xi Yi Jie He Za Zhi. 1991 Jul;11(7): 392–6, 387.
85. Sun Y et al. Zhongguo Zhong Xi Yi Jie He Za Zhi. 2000 Sep; 20(9):660–3.
86. Kang Z et al. J Tradit Chin Med. 1993 Dec;13(4):249–52.
87. Song H et al. Zhongguo Zhong Xi Yi Jie He Za Zhi. 2000 Feb; 20(2):107–9.
88. Ji SM et al. Zhongguo Zhong Xi Yi Jie He Za Zhi. 1993 Feb; 13(2):71–3, 67.
89. Xiao W et al. Zhongguo Zhong Yao Za Zhi. 2002 Apr; 27(4):241–4.
90. Yarnell E. World J Urol. 2002 Nov;20(5):285–93.
91. Boisnic S et al. Rev Stomat Chir Maxillofac. 2003 Sep; 104(4):201–5.
92. Peng SM et al. Zhongguo Zhong Xi Yi Jie He Za Zhi. 2002 Apr;22(4):264–6.
93. Usui T et al. J Endocrinol. 2002 Nov;175(2):289–96.
94. Matsuda H et al. Bioorg Med Chem Lett. 2001 Jul 23; 11(14):1839–42.
95. Hikaka S et al. J Periodontal Res. 1996 Aug;31(6):408–13.

96. Iida K et al. Planta Med. 1995 Oct;61(5):425–8.
97. Lee J et al. Life Sci. 2006 Nov 25;79(26):2480–5.
98. Misiti F et al. Brain Res Bull. 2006 Dec 11;71(1–3):29–36.
99. Yang Y et al. Biochem Biophys Res Commun. 2007 Feb 9;
     353(2):225–30.
100. Huang ZH et al. Zhongguo Zhong Xi Yi Jie He Za Zhi.
     1997 Aug;17(8):459–61.
101. Fok TF. J Perinatol. 2001 Dec;21 Suppl 1:S98–100.
102. Gu J et al. Chin Med J (Engl). 2000 Jun;113(6):529–31.
103. Tian J et al. J Tradit Chin Med. 1997 Sep;17(3):168–73.
104. Zhou H, Jiao D. Zhong Xi Yi Jie He Za Zhi. 1990 Mar;
     10(3):150–1, 131–2.
105. Wang DZ et al. Zhong Xi Yi Jie He Za Zhi. 1991 Sep;
     11(9):524–6, 515.
106. Willems M et al. Neth J Med. 2003 Jan;61(1):22–4.
107. Choi GJ et al. Crop Protection. 2004 Dec;23(12):1215–21.
108. Midiwo JO, Rukunga GM. Phytochemistry. 1985;24(6):
     1390–1.
109. Baskan S et al. Talanta. 2007 Feb 15;71(2):747–50.
110. Gunaydin K et al. Nat Prod Lett. 2002 Feb;16(1):65–70.

Ranunculaceae

1.   Seegal BC, Holden M. Science. 1945;101(2625):413–4.
2.   Martin ML et al. Planta Med. 1990 Feb;56(1):66–9.
3.   Mares D. Mycopathologia. 1987 Jun;98(3):133–40.
4.   Mares D, Fasulo MP. Cytobios. 1990;61(245):89–95.
5.   Baer H et al. J Biol Chem. 1946 Jan 1;162(1):65–8.
6.   Minakata H et al. Mutat Res. 1983 Mar;116(3–4):317–22.
7.   Cappelletti EM et al. J Ethnopharmacol. 1982 Sep;6(2):161–90.
8.   Popp M et al. Maturitas. 2003 Mar 14;44 Suppl 1:S1–7.
9.   Chen SN et al. J Nat Prod. 2007 Jun;70(6):1016–23.
10. Mimaki Y et al. J Nat Prod. 2006 May;69(5):829–32.
11. Jiang B et al. J Agric Food Chem. 2006 May 3;54(9):3242–53.
12. Wang HK et al. J Agric Food Chem. 2005 Mar 9;53(5):1379–86.
13. Chen SN et al. J Nat Prod. 2002 Oct;65(10):1391–7.
14. Shao Y et al. J Nat Prod. 2000 Jul;63(7):905–10.
15. Panossian A et al. Phytochem Anal. 2004 Mar–Apr;15(2):
     100–8.
16. He K et al. J Chromatogr A. 2006 Apr 21;1112(1–2):241–54.
17. Jarry H et al. Planta Med. 1985 Aug;51(4):316–9.
18. Jiang B et al. Phytomedicine. 2006 Jul;13(7):477–86.
19. Kennelly EJ et al. Phytomedicine. 2002 Jul;9(5):461–7.
20. Nuntanakorn P et al. Phytochem Anal. 2007 May–Jun;
     18(3):219–28.
21. Nuntanakorn P et al. J Nat Prod. 2006 Mar;69(3):314–8.
22. Fabricant DS et al. J Nat Prod. 2005 Aug;68(8):1266–70.
23. Stromeier S et al. Planta Med. 2005 Jun;71(6):495–500.
24. Li W et al. Rapid Commun Mass Spectrom. 2003;17(9):
     978–82.
25. Chen SN et al. Phytochemistry. 2002 Oct;61(4):409–13.
26. Kruse SO et al. Planta Med. 1999 Dec;65(8):763–4.
27. Jiang B et al. J Ethnopharmacol. 2005 Jan 15;96(3):521–8.
28. Grippo AA et al. Am J Health Syst Pharm. 2006 Apr 1;
     63(7):635–44.
29. Martindale, The Extra Pharmacopoeia 26th Ed. Pharmaceu-
     tical Press London March 1973 p. 325.
30. Liu ZP et al. J Med Food. 2001 Autumn;4(3):171–8.
31. Wuttke W et al. J Steroid Biochem Mol Biol. 2002
     Dec;83(1–5):133–47.

32. Wober J et al. J Steroid Biochem Mol Biol. 2002 Dec;83(1–5):
     227–33.
33. Liu Z et al. Wei Sheng Yan Jiu. 2001 Mar;30(2):77–80.
34. Lupu R et al. Int J Oncol. 2003 Nov;23(5):1407–12.
35. Oerter Klein K et al. J Clin Endocrinol Metab. 2003 Sep;
     88(9):4077–9.
36. Amato P et al. Menopause. 2002 Mar–Apr;9(2):145–50.
37. Onorato J, Henion JD. Anal Chem. 2001 Oct 1;73(19):
     4704–10.
38. Bolle P et al. J Steroid Biochem Mol Biol. 2007 Nov–Dec;
     107(3–5):262–9.
39. Stute P et al. Maturitas. 2007 Aug 20;57(4):382–91.
40. Jarry H et al. Maturitas. 2003 Mar 14;44 Suppl 1:S31–8.
41. Burdette JE et al. J Agric Food Chem. 2003 Sep 10;51(19):
     5661–70.
42. Rhyu MR et al. J Agric Food Chem. 2006 Dec 27;54(26):
     9852–7.
43. Viereck V et al. J Bone Miner Res. 2005 Nov;20(11):2036–43.
44. Qiu SX et al. Chem Biol. 2007 Jul;14(7):860–9.
45. Briese V et al. Maturitas. 2007 Aug 20;57(4):405–14.
46. Bai W et al. Maturitas. 2007 Sep 20;58(1):31–41.
47. Oktem M et al. Adv Ther. 2007 Mar–Apr;24(2):448–61.
48. Radowicki S et al. Ginekol Pol. 2006 Sep;77(9):678–83.
49. Sammartino A et al. Gynecol Endocrinol. 2006 Nov;
     22(11):646–50.
50. Vermes G et al. Adv Ther. 2005 Mar–Apr;22(2):148–54.
51. Liske E et al. J Womens Health Gend Based Med. 2002 Mar;
     11(2):163–74.
52. Pockaj BA et al. Cancer Invest. 2004;22(4):515–21.
53. Wuttke W et al. Maturitas. 2003 Mar 14;44 Suppl 1:S67–77.
54. Nappi RE et al. Gynecol Endocrinol. 2005 Jan;20(1):30–5.
55. Wuttke W et al. Menopause. 2006 Mar–Apr;13(2):185–96.
56. Hernandez Munoz G, Pluchino S. Maturitas. 2003 Mar 14;
     44 Suppl 1:S59–65.
57. Wehmann-Willenbrock E, Riedel HH. Zentralbl Gynakol.
     1988;110(10):611–8.
58. Frei-Kleiner S et al. Maturitas. 2005 Aug 16;51(4):397–404.
59. Osmers R et al. Obstet Gynecol. 2005 May;105(5 Pt 1):
     1074–83.
60. Rotem C, Kaplan B. Gynecol Endocrinol. 2007 Feb;23(2):
     117–22.
61. Uebelhack R et al. Obstet Gynecol. 2006 Feb;107(2 Pt 1):
     247–55.
62. Verhoeven MO et al. Menopause. 2005 Jul–Aug;12(4):
     412–20.
63. Pockaj BA et al. J Clin Oncol. 2006 Jun 20;24(18):2836–41.
64. Jacobson JS et al. J Clin Oncol. 2001 May 15;19(10):2739–45.
65. Newton KM et al. Ann Intern Med. 2006 Dec 19;145(12):
     869–79.
66. Low Dog T. Am J Med. 2005 Dec 19;118 Suppl 12B:98–108.
67. Viereck V et al. Trends Endocrinol Metab. 2005 Jul;16(5):
     214–21.
68. Fugate SE, Church CO. Ann Pharmacother. 2004 Sep;38(9):
     1482–99.
69. Kronenberg F, Fugh-Berman A. Ann Intern Med. 2002 Nov 19;
     137(10):805–13.
70. Cheema D et al. Arch Gynecol Obstet. 2007 Nov;276(5):
     463–9.
71. Lieberman S. J Womens Health. 1998 Jun;7(5):525–9.
72. Borrelli F, Ernst E. Eur J Clin Pharmacol. 2002 Jul;58(4):
     235–41.

73. Geller SE, Studee L. Menopause. 2007 May–Jun;14(3 Pt 1): 541–9.

74. Mahady GB. Treat Endocrinol. 2005;4(3):177–84.

75. Huntley AL, Ernst E. Menopause. 2003 Sep–Oct;10(5): 465–76.

76. Burke BE et al. Biomed Pharmacother. 2002 Aug;56(6): 283–8.

77. Duker EM et al. Planta Med. 1991 Oct;57(5):420–4.

78. Bodinet C, Freudenstein J. Menopause. 2004 May–Jun;11(3): 281–9.

79. Hostanska K et al. Biol Pharm Bull. 2004 Dec;27(12): 1970–5.

80. Sakurai N et al. Bioorg Med Chem. 2003 Mar;11(6):1137–40.

81. Garita-Hernandez M et al. Planta Med. 2006 Mar;72(4): 317–23.

82. Hostanska K et al. Breast Cancer Res Treat. 2004 Mar;84(2): 151–60.

83. Einbond LS et al. Breast Cancer Res Treat. 2004 Feb;83(3): 221–31.

84. Gaube F et al. BMC Pharmacol. 2007 Sep;20;7(1):11.

85. Einbond LS et al. Int J Cancer. 2007 Nov 1;121(9):2073–83.

86. Einbond LS et al. Anticancer Res. 2007 Mar–Apr;27(2): 697–712.

87. Bodinet C, Freudenstein J. Breast Cancer Res Treat. 2002 Nov;76(1):1–10.

88. Zierau O et al. J Steroid Biochem Mol Biol. 2002 Jan;80(1): 125–30.

89. Hostanska K et al. In Vivo. 2007 Mar–Apr;21(2):349–55.

90. Einbond LS et al. Planta Med. 2006 Oct;72(13):1200–6.

91. Rockwell S et al. Breast Cancer Res Treat. 2005 Apr;90(3): 233–9.

92. Rice S et al. Maturitas. 2007 Apr 20;56(4):359–67.

93. Jarry H et al. Phytomedicine. 2005 Mar;12(3):178–82.

94. Jarry H et al. Planta Med. 2007 Feb;73(2):184–7.

95. Hostanska K et al. Anticancer Res. 2005 Jan–Feb;25(1A): 139–47.

96. Watanabe K et al. Chem Pharm Bull (Tokyo). 2002 Jan;50(1): 121–5.

97. Kapadia GJ et al. Pharmacol Res. 2002 Mar;45(3):213–20.

98. Walji R et al. Support Care Cancer. 2007 Aug;15(8):913–21.

99. Antoine C et al. Climacteric. 2007 Feb;10(1):23–6.

100. Zepelin HH et al. Int J Clin Pharmacol Ther. 2007 Mar; 45(3):143–54.

101. Rebbek TR et al. Int J Cancer. 2007 Apr 1;120(7):1523–8.

102. Wojcikowski K et al. J Altern Complement Med. 2007 Jan–Feb;13(1):103–9.

103. Burdette JE et al. J Agric Food Chem. 2002 Nov 20;50(24): 7022–8.

104. Lai GF et al. J Asian Nat Prod Res. 2005 Oct;7(5):695–9.

105. Takahira M et al. Biol Pharm Bull. 1998 Aug;21(8):823–8.

106. Sakurai N et al. Bioorg Med Chem Lett. 2004 Mar 8; 14(5):1329–32.

107. Kim CD et al. Immunopharmacol Immunotoxicol. 2004 May;26(2):299–308.

108. Siedle B et al. Pharmazie. 2003 May;58(5):337–9.

109. Loser B et al. Planta Med. 2000 Dec;66(8):751–3.

110. Verhoeven MO et al. Fertil Steril. 2007 Apr;87(4)849–57.

111. Spangler L et al. Maturitas. 2007 Jun 20;57(2):195–204.

112. Chung DJ et al. Yonsei Med J. 2007 Apr 30;48(2):289–94.

113. Ehrlich M et al. Dermatol Surg. 2006 May;32(5):618–25.

114. Kusano A et al. Biol Pharm Bull (Tokyo). 2001 Oct;24(10): 1198–201.

115. Beuscher N. Z Phytother. 1995;16:301–10.

116. Reed S et al. Menopause. 2008 Jan–Feb;15(1):51–8.

117. Hirschberg AL et al. Menopause. 2007 Jan–Feb;14(1): 89–96.

118. Raus K et al. Menopause. 2006 Jul–Aug;13(4):678–91.

119. Dog TL et al. Menopause. 2003 Jul–Aug;10(4):299–313.

120. Huntley A. Expert Opin Drug Saf. 2004 Nov;3(6):615–23.

121. Huntley A, Ernst E. Menopause. 2003 Jan–Feb;10(1): 58–64.

122. Dugoua JJ et al. Can J Clin Pharmacol. 2006 Fall;13(3): e257–61.

123. Whiting PW et al. Med J Aust. 2002 Oct 21;177(8):440–3.

124. Dunbar K, Solga SF. Liver Int. 2007 Sep;27(7):1017–8.

125. Levitsky J et al. Dig Dis Sci. 2005 Mar;50(3):538–9.

126. Lynch CR et al. Liver Transplant. 2006 Jun;12(6):989–92.

127. Gori L, Firenzuoli F. Forsch Komplementarmed. 2007 Apr; 14(2):109–10.

128. Thomsen M, Schmidt M. J Altern Complement Med. 2003 Jun;9(3):337–40.

129. Meyer S et al. Dermatology. 2007;214(1):94–6.

130. Cohen SM et al. Menopause. 2004 Sep–Oct;11(5):575–7.

131. Light TD, Light JA. Am J Transplant. 2003 Dec;3(12): 1608–9.

132. Minciullo PL et al. Phytomedicine. 2006 Jan;13(1–2):115–8.

133. Shuster J. Hosp Pharm. 1996;31:1553–1554.

134. Ingraffea A et al. J Am Acad Dermatol. 2007 May;56(5 Suppl):S124–6.

135. Fuchikami H et al. Drug Metab Dispos. 2006 Apr;34(4): 577–82.

136. Tukamoto S et al. Evid Based Complement Alternat Med. 2005 Jun;2(2):223–6.

137. Gurley B et al. J Clin Pharmacol. 2006 Feb;46(2):201–13.

138. Gurley B et al. Clin Pharmacol Ther. 2005 May;77(5):415–26.

139. Gurley B et al. Drug Metab Dispos. 2006 Jan;34(1):69–74.

140. American Herbal Pharmacopoeia and Therapeutic Compendium; American Herbal Pharmacopoeia:Santa Cruz,CA,2001 p. 1.

141. Van Berkel GJ et al. Anal Chem. 2007 Apr 1;79(7):2778–89.

142. Unger M et al. Electrophoresis. 2005 Jun;26(12):2430–6.

143. McNamara CE et al. J Nat Prod. 2004 Nov;67(11):1818–22.

144. Abourshed EA, Khan IA. J Pharm Sci. 2001 Jul;90(7):817–22.

145. Gentry EJ et al. J Nat Prod. 1998 Oct;61(10):1187–93.

146. Hwang BY et al. Planta Med. 2003 Jul;69(7):623–7.

147. Weber HA et al. J Agric Food Chem. 2003 Dec 3;51(25): 7352–8.

148. Edwards DJ, Draper EJ. J Am Pharm Assoc (2003). 2003 May–Jun;43(3):419–23.

149. Govindan M, Govindan G. Fitoterapia. 2000 Jun;71(3):232–5.

150. Serafim TL et al. Cancer Chemother Pharmacol. 2008 May; 61(6):1007–18.

151. Zeng X, Zeng X. Biomed Chromatogr. 1999 Nov;13(7): 442–4.

152. Abidi P et al. J Lipid Res. 2006 Oct;47(10):2134–47.

153. Mahady GB et al. Phytother Res. 2003 Mar;17(3):217–21.

154. Scazzocchio F et al. Planta Med. 2001 Aug;67(6):561–4.

155. Periera Da Silva A et al. Phytother Res. 2000 Dec;14(8):612–6.

156. Lau CW et al. Cardiovasc Drug Rev. 2001 Sep;19(3):234–44.

157. Inbaraj JJ et al. Chem Res Toxicol. 2006 Jun;19(6):739–44.

158. Inbaraj JJ et al. Chem Res Toxicol. 2001;14(11):1529.

159. Chignell CF et al. Photochem Photobiol. 2007 Jul–Aug; 83(4):938–43.

160. Bhowmick SK et al. Clin Pediatr (Phila). 2007 Nov;46(9): 831–4.

161. Palanisamy A et al. J Toxicol Clin Toxicol. 2003;41(6):865–7.
162. Raner GM et al. Food Chem Toxicol. 2007 Dec;45(12):
     2359–65.
163. Etheridge AS et al. Planta Med. 2007 Jul;73(8):731–41.
164. Foster BC et al. Phytomedicine. 2003 May;10(4):334–42.
165. Chatterjee P, Franklin MR. Drug Metab Dispos. 2003 Nov;
     31(11):1391–7.
166. Budzinski JW et al. Phytomedicine. 2000 Jul;7(4):273–82.
167. Gurley BJ et al. Clin Pharmacol Ther. 2008 Jan;83(1):61–9.
168. Gurley BJ et al. Clin Pharmacol Ther. 2005 May;77(5):415–26.
169. Gurley BJ et al. Drug Metab Dispos. 2007 Feb;35(2):240–5.
170. Sandhu RS et al. J Clin Pharmacol. 2003 Nov;43(11):1283–8.
171. Tomczyk M, Gudej J. Rocz Akad Med Bialymst. 2002;47:
     213–7.
172. Texier A et al. Phytochemistry. 1984 Jan;23(12):2903–5.
173. Pourrat H et al. Ann Pharm Fr. 1982;40(4):373–6.
174. Pourrat H et al. Ann Pharm Fr. 1979;37(9–10):441–4.
175. Tomczyk M, Gudej J. Z Naturforsch [C]. 2003 Sep–Oct;
     58(9–10):762–4.
176. Jaric S et al. J Ethnopharmacol. 2007 Apr 20;111(1):160–75.
177. Oumeish OY. Clin Dermatol. 1999 Jan;17(1):13–20.

Rhamnaceae

1. Martindale, The Extra Pharmacopoeia 26th Ed. Pharmaceutical Press London March 1973 p. 1626.
2. Fairbairn JW et al. J Pharm Sci. 1977 Sep;66(9):1300–3.
3. Fairbairn JW, Simic S. J Pharm Pharmacol. 1970 Oct;22(10):
   778–80.
4. No authors listed. Analyst. 1968 Nov;93(1112):749–55.
5. Sydiskis RJ et al. Antimicrob Agents Chemother. 1991 Dec;
   35(12):2463–6.
6. Lin LT et al. Phytother Res. 2002 Aug;16(5):440–4.
7. Fork FT et al. Gastrointest Radiol. 1982;7(4):383–9.
8. Wicke L. Wien Med Wochenschr. 1981 Mar 15;131(5):133–4.
9. Reither M. Rontgenblatter. 1980 Aug;33(8):418–21.
10. Hangartner PJ et al. Endoscopy. 1989 Nov;21(6):272–5.
11. de Witte P. Pharmacol. 1993 Oct;47(Suppl 1):86–97.
12. de Witte P et al. Planta Med. 1991 Oct;57(5):440–3.
13. Nadir A et al. Am J Gastroenterol. 2000 Dec;95(12):3634–7.
14. Giavina-Bianchi PF et al. Ann Allergy Asthma Immunol.
    1997 Nov;79(5):449–54.
15. Fugh-Berman A. Lancet. 2000 Jan 8;355(9198):134–8.

Rosaceae

1. Tomlinson CTM et al. Biochem Syst Ecol. 2003 Apr;31(4):
   439–41.
2. Bilia AR et al. Phytochemistry. 1993 Mar;32(4):1078–9.
3. Bajer T et al. J Sep Sci. 2007 Jan;30(1):122–7.
4. Correia H et al. Biomed Chromatogr. 2006 Jan;20(1):88–94.
5. Bate-Smith EC. Phytochemistry. 1973 Jul;12(7):1809–12.
6. Jones E, Hughes RE. Phytochemistry. 1983 Jan;22(11):2493–99.
7. Venskutonis PR et al. Fitoterapia. 2007 Feb;78(2):166–8.
8. Correia HS et al. Biofactors. 2007;29(2–3):91–104.
9. Ivanova D et al. J Ethnopharmacol. 2005 Jan 4;96(1–2):
   145–50.
10. Kwon DH et al. Phytother Res. 2005 Apr;19(4):355–8.
11. Copeland A et al. Fitoterapia. 2003 Feb;74(1–2):133–5.
12. Swanston-Flatt SK et al. Diabetologia. 1990 Aug;33(8):462–4.
13. Trouillas P et al. Food Chem. 2003 Mar;80(3):399–407.
14. Djipa CD et al. J Ethnopharmacol. 2000 Jul;71(1–2):307–13.
15. Shrivastava R et al. Phytother Res. 2007 Apr;21(4):369–73.
16. D'Agostino M et al. Phytother Res. 1998;12(S1):S162–3.
17. Olafsdottir ES et al. Biochem Syst Ecol. 2001 Oct;29(9):
    959–62.
18. Hamad I et al. J Biotechnol. 2007 Sep;131(2 Suppl 1):S40–41.
19. Kiselova Y et al. Phtyother Res. 2006 Nov;20(11):961–5.
20. Tunon H et al. J Ethnopharmacol. 1995 Oct;48(2):61–76.
21. Jonadet M et al. J Pharmacol. 1986 Jan–Mar;17(1):21–7.
22. Jiminez F et al. J Invest Dermatol. 2006 Jun;126(6):1272–80.
23. Shrivastava R, John GW. Clin Drug Investig. 2006;26(10):
    567–73.
24. Said O et al. J Ethnopharmacol. 2002 Dec;83(3):251–65.
25. Peshel W et al. Fitoterapia. 2008 Jan;79(1):6–20.
26. Urbonaviciute A et al. J Chromatogr A. 2006 Apr 21;
    1112(1–2):339–44.
27. Jakstas V et al. Medicina (Kaunas). 2004;40(8):750–2.
28. Rayyan S et al. Phytochem Anal. 2005
    Sep–Oct;16(5):334–41.
29. Urbanek M et al. Electrophoresis. 2002 Apr;23(1–2):1045–52.
30. Ficarra P et al. Farmaco. 1990 Feb;45(2):247–55.
31. Svedstrom U et al. Phytochemistry. 2002 Aug;60(8):821–5.
32. Svedstrom U et al. J Chromatogr A. 2006 Apr 21;1112(1–2):
    103–111.
33. Rohr GE et al. J Chromatogr A. 1999 Mar 12;835(1–2):59–65.
34. Bilia AR et al. J Pharm Biomed Anal. 2007 May 9;44(1):70–8.
35. Svedstrom U et al. J Chromatogr A. 2002 Aug 30;968(1–2):
    53–60.
36. Ahumada C et al. J Pharm Pharmacol. 1997 Mar;49(3):329–31.
37. Djumlija LC. Aust J Med Herbalism. 1994 Sep;6(2):37–42.
38. WHO Monographs on Selected Medicinal Plants—Vol 2.
    WHO Geneva 2004 p. 66–82.
39. Wagner H, Grevel J. Planta Med. 1982 Jun;45(6):98–101.
40. Cuyckens F, Claeys M. Rapid Commun Mass Spectrom. 2002;
    16(24):2341–8.
41. Ficarra P et al. Farmaco. 1990 Feb;45(2):237–45.
42. Kirakosyan A et al. J Agric Food Chem. 2003 Jul 2;51(14):
    3973–6.
43. Kalny P et al. Sci Total Environ. 2007 Aug 1;381(1–3):99–104.
44. Martindale, The Extra Pharmacopoeia 26th Ed. Pharmaceu-
    tical Press London March 1973.
45. Vierling W et al. Phytomedicine. 2003 Jan;10(1):8–16.
46. Kirakosyan A et al. Physiol Plant. 2004 Jun;121(2):182–6.
47. Kiselova Y et al. Phytother Res. 2006 Nov;20(11):961–5.
48. Sroka Z et al. Z Naturforsch [C]. 2001 Sep–Oct;56(9–10):
    739–44.
49. Rakotoarison DA et al. Pharmazie. 1997 Jan;52(1):60–4.
50. Quettier-Deleu C et al. Pharmazie. 2003 Aug;58(8):577–81.
51. Rajalakshmi K et al. Indian J Exp Biol. 2000 May;38(5):
    509–11.
52. Chatterjee SS et al. Arzneimittelforschung. 1997 Jul;47(7):
    821–5.
53. Bahorun T et al. Arzneimittelforschung. 1996 Nov;46(11):
    1086–9.
54. Bahorun T et al. Planta Med. 1994 Aug;60(4):323–8.
55. Chang WT et al. Am J Chin Med. 2005;33(1):1–10.
56. Ververis M et al. Life Sci. 2004;74:1945–55.
57. Long SR et al. Phytomedicine. 2006 Nov;13(9–10):643–50.
58. Zhu XX et al. Zhongguo Zhong Yao Za Zhi. 2006
    Apr;31(7):566–9.

59. Brixius K et al. Cardiovasc Drugs Ther. 2006 Jun;20(3):177–84.
60. Siegel G et al. Phytother Res. 1996;10(Suppl 1):S195–8.
61. Corder R et al. Clin Sci (Lond). 2004 Nov;107(5):513–7.
62. Lipnicka P et al. Folia Med Cracov. 2003;44(1–2):187–99.
63. Lacaille-Dubois MA et al. Phytomedicine. 2001;8(1):47–52.
64. Schwinger RH et al. J Cardiovasc Pharmacol. 2000 May; 35(5):700–7.
65. Brixius K et al. Herz-Kreislauf. 1998 Jan;30(1):28–33.
66. Vibes J et al. Prostaglandins Leukot Essent Fatty Acids. 1994 Apr;50(4):173–5.
67. Chang WT et al. Am J Chin Med. 2005;33(1):1–10.
68. Degenring FH et al. Phytomedicine. 2003;10(5):363–9.
69. Lalukota K et al. Eur J Heart Fail. 2004 Dec;6(7):953–5.
70. Habs M. Forsch Komplementarmed Klass Naturheilkd. 2004 Aug;11 Suppl 1:36–9.
71. Rietbrock N et al. Arneimittelforschung. 2001 Oct;51(10): 793–8.
72. Zapfe G. Phytomedicine. 2001 Jul;8(4):262–6.
73. Weikl A et al. Fortschr Med. 1996 Aug 30;114(24):291–6.
74. Tauchert M. Am Heart J. 2002 May;143(5):910–5.
75. Leuchtgens H. Fortschr Med. 1993 Jul 20;111(20–21):352–4.
76. Cleland JG et al. Eur J Heart Fail. 2007 Jun–Jul;9(6–7):740–5.
77. Pittler MH et al. Am J Med. 2003 Jun 1;114(8):665–74.
78. Weihmayr T, Ernst E. Fortschr Med. 1996 Jan 20;114(1–2): 27–9.
79. Walker A et al. Br J Gen Pract. 2006 Jun;56(527):437–43.
80. Walker AF et al. Phytother Res. 2002 Feb;16(1):48–54.
81. Hempel B et al. Arzneimittelforschung. 2005;55(8):443–50.
82. Kroll M et al. Phytomedicine. 2005 Jun;12(6–7):395–402.
83. Belz GG et al. Phytomedicine. 2002 Oct;9(7):581–8.
84. Belz GG, Loew D. Phytomedicine. 2003;10 Suppl 4:61–7.
85. Tauchert M et al. Herz. 1999 Oct;24(6):465–74.
86. Loew D. Wien Med Wochenschr. 1999;149(8–10):226–8.
87. Blesken R. Fortschr Med. 1992 May 30;110(15):290–2.
88. Holubarsch CJ et al. Eur J Heart Fail. 2000 Dec;2(4):431–7.
89. Von Eiff M et al. Acta Ther. 1994;20:47–66.
90. Rogers KL et al. Eur J Pharm Sci. 2000 Feb;9(4):355–63.
91. Saenz MT et al. Z Naturforsch [C]. 1997 Jan–Feb;52(1–2): 42–4.
92. Leskovac A et al. Planta Med. 2007 Sep;73(11):1169–75.
93. Hanus M et al. Curr Med Res Opin. 2004 Jan;20(1):63–71.
94. Bourin M et al. Fundam Clin Pharmacol. 1997;11(2):127–32.
95. Zuo Z et al. Life Sci. 2006 Nov 25;79(26):2455–62.
96. Schlegelmilch R, Heywood R. J Am Coll Toxicol. 1994;13: 103–11.
97. Daniele C et al. Drug Saf. 2006;29(6):523–35.
98. Valli G, Giardina EV. J Am Coll Cardiol. 2002;39(7):1083–95.
99. Tankanow R et al. J Clin Pharmacol. 2003 Jun;43(6):637–42.
100. Krasnov EA et al. Chem Nat Comp. 2006 Mar;42(2):148–51.
101. Shelyuto VL et al. Chem Nat Comp. 1977 Jan;13(1):100–1.
102. Lamaison JL et al. Plant Med Phytother. 1991;25:1–5.
103. Kudriashov BA et al. Izv Akad Nauk SSSR Biol. 1991 Nov–Dec;(6):939–43.
104. Jones E, Hughes RE. Phytochemistry. 1983 Jan;22(11):2493–9.
105. Kahkonen MP et al. J Agric Food Chem. 1999 Oct;47(10): 3954–62.
106. Ryzhikov MA, Ryzhikova VO. Vopr Pitan. 2006;75(2): 22–6.
107. Sroka Z et al. Z Naturforsch [C]. 2001 Sep–Oct;56(9–10): 739–44.
108. Trouillas P et al. Food Chem. 2003 Mar;80(3):399–407.
109. Calliste CA et al. J Agric Food Chem. 2001 Jul;49(7): 3321–7.

110. Shilova IV et al. Bull Exp Biol Med. 2006 Aug;142(2): 216–8.
111. Halkes SBA et al. Phytother Res. 1997 Nov;11(7):518–20.
112. Tunon H et al. J Ethnopharmacol. 1995 Oct;48(2):61–76.
113. Spiridonov NA et al. Phytother Res. 2005 May;19(5):428–32.
114. Rauha JP et al. Int J Food Microbiol. 2000 May 25;56(1):3–12.
115. Liapina LA, Koval'chuk GA. Izv Akad Nauk Ser Biol. 1993 Jul–Aug;(4):625–8.
116. Lamaison JL et al. Ann Pharm Fr. 1990;48(6):335–40.
117. Peresun'ko AP et al. Vopr Onkol. 1993;39(7–12):291–5.
118. Abebe W. J Clin Pharm Ther. 2002 Dec;27(6):391–40.
119. Kim MJ. Thromb Res. 2005 Jan;117(1):197–200.
120. Horsley SB, Meinwald J. Phytochemistry. 1981 Jan;20(5): 1127–8.
121. Santamour FS, Riedel LGH. Biochem Syst Ecol. 1994 Mar; 22(2):197–201.
122. Buchalter L. J Pharm Sci. 1969 Oct;58(10):1272–3.
123. Yamaguchi K et al. Oncol Rep. 2006 Jan;15(1):275–81.
124. Omar S et al. J Ethnopharmacol. 2000 Nov;73(1):161–70.
125. Vrhovsek U et al. J Agric Food Chem. 2006 Jun 14;54(12): 4469–75.
126. Gudej J, Tomczyk M. Arch Pharm Res. 2004 Nov;27(11): 1114–9.
127. Bate-Smith EC. Phytochemistry. 1973 Apr;12(4):907–12.
128. Gudej J. Acta Pol Pharm. 2003 Jul–Aug;60(4):313–5.
129. Skupien K et al. Cancer Lett. 2006 May 18;236(2):282–91.
130. Venskutonis PR et al. Fitoterapia. 2007 Feb;78(2):162–5.
131. Patel AV et al. Curr Med Chem. 2004 Jun;11(11):1501–12.
132. Gallaher RN et al. J Food Comp Anal. 2006 Aug;19(Suppl 1): S53–7.
133. Rojas-Vera J et al. Phytother Res. 2002 Nov;16(7):665–8.
134. Parsons M et al. J Aust Coll Midwives. 1999;3:20–5.
135. Simpson M et al. J Midwif Women's Health. 2001;46(2):51–9.
136. Wang SY, Lin HS. J Agric Food Chem. 2000 Feb;48(2):140–6.
137. Johansson S et al. J Nat Prod. 2002 Jan;65(1):32–41.
138. Kreander K et al. J Pharm Pharmacol. 2006 Nov;58(11): 1545–52.

Rubiaceae

1. Itoh A et al. Phytochemistry. 1999 Nov;52(6):1169–76.
2. Itoh A et al. Phytochemistry. 1991;30(9):3117–23.
3. Quang LS, Woolf AD. Curr Opin Pediatr. 2000 Apr;12(2): 153–62.
4. Martindale, The Extra Pharmacopoeia 26th Ed. Pharmaceutical Press London March 1973 p. 711–4.
5. Souza MM et al. Braz J Biol. 2006 Feb;66(1A):151–9.
6. Litovitz T. Pediatrics. 1988 Sep;82(3 Pt 2):514–6.
7. Manoguerra AS, Cobaugh DJ. Clin Toxicol (Phila). 2005; 43(1):1–10.
8. Boyd EM, Knight LM. J Pharm Pharmacol. 1964 Feb;16: 118–24.
9. Tan GT et al. Biochem Biophys Res Commun. 1992 May 29; 185(1):370–8.
10. Murali PM et al. Respir Med. 2006 Jan;100(1):39–45.
11. Czajka PA, Russell SL. Pediatrics. 1985 Jun;75(6):1101–4.
12. Thyagarajan D et al. Med J Aust. 1993 Dec 6–20;159(11–12): 757–60.
13. Dresser LP et al. J Neurol Neurosurg Psychiatry. 1993 May; 56(5):560–2.

14. Andersen JM et al. J Pediatr Gastroenterol Nutr. 1997 May; 24(5):612–5.
15. Ho PC et al. Clin Cardiol. 1998 Oct;21(10):780–3.
16. Kuntzer T et al. J Neurol. 1989 May;236(4):246–8.
17. Silber TJ. J Adolesc Health. 2005 Sep;37(3):256–60.
18. Yamashita M et al. Vet Hum Toxicol. 2002 Oct;44(5):257–9.
19. Hassan SM. J Pharm Belg. 1983;38(6):305–8.
20. Kelly NR et al. Clin Pediatr (Phila). 2007 May;46(4):320–4.
21. Asano T et al. Biol Pharm Bull. 2001 Jun;24(6):678–82.
22. Ravishankara MN et al. Planta Med. 2001 Apr;67(3):294–6.
23. McCalley DV. J Chromatogr A. 2002 Aug 16;967(1):1–19.
24. Bartok T et al. J Mass Spectrom. 2000 Jun;35(6):711–7.
25. Kinsley-Scott TR, Norton SA. J Am Acad Dermatol. 2003 Sep; 49(3):499–502.
26. Smith NK. J R Soc Med. 1997 Oct;90(10):589–90.
27. Howard MA et al. Proc (Bayl Univ Med Cent). 2003 Jan; 16(1):21–6.
28. Pinn G. Aust Fam Physician. 1998 Oct;27(10):922–3.
29. Knauer A et al. Wien Klin Wochenschr. 2003;115 Suppl 3:39–44.
30. Folley M, Tilley L. Pharmacol Ther. 1998 Jul;79(1):55–87.
31. Nattel S, Singh BN. Am J Cardiol. 1999 Nov 4;84(9 Suppl 1):11–19.
32. Prinz A. Wien Klin Wochenschr. 1990 Dec 21;102(24):721–3.
33. Bruce-Chwatt LJ. Br Med J (Clin Res Ed). 1988 May 28;296(6635):1486–7.
34. Rojas JJ et al. BMC Complement Altern Med. 2006 Feb 17;6:2.
35. Furusawa S et al. J Pharm Pharmacol. 2001 Jul;53(7):1029–39.
36. Solary E et al. Leukaemia. 2000 Dec;14(12):2085–94.
37. Genne P et al. Leukaemia. 1994 Jan;8(1):160–4.
38. el Benna J, Labro MT. J Antimicrob Chemother. 1990 Jun; 25(6):949–57.
39. Mitsui N et al. Chem Pharm Bull (Tokyo). 1989 Feb;37(2): 363–6.
40. Pedersen-Bjergaard U et al. Eur J Clin Pharmacol. 1998 Nov–Dec;54(9–10):701–6.
41. Bird MR et al. Pathology. 1995 Apr;27(2):136–9.
42. Ergun F, Sener B. J Fac Pharm Gazi Univ (Ankara). 1986; 3(1):59–63.
43. Deliorman D et al. Pharm Biol. 2001 Jun;39(3):234–5.
44. Tzakou O et al. Fitoterapia. 1990;61(1):93.
45. Baser KHC et al. JEOR. 2004 Jul–Aug;16:305–7.
46. Roberg M. Arch Pharm. 1937;275(3):145–66.
47. Morimoto M et al. Phytochemistry. 2002 May;60(2):163–6.
48. Hultin E, Torssell K. Phytochemistry. 1965 May;4(3):425–33.
49. Mhaske SB, Argade NP. Tetrahedron. 2006 Oct;62(42): 9787–826.
50. Jones E, Hughes RE. Phytochemistry. 1983 Jan;22(11): 2493–9.
51. Romero CD et al. J Ethnopharmacol. 2005 Jun;99(2):253–7.
52. Belew C. J Nursemidwifery. 1999 May;44(3):231–52.

Rutaceae

1. Kaiser R et al. J Agric Food Chem. 1975 May;23(5):943–50.
2. El-Shafae AM, El-Domiaty MM. J Pharm Biomed Anal. 2001 Nov;26(4):539–45.
3. Lis-Balchin M et al. J Pharm Pharmacol. 2001 Apr;53(4): 579–82.
4. Simpson D. Scott Med J. 1998 Dec;43(6):189–91.

5. Martindale, The Extra Pharmacopoeia 26th Ed. Pharmaceutical Press London March 1973.
6. Steenkamp V et al. J Ethnopharmacol. 2006 Jan;103(1):71–5.
7. Viljoen AM et al. S Afr J Bot. 2007 Apr;73(2):319–20.
8. De Feo V et al. Phytochemistry. 2002 Nov;61(5):573–8.
9. Stashenko EE et al. J Biochem Biophys Methods. 2000 Jul 5; 43(1–3):379–90.
10. Koblovska R et al. Phytochem Anal. 2008 Jan–Feb;19(1): 67–70.
11. Proestos C et al. Food Chem. 2006 Apr;95(4):664–71.
12. Chen CC et al. J Nat Prod. 2001 Jul;64(7):990–2.
13. Ivanova A et al. Fitoterapia. 2005 Jun;76(3–4):344–7.
14. Hale AL et al. J Agric Food Chem. 2004 Jun 2;52(11):3345–9.
15. Milesi S et al. Plant Sci. 2001 Jun;161(1):189–99.
16. Gray AI, Waterman PG. Phytochemistry. 1978 Jan;17(5): 845–64.
17. Jager AK et al. J Ethnopharmacol. 2006 Apr 21;105(1–2): 294–300.
18. Oliva A et al. J Agric Food Chem. 2003 Feb 12;51(4):890–6.
19. Paulini H et al. Planta Med. 1991 Feb;57(1):82–3.
20. Grundon MF, Okely HM. Phytochemistry. 1979 Sep; 18(10):1768–9.
21. Lans C. J Ethnobiol Ethnomed. 2007 Mar 15;3:13.
22. Al-Heali FM, Rahemo Z. Turkiye Parazitol Derg. 2006;30(4): 272–4.
23. Alzoreky NS, Nakahara K. Int J Food Microbiol. 2003 Feb 15;80(3):223–30.
24. Ojala T et al. J Ethnopharmacol. 2000 Nov;73(1–2):299–305.
25. Valsaraj R et al. J Ethnopharmacol. 1997 Oct;58(2):75–83.
26. Adsersen A et al. J Ethnopharmacol. 2006 Apr 6;104(3): 418–22.
27. Risa J et al. J Ethnopharmacol. 2004 Aug;93(2):177–82.
28. Bethge EW et al. Gen Physiol Biophys. 1991 Jun;10(3): 225–44.
29. Bohuslavizki KH et al. Gen Physiol Biophys. 1992 Oct;11(5): 507–12.
30. Rethy B et al. Planta Med. 2007 Jan;73(1):41–8.
31. Bamigboye AA, Smyth R. Cochrane Database Syst Rev. 2007 Jan;24;(1):CD001066.
32. Bernado LC et al. Cell Mol Biol (Noisy-le-Grand). 2002 Jul; 48(5):517–20.
33. Paulini H et al. Mutagenesis. 1987 Jul;2(4):271–3.
34. Paulini H, Schimmer O. Mutagenesis. 1989 Jan;4(1):45–50.
35. Schimmer O, Kuhne I. Mutat Res. 1990 Jan;243(1):57–62.
36. Natarajan AT et al. Mutat Res. 1981 Nov;84(1):113–24.
37. Heskel NS et al. Contact Dermatitis. 1983 Jul;9(4):278–80.
38. Wessner D et al. Contact Dermatitis. 1999 Oct;41(4):232.
39. Schempp CM et al. Hautarzt. 1999 Jun;50(6):432–4.
40. Eickhorst K et al. Dermatitis. 2007 Mar;18(1):52–5.
41. Furniss D, Adams T. J Burn Care Res. 2007 Sep–Oct;28(5): 767–9.
42. Seak CJ, Lin CC. Clin Toxicol (Phila). 2007;45(2):173–5.
43. Ciganda C, Laborde A. J Toxicol Clin Toxicol. 2003;41(3): 235–9.
44. Gibbons S et al. Phytother Res. 2003 Mar;17(3):274–5.
45. Fish F, Waterman PG. J Pharm Pharmacol. 1973 Dec;25 Suppl:115P-6.
46. Fish F et al. Lloydia. 1975 May–Jun;38(3):268–70.
47. Crombie L. Nature. 1954 Oct;174(4435):833.
48. Rao KV, Davies R. J Nat Prod. 1986 Mar–Apr;49(3):340–2.
49. Brinker F. Br J Phytother. 1991–2;2(4):160–70.
50. Ju Y et al. Phytother Res. 2001 Aug;15(5):441–3.

51. Simeray J et al. Phytochemistry. 1985 Oct;24(11):2720–1.
52. Dreyer DL. Tetrahedron. 1967 Jan;23(12):4613–22.
53. Saqib QN et al. Phytother Res. 2006 Jan 11;4(6):216–9.
54. Bafi-Yeboa NF et al. Phytomedicine. 2005 May;12(5):370–7.
55. Melliou E et al. J Nat Prod. 2005 Jan;68(1):78–82.
56. Gray AI, Waterman PG. Phytochemistry. 1978 Jan;17(5): 845–64.
57. Li CY et al. J Nat Prod. 2005 Nov;68(11):1622–4.
58. Smith ML et al. Photochem Photobiol. 2004 Jun;79(6):506–9.

Salicaceae

1. Morse AM et al. Phytochemistry. 2007 Aug;68(15):2043–52.
2. Pearl IA, Darling SF. Phytochemistry. 1971 Feb;10(2):483–4.
3. Pearl IA, Darling SF. Phytochemistry. 1971 Feb;10(12): 3161–66.
4. Hubbes M. Science. 1962 Apr 13;136(3511):156.
5. Fernandez MP et al. J Chromatogr A. 2001 Jul 13;922(1–2): 225–33.
6. Oka M et al. Phytomedicine. 2007 Aug;14(7–8):465–72.
7. Faustova NM et al. Zh Mikrobiol Epidemiol Immunobiol. 2006 May–Jun;(3):3–7.
8. Schempp H et al. Arzneimittelforschung. 2000 Apr;50(4): 362–72.
9. Rohnert U et al. Z Naturforsch [C]. 1998 Mar–Apr;53(3–4): 233–40.
10. von Kruedener S et al. Arzneimittelforschung. 1996 Aug;46(8): 809–14.
11. Meyer B et al. Arzneimittelforschung. 1995 Feb;45(2):174–6.
12. Gundermann KJ, Muller J. Wien Med Wochenschr. 2007; 157(13–14):343–7.
13. Klein-Galczinsky C. Wien Med Wochenschr. 1999;149(8–10): 248–53.
14. Turner NJ, Hebda RJ. J Ethnopharmacol. 1990 Apr;29(1): 59–72.
15. van Kreudener S et al. Arzneimittelforschung. 1995 Feb; 45(2):169–71.
16. Aalto-Korte K et al. Contact Dermatitis. 2005 Feb;52(2):93–5.
17. Jolanki R et al. Contact Dermatitis. 1997 Dec;37(6):304–5.
18. Claus EP. Pharmacognosy 4th Ed. Henry Kimpton. London 1961 p. 146.
19. Greenaway W et al. J Chromatogr A. 1989 Jan;472:393–400.
20. Wollenweber E. Biochem Syst Ecol. 1975;3(1):35–45.
21. Greenaway W, Whatley FR. J Chromatogr A. 1991 Jan;543: 113–21.
22. Isidorov VA, Vinogorova VT. Z Naturforsch [C]. 2003 May–Jun;58(5–6):355–60.
23. Jerkovic I, Mastelic J. Phytochemistry. 2003 May;63(1): 109–13.
24. Levin ED et al. Phytochemistry. 1988;27(10):3241–3.
25. Whatley FR et al. Z Naturforsch [C]. 1989 May–Jun;44(5–6): 353–6.
26. Popova M et al. Phytochem Anal. 2004 Jul–Aug;15(4):235–40.
27. Poblocka-Olech L et al. J Sep Sci. 2007 Nov;30(17):2958–66.
28. Kammerer B et al. Phytochem Anal. 2005 Nov–Dec;16(6): 470–8.
29. Du Q et al. Nat Prod Res. 2007 May;21(5):451–4.
30. Jurgenliemk G et al. Pharmazie. 2007 Mar;62(3):231–4.
31. Bridle P et al. Phytochemistry. 1970;9(5):1097–8.
32. Karacsonyi S et al. Carbohydr Res. 1975 Nov;44(2):285–90.
33. Vane JR. J Physiol Pharmacol. 2000 Dec;51(4 Pt 1):573–86.
34. Appelboom T. Rheumatology (Oxford). 2002 Apr;41 Suppl 1: 28–34.
35. Jerie P. Cas Lek Cesk. 2006;145(12):901–4.
36. Chrubasik JE et al. Phytother Res. 2007 Jul;21(7):675–83.
37. Marz RW, Kemper F. Wien Med Wochenschr. 2002; 152(15–16):354–9.
38. Nahrstedt A et al. Wien Med Wochenschr. 2007;157(13–14): 348–51.
39. Khayyal MT et al. Arzneimittelforschung. 2005;55(11): 677–87.
40. Wuthold K et al. J Chromatogr Sci. 2004 Jul;42(6):306–9.
41. Chrubasik S et al. Arthritis Rheum. 2003 Jan;48(1):278–80.
42. Kahkonen MP et al. J Agric Food Chem. 1999 Oct;47(10): 3954–62.
43. Fiebich BL, Chrubasik S. Phytomedicine. 2004;11(2–3): 135–8.
44. Williamson EM. Phytomedicine. 2001 Sep;8(5):401–9.
45. Wagner I et al. Clin Pharmacol Ther. 2003 Mar;73(3):272–4.
46. Chrubasik S et al. Rheumatology. 2001 Dec;40(12):1388–93.
47. Chrubasik S et al. Phytomedicine. 2001 Jul;8(4):241–51.
48. Chrubasik S et al. Am J Med. 2000 Jul;109(1):9–14.
49. Schmid B et al. Phytother Res. 2001 Jun;15(4):344–50.
50. Biegert C et al. J Rheumatol. 2004 Nov;31(11):2121–30.
51. Gagnier JJ et al. Spine. 2007 Jan 1;32(1):82–92.
52. Hostanska K et al. Cancer Detect Prev. 2007;31(2):129–39.
53. Nizard C et al. Ann N Y Acad Sci. 2004 Jun;1019:223–7.
54. Shrivastava R et al. Clin Drug Investig. 2006;26(5):287–96.
55. Krivoy N et al. Planta Med. 2001 Apr;67(3):209–12.
56. Pirker R et al. J Chromatogr B Analyt Technol Biomed Life Sci. 2004 Oct 5;809(2):257–64.
57. Schmid B et al. Eur J Clin Pharmacol. 2001 Aug;57(5): 387–91.
58. Boullata JI et al. Ann Pharmacother. 2003 Jun;37(6):832–5.
59. Heck AM et al. Am J Health Syst Pharm. 2000 Jul 1; 57(13):1221–7.

Scrophulariaceae

1. Wiegrebe H, Witchl M. J Chromatogr. 1993 Feb;5; 630(1–2):402–7.
2. Ikeda Y et al. J Chromatogr A. 1996 Oct 11;746(2):255–60.
3. Moore WN, Taylor LT. J Nat Prod. 1996 Jul;59(7):690–3.
4. Orosz F et al. Anal Biochem. 1986 Jan;156(1):171–5.
5. Ikeda Y et al. J Nat Prod. 1995 Jun;58(6):897–901.
6. Usai M et al. Nat Prod Res. 2007 Jul 20;21(9):798–804.
7. Lugt CB. Planta Med. 1973 Mar;23(2):176–81.
8. Groeneveld HW et al. Planta Med. 1992 Jun;58(3):239–44.
9. Choi DY et al. J Biomed Sci. 2005 Dec;12(6):949–59.
10. Oh JW et al. J Pharm Pharmacol. 2005 Jul;57(7):903–10.
11. Martindale, The Extra Pharmacopoeia 26th Ed. Pharmaceutical Press London March 1973.
12. Hollman A. BMJ. 1996 Apr 6;312(7035):912.
13. Hauptman PJ, Kelly RA. Circulation. 1999 Mar 9;99(9): 1265–70.
14. Norn S, Kruse PR. Dan Medicinhist Arbog. 2004;119–32.
15. Lopez-Lazaro M et al. Planta Med. 2003 Aug;69(8):701–4.
16. Lindholm P et al. J Biomol Screen. 2002 Aug;7(4):333–40.
17. Ramlakhan SL, Fletcher AK. Eur J Emerg Med. 2007 Dec; 14(6):356–9.

18. Lacassie E et al. J Forensic Sci. 2000 Sep;45(5):1154–8.
19. Blazics B, Kery A. http://www.thieme-connect.de/ejournals/abstract/plantamedica/doi/10.1055/s-2007-987047.
20. Kozlowski J, Krajewska A. Farm Pol. 1982;38(10):471–4.
21. Salama O, Sticher O. Planta Med. 1983 Feb;47(2):90–4.
22. Sticher O, Salama O. Planta Med. 1981 Jun;42(6):122–3.
23. Plouvier V, Favre-Bonvin J. Phytochemistry. 1971 Aug;10(8):1697–1722.
24. Tomas-Barberan FA et al. Phytochemistry. 1988 Jan;27(8):2631–45.
25. Ersoz T et al. J Nat Prod. 2000;63(10):1449–50.
26. Sticher O et al. Planta Med. 1982 Jul;45(7):159.
27. Salama O et al. Phytochemistry. 1981 Jan;20(11):2603–4.
28. Salama O et al. Planta Med. 1981 Jun;42(6):123–4.
29. Chudnicka A, Matysik G. J Ethnopharmacol. 2005 Jun;99(2):281–6.
30. Jones E, Hughes RE. Phytochemistry. 1983 Jan;22(11):2493–9.
31. Trovato A et al. Boll Chim Farm. 1996 Apr;135(4):263–6.
32. Sesterhenn K et al. Plant Cell Rep. 2007 Mar;26(3):365–71.
33. Weinges K, Von Der Eltz H. Leibigs Annalen. 1832–1997;1978(12):1968–73.
34. Miyase T, Mimatsu A. J Nat Prod. 1999 Aug;62(8):1079–84.
35. Swiatek L. Pol J Pharmacol Pharm. 1973;25(5):461–4.
36. Jones E, Hughes RE. Phytochemistry. 1983 Jan;22(11):2493–9.
37. Zhou FY et al. Carbohydr Res. 2006 Nov;341(15):2469–77.
38. Stevenson PC et al. Phytother Res. 2002 Feb;16(1):33–5.
39. Fernandez MA et al. J Ethnopharmacol. 1996 Jul;53(1):11–14.
40. Slagowska A et al. Pol J Pharmacol Pharm. 1987 Jan–Feb;39(1):55–61.
41. Klimek B. Phytochemistry. 1996 Dec;43(6):1281–4.
42. Khuroo MA et al. Phytochemistry. 1988 Jan;27(11):3541–4.
43. Swiatek L et al. Planta Med. 1982 Jul;45(7):153.
44. Mehrotra R et al. J Nat Prod. 1989 May–Jun;52(3):640–3.
45. Miyase T et al. Chem Pharm Bull (Tokyo). 1997 Dec;45(12):2029–33.
46. Warashina T et al. Phytochemistry. 1992 Mar;31(3):961–5.
47. Turker AU, Gurel E. Phytother Res. 2005 Sep;19(9):733–9.
48. Pardo F et al. J Chem Ecol. 1998;24:645–53.
49. Turker AU, Camper ND. J Ethnopharmacol. 2002 Oct;82(2–3):117–25.
50. McCutheon AR et al. J Ethnopharmacol. 1992 Oct;37(3):213–23.
51. Zgorniak-Nowosielska I et al. Arch Immunol Ther Exp (Warz). 1991;39(1–2):103–8.
52. McCutcheon AR et al. J Ethnopharmacol. 1994 Dec;44(3):157–69.
53. Lin LT et al. Phytother Res. 2002 Aug;16(5):440–4.
54. Galasinksi W et al. Acta Pol Pharm. 1996 Sep–Oct;53(5):311–8.
55. Sarrell EM et al. Pediatrics. 2003 May;111(5):574–9.
56. Sarrell EM et al. Arch Pediatr Adolesc Med. 2001 Jul;155(7):796–9.
57. Romaguera C et al. Contact Dermatitis. 1985 Mar;12(3):176.
58. Claus EP. Pharmacognosy 4th Ed. Henry Kimpton. London 1961.
59. Albach DC et al. Phytochemistry. 2004 Jul;65(14):2129–34.
60. Grayer-Barkmeijer RJ. Biochem Syst Ecol. 1973 May;1(2):101–10.

Solanaceae

1. Hartmann T et al. Planta Med. 1986 Oct;52(5):390–5.
2. Talaty N et al. Analyst. 2005 Dec;130(12):1624–33.
3. Ylinen M et al. Planta Med. 1986 Apr;52(2):85–7.
4. Phillipson JD, Handa SS. Phytochemistry. 1976;15(5):605–8.
5. Bekkouche K et al. Phytochemistry. 2001 Oct;58(3):455–62.
6. Shvets SA et al. Adv Exp Med Biol. 1996;404:475–83.
7. Martindale, The Extra Pharmacopoeia 26th Ed. Pharmaceutical Press London March 1973.
8. Betterman H et al. Auton Neurosci. 2001 Jul 20;90(1–2):132–7.
9. Mazzanti G et al. Pharmacol Res Commun. 1988 Dec;20 Suppl 5:49–53.
10. Schneider F et al. J Toxicol Clin Toxicol. 1996;34(1):113–7.
11. Southgate HJ et al. J R Soc Health. 2000 Jun;120(2):127–30.
12. Caksen H et al. Hum Exp Toxicol. 2003 Dec;22(12):665–8.
13. Jellema K et al. Ned Tijdschr Geneeskd. 2002 Nov 16;146(46):2173–6.
14. Heindl S et al. Dtsch Med Wochenschr. 2000 Nov 10;125(45):1361–5.
15. Jaspersen-Schib R et al. Schweiz Med Wochenschr. 1996 Jun 22;126(25):1085–98.
16. Joshi P et al. Postgrad Med J. 2003 Apr;79(930):239–40.
17. Wilhelm H et al. Fortschr Ophthalmol. 1991;88(5):588–91.
18. Calixto JB et al. Pharmacol Ther. 2005 May;106(2):179–208.
19. Ben-Chaim A et al. Theor Appl Genet. 2006 Nov;113(8):481–90.
20. Thompson RQ et al. Anal Bioanal Chem. 2005 Apr;381(7):1441–51.
21. Surh YJ, Lee SS. Food Chem Toxicol. 1996 Mar;34(3):313–6.
22. Higashiguchi F et al. J Agric Food Chem. 2006 Aug 9;54(16):5948–53.
23. Garces-Claver A et al. J Agric Food Chem. 2007 Aug 22;55(17):6951–7.
24. De Masi L et al. Mol Nutr Food Res. 2007 Aug;51(8):1053–62.
25. Garces-Claver A et al. J Agric Food Chem. 2006 Dec 13;54(25):9303–11.
26. Antonious GF, Jarret RL. J Environ Sci Health B. 2006;41(5):717–29.
27. Barbero GF et al. J Agric Food Chem. 2006 May 3;54(9):3231–6.
28. Kozukue N et al. J Agric Food Chem. 2005 Nov 16;53(23):9172–81.
29. Ochi T et al. J Nat Prod. 2003 Aug;66(8):1094–6.
30. Kirschbaum-Titze P et al. J Agric Food Chem. 2002 Feb 27;50(5):1264–6.
31. Materska M et al. Phytochemistry. 2003 Aug;63(8):893–8.
32. Materska M, Perucka I. J Agric Food Chem. 2005 Mar 9;53(5):1750–6.
33. Schweiggert U et al. Rapid Commun Mass Spectrom. 2005;19(18):2617–28.
34. Lee JH et al. Chem Pharm Bull (Tokyo). 2007 Aug;55(8):1151–6.
35. Lee JH et al. Chem Pharm Bull (Tokyo). 2006 Oct;54(10):1365–9.
36. Iorizzi M et al. J Agric Food Chem. 2001 Apr;49(4):2022–9.
37. Catchpole OJ et al. J Agric Food Chem. 2003 Aug 13;51(17):4853–60.
38. De Lucca AJ et al. Med Mycol. 2002 Apr;40(2):131–7.
39. Yahara S et al. Phytochemistry. 1994 Oct;37(3):831–5.
40. Ching LS, Mohamed S. J Agric Food Chem. 2001 Jun;49(6):3101–5.

41. Dasgupta P, Fowler CJ. Br J Urol. 1997 Dec;80(6):845–52.
42. Johnson W. J Int Toxicol. 2007;26 Suppl 1:3–106.
43. Suhaj M. J Food Comp Anal. 2006 Sep;19(6):531–7.
44. Antonious GF et al. J Environ Sci Health B. 2006;41(7): 1237–43.
45. Luqman S, Rizvi SI. Phytother Res. 2006 Apr;20(4):303–6.
46. Rosa A et al. J Agric Food Chem. 2002 Dec 4;50(25):7396–401.
47. Stander S et al. Exp Dermatol. 2004 Mar;13(3):129–39.
48. Bortolotti M et al. Aliment Pharmacol Ther. 2002 Jun;16(6):1075–82.
49. Bunker CB et al. Agents Action. 1991 May;33(1–2):195–6.
50. Reilly DM, Green MR. Acta Derm Venereol (Stockh). 1999 May;79(3):187–90.
51. Hahn K et al. Neurology. 2007 Apr 17;68(16):1251–6.
52. Rizvi SI, Luqman S. Cell Mol Biol Lett. 2003;8(4):919–25.
53. Reilly CA et al. Toxicol Sci. 2003;73:170–81.
54. Calixto JB et al. Expert Opin Emerg Drugs. 2001 Oct;6(2): 261–79.
55. Frerick H et al. Pain. 2003 Nov;106(1–2):59–64.
56. Keitel W et al. Arzneimittelforschung. 2001 Nov;51(11): 896–903.
57. Gagnier JJ et al. Spine. 2007 Jan 1;32(1):82–92.
58. Gagnier JJ et al. Cochrane Database Syst Rev. 2006 Apr 19;(2): CD004504.
59. Kim KS et al. Paediatr Anaesth. 2006 Oct;16(10):1036–41.
60. Kim KS, Nam YM. Anesth Analg. 2006 Sep;103(3):709–13.
61. Tandan R et al. Diabetes Care. 1992 Jan;15(1):8–14.
62. Watson CP et al. Pain. 1989 Aug;38(2):177–86.
63. Sicuteri F et al. Clin J Pathol. 1989;5:49–53.
64. Watson CP et al. Pain. 1988 Jun;33(3):333–40.
65. Deal CL et al. Clin Ther. 1991; 13:383–95.
66. McCarthy GM, McCarty DJ. J Rheumatol. 1992 Apr; 19(4):604–7.
67. Cheshire WP, Synder CR. Pain. 1990 Sep;42(3):307–11.
68. Jensen-Jarolim E et al. J Nutr. 1998 Mar;128(3):577–81.
69. Yeoh KG et al. Dig Dis Sci. 1995 Mar;40(3):580–2.
70. Rodriguez-Stanley S et al. Aliment Pharmacol Ther. 2000 Jan; 14(1):129–34.
71. Yeoh KG et al. J Clin Gastroenterol. 1995;21:87–90.
72. Horowitz M et al. J Gastroenterol Hepatol. 1992 Jan–Feb; 7(1):52–6.
73. Gonzalez R et al. Dig Dis Sci. 1998;43(6):1165–71.
74. Agarwal MK et al. Indian J Gastroenterol. 2002 Sep–Oct; 21(5):179–82.
75. Milke P et al. Dig Dis. 2006;24(1–2):184–8.
76. v Schonfeld J, Evans DF. Z Gastroenterol. 2007 Feb;45(2): 171–5.
77. Kumar N et al. Br Med J. 1984 Jun 16;288(6433):1803–4.
78. Kang JY et al. Dig Dis Sci. 1995 Mar;40(3):576–9.
79. Huynh HT, Teel RW. Anticancer Res. 2005 Jan–Feb; 25(1A):117–20.
80. van Wyk CW et al. Indian J Exp Biol. 1995 Apr;33(4):244–8.
81. Morre DJ, Morre DM. J Pharm Pharmacol. 2003 Jul; 55(7):987–94.
82. Surh YJ. Food Chem Toxicol. 2002 Aug;40(8):1091–7.
83. Han SS et al. Arch Pharm Res. 2002 Aug;25(4):475–9.
84. Modly CE et al. Drug Metab Dispos. 1986 Jul–Aug;14(4): 413–6.
85. Tsou MF et al. Anticancer Res. 2006 May–Jun;26(3A):1965–71.
86. Lee YS et al. Free Rad Res. 2004 Apr;38(4):405–12.
87. Morre D et al. Eur J Cancer. 1996;32:1995–2003.
88. Kim JD et al. Cancer Lett. 1997;120:235–41.
89. Zhang J et al. Leuk Res. 2003 Mar;27(3):275–83.
90. Richeux F et al. Arch Toxicol. 1999 Sep;73(7):403–9.
91. Min JK et al. Cancer Res. 2004 Jan 15;64(2):644–51.
92. Molnar J et al. In Vivo. 2004 Mar–Apr;18(2):237–44.
93. Mathew A et al. Eur J Cancer Prev. 2000 Apr;9(2):89–97.
94. Serra I et al. Int J Cancer. 2002 Dec 1;102(4):407–11.
95. Pandey M, Shukla VK. Eur J Cancer Prev. 2002 Aug;11(4): 365–8.
96. Duffy VB et al. J Am Diet Assoc. 1997 Sep;97(9 Suppl 1):A26.
97. Berger A et al. J Pain Sympt Manag. 1995 Apr;10(3):243–8.
98. Franco-Cereceda A, Rudehill A. Acta Physiol Scand. 1989 Aug;136(4):575–80.
99. Ahuja KD et al. Eur J Clin Nutr. 2007 Mar;61(3):326–33.
100. Ahuja KD, Ball MJ. Br J Nutr. 2006 Aug;96(2):239–42.
101. Yoshioka M et al. Br J Nutr. 1998 Dec;80(6):503–10.
102. Yoshioka M et al. J Nutr Sci Vitaminol (Tokyo). 1995;41: 647–56.
103. Altomare DF et al. Dis Colon Rectum. 2006 Jul;49(7): 1018–23.
104. Rau O et al. Pharmazie. 2006 Nov;61(11):952–6.
105. Yoshioka M et al. Br J Nutr. 2004 Jun;91(6):991–5.
106. Matsumoto T et al. J Nutr Sci Vitaminol (Tokyo). 2000 Dec; 46(6):309–15.
107. Yoshioka M et al. J Nutr Sci Vitaminol (Tokyo). 1995 Dec; 41(6):647–56.
108. Hachiya S et al. Biosci Biotechnol Biochem. 2007 Mar; 71(3):671–6.
109. Lim K et al. Med Sci Sports Exerc. 1997 Mar;29(3):355–61.
110. Yoshioka M et al. Br J Nutr. 1999 Aug;82(2):115–23.
111. Yoshioka M et al. Br J Nutr. 2001 Feb;85(2):203–11.
112. Ahuja KD et al. Am J Clin Nutr. 2006 Jul;84(1):63–9.
113. Chaiyata P et al. J Med Assoc Thai. 2003 Sep;86(9):854–60.
114. Domotor A et al. Eur J Pharmacol. 2006 Mar;18;534(1–3): 280–3.
115. Sharpe PA et al. J Am Diet Assoc. 2006 Dec;106(12): 2045–51.
116. Stepanovic S et al. J Med Microbiol. 1998 Nov;47(11): 1027–30.
117. De Lucca AJ et al. Med Mycol. 2002 Apr;40(2):131–7.
118. Renault S et al. Med Mycol. 2003 Feb;41(1):75–81.
119. Frischkorn CG et al. Naturwissenschaften. 1978 Sep; 65(9):480–3.
120. Jones NL et al. FEBS Microbiol Lett. 1997 Jan 15;146(2): 223–7.
121. Cichewicz RH, Thorpe PA. J Ethnopharmacol. 1996 Jun; 52(2):61–70.
122. Molina-Torres J et al. J Ethnopharmacol. 1999 Mar; 64(3):241–8.
123. Rau E. Adv Ther. 2001 Jul–Aug;17(4):197–203.
124. Graham DY et al. Am J Gastroenterol. 1999 May;94(5): 1200–2.
125. Calvet X et al. J Am J Gastroenterol. 2000 Mar;95(3):820–1.
126. Degim IT et al. Int J Pharm. 1999;179:21–5.
127. Flynn DL et al. Prostaglandins Leukot Med. 1986 Oct; 24(2–3):195–8.
128. Honda I et al. Am Rev Respir Dis. 1991 Jun;143(6):1416–8.
129. Kim DY, Chancellor MB. J Endourol. 2000 Feb;14(1): 97–103.
130. Stander S et al. J Am Acad Dermatol. 2001 Mar;44(3): 471–8.
131. Marabini S et al. Eur Arch Otorhinolaryngol. 1991;248(4): 191–4.

132. Perez-Galvez A et al. Br J Nutr. 2003 Jun;89(6):787–93.
133. Tuntipopipat S et al. J Nutr. 2006 Dec;136(12):2970–4.
134. Williams SR et al. Ann Emerg Med. 1995 May;25(5):713–5.
135. Feldman H, Levy PD. Am J Emerg Med. 2003 Mar;21(2):159.
136. Greer JM et al. Cutis. 1993 Feb;51(2):112–4.
137. Blanc P et al. Chest. 1991 Jan;99(1):27–32.
138. Azizan A, Blevins RD. Arch Environ Contam Toxicol. 1995 Feb;28(2):248–58.
139. Richeux F et al. Toxicology. 2000 May 19;147(1):41–9.
140. Oikawa S et al. Free Radic Res. 2006 Sep;40(9):966–73.
141. Surh YJ et al. Mutat Res. 1998 Jun 18;402(1–2):259–67.
142. Olajos EJ, Salem H. J Appl Toxicol. 2001 Sep–Oct;21(5): 355–91.
143. Zollman TM et al. Ophthalmology. 2000 Dec;107(12): 2186–9.
144. Vesaluoma M et al. Invest Ophthalmol Vis Sci. 2000 Jul; 41(8):2138–47.
145. Nazari F et al. Phytochem Anal. 2007;18(4):333–40.
146. Berkov S et al. Fitoterapia. 2006 Apr;77(3):179–82.
147. Philipov S, Berkov S. Z Naturforsch [C]. 2002 May–Jun; 57(5–6):559–61.
148. Miraldi E et al. Fitoterapia. 2001 Aug;72(6):644–8.
149. Mroczek T et al. J Chromatogr A. 2006 Feb 24;1107(1–2): 9–18.
150. Desai NN et al. Biochem J. 1981 Aug 1;197(2):345–53.
151. Reid KA et al. J Ethnopharmacol. 2006 Jun 15;106(1): 44–50.
152. Eftekhar F et al. Fitoterapia. 2005 Jan;76(1):118–20.
153. Sasaki T et al. Br J Cancer. 2002 Oct 7;87(8):918–23.
154. Charpin D et al. Thorax. 1979 Apr;34(2):259–61.
155. Barnett AE et al. Br Med J. 1977 Dec 24–31;2(6103):1635.
156. Nogue S et al. J Int Med Res. 1995 Mar–Apr;23(2):132–7.
157. Spina SP, Taddei A. CJEM. 2007 Nov;9(6):467–8.
158. Montcriol A et al. Ann Fr Anesth Reanim. 2007 Sep;26(9): 810–3.
159. Diker D et al. Eur J Intern Med. 2007 Jul;18(4):336–8.
160. Marc B et al. Presse Med. 2007 Oct;36(10 Pt 1):1399–403.
161. Torbus O et al. Wiad Lek. 2002;55 Suppl 1 (Pt 2):950–7.
162. Ertekin V et al. J Emerg Med. 2005 Feb;28(2):227–8.
163. Birmes P et al. Presse Med. 2002 Jan 19;31(2):69–72.
164. Wilhelm H et al. Fortschr Ophthalmol. 1991;88(5):588–91.
165. Forrester MB. J Toxicol Environ Health A. 2006 Oct; 69(19):1757–62.
166. Jaspersen-Schib R et al. Schweiz Med Wochenschr. 1996 Jun 22;126(25):1085–98.
167. Friedman M. J Chromatogr A. 2004 Oct 29;1054(1–2):143–55.
168. Boumba VA et al. Vet Hum Toxicol. 2004 Apr;46(2):81–2.
169. Khalil SA, El-Masry S. J Pharm Sci. 1976 Apr;65(4):614–5.
170. Asano N et al. Carbohydr Res. 1996 Apr;284(2):169–78.
171. Salej B et al. Chem Pharm Bull (Tokyo). 2006 Apr;54(4): 538–41.
172. Ma CY et al. J Nat Prod. 2002 Feb;65(2):206–9.
173. Ma CY, Williams ID. J Nat Prod. 1999 Oct;62(10):1445–7.
174. Pamoutsaki IA et al. Ann Otol Rhinol Laryngol. 2002 Jun;111(6):553–7.
175. Miyazaki M. Yakushigaku Zasshi. 1994;29(3):469–83.
176. Lee MR. J R Coll Physicians Edinb. 2006 Dec;36(4):366–73.
177. Zhang L et al. Proc Natl Acad Sci USA. 2004 Apr 27; 101(17):6786–91.
178. Khan FZ et al. Pak J Pharm Sci. 1992 Jan;5(1):55–61.
179. Doneray H et al. Eur J Emerg Med. 2007 Dec;14(6):348–50.
180. Stefanek J et al. Vnitr Lek. 2000 Nov;46(11):808–10.

181. Manriquez O et al. Vet Hum Toxicol. 2002 Feb;44(1):31–2.
182. Jaspersen-Schib R et al. Schwiez med Wochenschr. 1996 Jun 22;126(25):1085–98.
183. Oztekin-Mat A. Ann Pharm Fr. 1994;52(5):260–5.
184. Betz P et al. Arch Kriminol. 1991 Nov–Dec;88(5–6):175–82.
185. Vidovic D et al. Kijec Vjesn. 2005 Jan–Feb;127(1–2):22–3.
186. Wilhelm H et al. Fortschr Ophthalmol. 1991;88(5):588–91.

Tiliaceae

1. Martindale, The Extra Pharmacopoeia 26th Ed. Pharmaceutical Press London March 1973 p. 269.
2. Buchbauer G et al. Flav Frag J. 1995 May–Jun;10(3):221–4.
3. Buchbauer G et al. Flav Frag J. 1992 Dec;7(6):329–32.
4. Toker G et al. J Pharm Biomed Anal. 2001 Aug;26(1):111–21.
5. Exarchou V et al. J Chromatogr A. 2006 Apr 21;1112(1–2): 293–302.
6. Fiamegos YC et al. J Chromatogr A. 2004 Jul 2;1041(1–2):11–8.
7. Kram G, Franz G. Planta Med. 1983 Nov;49(11):149–53.
8. Manuele MG et al. Life Sci. 2006 Oct 19;79(21):2043–8.
9. Ozcan M et al. Food Chem. 2008 Feb;106(3):1120–7.
10. Celechovska O et al. Ceska Slov Farm. 2004 Nov;53(6):336–9.
11. Liu XL et al. Acta Pharm Sinica. 2001;22:929–33.
12. Cassady JM et al. J Nat Prod. 1979;42(3):274–8.
13. Barreiro Arcos ML et al. Phytother Res. 2006 Jan;20(1):34–40.
14. Medina JH et al. Biochem Biophys Res Commun. 1988 Apr 29;152(2):534–9.
15. Anesini C et al. Fitoterapia. 1999 Aug;70(4):361–7.
16. Pazdzioch-Czochra M, Widenska A. Anal Chim Acta. 2002 Feb;452(2):177–84.
17. Romero-Jimenez M et al. Mutat Res. 2005 Aug 1;585(1–2): 147–55.
18. Hirvonen T et al. Ann Epidemiol. 2006 Jul;16(7):503–8.
19. Rodriguez-Fragoso L et al. Toxicol Appl Pharmacol. 2008 Feb 15;227(1):125–35.
20. Loureiro G et al. Allergol Immunopathol (Madr). 2005 Jul–Aug;33(4):192–8.
21. Krakowiak A et al. Contact Dermatitis. 2004 Jul;51(1):34.
22. Rudzki E et al. Contact Dermatitis. 2003 Sep;49(3):162.
23. Picardo M et al. Contact Dermatitis. 1988 Jul;19(1):72–3.
24. Hurrell RF et al. Br J Nutr. 1999 Apr;81(4):289–95.

Turneraceae

1. Zhao J et al. J Nat Prod. 2007 Feb;70(2):289–92.
2. Kumar S et al. J Med Food. 2006 Summer;9(2):254–60.
3. Alcaraz-Melendez L et al. Fitoterapia. 2004 Dec;75(7–8): 696–701.
4. Godoi AF et al. J Chromatogr A. 2004 Feb 20;1027(1–2):127–30.
5. Piacente S et al. Z Naturforsch [C]. 2002 Nov–Dec;57(11–12): 983–5.
6. Bicchi C et al. Flav Frag J. 2002;18(1):59–61.
7. Spencer KC, Seigler DS. Planta Med. 1981 Oct;43(10):175–8.
8. Dominguez XA, Hinojosa M. Planta Med. 1976 Aug;30(1): 68–71.
9. Ramirez-Orduna R et al. Small Rumin Res. 2005 Feb;57(1): 1–10.
10. Aspiazu J et al. Nucl Instr Meth Phys Res B. 1995 Aug;101(4): 453–8.

11. Mendes FR, Carlini EA. J Ethnopharmacol. 2007 Feb 12;109(3): 493–500.
12. Zava DT et al. Proc Soc Exp Biol Med. 1998 Mar;217(3): 369–78.
13. Hernandez T et al. J Ethnopharmacol. 2003 Oct;88(2–3):181–8.
14. Ito TY et al. J Sex Marital Ther. 2006 Oct–Dec;32(5):369–78.
15. Ito TY et al. J Sex Marital Ther. 2001 Oct–Dec;27(5):541–9.
16. Polan ML et al. J Womens Health (Larchmt). 2004 May; 13(4):427–30.
17. Rowland DL, Tai W. J Sex Marital Ther. 2003 May–Jun;29(3): 185–205.
18. Andersen T, Fogh J. J Hum Nutr Diet. 2001 Jun;14(3):243–50.

Ulmaceae

1. Beveridge RJ et al. Carbohydr Res. 1971 Aug;19(1):107–16.
2. Beveridge RJ et al. Carbohydr Res. 1969 Apr;9(4):429–39.
3. Hough L et al. Nature. 1950 Jan 7;165(4184):34–5.
4. Martindale, The Extra Pharmacopoeia 26th Ed. Pharmaceutical Press London March 1973 p. 1088.
5. Claus EP. Pharmacognosy. 4th Ed. Henry Kimpton. London 1961 p. 86.
6. Langmead L et al. Aliment Pharmacol Ther. 2002 Feb; 16(2):197–205.
7. Choi HR et al. Phytother Res. 2002 Jun;16(4):364–7.
8. Tai J, Cheung S. Phytother Res. 2005 Feb;19(2):107–12.
9. Felton JS et al. Toxicol. 2004 May;198(1):135–45.
10. Ottenweller J et al. J Altern Complement Med. 2004;10:687–91.
11. Zick SM et al. J Altern Complement Med. 2006 Dec;12(10): 971–80.
12. Leonard SS et al. J Ethnopharmacol. 2006 Jan 16;103(2): 288–96.
13. Spaulding-Albright N. J Am Diet Assoc. 1997 Oct;97(10): S208–15.
14. Kaegi E. Can Med Assoc J. 1998;158(7):897–902.
15. Langmead L et al. Digest Liver Dis. 2000 May;32:A48.
16. Brown AC et al. Altern Med Rev. 2004 Sep;9(3):297–307.
17. Gallagher R. J Pain Sympt Manag. 1997 Jul;14(1):1–2.

Urticaceae

1. Budzianowski J et al. J Nat Prod. 1985 Mar;48(2):336.
2. Budzianowski J. Phytochemistry. 1990:29(10):3299–301.
3. Colombo P et al. Int Arch Allergy Immunol. 2003 Mar; 130(3):173–9.
4. Bullita S et al. Genet Resour Crop Evol. 2007 Nov;54(7): 1447–64.
5. Guil JL et al. J Chromatogr A. 1996 Jan;719(1):229–35.
6. Guarrera PM. Fitoterapia. 2005 Jan;76(1):1–25.
7. Uncini Manganelli RE et al. J Ethnopharmacol. 2005 Apr 26; 98(3):323–7.
8. Ji TF et al. Zhong Yao Cai. 2007 Jun;30(6):662–4.
9. Exarchou V et al. J Chromatogr A. 2006 Apr 21;1112(1–2): 293–302.
10. Akbay P et al. Phytother Res. 2003 Jan;17(1):34–7.
11. Emmelin N, Feldberg W. J Physiol. 1947 Oct 15;106(4): 440–55.
12. Smallman BN, Maneckjee A. Biochem J. 1981 Jan 15; 194(1):361–4.
13. Collier HO, Chesher GB. Br J Pharmacol. 1956 Jun;11(2):186–9.
14. Budzianowski J. Planta Med. 1991 Oct;57(5):507.
15. Fiamegos YC et al. J Chromatogr A. 2004 Jul 2;1041(1–2):11–8.
16. Chaurasia N, Wichtl M. Planta Med. 1987 Oct;53(5):432–4.
17. Sovova H et al. J Supercrit Fluids. 2004 Jul;30(2):213–24.
18. Guil-Guerrero JL et al. J Food Comp Anal. 2003 Apr;16(2): 111–9.
19. Czarnetzki BM et al. Int Arch Allergy Appl Immunol. 1990; 91(1):43–6.
20. Sajfrtova M et al. J Supercrit Fluids. 2005 Sep;35(2):111–8.
21. Ganzera M et al. Electrophoresis. 2005 May;26(9):1724–31.
22. Schottner M et al. Planta Med. 1997 Dec;63(6):529–32.
23. Wagner H et al. Planta Med. 1989 Oct;55(5):452–4.
24. Musa Oczan M et al. Food Chem. 2008 Feb;106(3):1120–7.
25. Basgel S, Erdemoglu SB. Sci Total Environ. 2006 Apr; 359(1–3):82–9.
26. Fijalek Z et al. Pharmazie. 2003 Jul;58(7):480–2.
27. Chrubasik JE et al. Phytomedicine. 2007 Jun 27;14(6): 423–35.
28. Gozum S et al. Cancer Nurs. 2007 Jan–Feb;30(1):38–44.
29. Kultur S. J Ethnopharmacol. 2007 May 4;111(2):341–64.
30. Wagner H. Environ Health Perspect. 1999 Oct;107(10): 779–81.
31. No authors. Altern Med Rev. 2007 Sep;12(3):280–4.
32. Klingelhoefer S et al. J Rheumatol. 1999 Dec;26(12):2517–22.
33. Hudec J et al. J Agric Food Chem. 2007 Jul 11;55(14): 5689–96.
34. Mavi A et al. Biol Pharm Bull. 2004 May;27(5):702–5.
35. Pieroni A et al. Phytother Res. 2002 Aug;16(5):467–73.
36. Karakaya S et al. Int J Food Sci Nutr. 2001 Nov;52(6):501–8.
37. Gulcin I et al. J Ethnopharmacol. 2004 Feb;90(2–3):205–15.
38. Chrubasik JE et al. Phytomedicine. 2007 Aug;14(7–8): 568–79.
39. Hryb DJ et al. Planta Med. 1995 Feb;61(1):31–2.
40. Gansser D, Spiteller G. Z Naturforsch [C]. 1995 Jan–Feb; 50(1–2):98–104.
41. Hirano T et al. Planta Med. 1994 Feb;60(1):30–3.
42. Gansser D, Spiteller G. Planta Med. 1995 Apr;61(2):138–40.
43. Safarinejad Mr. J Herb Pharmacother. 2005;5(4):1–11.
44. Schneider T, Rubben H. Urologe A. 2004 Mar;43(3):302–6.
45. Lopatkin N et al. Urologiia. 2006 Mar–Apr;(2):14–9.
46. Popa G et al. MMW Fortschr Med. 2005 Oct 6;147 Suppl 3: 103–8.
47. Lopatkin N et al. World J Urol. 2005 Jun;23(2):139–46.
48. Schneider HJ et al. Fortschr Med. 1995 Jan 30;113(3):37–40.
49. Bondarenko B et al. Phytomedicine. 2003;10 Suppl 4:53–5.
50. Lopatkin N et al. Int Urol Nephrol. 2007;39(4):1137–46.
51. Engelmann U et al. Arzneimittelforschung. 2006;56(3): 222–9.
52. Sokeland J. BJU Int. 2000 Sep;86(4):439–42.
53. Sokeland J, Albrecht J. Urologe A. 1997 Jul;36(4):327–33.
54. Melo EA et al. Int Braz J Urol. 2002 Sep–Oct;28(5):418–25.
55. Krezski T et al. Clin Ther. 1993 Nov–Dec;15(6):1011–20.
56. Madersbacher S et al. Urologe A. 2005 May;44(5):513–20.
57. Dvorkin L, Song KY. Ann Pharmacother. 2002 Sep;36(9): 1443–52.
58. Dreikorn K. Curr Urol Rep. 2000 Aug;1(2):103–9.
59. Koch E. Planta Med. 2001 Aug;67(6):489–500.
60. Davidov MI et al. Urol Nefrol (Mosk). 1995 Sep–Oct;(5):19–20.
61. Turker AU, Usta C. Nat Prod Res. 2008 Jan;22(2):136–46.

62. Al-Bakri AG, Afifi FU. J Microbiol Meth. 2007 Jan;68(1): 19–25.
63. Steenkamp V et al. J Ethnopharmacol. 2004 Dec;95(2–3):353–7.
64. Tosun F et al. J Ethnopharmacol. 2004 Dec;95(2–3):273–5.
65. Gul N et al. Basic Clin Pharmacol Toxicol. 2004 Nov;95(5): 215–9.
66. De Bolle MF et al. Electrophoresis. 1991 Jun;12(6):442–4.
67. van der Meer FJ et al. Antiviral Res. 2007 Oct;76(1):21–9.
68. Balzarini J et al. Mol Pharmacol. 2007 Jan;71(1):3–11.
69. De Clerq E. Med Res Rev. 2000 Sep;20(5):323–49.
70. Balzarini J et al. Antiviral Res. 1992 Jun;18(2):191–207.
71. Balzarini J et al. J Biol Chem. 2005 Dec 9;280(49):41005–14.
72. Galelli A, Truffa-Bachi P. J Immunol. 1993 Aug 15;151(4): 1821–31.
73. Van der Weijden GA et al. J Clin Periodontol. 1998 May;25(5): 399–403.
74. Galitskii LA et al. Probl Tuberk. 1997;(4):35–8.
75. Teucher T et al. Arzneimittelforschung. 1996 Sep;46(9): 906–10.
76. Obertreis B et al. Arzneimittelforschung. 1996 Apr;46(4): 389–94.
77. Setty AR, Sigal LH. Semin Arthritis Rheum. 2005 Jun;34(6): 773–84.
78. Schulze-Tanzil G et al. Histol Histopathol. 2002 Apr; 17(2):477–85.
79. Broer J, Behnke B. J Rheumatol. 2002 Apr;29(4):659–66.
80. Riehemann K et al. FEBS Lett. 1999 Jan 8;442(1):89–94.
81. Obertreis B et al. Arzneimittelforschung. 1996 Jan; 46(1):52–6.
82. Alford L. Altern Ther Health Med. 2007 Nov–Dec;13(6):58.
83. Randall C et al. Complement Ther Med. 1999 Sep;7(3): 126–31.
84. Randall C et al. J R Soc Med. 2000 Jun;93(6):305–9.
85. Rau O et al. Pharmazie. 2006 Nov;61(11):952–6.
86. Onal S et al. Prep Biochem Biotechnol. 2005;35(1):29–36.
87. Otoom SA et al. J Herb Pharmacother. 2006;6(2):31–41.
88. Ziyyat A et al. J Ethnopharmacol. 1997 Sep;58(1):45–54.
89. Fodor JI, Keve T. Acta Pharm Hung. 2006;76(4):200–7.
90. Sajid TM et al. Pak J Pharm Sci. 1991 Jul;4(2):145–52.
91. Pierre S et al. Platelets. 2005 Dec;16(8):469–73.
92. Mekhfi H et al. J Ethnopharmacol. 2004 Oct;94(2–3): 317–22.
93. Wessler I et al. Jpn J Pharmacol. 2001 Jan;85(1):2–10.
94. Kirchhoff HW. Z Phytother. 1983;4:621–6.
95. Harput US et al. Phytother Res. 2005 Apr;19(4):346–8.
96. Durak I et al. Cancer Biol Ther. 2004 Sep;3(9):855–7.
97. Kapadia GJ et al. Pharmacol Res. 2002 Mar;45(3):213–20.
98. Konrad L et al. Planta Med. 2000 Feb;66(1):44–7.
99. Lichius JJ et al. Pharmazie. 1999 Oct;54(10):768–71.
100. Mittman P. Planta Med. 1990 Feb;56(1):44–7.
101. Patten G. Aust J Med Herb. 1993 Dec;5(1):5–13.
102. Basaran AA et al. Teratog Carcinog Mutagen. 1996;16(2): 125–38.
103. McGovern TW, Barkley TM. Cutis. 1998 Aug;62(2):63–4.
104. Oliver F et al. Clin Exp Dermatol. 1991 Jan;16(1):1–7.
105. Edwards EK Jr, Edwards EK Sr. Contact Dermatitis. 1992 Apr;27(4):264.
106. Vega-Maray AM et al. Ann Allergy Asthma Immunol. 2006 Sep;97(3):343–9.
107. Weber RW. Ann Allergy Asthma Immunol. 2003 Apr; 90(4):A6.

Valerianaceae

1. Zizovic I et al. J Supercrit Fluids. 2007 Dec;43(2):249–58.
2. Circosta C et al. J Ethnopharmacol. 2007 Jun 13;112(2):361–7.
3. Paul C et al. Phytochemistry. 2001 May;57(2):307–13.
4. Letchamo W et al. J Agric Food Chem. 2004 Jan 16; 52(12):3915–9.
5. Dharmaratne HR et al. Planta Med. 2002 Jul;68(7):661–2.
6. Mikell JR et al. Pharmazie. 2001 Dec;56(12):946–8.
7. Gao XQ, Bjork L. Fitoterapia. 2000 Feb;71(1):19–24.
8. Tori M et al. Phytochemistry. 1996 Feb;41(3):977–9.
9. Granchier F et al. Phytochemistry. 1995 Nov;40(5):1421–4.
10. Bos R et al. Phytochemistry. 1986 Apr;25(5):1234–5.
11. Bos R et al. Phytochemistry. 1985 Dec;25(1):133–5.
12. Bos R et al. Phytochemistry. 1983 Jan;22(6):1505–6.
13. Corsi G et al. Biochem Syst Ecol. 1984 Jan;12(1):57–62.
14. Johnson RD, Waller GR. Phytochemistry. 1971 Dec; 10(12):3334–5.
15. Bos R et al. J Chromatogr A. 2002 Aug 16;967(1):131–46.
16. Lin LJ et al. Pharm Res. 1991 Sep;8(9):1094–102.
17. Marder M et al. Pharm Biochem Behav. 2003 Jun;75(3):537–45.
18. Fernandez S et al. Pharmacol Biochem Behav. 2004 Feb; 77(2):399–404.
19. Schumacher B et al. J Nat Prod. 2002 Oct;65(10):1479–85.
20. Goppel M, Franz G. Pharmazie. 2004 Jun;59(6):446–52.
21. Navarrete A et al. J AOAC Int. 2006 Jan–Feb;89(1):8–15.
22. Wojdylo A et al. Food Chem. 2007 Jan;105(3):940–9.
23. Pullela SV et al. Planta Med. 2005 Oct;71(10):960–1.
24. Hromadkova Z et al. Ultrason Sonochem. 2002 Jan;9(1):37–44.
25. Santos MS et al. Planta Med. 1994 Oct;60(5):475–6.
26. Houghton PJ. J Pharm Pharmacol. 1999 May;51(5):505–12.
27. WHO Monographs on Selected Medicinal Plants—Vol 1. WHO Geneva 1999 p. 267–76.
28. Grippo AA et al. Am J Health Syst Pharm. 2006 Apr 1; 63(7):635–44.
29. Arce S et al. J AOAC Int. 2005 Jan–Feb;88(1):221–5.
30. Weber G, Konieczynski P. Anal Bioanal Chem. 2003 Apr;375(8):1067–73.
31. Martindale, The Extra Pharmacopoeia 26th Ed. Pharmaceutical Press London March 1973 p. 2046.
32. Mantle D et al. J Ethnopharmacol. 2000 Sep;72(1):47–51.
33. Bliwise DL, Ansari FP. Sleep. 2007 Jul 1;30(7):881–4.
34. Trauner G et al. Planta Med. 2008 Jan;74(1):19–24.
35. Granger RE et al. Biochem Pharmacol. 2005 Apr 1;69(7): 1101–11.
36. Ortiz JG et al. Neurochem Res. 1999 Nov;24(11):1373–8.
37. Muller CE et al. Life Sci. 2002 Sep 6;71(16):1939–49.
38. Lacher SK et al. Biochem Pharmacol. 2007 Jan 15;73(2): 248–58.
39. Koetter U et al. Phytother Res. 2007 Sep;21(9):847–51.
40. Dietz BM et al. Brain Res Mol Brain Res. 2005 Aug 18; 138(2):191–7.
41. Fernandez SP et al. Eur J Pharmacol. 2006 Jun;539(3): 168–76.
42. Marder M et al. Pharmacol Biochem Behav. 2003 Jun; 75(3):537–45.
43. Abourashed EA et al. Phytomedicine. 2004 Nov;11(7–8): 633–8.
44. Oxman AD et al. PLoS ONE. 2007 Oct 17;2(10):e1040.
45. Jacobs BP et al. Medicine (Baltimore). 2005 Jul;84(4): 197–207.
46. Diaper A, Hindmarsh I. Phytother Res. 2004 Oct;18(10): 831–6.

47. Coxeter PD et al. Complement Ther Med. 2003 Dec;11(4): 215–22.
48. Ziegler G et al. Eur J Med Res. 2002 Nov 25;7(11):480–6.
49. Dorn M. Forsch Komplementarmed Klass Naturheilkd. 2000 Apr;7(2):79–84.
50. Donath F et al. Pharmacopsychiatry. 2000 Mar;33(2):47–53.
51. Leathwood PD, Chauffard F. Planta Med. 1985 Apr;51(2): 144–8.
52. Balderer G, Borbely AA. Psychopharmacology (Berl). 1985; 87(4):406–9.
53. Leathwood PD et al. Pharmacol Biochem Behav. 1982 Jul; 17(1):65–71.
54. Schulz H et al. Pharmacopsychiatry. 1994 Jul;27(4):147–51.
55. Poyares DR et al. Prog Neuropsychopharmacol Biol Psychiatry. 2002 Apr;26(3):539–45.
56. Lindahl O, Lindwall L. Pharmacol Biochem Behav. 1989 Apr;32(4):1065–6.
57. Fussel A et al. Eur J Med Res. 2000 Sep 18;5(9):385–90.
58. Morin CM et al. Sleep. 2005 Nov 1;28(11):1465–71.
59. Schmitz M, Jackel M. Wien Med Wochenschr. 1998;148(13): 291–8.
60. Schellenberg R et al. Planta Med. 2004 Jul;70(7):594–7.
61. Muller SF, Klement S. Phytomedicine. 2006 Jun;13(6):383–7.
62. Cerny A, Schmid K. Fitoterapia. 1999 Jun;70(3):221–8.
63. Wheatley D. Hum Psychopharmacol. 2001 Jun;16(4):353–6.
64. Wheatley D. Phytother Res. 2001 Sep;15(6):549–51.
65. Sun J. J Altern Complement Med. 2003 Jun;9(3):403–9.
66. Meolie AL et al. J Clin Sleep Med. 2005 Apr 15;1(2):173–87.
67. Taibi DM et al. Sleep Med Rev. 2007 Jun;11(3):209–30.
68. Bent S et al. Am J Med. 2006 Dec;119(12):1005–12.
69. Pallesen S et al. Tidsskr Nor Laegeforen. 2002 Dec 10; 122(30):2857–9.
70. Kumar V. Phytother Res. 2006 Dec;20(12):1023–35.
71. Stevinson C, Ernst E. Sleep Med. 2000 Apr 1;1(2):91–99.
72. Brattstrom A. Wien Med Wochenstr. 2007;157(13–14):367–70.
73. Gutierrez S et al. Pharmacol Biochem Behav. 2004 May; 78(1):57–64.
74. Hallam KT et al. Hum Psychopharmacol. 2003 Dec;18(8): 619–25.
75. Glass JR et al. J Clin Psychopharmacol. 2003 Jun;23(3):260–8.
76. Kuhlmann J et al. Pharmacopsychiatry. 1999 Nov;32(6): 235–41.
77. Vonderheid-Guth B et al. Eur J Med Res. 2000 Apr 19; 5(4):139–44.
78. Gerhard U et al. Schweiz Rundsch Med Prax. 1996 Apr 9;85(15):473–81.
79. Kennedy DO et al. Phytother Res. 2006 Feb;20(2):96–102.
80. Cropley M et al. Phytother Res. 2002 Feb;16(1):23–7.
81. Muller D et al. Phytomedicine. 2003;10 Suppl 4:25–30.
82. Arushanian B et al. Eksp Kolin Farmakol. 2004 Nov–Dec; 67(6):23–5.
83. Andreatini R et al. Phytother Res. 2002 Nov;16(7):650–4.
84. Eadie MJ. Epilepsia. 2004 Nov;45(11):1338–43.
85. Jacobo-Herrera NJ et al. Phytother Res. 2006 Oct;20(10):917–9.
86. Murakami N et al. Bioorg Med Chem Lett. 2002 Oct 21; 12(20):2807–10.
87. Kapadia GJ et al. Pharmacol Res. 2002 Mar;45(3):213–20.
88. Romero-Jimenez M et al. Mutat Res. 2005 Aug;585(1): 147–55.
89. Shohet D et al. Pharmazie. 2001 Nov;56(11):860–3.
90. Bos R et al. Phytochem Anal. 1996;7(3):143–51.
91. Anderson GD et al. Phytother Res. 2005 Sep;19(9):801–3.
92. Vo LT et al. Clin Exp Pharmacol Physiol. 2003 Oct;30(10): 799–804.
93. Hui-lian W et al. Toxicol Appl Pharmacol. 2003 Apr 1; 188(1):36–41.
94. von der Hude W et al. Mutat Res. 1986 Jan–Feb;169(1–2): 23–7.
95. Bounthanh C et al. Planta Med. 1981;41:21–8.
96. Mkrtchyan A et al. Phytomedicine. 2005 Jun;12(6–7):403–9.
97. Holst L et al. Pharmacoepidemiol Drug Saf. 2008 Feb;17(2):151–9.
98. Dennehy CE et al. Am J Health Syst Pharm. 2005 Jul 15;62(14):1476–82.
99. De Smet PAGM. Clin Pharmacol Ther. 2004 Jul;76(1):1–17.
100. Willey LB et al. Vet Hum Toxicol. 1995 Aug;37(4):364–5.
101. Barreales M et al. An Med Interna. 2006 Oct;23(10):483–6.
102. Chen D et al. Am J Addict. 2002 Winter;11(1):75–7.
103. Garges HP et al. JAMA. 1998 Nov 11;280(18):1566–7.
104. Lefebvre T et al. J Pharm Pharm Sci. 2004 Aug 12; 7(2):265–73.
105. Hellum BH, Nilsen OG. Basic Clin Pharmacol Toxicol. 2007 Nov;101(5):350–8.
106. Hellum BH et al. Basic Clin Pharmacol Toxicol. 2007 Jan;100(1):23–30.
107. Strandell J et al. Phytomedicine. 2004 Feb;11(2–3):98–104.
108. Alkharfy KM, Frye RF. Xenobiotica. 2007 Feb;37(2):113–23.
109. Gurley BJ et al. Clin Pharmacol Ther. 2005 May;77(5): 415–26.
110. Donovan JL et al. Drug Metab Dispos. 2004 Dec;32(12): 1333–6.
111. Dergal JM et al. Drugs Aging. 2002;19(11):879–86.

Verbenaceae

1. Stainton RE. Br J Phytother. 1990;1(3–4):43–46.
2. Bilia AR et al. J Pharm Biomed Anal. 2008 Feb 13;46(3):463–70.
3. Tian J et al. Zhongguo Zhong Yao Za Zhi. 2005 Feb;30(4): 268–9.
4. Rosendal S et al. Phytochemistry. 1989 Jan;28(1):97–105.
5. Muller A et al. Chromatographia. 2004 Aug;60(3–4):193–7.
6. Calvo MI et al. Chromatographia. 1997 Sep;46(5):241–4.
7. Horodysky GR et al. J Biol Chem. 1969 Jun 25;244(12): 3110–6.
8. Chen GM et al. Zhong Yao Cai. 2006 Jul;29(7):677–9.
9. Kawashty SA, El-Garf IA. Biochem Syst Ecol. 2000 Nov 1;28(9):919–21.
10. De-Oliveira AC et al. Toxicol. 1997 Dec 26;124(2):135–40.
11. Zhang T et al. Zhongguo Zhong Yao Za Zhi. 2000 Nov; 25(11):676–8.
12. Deepak M, Handa SS. Phytother Res. 2000 Sep;14(6):463–5.
13. Liu CH, Liu Y. Zhongguo Zhong Yao Za Zhi. 2002 Dec; 27(12):916–8.
14. Deepak M, Handa SS. Phytochemistry. 1998 Sep;49(1):269–71.
15. Guil JL et al. J Chromatogr A. 1996 Jan;719(1):229–35.
16. Jones E, Hughes RE. Phytochemistry. 1983 Jan;22(11):2493–9.
17. Winde E et al. Arch Pharm. 1961 Apr;294/66:220–9.
18. Guil Guerrero JL et al. J Food Comp Anal. 1998 Dec; 11(4):322–8.
19. Guarrera PM et al. J Ethnopharmacol. 2005 Jan 15;96(3): 429–44.
20. Calvo MI. J Ethnopharmacol. 2006 Oct 11;107(3):380–2.

21. Amenta R et al. Fitoterapia. 2000 Aug;71(Suppl 1):513–20.
22. Eddouks M et al. J Ethnopharmacol. 2002 Oct;82(2):97–103.
23. Mantle D et al. Comp Biochem Physiol. 1998 Dec;121(4): 385–91.
24. Li RW et al. J Ethnopharmacol. 2003 Mar;85(1):25–32.
25. Lai SW et al. Neuropharmacol. 2006 May;50(6):641–50.
26. Hernandez NE et al. J Ethnopharmacol. 2000 Nov;73(1–2): 317–22.
27. Zava DT et al. Proc Soc Exp Biol Med. 1998 Mar;217(3): 369–78.
28. Dudai N et al. Planta Med. 2005 May;71(5):484–8.
29. Hiroven T et al. Ann Epidemiol. 2006 Jul;16(7):503–8.
30. Zaida F et al. Ann Nutr Metab. 2006;50(3):237–41.
31. Hurrell RF et al. Br J Nutr. 1999 Apr;81(4):289–95.
32. Del Pozo MD et al. Contact Dermatitis. 1994 Sep;31(3):200–1.
33. Kuruuzum-Uz A et al. Phytochemistry. 2003 Aug;63(8): 959–64.
34. Asker E et al. Acta Crystallog Sec E. 2006 Sep;62(9):4159–61.
35. Hajdu Z et al. Phytother Res. 2007 Apr;21(4):391–4.
36. Hirobe C et al. Phytochemistry. 1997 Oct;46(3):521–4.
37. Sorensen JM, Katsiotis ST. Planta Med. 2000 Apr;66(3): 245–50.
38. Jarry H et al. Maturitas. 2006 Nov 1;55(Suppl 1):S26–36.
39. Li S et al. Tetrahed Lett. 2002 Jul;43(29):5131–4.
40. Hoberg E et al. Planta Med. 2000 May;66(4):352–5.
41. Hoberg E et al. Phytochemistry. 2003 Jun;63(3):375.
42. Liu J et al. Phytomedicine. 2004 Jan;11(1):18–23.
43. Tsoulogiannis IN, Spandidos DA. Hormones (Athens). 2007 Jan–Mar;6(1):80–2.
44. Wuttke W et al. Phytomedicine. 2003 May;10(4):348–57.
45. Meier B et al. Phytomedicine. 2000 Oct;7(5):373–81.
46. Liu J et al. J Agric Food Chem. 2001 May;49(5):2472–9.
47. Oerter Klein K et al. J Clin Endocrinol Metab. 2003 Sep; 88(9):4077–9.
48. Jarry H et al. Planta Med. 2003 Oct;69(10):945–7.
49. Webster DE et al. J Ethnopharmacol. 2006 Jun 30;106(2): 216–21.
50. Milewicz A, Jedrzejuk D. Maturitas. 2006 Nov;55 (Suppl 1): S47–54.
51. Prilepskaya VN et al. Maturitas. 2006 Nov;55 (Suppl 1): S55–63.
52. Schellenberg R. BMJ. 2001 Jan 20;322(7279):134–7.
53. Berger D et al. Arch Gynecol Obstet. 2000 Nov;264(3):150–3.
54. Loch EG et al. J Womens Health Gend Based Med. 2000 Apr; 9(3):315–20.
55. Lauritzen C et al. Phytomedicine. 1997;4:183–9.
56. Atmaca M et al. Hum Psychopharmacol. 2003 Apr;18(3): 191–5.
57. Halaska M et al. Breast. 1999 Aug;8(4):175–81.
58. Halaska M et al. Ceska Gynekol. 1998 Oct;63(5):388–92.
59. Milewicz A et al. Arzneimittelforschung. 1993 Jul;43(7): 752–6.
60. Gerhard II et al. Forsch Komplementarmed. 1998;5(6): 272–8.
61. Westphal LM et al. Clin Exp Obstet Gynecol. 2006;33(4): 205–8.
62. Rotem C, Kaplan B. Gynecol Endocrinol. 2007 Feb;23(2): 117–22.
63. Amman W. Ther Ggw. 1967 Jan;106(1):124–6.
64. Amman W. Z Allgemeinmed. 1975 Dec 20;51(35):1645–8.

65. Amman W. ZFA (Stuttgart). 1979 Jan 10;55(1):48–51.
66. Amman W. ZFA (Stuttgart). 1982 Feb 10;58(4):228–31.
67. Bautze HJ. Medizinische. 1953 Feb 7;21(6):189–90.
68. Gallagher J et al. Eur J Obstet Gynecol Reprod Biol. 2008 Apr;137(2):257–8.
69. Tamagno G et al. Eur J Obstet Gynecol Reprod Biol. 2007 Nov;135(1):139–40.
70. Merz PG et al. Exp Clin Endocrinol Diabetes. 1996;104(6): 447–53.
71. Saglam H et al. Phytother Res. 2007 Nov;21(11):1059–60.
72. Ohyama K et al. Int J Biochem Cell Biol. 2005 Jul;37(7): 1496–510.
73. Weisskopf M et al. Planta Med. 2005 Oct;71(10):910–6.
74. Dixon-Shanies D, Shaikh N. Oncol Rep. 1999 Nov–Dec; 6(6):1383–7.
75. Ohyama K et al. Biol Pharm Bull. 2003 Jan;26(1):10–18.
76. Dericks-Tan JS et al. Exp Clin Endocrinol Diabetes. 2003 Feb;111(1):44–6.
77. Mehlhorn H et al. Parasitol Res. 2005 Mar;95(5):363–5.
78. Daniele C et al. Drug Saf. 2005;28(4):319–32.
79. Cahill DJ et al. Hum Reprod. 1994 Aug;9(8):1469–70.

Violaceae

1. Cu JQ et al. Phytochemistry. 1992 Feb;31(2):571–3.
2. Burdock GA et al. Food Chem. 2001 Oct;75(1):1–27.
3. Drozdova IL, Bubenchikov RA. Pharm Chem J. 2005 Apr; 39(4):197–200.
4. Ireland DC et al. Biochem J. 2006 Nov 15;400(1):1–12.
5. Svangard E et al. J Nat Prod. 2007 Apr;70(4):643–7.
6. Trabi M et al. J Nat Prod. 2004 May;67(5):806–10.
7. Al-Heali FM, Rahemo Z. Turkiye Parazitol Derg. 2006; 30(4):272–4.
8. Arora DS, Kaur GJ. J Nat Med. 2007 Jul;61(3):313–7.
9. Ireland DC et al. Biopolymers. 2008;90(1):51–60.
10. Amer A, Mehlhorn H. Parasitol Res. 2006 Sep;99(4):478–90.
11. Rimkiene S et al. Medicina (Kaunas). 2003;39(4):411–6.
12. Witkowska-Banaszczak E et al. Fitoterapia. 2005 Jul; 76(5):458–61.
13. Svangard E et al. J Nat Prod. 2004 Feb;67(2):144–7.
14. Molnar P et al. Phytochemistry. 1980 Jan;19(4):623–7.
15. Hansmann P, Kleinig H. Phytochemistry. 1982 Jan; 21(1):238–9.
16. Molnar P et al. Phytochemistry. 1985 Dec;25(1):195–9.
17. Osawa Y et al. Phytochemistry. 1971 Jul;10(7):1591–3.
18. Saito N et al. Phytochemistry. 1983 Jan;22(1):1007–9.
19. Goun EA et al. J Ethnopharmacol. 2002 Aug;81(3):337–42.
20. Ivancheva S, Stantcheva B. J Ethnopharmacol. 2000 Feb; 69(2):165–72.
21. Amenta R et al. Fitoterapia. 2000 Aug;71(Suppl 1):S13–20.
22. Gorchakova T et al. Atheroscler Suppl Comp. 2005 Apr; 6(1):66–7.
23. Mantle D et al. J Ethnopharmacol. 2000 Sep;72(1):47–51.
24. Goransson U et al. Anal Biochem. 2003 Jul 1;318(1):107–17.
25. Klovekorn W et al. Int J Clin Pharmacol Ther. 2007 Nov; 45(11):583–91.
26. WHO Drug Information Vol 16, No. 01, 2002.

Zingiberaceae

1. Chavan P et al. Biotechnol Appl Biochem. 2008 May; 50(Pt1):61–9.
2. Wang Z et al. Anal Bioanal Chem. 2006 Nov;386(6):1863–8.
3. Yu Y et al. J Pharm Biomed Anal. 2007 Jan 4;43(1):24–31.
4. Wolmuth H et al. J Agric Food Chem. 2006 Feb 22;54(4): 1414–9.
5. Jiang H et al. Rapid Commun Mass Spectrom. 2005;19(20): 2957–64.
6. Sekiwa-Iijima Y et al. J Agric Food Chem. 2001 Dec; 49(12):5902–6.
7. Millar JG. J Nat Prod. 1998 Aug;61(8):1025–6.
8. Jolad SD et al. Phytochemistry. 2004 Jul;65(13):1937–54.
9. Ma J et al. Phytochemistry. 2004 Apr;65(8):1137–43.
10. Rai S et al. J Sep Sci. 2006 Oct;29(15):2292–5.
11. Lee S et al. J AOAC Int. 2007 Sep–Oct;90(5):1219–26.
12. Schwertner HA, Rios DC. J Chromatogr B Analyt Technol Biomed Life Sci. 2007 Sep 1;856(1–2):41–7.
13. Jiang H et al. Rapid Commun Mass Spectrom. 2006;20(20): 3089–100.
14. Charles R et al. Fitoterapia. 2000 Dec;71(6):716–8.
15. Sekiwa Y et al. J Agric Food Chem. 2000 Feb;48(2):373–7.
16. Jolad SD et al. Phytochemistry. 2005 Jul;66(13):1614–35.
17. Kuo PC et al. Arch Pharm Res. 2005 May;28(5):518–28.
18. Tao QF et al. J Nat Prod. 2008 Jan;71(1):12–7.
19. Jiang H et al. Rapid Commun Mass Spectrom. 2007; 21(4):509–18.
20. Saha S et al. J Chromatogr A. 2003 Mar 28;991(1):143–50.
21. Siddaraju MN, Dharmesh SM. Mol Nutr Food Res. 2007 Mar; 51(3):324–32.
22. Chrubasik S et al. Phytomedicine. 2005 Sep;12(9):684–701.
23. Kim M et al. Biochim Biophys Acta. 2007 Dec;1770(12): 1627–35.
24. Choi KH, Laursen RA. Eur J Biochem. 2000 Mar;267(5): 1516–26.
25. Moreschi SR et al. J Agric Food Chem. 2004 Mar 24; 52(6):1753–8.
26. Badria FA. J Med Food. 2002 Fall;5(3):153–7.
27. Pape C, Luning K. J Pineal Res. 2006 Sep;41(2):157–65.
28. Ghayur MN, Gilani AH. Dig Dis Sci. 2005 Oct;50(10): 1889–97.
29. Yoshikawa M et al. Chem Pharm Bull (Tokyo). 1994 Jun; 42(6):1226–30.
30. Swain AR et al. J Am Diet Assoc. 1985;85:950–60.
31. Ma X, Gang DR. Phytochemistry. 2006 Oct;67(20):2239–55.
32. Shadmani A et al. Pak J Pharm Sci. 2004 Jan;17(1):47–54.
33. Catchpole OJ et al. J Agric Food Chem. 2003 Aug 13; 51(17):4853–60.
34. Shi Q et al. Zhong Yao Cai. 1999 Mar;22(3):134–5.
35. Yoshikawa M et al. Yakugaku Zasshi. 1993 Apr;113(4): 307–15.
36. Jiang H et al. Phytochemistry. 2006 Aug;67(15):1673–85.
37. Wolmuth H et al. J Agric Food Chem. 2005 Jul 13; 53(14):5772–8.
38. Gong F et al. J Agric Food Chem. 2004 Oct 20;52(21):6378–83.
39. Bhattarai S et al. J Pharm Sci. 2001 Oct;90(10):1658–64.
40. Uma Pradeep K et al. Plant Foods Hum Nutr. 1993 Sep; 44(2):137–48.
41. Uchibayashi M. Yakushigaku Zasshi. 2001;36(1):58–60.
42. Martindale, The Extra Pharmacopoeia 26th Ed. Pharmaceutical Press London March 1973 p. 1241–2.
43. Grzanna R et al. J Med Food. 2005 Summer;8(2):125–32.
44. Masuda Y et al. Biofactors. 2004;21(1–4):293–6.
45. Pezo D et al. Anal Bioanal Chem. 2006 Aug;385(7):1241–6.
46. Shin SG et al. J Agric Food Chem. 2005 Sep 21;53(19):7617–22.
47. Ippoushi K et al. Planta Med. 2005 Jun;71(6):563–6.
48. Ninfali P et al. Br J Nutr. 2005 Feb;93(2):257–66.
49. Surh YJ et al. J Environ Pathol Toxicol Oncol. 1999;18(2): 131–9.
50. Blomhoff R. Tidsskr Nor Laegeforen. 2004 Jun 17;124(12): 1643–5.
51. Wang CC et al. In Vivo. 2003 Nov–Dec;17(6):641–5.
52. Halvorsen BL et al. J Nutr. 2002 Mar;132(3):461–71.
53. Baliga MS et al. Nahrung. 2003 Aug;47(4):261–4.
54. Asnani V, Verma RJ. Acta Pol Pharm. 2007 Jan–Feb; 64(1):35–7.
55. Chung WY et al. Redox Rep. 2003;8(1):31–3.
56. Patro BS et al. Chembiochem. 2002 Apr;68(4):364–70.
57. Shobana S, Naidu KA. Prostaglandins Leukot Essent Fatty Acids. 2000 Feb;62(2):107–10.
58. Eguchi A et al. Free Radic Res. 2005 Dec;39(12):1367–75.
59. Asnani V, Verma RJ. Acta Pol Pharm. 2006 Mar–Apr; 63(2):117–9.
60. Jolad SD et al. Phytochemistry. 2004 Jul;65(13):1937–54.
61. Nurtjahja-Tjendraputra E et al. Thromb Res. 2003; 111(4–5):259–65.
62. Tjendraputra E et al. Bioorg Chem. 2001 Jun;29(3):156–63.
63. Srivastava KC. Prostaglandins Leukot Med. 1986 Dec; 25(2–3):187–98.
64. Lantz RC et al. Phytomedicine. 2007 Feb;14(2–3):123–8.
65. Kiuchi F et al. Chem Pharm Bull (Tokyo). 1992 Feb; 40(2):387–91.
66. Phan PV et al. J Altern Complement Med. 2005 Feb;11(1): 149–54.
67. Frondoza CG et al. In Vitro Cell Dev Biol Anim. 2004 Mar–Apr; 40(3–4):95–101.
68. Chang CP et al. J Ethnopharmacol. 1995 Aug 11;48(1):13–19.
69. Iwasaki Y et al. Nutr Neurosci. 2006;9:169–78.
70. Dedov VN et al. Br J Pharmacol. 2002 Nov;137(6):793–8.
71. Srivastava KC, Mustafa T. Med Hypotheses. 1989 May; 29(1):25–8.
72. Ali BH et al. Food Chem Toxicol. 2008 Feb;46(2):409–20.
73. Grzanna R et al. J Altern Complement Med. 2004 Dec; 10(6):1009–13.
74. Minghetti P et al. Planta Med. 2007 Dec;73(15):1525–30.
75. Kim JK et al. Free Radic Res. 2007 May;41(5):603–14.
76. Nonn L et al. Carcinogenesis. 2007 Jun;28(6):1188–96.
77. Srivastava KC, Mustafa T. Med Hypotheses. 1992 Dec; 39(4):342–8.
78. Wigler I et al. Osteoarthritis Cartilage. 2003 Nov;11(11): 783–9.
79. Altman RD, Marcussen KC. Arthritis Rheum. 2001 Nov; 44(11):2531–8.
80. Chopra A et al. J Clin Rheumatol. 2004 Oct;10(5):236–45.
81. Bliddal H et al. Osteoarthritis Cartilage. 2000 Jan;8(1):9–12.
82. Hollyer T et al. BMC Complement Altern Med. 2002 May 17;2:5.
83. Abdel-Aziz H et al. Eur J Pharmacol. 2006 Jan 13;530(1–2): 136–43.
84. Yang Y et al. Phytomedicine. 2002 Mar;9(2):146–52.
85. Holtmann S et al. Acta Otolaryngol. 1989 Sep–Oct; 108(3–4):168–74.
86. Scurr JH, Gulati OP. Phytother Res. 2004 Sep;18(9):687–95.

87. Huang QR et al. Chem Pharm Bull (Tokyo). 1991 Feb; 39(2):397–9.
88. Mascolo N et al. J Ethnopharmacol. 1989 Nov;27(1–2): 129–40.
89. Mahesh R et al. Pharmazie. 2005 Feb;60(2):83–96.
90. Stewart JJ et al. Pharmacology. 1991;42(2):111–20.
91. Micklefield GH et al. Int J Clin Pharmacol Ther. 1999 Jul; 37(7):341–6.
92. Phillips S et al. Anaesthesia. 1993 May;48(5):393–5.
93. Lien HC et al. Am J Physiol Gastrointest Liver Physiol. 2003 Mar;284(3):G481–9.
94. Power ML et al. J Reprod Med. 2007 Oct;52(10):922–8.
95. Keating A, Chez RA. Althern Ther Health Med. 2002 Sep–Oct;8(5):89–91.
96. Vutyavanich T et al. Obstet Gynecol. 2001 Apr;97(4): 577–82.
97. Willetts KE et al. Aust N Z J Obstet Gynaecol. 2003 Apr; 43(2):139–44.
98. Portnoi G et al. Am J Obstet Gynecol. 2003 Nov;189(5): 1374–7.
99. Chittumma P et al. J Med Assoc Thai. 2007 Jan;90(1): 15–20.
100. Smith C et al. Obstet Gynecol. 2004 Apr;103(4):639–45.
101. Sripramote M, Lekyananda N. J Med Assoc Thai. 2003 Sep;86(9):846–53.
102. Pongrojpaw D et al. J Med Assoc Thai. 2007 Sep;90(9): 1703–9.
103. Fischer-Rasmussen W et al. Eur J Obstet Gynecol Reprod Biol. 1991 Jan 4;38(1):19–24.
104. Nanthakomon T, Pongrojpaw D. J Med Assoc Thai. 2006 Oct;89 Suppl 4:S130–6.
105. Apariman S et al. J Med Assoc Thai. 2006 Dec;89(12): 2003–9.
106. Pongrojpaw D, Chiamchanya C. J Med Assoc Thai. 2003 Mar;86(3):244–50.
107. Phillips S et al. Anaesthesia. 1993 Aug;48(8):715–7.
108. Bone ME et al. Anaesthesia. 1990 Aug;45(8):669–71.
109. Chaiyakunapruk N et al. Am J Obstet Gynecol. 2006 Jan; 194(1):95–9.
110. Eberhart LH et al. Anesth Analg. 2003 Apr;96(4):995–8.
111. Visalyaputra S et al. Anaesthesia. 1998 May;53(5):506–10.
112. Arfeen Z et al. Anaesth Intensive Care. 1995 Aug;23(4): 449–52.
113. Tavlan A et al. Clin Drug Investig. 2006;26(4):209–14.
114. Morin AM et al. Anasthesiol Intensivmed Notfallmed Schmerzther. 2004 May;39(5):281–5.
115. Meyer K et al. Dermatol Nurs. 1995 Aug;7(4):242–4.
116. Manusirivithaya S et al. Int J Gynecol Cancer. 2004 Nov–Dec;14(6):1063–9.
117. Wood CD et al. Clin Res Pr Drug Regul Aff. 1988;6(2): 129–36.
118. Mowrey DB, Clayson DE. Lancet. 1982 Mar 20;319(8273): 655–7.
119. Schmid R et al. J Travel Med. 1994 Dec 1;1(4):203–6.
120. Grontved A et al. Acta Otolaryngol. 1988 Jan–Feb; 105(1–2):45–9.
121. Grontved A, Hentzer E. ORL J Otorhinolaryngol Relat Spec. 1986;48(5):282–6.
122. Boone SA, Shields KM. Ann Pharmacother. 2005 Oct;39(10):1710–3.
123. Borrelli F et al. Obstet Gynecol. 2005 Apr;105(4):849–56.
124. Betz O et al. Forsch Komplementaramed Klass Naturhee-ilkd. 2005 Feb;12(1):14–23.
125. Aikins Murphy P. Obstet Gynecol. 1998 Jan;91(1):149–55.
126. Jewell D, Young G. Cochrane Database Syst Rev. 2002;(1): CD000145.
127. Ernst E, Pittler MH. Br J Anaesth. 2000 Mar;84(3):367–71.
128. Bryer E. J Midwifery Womens Health. 2005 Jan–Feb; 50(1):e1–3.
129. Rhode J et al. BMC Complement Altern Med. 2007 Dec 20;7(1):44.
130. Lee SH et al. Mol Carcinog. 2008 Mar;47(3):197–208.
131. Shukla Y et al. Mol Nutr Food Res. 2007 Dec;51(12): 1492–502.
132. Campbell CT et al. Toxicol Lett. 2007 Sep;173(3):151–60.
133. Lee HS et al. J Nutr Biochem. 2008 May;19(5):313–9.
134. Ishiguro K et al. Biochem Biophys Res Commun. 2007 Oct 12;362(1):218–23.
135. Vijaya Padma V et al. Basic Clin Pharmacol Toxicol. 2007 May;100(5):302–7.
136. Chen CY et al. J Agric Food Chem. 2007 Feb 7;55(3): 948–54.
137. Park YJ et al. Yonsei Med J. 2006 Oct 31;47(5):688–97.
138. Wei QY et al. J Ethnopharmacol. 2005 Nov 14;102(2): 177–84.
139. Lee S, Surh YJ. Cancer Lett. 1998 Dec 25;134(2):163–8.
140. Keum YS et al. Cancer Lett. 2002 Mar 8;177(1):41–7.
141. Wang G et al. Cell Mol Life Sci. 2005 Apr;62(7–8):881–93.
142. Kim EC et al. Biochem Biophys Res Commun. 2005 Sep 23;335(2):300–8.
143. Lu P et al. Zhongguo Zhong Yao Za Zhi. 2003 Sep;28(9): 873–5.
144. Kapadia GJ et al. Pharmacol Res. 2002 Mar;45(3):213–20.
145. Vimala S et al. Br J Cancer. 1999 Apr;80(1–2):110–6.
146. Surh YJ et al. Mutat Res. 1998 Jun 18;402(1–2):259–67.
147. Sagar SM et al. Curr Oncol. 2006 Jun;13(3):99–107.
148. Nabekura T et al. Biochem Biophys Res Commun. 2005 Feb 18;327(3):866–70.
149. Shukla Y, Singh M. Food Chem Toxicol. 2007 May; 45(5):683–90.
150. Song Y et al. Zhongguo Zhong Yao Za Zhi. 2007 Oct; 32(19):2062–5.
151. Guh JH et al. J Pharm Pharmacol. 1995 Apr;47(4):329–32.
152. Srivastava KC. Prostaglandins Leukot Med. 1984 Feb; 13(2):227–35.
153. Nicoll R, Henein MY. Int J Cardiol. 2007 Nov 23;[epub ahead of print].
154. Verma SK, Bordia A. Indian J Med Sci. 2001 Feb;55(2):83–6.
155. Verma SK et al. Indian J Med Res. 1993 Oct;98:240–2.
156. Bordia A et al. Prostaglandins Leukot Essent Fatty Acids. 1997 May;56(5):379–84.
157. Srivastava SK. Prostaglandins Leukot Essent Fatty Acids. 1989 Mar;35(3):183–5.
158. Bakon J. Med Hypotheses. 1991 Mar;34(3):230–1.
159. Janssen PL et al. Eur J Clin Nutr. 1996 Nov;50(11):772–4.
160. Schnitzler P et al. Antimicrob Agents Chemother. 2007 May;51(5):1859–62.
161. Koch C et al. Phytomedicine. 2008 Jan;15(1–2):71–8.
162. Denyer CV et al. J Nat Prod. 1994 May;57(5):658–62.
163. Sookkongwaree K et al. Pharmazie. 2006 Aug;61(8): 717–21.
164. Norajit K et al. Molecules. 2007 Aug 23;12(8):2047–60.
165. Paramasivam S et al. J Environ Biol. 2007 Apr;28(2):271–4.
166. Betoni JE et al. Mem Inst Oswaldo Cruz. 2006 Jun;101(4): 387–90.

167. Gupta S, Ravishankar S. Foodborne Pathog Dis. 2005 Winter;2(4):330–40.
168. Thongson C et al. Lett Appl Microbiol. 2004;39(5):401–6.
169. Nguefack J et al. Lett Appl Microbiol. 2004;39(5):395–400.
170. Konning GH et al. Fitoterapia. 2004 Jan;75(1):65–7.
171. Akoachere JF et al. East Afr J Med. 2002 Nov;79(11): 588–92.
172. Friedman M et al. J Food Prot. 2002 Oct;65(10):1545–60.
173. Nostro A et al. Phytother Res. 2006 Mar;20(3):187–90.
174. O'Mahony R et al. World J Gastroenterol. 2005 Dec 21; 11(47):7499–507.
175. Mahady GB et al. Phytother Res. 2005 Nov;19(11):988–91.
176. Weseler A et al. Pharmazie. 2005 Jul;60(7):498–502.
177. Mahady GB et al. Anticancer Res. 2003 Sep–Oct;23(5A): 3699–702.
178. Nagoshi C et al. Biol Pharm Bull. 2006 Mar;29(3):443–7.
179. Leal PF et al. J Agric Food Chem. 2003 Apr 23;51(9): 2520–5.
180. Flicker C et al. Phytother Res. 2003 Sep;17(8):897–902.
181. Flicker C et al. Mycoses. 2003 Feb;46(1–2):29–37.
182. Sanderson L et al. J Helminthol. 2002 Sep;76(3):241–7.
183. Adewunmi CO et al. Planta Med. 1990 Aug;56(4):374–6.
184. Goto C et al. Parasitol Res. 1990;76(8):653–6.
185. Kato A et al. J Agric Food Chem. 2006 Sep 6;54(18):6640–4.
186. Kim DS et al. Planta Med. 2002 Apr;68(4):375–6.
187. Kang SC et al. Phytother Res. 2006 Nov;20(11):1017–9.
188. Bandell M et al. Neuron. 2004 Mar 25;41(6):849–57.
189. Wilasrusmee C et al. Am Surg. 2002 Oct;68(10):860–4.
190. Prescott J, Stevenson RJ. Physiol Behav. 1996 Dec;60(6): 1473–80.
191. Prescott J, Stevenson RJ. Physiol Behav. 1996 Aug;60(2): 617–24.
192. Katagiri F et al. Biol Pharm Bull. 2004 Oct;27(10):1679–82.
193. Gonlachanvit S et al. J Pharmacol Exp Ther. 2003 Dec; 307(3):1098–103.
194. Cady RK et al. Med Sci Monit. 2005 Sep;11(9):P165–9.
195. Kobayashi H et al. Drugs Exp Clin Res. 2004;30(5–6): 197–202.
196. Kobayashi H et al. Int J Tissue React. 2004;26(3–4):113–7.
197. Roberts AT et al. J Med Food. 2007 Mar;10(1):184–8.
198. Greenway FL et al. Int J Obes (Lond). 2006 Dec;30(12): 1737–41.
199. Schwertner HA et al. Obstet Gynecol. 2006 Jun;107(6): 1337–43.
200. Masteikova R et al. Ceska Slov Farm. 2006 Nov;55(6): 268–71.
201. Borrelli F et al. Obstet Gynecol. 2005 Sep;106(3):640–1.
202. Ramos Ruiz A et al. J Ethnopharmacol. 1996 Jul 5;52(3): 123–7.
203. Tantaoui-Elaraki A, Beraoud L. J Environ Pathol Toxicol Oncol. 1994;13(1):67–72.
204. Hashim S et al. Nutr Cancer. 1994;21(2):169–75.
205. Sivaswamy SN et al. Indian J Exp Biol. 1991 Aug;29(8): 730–7.
206. Soudamini KK et al. Indian J Physiol Pharmacol. 1995 Oct;39(4):347–53.
207. Nagabhushan M et al. Cancer Lett. 1987 Aug;36(2): 221–33.
208. Nakamura H, Yamamoto T. Mutat Res. 1982 Feb;103(2): 119–26.
209. Kanerva L et al. Contact Dermatitis. 1996 Sep;35(3): 157–62.
210. Futrell JM, Rietschel RL. Cutis. 1993 Nov;52(5):288–90.
211. Toorenenbergen AW, Dieges PH. J Allergy Clin Immunol. 1985 Sep;17(3):477–81.
212. Lumb AB. Thromb Haemost. 1994 Jan;71(1):110–1.
213. Desai HG et al. Indian J Med Res. 1990 Apr;92:139–41.
214. Brandin H et al. Phytother Res. 2007 Mar;21(3):239–44.
215. Koo KL et al. Thromb Res. 2001 Sep 1;103(5):387–97.
216. Shalansky S et al. Pharmacotherapy. 2007 Sep;27(9): 1237–47.
217. Jiang X et al. Br J Clin Pharmacol. 2005 Apr;59(4):425–32.
218. Jiang X et al. J Clin Pharmacol. 2006 Nov;46(11):1370–8.
219. Vaes LP, Chyka PA. Ann Pharmacother. 2000 Dec;34(12): 1478–82.
220. Young HY et al. Am J Chin Med. 2006;34(4):545–51.
221. Kruth P et al. Ann Pharmacother. 2004 Feb;38(2):257–60.

PRIMARY REFERENCES

Barker, J—*The Medicinal Flora of Britain and N. W. Europe.* Winter Press, U. K. 2001.

BHP—*British Herbal Pharmacopoeia.* British Herbal Medicine Association, 1983.

BHC—*British Herbal Compendium.* British Herbal Medicine Association, 1992.

Bodkin, F—*Encyclopaedia Botanica.* Angus and Robertson, Australia, 1986.

Culpeper, N—*Culpeper's Complete Herbal and English Physician.* Facsimile edition, Gareth Powell, 1979.

German Commission E—Monographs. Integrative Medicine Communications 2000.

Grieve, M—*A Modern Herbal.* Dover Publications, New York, 1971.

Lewis and Elvin Lewis—*Medical Botany.* 1977.

Messegue, M—*Health Secrets of Plants and Herbs. Collins, 1979.*

Millspaugh, C—*American Medicinal Plants.* Dover Publications, New York, 1974.

Polunin, O—*Flowers of Europe.* Oxford University Press 1969.

Weiss, R—*Herbal Medicine.* AB Arcanum, Beaconsfield, England 1988.

Wohlmuth, H—*Introduction to Botany and Plant Identification.* Mac-Platypus Productions, 1993.

Wren, C—*Potter's New Cyclopaedia of Botanical Drugs and Preparations.* C W Daniel Co Ltd., 1988.

THERAPEUTIC INDEX

Bold entries refer to actions
 * *in vitro* on whole herb
** *in vitro* on isolated constituents

abdominal discomfort, 244, 444
abdominal pain. *See* under pain
abrasions, 21, 125, 255, 387
abscesses
   mammary, topical, 329
   topical, 346
acaricidal, 19, 22, 81, 94, 124
acid secretion, postprandial, 184
Acinetobacter**, 49
acne
   teenage, 445
   topical, 62, 83, 225, 226, 228, 329, 445
Adaptogen, 31, 34
addiction cravings, 332
Addison's disease, 183, 186
adenitis, 328
adenoviruses*, 312
ADHD. *See* Attention Deficit Hyperactivity Disorder
adjustment mood disorder, 331, 376
adrenal insufficiency, 38, 183
Adrenal tonic, 113
adrenocortical insufficiency, 183, 186
Adrenocorticotropic, 182
agoraphobia, 331
AIDS, 21, 34, 52, 70, 71, 86, 143, 150, 221

alcoholism, 57, 257, 386
allergic conditions, 158
alopecia
   androgenic, 42, 43, 128, 211, 445
   areata, 237, 252
   neurotica, 54
Alterative, 70, 74, 101, 103, 191, 226, 227, 281, 328, 356
alternating bowel habit, 277
alveolar osteitis, 277
Alzheimer's disease, 442, 456
Amanita phalloides, 85, 87
amenorrhoea
   atonic, 392
   secondary, 445
amoebiasis, 172
anaemia, 17, 38, 39, 65, 111, 117, 196, 356
anal fissures, 177, 342, 354, 368
analgesic
   topical, 29, 54, 108, 165, 189, 315, 420, 433
Analgesic, 29, 140, 250, 292, 314, 322, 400, 433
   mild, 250
anaphrodisiac in men, 129
angina, 35, 55, 105, 209, 212, 281, 375, 376
Anhidrotic, 412
Anisakis, 455

mouth. *See* inflammation, oral mucosal
muscle, 54
musculoskeletal, 115, 322
nasopharynx, 89, 254
nerve, 119
oral, 61, 98
pharynx, 98
respiratory tract, 79
rheumatic, 122
skin. *See* skin inflammation
urinary tract, 13, 89
inflammatory bowel conditions, 427
inflammatory bowel disease, 129, 177, 195, 323, 340, 415
influenza virus*, 61, 110, 132, 143, 163, 270, 295, 409
injuries, 61, 115, 141, 216, 346, 380, 399, 430, 446
inotropic, 284, 375, 376, 437
insect bites. *See* under bites
insect repellent, 448
Insect repellent, 236
insecticide, 260
insomnia
    due to neuralgia, 190
    nervous, 190
insulin levels, reduce, 287
insulin sensitivity, peripheral, 341
intermittent claudication, 376, 394
intrauterine foetal growth retardation, 37
irregular pulse, 376
irritability, 444
irritable bowel, 235, 286, 290
irritable bowel syndrome, 66, 82, 129, 135, 176, 201, 244, 246, 277, 339, 342, 415
    rectal pain, 415
Irritant, 316
ischaemic-reperfusion injury, 209
itches. *See* under skin

Japanese encephalitis virus*, 184
jaundice
    infantile cholestatic, 354
    neonatal, 354
joint distortions, 115
joint inflammation. *See* under inflammation
joint pain. *See* under pain

keloids, 17
keratitis herpetic, 61
kidney stone. *See* lithiasis
kinetosis. *See* motion sickness
Klebsiella*, 56, 163, 225, 251, 269
Klebsiella**, 56, 61, 160, 251, 254, 263, 269, 409

labour. *See also* childbirth
    false pains, 105, 136, 388, 474
    placenta expulsion, 59
lacerations, 298
lactation, 442
    cessation, 445
    increase, 180, 195, 196, 434, 442, 445, 474
    miscarriage, 113, 195
larvicidal, 28, 124, 255
laryngitis
    topical, 384
    with aphonia, 399
Laxative, 63, 75, 96, 101, 103, 174, 176, 194, 201, 223, 226, 227, 275, 286, 300, 308, 352, 356, 364, 368, 448, 449
    mild, 224
Legionella**, 185
Leishmania*, 92, 276
Leishmania**, 92, 185, 260, 270, 276, 339
leishmaniasis, 102
leprosy, 201
Leptospira*, 81
leptospirosis, 282
leucopenia, 38, 72, 102
leucorrhoea
    topical, 25, 164, 283, 304, 306, 373
leukaemia, 110
leukaemia, 35
leukaemia*, 35, 61, 110, 142, 183, 270, 309, 455
    monoblastic, 183
leukaemia**, 58, 86, 92, 102, 110, 119, 127, 142, 153, 183, 270, 294, 352, 381, 416, 455
    lymphocytic, 142
    myeloid, 110
lice. *See also* head lice
lichen planus, 277
lipid reduction, 339, 341
lipoprotein oxidation, 416
Listeria*, 391
Listeria**, 19, 225, 260, 263, 455
lithiasis, urinary, 89, 97, 107, 148, 161, 277, 377, 434, 438.
    See also under urinary calculus
liver
    alcohol abuse, 86
    cirrhosis, 186
    congestion, 211
    disease, 341
        cholestatic, 341
    disorders, 17, 397, 475
    drug abuse, 86, 177, 278, 369
    dysfunction, 410
    failure sub-acute, 184

Printed in the USA
CPSIA information can be obtained
at www.ICGtesting.com
LVHW081936090924
790534LV00008B/841